FIFTH EDITION

HEARING IN CHILDREN

FIFTH EDITION

Hearing in Children

Jerry L. Northern, Ph.D.

Professor Emeritus
Department of Otolaryngology
University of Colorado
School of Medicine
Denver, Colorado

Vice-President, Professional Services
HEARx LTD
West Palm Beach, Florida

Marion P. Downs, D.H.S., D.S.

Professor Emerita
Department of Otolaryngology
University of Colorado
School of Medicine
Denver, Colorado

LIPPINCOTT WILLIAMS & WILKINS
A **Wolters Kluwer** Company
Philadelphia · Baltimore · New York · London
Buenos Aires · Hong Kong · Sydney · Tokyo

Editor: Timothy L. Julet
Managing Editor: Linda S. Napora
Marketing Manager: Christen DeMarco
Production Editor: Paula C. Williams
Printer: R. R. Donnelley & Sons Company

Printed in the United States of America

Library of Congress Cataloging-in-Publication Data
Northern, Jerry L.
    Hearing in children/Jerry L. Northern, Marion P. Downs--5th ed.
        p. cm.
    Includes bibliographical references and index.
    ISBN 0-683-30764-9
        1. Hearing disorders in children. I. Downs, Marion P. II. Title.
RF291.5.C45 N67 2001
618.92′0978--dc21

                                                2001038193

*The publishers have made every effort to trace the copyright hold-
ers for borrowed material. If they have inadvertently overlooked
any, they will be pleased to make the necessary arrangements at
the first opportunity.*

To purchase additional copies of this book call our customer service
department at **(800) 638-3030** or fax orders to **(301) 824-7390.** International customers should call **(301) 714-2324.**

***Visit Lippincott Williams & Wilkins on the Internet:
http://www.lww.com.*** Lippincott Williams & Wilkins customer
service representatives are available from 8:30 am to 6:00 pm,
EST, Monday through Friday, for telephone access.

05 06 07
2 3 4 5 6 7 8 9 10

Foreword

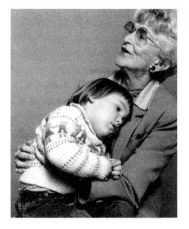

Pediatric audiology came quietly into being in the early 1940s, spurred by dedicated educators of the deaf who studied the auditory behaviors of normal-hearing children. These educators were Lord and Lady Ewing in England. They combined the use of gross noisemakers with their own sophisticated skills of observation, developing those simple techniques into an art.

And what an art! A case can still be made that the highest form of pediatric audiology is a known sound stimulus in the hand of a zealous, practiced observer which is pointed at an infant's ear. Many thousands of hearing-impaired individuals are enjoying more successful lives as a result of having been identified early in life by such techniques. But there are not enough of those fortunate ones. In this book, we find the full 21st century response to the need for pediatric audiology that utilizes state-of-the-art technology to ensure that *all* children will have available to them the identification of their problems at the earliest possible time.

For the goal is *all!* Not just the child with parents who can afford testing and monitoring. Not just those who happen to fall into a category that places them *at risk* for deafness. Not just the ones that happen to be in the right place at the right time to be screened. But *all children!* They are all entitled to be touched by the screening hand of modern technology. There is too much at stake to miss any.

Not only those severe and profound losses so devastating to speech and language, but even the mildest losses with their sequelae in delayed expressive language must be identified early enough to allow interventions that will lessen their problems. The development of cochlear implants makes it even more critical that losses be identified early. We can now envision a world in which a deaf baby can be undergo implantation at birth and, with the plasticity of the young brain, can utilize the implant code to become a functional hearing person.

The field of preventive medicine gives us an analog: it has been said that "medicine is unique among the sciences in that it strives incessantly to defeat the object of its own invention." This object, of course, is disease, and there is a parallel in audiology. Since our beginnings in the mid-1940s, we have measured, described, researched, cataloged, analyzed, and synthesized the entity of hearing loss exhaustively. Now, having defined it, we must busy ourselves with preventing the devastation of its effects on children. In such terms, preventive audiology becomes a viable endeavor—a discipline devoted to preventing the effects of ear disease on the individual who suffers from it. Such prevention can only be accomplished by early detection of the condition and by proper provision for remedial therapy and education.

Marion P. Downs, D.H.S., D.S.

Preface

What started out to be a quick update and rewrite of the fourth edition steadily extended into a 2-year thorough overhaul of *Hearing in Children*. The 1990s was an exciting period of change in all aspects of pediatric audiology that is reflected in the extensive updates included in every chapter of this fifth edition. Many of the advances in medical knowledge and technical aspects have been included in this new edition. The reader will find updates and discussions of new hearing testing and hearing screening technologies, inclusion of guidelines and position statements, and hearing aid fitting and management issues—all of which have contributed to the raising of standards to new and higher benchmarks in pediatric hearing health care. This improvement in focus and attention for the child with hearing difficulties and associated special needs has been noted by physicians, allied health professionals, educators, and audiologists.

This fifth edition of *Hearing in Children* presents a wealth of new materials, including a totally new chapter devoted to the growing problems resulting from childhood otitis media. Numerous discussions reflect the new emphasis on the role of the child's family in all aspects of the habilitation process. Considerable information is presented on early identification and early intervention as documented by the Joint Committee on Infant Hearing Year 2000 Position Statement. In researching and editing this new edition of *Hearing in Children*, we deleted more than 600 out-of-date references to make room for the inclusion of new information from 465 current reference works. We have been diligent, once again, to delete sufficient material so that the update of new text results in a readable and easy-to-use reference textbook for professional clinicians and graduate students.

As I now join my colleague Marion Downs at the emeritus level of our careers, I look back and realize that we have lost many of our colleagues who have worked with us to help with previous editions of *Hearing in Children*. We remember with fondness and great appreciation the contributions and friendship given to us from Kathleen O. Blane, F. Blair Simmons, Aram Glorig, La Vonne Bergstrom, and Laslo Stein.

We have watched with pride and pleasure as pediatric audiology has grown into a specialty area of expertise. Our hopes and expectations for the future to focus on the special audiologic needs of infants and children with hearing impairments, described in our first edition nearly 30 years ago, have blossomed into a substantial body of knowledge and skills resulting in a high standard of clinical services. The fact that audiologists continue to press for earlier identification of hearing loss in all babies, while developing improved methods of management of children with hearing impairment, is clearly the best outcome to us after our long careers in providing pediatric clinical services, writings, and teachings. The successes achieved in pediatric audiology are the result of contributions from uncountable clinicians and researchers over the years. We are pleased to be just a small part of that progress.

J.L.N.

Acknowledgments

First Edition. A book of this magnitude cannot be assembled and written without the help of many other people. We pay special tribute to and thank five of our colleagues and good friends who gave graciously of their valuable time and personal material for our benefit: La Vonne Bergstrom, MD; Isamu Sando, MD; Janet M. Stewart, MD; Marlin Weaver, MD; and Winfield McChord, Jr., MS.

Many others responded to our needs, willingly and unselfishly, to provide requested information at a moment's notice: Carol Amon, MA; Owen Black, MD; Carol Cox, MA; Kathleen O. Foust, MA; William K. Frankenberg, MD; Aram Glorig, MD; W. G. Hemenway, MD; Brian Hersch, MD; Mrs. Page T. Jenkins; Pat Tesauro, MA; Darrel Teter, PhD; and Harold Weber, MA. Connie H. Knight, MA, Audiologist at the Georgia Retardation Center, Atlanta, was our Research Associate and gathered much of the material presented in the "Index of Selected Birth Defect Syndromes." Sharon Mraz was our Editorial Assistant. Patricia Jenkins Thompson, MA, diligently proofread and critiqued our efforts.

Y. Oishi, MD, served as our primary photographer; Miriam Eliachar illustrated the chapter pictures and embryology figures; and Anita McGuire typed the entire manuscript. We also acknowledge the cooperation of the publishing staff at Williams & Wilkins, especially William R. Hensyl, who encouraged us to write this textbook.

Finally, we extend our appreciation and thanks to our spouses, families, children, and friends, who will long remember (as will we!) this period during which we were too busy, too preoccupied, or too tired—our Year of the Book, 1973.

Second Edition. Once again numerous colleagues came to our aid to provide advice, share materials, and labor in the libraries to help prepare the Second Edition of *Hearing in Children.* We express our warmest thanks to Jeff Adams, Marlin Cohrs, Roni Halpern, Donna Lutz, Winfield McChord, Deborah Smith, Steven Staller, Darrel Teter, Harold Weber, and Janet Zarnoch. We are particularly grateful for the contributions of Mrs. Kathleen Bryant, Speech Pathologist at the University of Colorado Medical Center. Patsy Tormey, our helpful secretary, typed the manuscript and quietly tolerated our many revisions. Ruby Richardson at Williams & Wilkins nudged us gently, but firmly, throughout this revision. Finally, we appreciate the helpful comments and critique provided by our professional friends who took time to respond to a lengthy questionnaire regarding the first edition. Their guidance and suggestions greatly influenced the second edition of *Hearing in Children.*

Third Edition. We are grateful to a new cadre of friends, students, and associates who responded to our requests for help with the third edition. We thank David Asher, James R. Curran, Sandra Abbott Gabbard, Marianne Geisler, Christine Gerhardt, Katherine Pike Gerkin, Kathryn Grose, Deanie Johnson, Deborah Kinder, Sharon A. Mitchell, Patrick Sullivan, MD, and Ann Wilson. Patsy Tormey-

Meredith typed the manuscripts again, but this time during maternity leave. We were delighted to work again with William R. Hensyl, of Williams & Wilkins, who was the original perpetrator of *Hearing in Children*.

Fourth Edition. We are indebted to many of our colleagues for their supportive efforts. Especially helpful through their review, critical commentary, and useful suggestions were: Julia M. Davis, Sandy Friel-Patti, Judith S. Gravel, M. Suzanne Hasenstab, Deborah Hayes, John and Claire Jacobson, Susan Jerger, Robert W. Keith, and Laszlo Stein. We thank them for their time and effort. Once again, we are most thankful to our ever-dependable secretary/friend Patsy Tormey-Meredith, for bearing with us again in typing (and retyping) the manuscript. A special thanks is extended to the University Hospital audiology staff for their patience, understanding, and support during the many months spent preparing this new edition.

Fifth Edition. One of the great pleasures in working in the field of audiology has been the close association with colleagues who have stepped forward once again to help with this new edition. I especially acknowledge the contributions of three anonymous reviewers who made many worthwhile suggestions for improvements in this new edition. I also pay special thanks to Harvey Dillon, Kiara Ebinger, Sandra Abbott Gabbard, Parker Haberly, Robert Keith, Patsy Meredith, H. Gus Mueller, and Laszlo Stein, for generously helping and providing materials. Miriam Eliachar, from Jerusalem, willingly created a number of new illustrations in her signature style. I am especially grateful to my esteemed colleague, Deborah Hayes of the Denver Children's Hospital, for her review and comments for each revised chapter and her responsiveness to my requests that were always on a moment's notice. I certainly could not forget to acknowledge the support from my closest colleague for more than 35 years, Marion Downs, who serves as the highest role model for all of us who work with children with hearing disabilities. Most importantly, a huge thanks and a lot of love to my wife, Deborah, who encouraged and supported me daily and was so understanding of my time and energy commitment throughout the process of rewriting this Fifth Edition of *Hearing in Children*.

A Note From Marion P. Downs: *I am immensely grateful to Jerry Northern for letting my name continue as co-author of this new edition. I have contributed only a few meager paragraphs, and the entire burden has been his to update and revise most of the former revisions of* Hearing in Children. *It has been a prodigious effort on his part because even as we write, technology is overtaking us and making many words obsolete! I congratulate him and thank him for continuing our cherished volumes with such fortitude!*

Contents

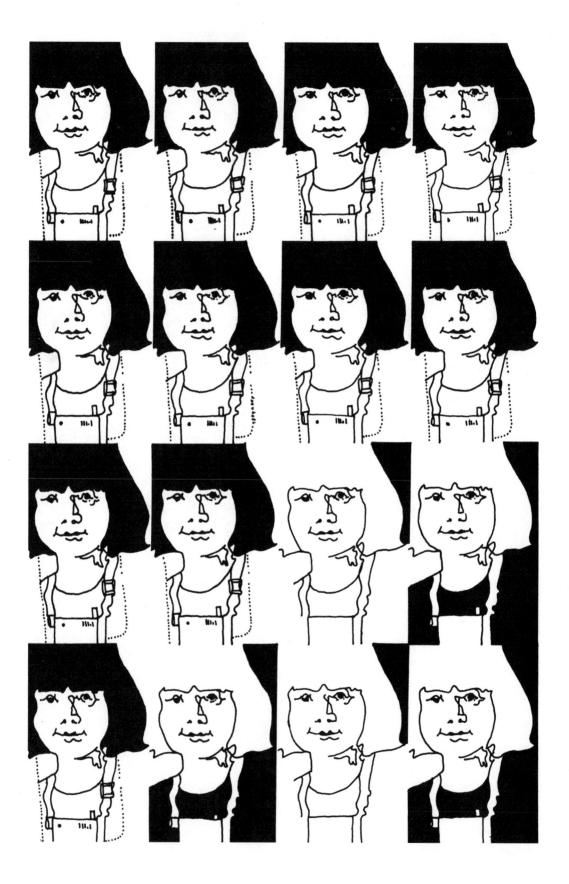

CHAPTER 1

Hearing and Hearing Loss in Children

Long ago the function of hearing became the building block on which our intricate human communication system was constructed. If predawn humans had not inherited an ear, they might have resorted to signing with their fingers or scratching marks on the sand to share their thoughts. The result would have been an awkward method of communication that could have slowed, for millennia, our so-called progress. For good or bad, we have developed the ear and the vocal mechanism as the media through which language is customarily learned and communicated. An illustration of the interdependence of the ear and speech is found in the direct relationship between the frequencies that make speech intelligible and the differential sensitivity of the human ear. Human ears hear best at precisely those frequencies at which humans formulate speech. The question of which of these factors came first is an ontogenic mystery that no one has solved.

The structure of language is unique to Homo sapiens, although experimenters have demonstrated that signed symbols and other visual language forms can be taught to chimpanzees and believe that the beginnings of true, rudimentary language are evidenced in these primates (e.g., Savage-Rumbaugh, Taylor, & Shanker, 1998). Other investigators insist that the conceptual system learned by these primates is not linguistic, that is, that primates do not "think in words"; instead, they use a signalization system that is far removed from the higher symbolization and syntax of human language (Johnson, 1995; Churchland, 1997). Nevertheless, neither group would question

that between the laboriously learned signal responses of the chimpanzee and the first voluntary sentence of the 18-month-old baby lies "a whole day of creation" (Langer, 1957).

The human baby appears to be born with "preexistent knowledge" of language, what Chomsky (1966, 1995) calls a "language organ," that is, specialized neural wiring that exists only in humans awaiting auditory experience with a symbol-based communication system (either oral or sign language) to trigger it into performing. It follows that language can be termed a "biobehavioral" function. These structures are dependent on auditory stimulation for their emergence in the normally developing child. Thus, there exists a crucial interdependence between language development and the ability to hear.

Both the appearance of language and the development of hearing are time-locked functions. The determining periods for hearing development begin very early. The infant is born with billions of neurons with trillions of connections that, in the case of the auditory cortex, await auditory stimulation to strengthen them (Chugani, 1997). If there is no stimulation, as in the case of deafness, the synapses wither through a process called "pruning." Obviously, for the acoustic speech stimulation to affect the infant's neuronal development, the speech spectrum must be audible. Audibility, or the ability to hear, is vital in the process of normal speech and oral language development. A deaf infant who ages without the ability to hear speech has fewer and fewer synapses available to develop auditory perceptions and their associated language skills. Ultimately, it becomes impossible for such a child to acquire "hearing" as we know it. Moreover, this child can only hope to generate language through visual symbols without extensive and long-term habilitation efforts.

It is now possible to demonstrate these facts empirically. Kuhl (1988) found through electrophysiologic measurements that an infant's "auditory map" is completely formed by 12 months of age. However, even earlier than 12 months—at 6 months of age—the infant has already learned all the basic sounds of his or her native language. Almost from birth, infants are sensitized to the subtle auditory cues of their linguistic community (Carney, 1999). Researchers have determined that by 8 months of age, a Japanese infant is able to distinguish all the sounds that are made in every known language, including /r/ and /l/. However, the adult Japanese is not able to make these distinctions. The perceptions for differentiating them have been "pruned" and are lost almost irretrievably. A baby who is deprived of appropriate language stimulation during the first 2 or 3 years of life will never fully attain his or her best potential language function, whether the deprivation is from lack of hearing or from lack of high-quality language experience.

The importance of early hearing to language is demonstrated by the story of the deaf-blind Helen Keller, whose remarkable achievement in mastering language skills has become legend. Her proficiency in language can be understood when one realizes that she acquired both deafness and blindness from meningitis in 1882 at 19 months of age (Wepman, 1987). Helen Keller is an example of Lenneberg's (1967) apt description: "It seems as if even a short exposure to language, a brief moment during which the curtain has been lifted and oral communication established, is sufficient to give a child some

foundation on which much later language may be based." Helen Keller gave us insight into the importance of hearing to everyday life when she said, "I am just as deaf as I am blind. The problems of deafness are deeper and much more complex, if not more important, than those of blindness. Deafness is a much worse misfortune, for it means the loss of the most vital stimulus—the sound of the voice that brings language, sets thought astir, and keeps us in the intellectual company of man."

It is the importance of oral communication that makes us so uniquely "human." Of course, we can write, draw, and read as well as use gestures and sign language to communicate ideas. Most commonly, however, we choose to talk, we listen, and we "think" using language and speech. It is for these reasons that it is urgent to attack and resolve promptly the hearing problems of children, with all the skill, knowledge, and insights of which we are capable. The prevention of hearing loss in children protects the right of children to their essential humanity, which lies in optimal language function.

HEARING LOSS—THE HIDDEN DISABILITY

Hearing loss in children is a silent, hidden disability. Hearing loss is hidden because children, especially infants and toddlers, cannot tell us that they are not hearing well. Hearing loss is a handicap because, if undetected and untreated, hearing loss in children can lead to delayed speech and language development, social and emotional problems, and academic failure. It is unnecessary for a child to suffer these consequences. By detecting hearing loss as early as possible, even as early as during the newborn period, effective treatment, which significantly reduces the handicap of hearing loss, can be applied. All too often, however, identification of a child's hearing loss is delayed because parents are unaware that any child, even a newborn infant, can undergo an accurate hearing test. Unfortunately, routine medical care seldom includes the simple hearing evaluation that could identify those children with hearing loss (American Academy of Audiology, 1992).

The magnitude of problems of hearing loss in children is reflected in the following facts:

- Three children in 1000 are born with congenital, significant, permanent, bilateral hearing loss.

- Three additional children in 1000 will acquire deafness in early childhood.

- Thirty-three infants are born each day in the United States with permanent hearing loss.

- Infants who spend time in the intensive care nursery during the newborn period are at a higher risk for hearing loss, with at least 1 in 50 showing significant hearing loss.

- It is estimated that 90% of very young children's knowledge is attributed to "incidental reception" of sounds around them. Thus, learning is hindered even with the slightest hearing loss.

- There is less than one-half the number of children with severe to profound hearing loss today than two decades ago. Conversely, there are now more than 10 times the number of children with mild to moderate hearing impairments.

- Ear infection, the most common infectious disease of childhood, is the most common cause of hearing loss. An estimated 5 million school days are missed every year due to otitis media.

- Nearly all children will develop some period of hearing loss related to ear infections during the period from birth through 10 years of age.

- Ten percent to 15% of children who receive hearing screening at school fail because they cannot hear within normal limits.

In 1989, the United States federal government accepted a new commitment aimed at reducing the harmful effects of childhood hearing loss. In a statement released by the United States Public Health Service, the former Surgeon General, C. Everett Koop, MD, observed that Helen Keller, who had the benefits of both sight and hearing until she was 19 months of age, often said that she regretted her deafness more than her blindness. A portion of Dr. Koop's statement regarding his belief that early identification of hearing problems in children is essential is presented below:

Deafness in infants is a serious concern because it interferes with the development of language—that which sets humans apart from all other living things. The longer a child's deafness goes undiscovered, the worse the outcome is likely to be. Language remediation, which is what specialists call the process of teaching hearing-impaired children to communicate, must begin as early as possible, because language develops so rapidly in the first few months of life. For example, by 6 weeks, a normally hearing infant is more attracted to human speech than to any other sound. A 6-month-old baby already has an ability to analyze language—to break it down into its parts—to put those parts back together again and to store language in its brain and retrieve it. By 18 months, most children are producing simple sentences.

Fortunately, many of the negative results of deafness in babies can be prevented or substantially lessened. Many research studies have demonstrated that early intervention with hearing-impaired children results in improved language development, increased academic success and increased lifetime earnings. Early intervention actually saves money, since hearing-impaired children who receive early help require less costly special education services later.

If it is to be effective, early intervention with deaf children should begin before the child's first birthday. Unfortunately, we are not doing a very good job of detecting infant deafness in the United States. A recent report to Congress and the President by the Commission on Education of the Deaf pointed out that the average age at which profoundly deaf children in this country are identified is $2\frac{1}{2}$ years. In contrast, the average at which such children are identified in Israel and Great Britain is 7 to 9 months.

Clearly, we must do a much better job of early identification if we are to reduce the unnecessary suffering, poor educational performance and lack of productivity that so often accompany deafness. Three groups of people must work together.

Parents are in the best position to identify their child's hearing difficulties. We need to do a better job of making parents aware of the danger signals and of the sources of help that are available to them.

Physicians need to become more responsive to parents' concerns about their child's hearing. Too often, those concerns are brushed aside or ignored. Yet, a recent study found that parents of hearing-impaired children knew about their baby's hearing loss an average of 7 months before it was diagnosed and that almost half of them were given poor advice, such as "don't worry about it" or "wait until the child starts school," when they told their doctors about their concerns.

State agencies can help by initiating high-risk screening programs, such as those currently in operation in Utah, Colorado, Oklahoma, Tennessee and several other states. Research indicates that such programs are able to identify up to 75% of infants who are born deaf or with hearing impairments.

Many others can help too, of course, from older brothers and sisters to grandparents and babysitters. We in the federal government are committed to doing our part. The 1986 Education of the Deaf Act, which authorized the creation of the Commission on the Education of the Deaf, was a first step. At the National Institutes of Health, a new research institute, the National Institute of Deafness and Communication Disorders, has been authorized and is now in formation.

I am optimistic. I foresee a time in this country, in the near future, in fact, when no child reaches his or her first birthday with an undetected hearing impairment. It's a tall order, yes, but if we all work together, I believe we can fill it.

According to the American Academy of Audiology (1992), more than 7000 professionally trained audiologists are available with appropriate skills and equipment to evaluate the hearing of any child at any age with a high degree of accuracy. The hearing of newborn infants can be tested by a sophisticated evoked potential technique, the auditory brainstem response, which accurately identifies even mild degrees of hearing loss. In children with a developmental age of 6 months or older, hearing can be assessed by traditional behavioral procedures that permit identification of any degree of hearing loss. Once hearing loss is identified, medical or audiologic intervention can be initiated immediately. At the first sign of hearing loss, children, even newborns, should receive a formal audiologic evaluation by a licensed audiologist.

HOW WE HEAR

Hearing is one of our most important senses, and yet the mysteries by which we perceive and understand complex sounds have yet to be revealed fully. The intricate actions and interactions of the hearing process have fascinated auditory researchers for more than a century. The microscopic, complicated, and interacting anatomy and neural connection mechanisms involved in hearing have challenged scientists. This complex sensory system is incredible when it is realized that the size of the entire hearing and balance anatomy is smaller than an adult's little fingernail and is totally embedded in the bones of the skull. The organ of hearing must process sounds that range from the soft rustle of leaves in the wind to the thunderous roar of a departing jet airplane. A simplified, introductory description of the pathways by which sounds reach the brain is presented below to aid in understanding the nature of hearing loss in children.

The basic description of hearing is most easily understood if the ear is divided into three major sections: the outer ear, the middle ear, and the inner ear. The outer ear consists of the external ear and the ear canal; the middle ear includes the eardrum (tympanic membrane) and a small air-space cavity that contains the three smallest bones of the body; the cochlea of the inner ear contains sensory cells that stimulate neural impulses of the auditory nerves to the brain (Fig. 1-1).

We hear sounds through two basic physiologic pathways. The traditional pathway of sound is the *air conduction route,* through which sound waves enter the external ear and ear canal, causing vibration of the tympanic membrane (Fig. 1-2A. The vibrations of the tympanic membrane are transmitted to the inner ear by the three small bones located in the middle ear. As the footplate of the third small bone (the stapes) vibrates, the vibration moves the fluids within the inner ear. Vibration of the inner ear fluid creates changes in the sensory cells, which in turn stimulate neural impulses that travel to the brain creating the sensation we recognize as "hearing."

There is a second route for sound, the *bone conduction pathway* (Fig. 1-2B). When a person hears his or her own voice from a tape or video recording, the typical response is that the voice sounds "strange." The recorded voice sounds "natural" to others, because they always listen to the person by air-conducted waves to their own hearing systems. For the individual, however, listening to his or her recorded voice is strange because people always hear their own voices by bone conduction when they speak. Because the inner ear is encased within the bones of the skull, vibrations carried through the mandible and jaw (and even through the throat) cause the fluids to move within the inner ear. Thus, vibrations of the skull are transmitted directly to the inner ear, effectively bypassing the external and middle portions of the ear. These bone-conducted vibrations stimulate the sen-

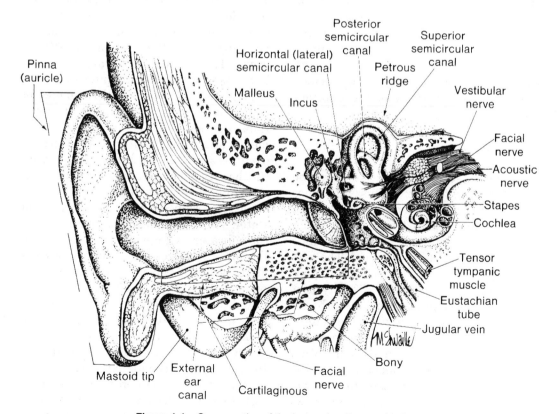

Figure 1-1. Cross-section of the human hearing mechanism.

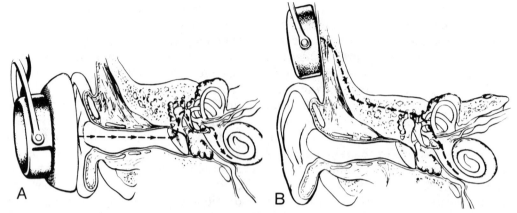

Figure 1-2. The two pathways of sound resulting in "hearing." *Broken arrows* show the routes of the air conduction hearing pathway (A) and the bone conduction hearing pathway (B).

sory cells of the inner ear, again resulting in the neural phenomenon we recognize as "hearing." Sounds transmitted by air-conducted vibrations and bone-conducted vibrations are perceived by the individual as precisely the same sound. It is the comparison of air-conducted and bone-conducted sounds during a hearing test that helps audiologists determine the type and location of a hearing problem. Chapter 2 provides a more thorough discussion of the physiology of cochlea and the neural activity of the auditory pathways.

NATURE OF SOUND

Psychologists and physicists describe sound very differently. This difference was emphasized in the early 1700s, when philosophers loved to debate the question of whether a falling tree makes noise if no one is nearby to hear the sound. The psychologist views sound as a personal quality of sensory perception. The physicist views sound as a propagating disturbance in the air initiated by a vibrating source. The physicist studies the generation, transmission, reception, and modification of sound waves as the science of acoustics. The psychologist studies the human reaction to sound waves that we know as "hearing." There is important information contained within both points of view which needs to be acknowledged to understand how we hear and communicate.

Sound waves in the air follow the physical rules of wave motion, much like the ripples created when a pebble is tossed in a pond. The vibrations produce wave motion. Sound waves are vibrating air particles, set into motion by an energy source, bumping each other to create repetitive waves. These sound waves are measured in terms of frequency and intensity.

Frequency is a physical parameter of sound defined as the number of vibrations per second. The vibrating movements of an object alternately increase *(compression)* and decrease *(rarefaction)* the density of surrounding air molecules, creating waves like those seen when a stone is dropped into a quiet pool of water. Thus, the pattern of movement of the vibrator is imprinted on the air in the form of waves. The number of complete cycles of waves that pass a given point in 1 second is the frequency of the sound. The sound of a single frequency is known as a *pure tone*. The fewer the cycles per second, the lower the frequency; as more cycles per second pass the given point, the higher the frequency measurement. Frequency was historically expressed as cycles per second (cps) and is now known by the internationally agreed upon term, hertz (Hz). A young child's hearing encompasses the frequencies from 20–20,000 Hz. Unfortunately, the ability to hear higher frequencies decreases with age, so adults seldom hear sounds above 8000 or 10,000 Hz.

The frequency of a sound determines the *pitch* of a tone. Pitch is the psychological perception of the frequency of a stimulus. As frequency is increased, the pitch of the sound also increases. A tuning fork produces a specific vibratory pattern determined by its mass and length that is a single pure tone frequency. Pure tones rarely exist in nature; instead, most sounds are complex because they consist of a spectrum of frequencies that differ in intensity and frequency. Although the middle C note on the musical scale is 256 Hz, the actual musical sound carries additional frequency harmonics related to the resonance of the instrument. The output pitch range of human speech is a broad range of frequencies from approximately 500–3500 Hz, which is nearly identical to the optimal frequency sensitivity of our hearing mechanism. Thus, our hearing is designed to receive the most important element of communication—speech (Fig. 1-3).

Intensity describes the physical measurement of the strength or magnitude of a sound. Intensity is determined by the force applied to the moving air molecules; greater forces cause larger sound waves. The psychological correlate of intensity is "loudness." The dynamic range of intensity in the human ability to hear is remarkable. The ratio of intensity of the faintest audible sound to the most intolerable sound is approximately 1–10,000,000! To deal conveniently with such a huge dynamic range, we use a logarithmic notation system with the unit of measure known as the *decibel (dB),* defined as one-tenth of a bel and named for Alexander Graham Bell.

The decibel is an arbitrary unit that expresses the ratio of a measured power or pressure to a specified reference value.

Because it is not an absolute measure, it has no meaning unless the reference value is identified. The usual physical reference value for sound pressure is 20 mPa, and the value is referred to as "dB SPL" (sound pressure level). In audiology measurements, the reference level for the decibel shown on audiograms is the biologic normal hearing baseline, or 0 "dB HL" (hearing level). For conversational speech, the average pressure level of the voice from 5 feet away is approximately 60 dB SPL. Because of the logarithmic nature of the decibel scale, every 10-dB increase represents a 10-fold multiplication of sound. Thus, 50 dB is 10 times more intense than 40 dB; 100 dB is a million times more intense than 40 dB. Furthermore, the 10-dB difference between 110 and 120 dB is much greater than the 10-dB difference between 40 and 50 dB.

Audiologists evaluate hearing by presenting single frequency tones to patients at varying intensities to establish auditory thresholds across a frequency range. Threshold is defined as the minimum effective stimulus that is capable of evoking a response. In audiometry, however, hearing thresholds are defined as the minimum intensity of a tone at which the patient will respond approximately 50% of the time. When the "hearing threshold" is identified at a particular test frequency, it is marked on a special chart known as an audiogram (Fig. 1-4). Audiologists determine pure tone thresholds by air conduction signals through earphones or bone-conducted signals through specialized vibration transducers that fit behind the ear against the skull.

NATURE OF HEARING LOSS

Hearing loss has no single cause, but rather occurs from a wide spectrum of possible causes including inherited or congenital problems, infections, diseases, or traumatic situations that affect different portions of the ear and hearing mechanism. Hearing losses are categorized as

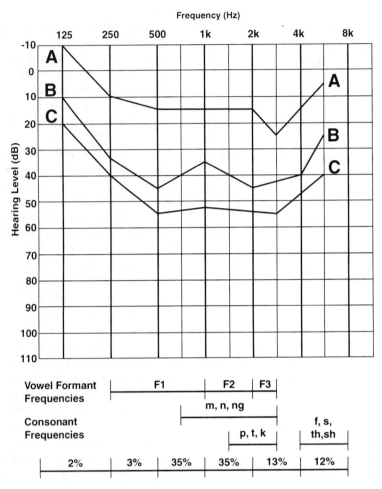

Figure 1-3. The area between curves A and B represents 80% of normal conversational speech levels. Conversational speech exceeds *curve A* 90% of the time, speech exceeds *curve B* only 50% of the time, and *curve C* merely 10% of the time. As hearing thresholds fall below curve B, difficulty understanding speech or even isolated words spoken in quiet surroundings are expected. (With permission from Chial, M. (1998). Yet another audiogram. *ASHA Hearing and Hearing Disorders: Research and Diagnostics Newsletter, 2*(1), 2–3.)

conductive or *sensorineural*. When a conductive hearing loss is overlaid on a sensorineural hearing loss, the resultant hearing problem is termed a *mixed hearing loss*. When auditory dysfunction is present in light of normal peripheral hearing mechanisms (i.e., normal hearing levels with no conductive or sensorineural hearing loss), the auditory dysfunction is categorized as a *central auditory problem*. Discussion of the causes of the various types of hearing loss is presented in Chapters 3 and 4.

Conductive Hearing Loss. Interference of any sort in the transmission of sound from the external auditory canal to the inner ear causes conductive hearing loss. In such cases, the inner ear is capable of normal function, but the sound vibration is unable to stimulate the cochlea via the normal air conduction pathway. The conductive-type loss is characterized by a hearing loss for air-conducted sounds, while sounds conducted to the inner ear directly by bone via the skull and temporal bone are heard normally.

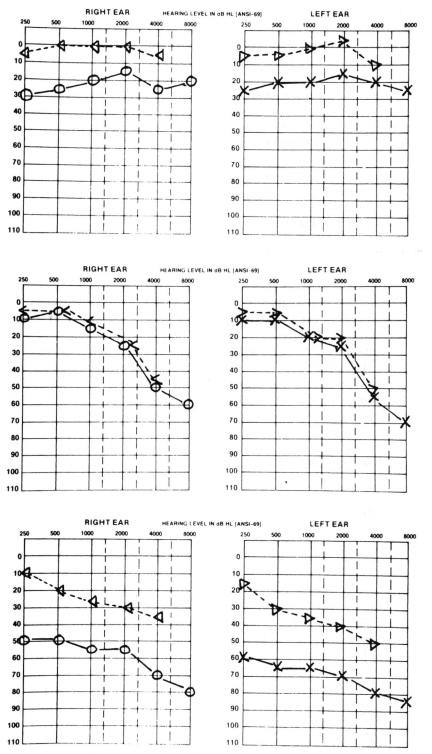

Figure 1-4 Audiograms showing bilateral conductive hearing loss *(top)*, bilateral sensorineural hearing loss *(center)*, and bilateral mixed-type hearing loss *(bottom)*.

Conductive hearing losses are the most common type of hearing loss found in children, often resulting from ongoing ear infections. When the ear canal or middle ear air-conduction pathway is totally blocked with wax or some other obstruction, a maximal conductive hearing loss exists. Conductive-type hearing loss is often associated with craniofacial malformations. Although some conductive hearing losses resolve spontaneously, most require medical or surgical treatment for hearing to return to normal.

Sensorineural Hearing Loss. Hearing impairment occurs when damage has been sustained by the sensory end organ or hair cells located within the cochlea, or the dysfunction may be a problem related to the auditory nerves in the higher pathways. Traditionally, damage to the sensory hair cells is not easily differentiated from auditory nerve damage, so the resultant hearing loss is included in the "sensorineural" category. Audiometric testing techniques such as electrocochleography, otoacoustic emissions, and auditory evoked potentials provide objective means to differente clearly between sensory and neural hearing impairment (see Chapter 7).

In sensorineural hearing losses, the air and bone conduction auditory thresholds are the same. Sensorineural hearing losses may easily be overlooked during the typical medical physical examination with an otoscope, because the external auditory canal and tympanic membrane are normal. Progressive sensorineural hearing loss may be due to a wide variety of causes such as bacterial and viral infections, familial inheritance, disease processes encroaching on the otic capsule, auditory nerve or membranous labyrinth, and even metabolic disorders. Sensorineural hearing loss is nearly always permanent and irreversible.

Mixed Hearing Loss. When both a sensorineural and a conductive loss are present, the result is termed a mixed hearing loss. The audiogram shows abnormal bone conduction thresholds, which are closer to normal hearing levels than the air conduction thresholds. This configuration is termed an air-bone gap. The air conduction-bone conduction threshold differences generally disappear when the conductive portion of the hearing loss is ameliorated. The mixed hearing loss, however, will improve only as much as the degree of air conduction-to-bone conduction gap, and hearing levels are not likely to return to normal limits.

Central Auditory Dysfunction. Childhood central auditory disorders can be classified into two groups: those with identifiable neuropathology and those of unknown etiologies that present as communication disorders. The vast majority of children whose conditions are diagnosed as central auditory disorders show communication disorder symptoms with normal hearing and no observable neuropathology (Stach, 1998). This type of auditory dysfunction is not usually accompanied by a decrease in auditory thresholds but tends to manifest itself in varying degrees as a decrease in auditory comprehension. For example, the child may have a normal audiogram but be unable to comprehend complex speech, which may lead to learning disabilities. Approximately 30% of all students diagnosed with learning disabilities have histories of chronic middle ear problems and conductive hearing loss (Upfold, 1988). The diagnosis and treatment of central auditory dysfunction is a complex topic and is discussed more fully in Chapter 5.

Degree and Severity of Hearing Loss. An important consideration in any hearing loss is its degree of impairment. The terms used to identify the degree of hearing loss are *mild, moderate, severe, profound,* and *anacusis* (or total hearing loss). Sometimes, borderline categories of hearing impairment are described with a combination of terms, such as "moderately severe" hearing loss. The term *hearing-impaired* is applied to all children with decreased hearing abilities from mild hearing loss to profound deafness. Children with hearing losses in the mild, moderate, and severe categories are likely to be described as hard-of-hearing. Children with hearing losses in the profound category are more likely to be classified as deaf. More information about how the degree of hearing loss affects a child's speech and language is provided later in this chapter.

Additional consideration regarding the severity of hearing loss is related to whether one ear *(unilateral)* or two ears *(bilateral)* are affected. The child with no hearing in one ear but with normal hearing in the other may function adequately in many situations. The child will fail the school screening test, however, and presents special challenges to the audiologist who tests his or her hearing. This youngster's auditory abilities will be lacking in circumstances where sound localization is needed or in instances when noise exists to compete with the signal of interest.

A complete description of a child's hearing loss should include whether it is unilateral or bilateral, the degree of auditory impairment, and the type of loss (conductive, sensorineural, or mixed). The cause of the hearing loss should also be included and the audiometric evaluation. Sample descriptions of hearing loss are "unilateral, severe sensorineural hearing loss due to mumps" and "bilateral, moderate conductive hearing loss due to middle ear fluid."

WHEN DOES HEARING LOSS IN CHILDREN BECOME A DISABILITY?

It is first necessary to ask if there is a definition for hearing loss in children. At what point does hearing in children cease to be normal and become abnormal? Where does "deafness" begin? These questions have never been satisfactorily researched or resolved. The problem is that no one has adequately defined the parameters of a hearing handicap or described the best method of securing the necessary data for such definition. Thus, it has been extremely difficult to estimate the prevalence of hearing handicaps, for unless there are agreed upon criteria, there is no way to determine the rate of occurrence. A review of a number of demographic studies reveals this dilemma. From these studies there emerge some basic certainties that will allow an estimate of the prevalence of hearing loss and an evaluation of its cost to society.

Demographic Studies of Children's Hearing. A classic survey reported by Jordan and Eagles (1961) obtained otoscopic examination results and auditory thresholds for approximately 4000 children between the ages of 5 and 10 years. When the individual pathologies were compared with the threshold audiometry, it was found that 50% of children with serous otitis media had hearing better than 15 dB HL. Another comparison revealed that of 30 children with nondraining perforations of the eardrum, 40% would not have been identified in the traditional hearing screening test. In other words, even a 15 dB HL screening criterion would have missed more than half the children with middle ear pathologies such as otitis media and perforated eardrums. These authors pointed out that audiometric screening—and even threshold audiometry—might not identify the majority of children with significant ear pathology. Does this mean that there is no relationship between ear disease and hearing loss? Most certainly not. It merely means that one of them has been incorrectly defined. Inasmuch as ear disease is an observable fact, while "hearing loss" is only a concept, the concept needs to be altered to fit the fact.

The Health Examination Survey of the Department of Health, Education and Welfare undertook, in 1963–1970, to collect hearing data on a representative sample of children 6–11 years of age (Leske, 1981). Ear, nose, and throat examinations, audiologic tests, and a parental health questionnaire were given to a sample of U.S. children. The estimate of the prevalence of "hearing handicaps" was obtained from the parent questionnaire, which inquired if their child had "trouble hearing." An equivalent of 1 million children between 6 and 11 years of age (4%) was judged to be hearing handicapped on the basis of this question. Yet the audiometric hearing tests collected by the survey revealed fewer than 1% of the children to be handicapped, using a criterion of average loss (500–2000 Hz) of 26 dB HL as a beginning hearing loss. The National Speech and Hearing Survey of 1968–1969 used the same criterion on a sample of children tested in grades 1 to 12 and found a prevalence of 0.73% (Hull, Mielke, Timmons, et al., 1971).

Evidently, a credibility gap existed in the survey between what parents thought and what the government team decreed as hearing handicap. Either the parents misjudged their children's ability to hear, or the scientific criterion of adequacy was in error. Which was the case? Resolving this question is critical to the activities of schools, government agencies, and health facilities whose task is to identify children with hearing loss.

The National Academy of Sciences conducted audiometric studies on 1639 children between the ages of 4 and 11 years in the Washington, DC, area (Kessner, Snow, & Singer, 1974). They chose as their criterion for a significant hearing loss the level of 15 dB or greater (500–2000 Hz). Based on their criterion for significant hearing loss, 2.2% of the children had bilateral hearing losses and 4.5% had unilateral hearing losses, for a total of 6.7% with significant hearing losses in one or both ears.

Other variables, in addition to ear disease and laterality, are important when looking at prevalence rates. The 1974 Na-

tional Academy of Science (Kessner et al.) study found the prevalence rates of both ear pathology and hearing loss to be almost twice as high in white children as in black children—a condition that may be unique to the Washington, DC, area. The most consistent demographic association was the education level of parents: the more education attained by the parents, the lower the prevalence of hearing loss in the children. There is a lesser but significant association with family income: the higher the income, the lower the rate of hearing loss.

The National Health Interview Survey of 1990 attempted to establish data on the prevalence of hearing impairment in the general population (Delgado, Johnson, Roy, & Trevino, 1990). Its criteria are derived from a descriptive rating obtained from the questions: "Does anyone in the family now have (1) deafness in both ears? (2) any trouble hearing with one or both ears? Currently using a hearing aid?" Affirmative answers were then probed for further information to determine the presence and degree of unilateral or bilateral hearing loss. Results from the national survey showed that 968,000 children (aged 3–17 years) had "hearing trouble," of which 143,000 (15%) "could not hear and understand normal speech." Although the national survey did not attempt to collect data on children younger than 3 years of age, the probing questions revealed that 1.1 million (5.6%) of these persons experienced the hearing problem before 3 years of age and 2.9 million (14.7%) developed the hearing loss between the ages of 3 and 18 years. Of the 143,000 persons who "could not hear and understand normal speech," the survey reported that 9438 (6.6%) of those persons developed the deafness before 3 years of age and 13,442 (9.4%) experienced the hearing problem between the ages of 3 and 18 years (Ries, 1994).

The Hispanic Health and Nutrition Examination Survey of 1990 included a comparative analysis of hearing in African-

American, Hispanic-American, and non-Hispanic white children. The results showed a significantly higher prevalence of hearing loss in Cuban-American and Puerto Rican children relative to the three ethnic study groups (Lee, Gomez-Marion, & Lee, 1996). In a follow-up report, the prevalence (per thousand) of overall hearing loss greater than 30 dB ranged from 6.4 in Mexican-Americans to 12.3 in Cuban-Americans. Moderate to profound unilateral hearing loss in the study ranged from 0 in Cuban-Americans to 5.2 in Puerto Ricans. Among these five ethnic groups, estimates were made that nearly 400,000 school-aged children in the United States have unilateral hearing loss (Lee, Gomez-Marion, & Lee, 1998).

Data extrapolated from the third National Health and Nutritional Examination Survey (1998) indicated that more than 7 million children have hearing loss. Based on a multi-stage probability study design that included an in-person interview and audiometric testing of 6166 nationally representative children aged 6 to 19 years, 14.9% of children had a hearing loss (defined as greater than 16 dB loss for either or both ears). High-frequency hearing loss was more prevalent than low-frequency hearing loss (12.7% versus 7.1%), and 4.9% of children had combined high- and low-frequency hearing loss. Most of the hearing loss noted was unilateral and mild (16–25 dB loss). Age, gender, and sociodemographic characteristics did not influence low-frequency hearing loss, but older male children and children from low-income families were more likely to have had high-frequency loss. Only 10.8% of children who had hearing loss on audiometric testing self-reported a hearing problem. Although this study did not seek to determine the cause of the hearing loss, it certainly reaffirms the necessity for regular hearing testing for all children and follow-up for those who fail the screening (Niskar et al., 1998). According to the National Institute on Deafness and Communicative Disorders (1997), there are approximately 3,000,000 children who are deaf or hard of hearing in the United States.

Minimal Criteria for Hearing Loss. There have been few studies that have attempted to establish normative data for normal hearing in children. The majority of available data about the hearing status of school-aged children is based solely on the results of hearing screening examinations. These studies are somewhat suspect because of deficient testing conditions and protocols, and thus cannot be used to establish absolute normative levels for hearing in children. Haapaniemi (1996) reported a scientific study of more than 1000 school-aged children in Finland. The Finnish study found that hearing levels in children had a tendency to improve with age up to 10 years (i.e., the mean threshold average for 10-year-olds was 3 dB better than in children of 7 years of age). Mean hearing thresholds were 0.4 dB–1.2 dB better in girls than in boys. This finding raises the question, do hearing levels really improve with age in childhood or is this improvement only the result of better attention and motivation? More normative studies of normal-hearing children will have to be conducted to answer this question adequately.

The American Academy of Otolaryngology's *Guide for the Evaluation of Hearing Handicap* gives directions to compensation agencies for rating the percentage of hearing loss in compensation cases involving adults. The rating schedule was never intended for use with children. Handicap is rated in terms of the ability to hear everyday speech in quiet and noise, but it is measured in terms of pure tone thresholds. The average of the thresholds at 500, 1000, 2000, and 3000 Hz was thought to reflect a realistic degree of the understanding of speech in both quiet and noise. Threshold at 3000 Hz is selected because of its importance in understanding speech in noise or when speech is distorted.

In the hearing handicap formula, only hearing loss averages greater than 25 dB are considered handicapping for compensation rating. This "low-fence" value of 25 dB has been used for many years to evaluate the hearing of adults, with the inherent assumption, apparently, that adults do not experience communication difficulties until their hearing impairment exceeds an average of 25 dB between 500 and 3000 Hz. Most audiologists realize that in real-life situations with environmental noise, the traditional low-fence of 25 dB does not adequately represent the "true" hearing handicap. It is possible that modern times are producing background noises so loud that they make hearing of speech increasingly difficult? And how realistic is it to apply this adult "low-fence" value to children's hearing needs? Davis, Elfenbein, Schum, and Bentler (1986) reported that hearing loss of any degree appeared to affect the psychoeducational development of children adversely, leading to the conclusion that even minimal hearing loss places children at risk for language and learning problems.

Bess, Dodd-Murphy, and Parker (1998) conducted a study of school-aged children in Nashville, TN, to determine the prevalence of minimal sensorineural hearing loss and to assess the relationship of the minimal loss to educational performance and functional status. Minimal hearing loss was defined as 20 dB HL or greater in the speech frequencies or a high-frequency loss of 20–40 dB at 1000, 2000, and 4000 Hz. They sampled 1218 children from the 3rd, 6th, and 9th grades and concluded that children with minimal sensorineural hearing loss experienced more difficulty than normal-hearing children on a series of educational and functional test measures. In fact, 31% of children with minimal sensorineural hearing loss had failed at least one grade. Edwards (1991, 1996) suggested that hearing aids might serve some of these children well and that other management intervention

strategies, such as enhancement of listening skills, auditory programming, and modification of the listening environment, might be helpful as well. The prevalence of minimal sensorineural hearing loss in the study was 5.4%, whereas the prevalence for all forms of hearing loss was 11.3%. Thus, the prevalence of hearing loss in the schools almost doubles when children with minimal sensorineural hearing loss are included. Even mild and moderate levels of hearing impairment interfere with the reception of a significant percentage of spoken language.

It is the authors' contention that children have a more critical need for hearing during their developmental and school years than do adults for understanding everyday speech. We believe strongly that 15 dB HL should be considered the lower limit of normal hearing for children and that impairment begins with each decibel of hearing loss greater than 15 dB HL (Figs. 1-5 and 1-6). Some may question why a 15-dB hearing loss may result in

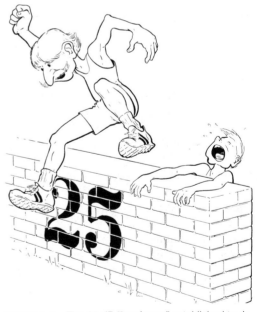

Figure 1-5. The 25 dB "low fence," established to define the beginning of hearing loss in adults, may be too severe to serve as the "low-fence" figure for children's hearing loss.

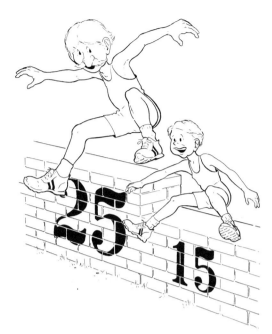

Figure 1-6. Normal hearing "low fence" for the beginning of hearing loss in children may be more appropriate at 15 dB HL because of their more critical need for hearing all the intricacies of speech.

speech and language delays. The reasons lie in the nature of speech sounds, with the major amount of speech energy residing in the voiced vowels and consonants. The unvoiced consonants /s, p, t, k, th, f, sh/ contain so little speech energy that they often fall below even normal hearing

thresholds in average rapid conversation. Persons who have learned speech and language normally can automatically use learned strategies for understanding speech in context (the brain can fill in the missing sounds). However, infants, toddlers, and young children who are just learning speech relationships need to hear *all* the sounds clearly to implant the perceptions solidly.

ACOUSTICS OF SPEECH

The sounds of the English language are generally classified as vowels or consonants. Vowel sounds tend to carry the most vocal energy (intensity) in speech, whereas the higher-frequency consonant sounds contribute to the intelligibility of speech. The relative importance of speech frequency bands for the understanding of spoken language is shown in Figure 1-7. Spoken language is further characterized by its *prosody*—described in terms of pitch and loudness, duration of spoken elements, as well as vocal stress and temporal patterns.

Vowels are characterized by periodicity produced by vocal fold vibration. Vowel quality is determined by energy in several frequency regions, called *formants,* whose center frequency depends on the

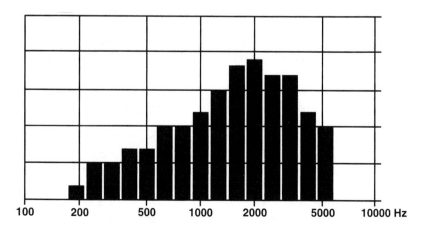

Figure 1-7. Graph showing the relative importance of individual speech bands for speech intelligibility. (Adapted from American National Standards Institute. (1969). *Specifications for audiometers.* ANSI S36-1969. New York: American National Standards Institute.)

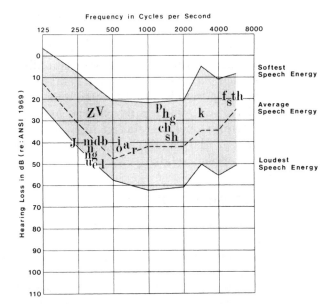

Figure 1-8. Average range of speech energy in dB HL is shown in audiogram form, with the average range of softest and loudest speech energy in conversation. (Adapted from Dudich et al., 1975; Skinner, M.W. (1978). The hearing of speech during language acquisition. *Otolaryngology Clinics of North America 11*, 631–650.)

shape of the vocal tract. The first three formants are the most important for correct recognition of English vowels. The frequency response of the first formant, F1, is about 250 Hz–1000 Hz; the second formant, F2, is found in the frequency region between 1000 Hz and 2000 Hz; and the third formant, F3, occurs between 2000 Hz and 3000 Hz. Vowels are usually more intense and relatively longer than consonants. The vocalized glides /w,j/ and semivowels /r,l/ resemble vowels in their acoustic representation (see Fig. 1–3).

General American English speech sounds are described in terms of the way they are produced. In traditional articulatory phonetics, the main divisions are (1) voicing, related to vocal fold vibration (e.g., voiced or voiceless); (2) place, related to articulators used to constrict the vocal tract (e.g., tongue or lips); and (3) manner, related to degree of nasal, oral, or pharyngeal cavity construction (e.g., plosives, fricatives, nasals). Thus /b/ in the word *be* is a voiced bilabial plosive. In contrast, acoustic phonetics identifies speech sounds in terms of acoustic parameters-frequency composition, relative intensities, and changes in duration. The acoustic energy of speech is surprisingly

small. Human vocal cords can convert only a fraction of the energy of the air stream flowing from the lungs into the acoustic energy required for speech.

Fricative consonants (i.e., /f/, /z/) are characterized by aperiodic noise and may be voiced or voiceless. Fricatives are classified in voiced-unvoiced cognate pairs. Each member of the pair is articulated in the same way and has similar acoustic characteristics except for the presence or absence of voicing. The frequency regions differentiate consonant pair, that is, the /3,ʃ/ pair has energy between 2500 and 4500 Hz, whereas the /z,s/ pair has energy in the frequency region of 3500 through 8000 Hz. The /h/, /f/, and /ə/ have less energy than the rest of the fricatives.

Plosive consonants, also known as stop consonants, are produced when air pressure is built up to the point of complete closure in the vocal tract and is then released abruptly, causing a burst of air. A silent period followed by a burst of air is distinctive in plosives and identifies them as different from other consonants. The unvoiced plosives are characterized by an aspiration period before the onset of the succeeding voiced vowels. The voiced plosives are characterized by the burst of air immediately preceding the onset of the succeeding vowel. Acoustic cues for differentiation among the various plosives are the frequency of the released burst and the second formants transitions. That is, changes in the center frequency of energy in the burst of /b/ and /p/ are relatively low frequency, those changes of /d/ and /t/ are relatively high frequency, and those changes in the center frequency burst of /k/ vary with the adjacent vowel. The relative contribution of the consonant frequencies to the understanding of speech is shown by the fact that nearly 70% of word recognition is determined by the speech energy between 500 and 2000 Hz. An additional 25% of word recognition energy occurs by energy falling above 2000 Hz.

Variation in Acoustic Parameters of Speech Sounds. Skinner (1978) suggested that infants would recognize speech sounds with relative ease if they were not spoken in rapid succession and if the acoustic features were constant. However, speech-sound acoustic cues vary (1) each time an individual speaker produces a speech sound, (2) from speaker to speaker, and (3) with changes in phonetic context as they are modified by adjacent speech sounds and stress patterns. Most children and adults recognize the ambiguous, sometimes even distorted, acoustic cues provided in everyday conversation with remarkable ease. Although there are multiple acoustic cues for recognizing speech sounds, other cues include the general speech situation or context, previous experience and expectations, and, most importantly, knowledge of the language. Speech recognition depends partially on the acoustic signal and partially on the listener's language experience. Through extensive listening experiences, the infant learns where the boundaries of speech sounds and words occur in connected speech. The process is called *segmentation* (see Chapter 5).

In different listening environments over time, the average intensity of speech varies between 20 and 60 dB HL, with an average of approximately 40 dB HL (Fig. 1-8). Shouting is about 65 dB HL; for whispering, the average intensity level may drop 10–20 dB below normal speech levels. The human vocal range constitutes a 700 to 1 ratio of intensities between the weakest and strongest speech sounds made while speaking at a normal conversational level (Fletcher, 1953). Ordinary background noise varies between approximately 35 and 68 dB SPL. For normal-hearing adults, the situation in which noise is 10–15 dB below the level of speech does not create difficulty in listening, because the listener can fill in missing acoustic cues. In contrast, the linguistically unsophisticated infant cannot fill in the missing acoustic details, and speech energy needs to be 30 dB louder than the background masking noise.

The frequency and intensity of general English sounds during conversational speech are plotted on an audiogram and compared with common environmental sounds in Figure 1-9. The diagrammatic audiogram shown in Figure 1-9 has proven useful in counseling parents about the audibility of speech in regard to their child's hearing loss. However, inasmuch as the data plotted on the audiogram are based on normal speech and normal hearing, the audiogram no doubt underestimates problems of speech understanding that arise from distortion contributed by sensorineural pathology as well as from environmental factors such as reverberation and competing noise (Chial, 1998).

Connected speech carries suprasegmental information, which depends on the rhythm of speech and consists of stress and intonation patterns as well as durational characteristics. Stressed speech sounds or words are longer in duration, more intense, and higher in fundamental frequency than unstressed speech sounds. Change in the fundamental frequency of voiced sounds contributes to intonation,

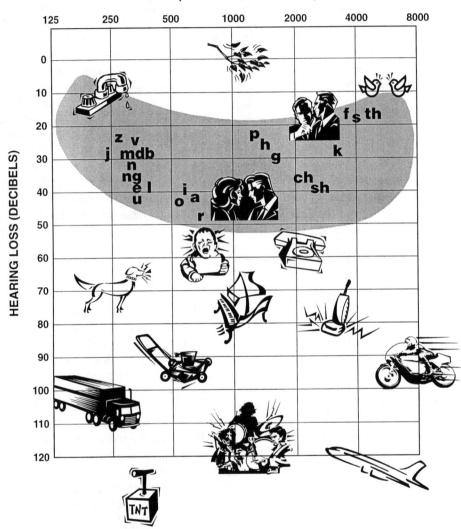

AUDIOGRAM OF FAMILIAR SOUNDS

PITCH (CYCLES PER SECOND)

Figure 1-9. Frequency spectrum of familiar sounds plotted on a standard audiogram. Shaded area represents the "speech banana" that contains most of the sound elements of spoken speech.

which helps the listener identify sentence type. There is little definitive information about the specific role of suprasegmental parameters, but within broad limits they can be specified for various grammatical configurations.

An ingenious scheme to show what happens with a mild 20-dB loss was de-vised by Dobie and Berlin (1979). They undertook to find out what kind of speech perception problems such a child would have in language learning situations. They recorded speech sample utterances in two ways. First they recorded the speech samples through correcting filters; then, they attenuated the samples by 20 dB to simulate how a person with a 20-dB conductive hearing loss would perceive the material. The perception of these treated utterances revealed that (1) there was a potential loss of transitional information, especially plural endings and related final-position fricatives, and (2) very brief utterances or high-frequency information could either be distorted or degraded if signal-to-noise conditions were less than satisfactory. Dobie and Berlin reasoned that on the basis of their findings, a child with a 20-dB hearing loss might be handicapped acoustically in the following ways:

• Morphologic markers might be lost or sporadically misunderstood. For example, "Where are Jack's gloves to be placed?" might be perceived as "Where Jack glove be place?"

• Very short words that are often elided in connected speech (see "are" and "to" above) will lose considerable loudness because of the critical relationship between intensity, duration, and loudness.

• Inflections or markers carrying subtle nuances, such as questioning and related intonation contouring, can at the very best be expected to come through inconsistently.

EFFECT OF HEARING LOSS ON SPEECH AND LANGUAGE

Hearing loss does not cause one specific kind of communication problem. The effects of a hearing loss depend on its severity, configuration, duration, and stability as well as the age of the person at onset. In the hearing-impaired child, the extent and type of early training; the type and timing of amplification; visual, emotional, and intellectual factors; and cultural and family support also influence language development. Age at identification and intervention are especially important factors in language development.

A child who sustains significant hearing loss after acquiring language (3 or 4 years of age) will have a less severe linguistic deficit than the child whose hearing loss is present at birth or develops within the first few months of life.

Children with hearing losses have limited opportunities to "overhear" information from various input sources, which leads to impoverished experiences with negative consequences for language rule formation, world knowledge, and vocabulary development (Carney & Moeller, 1998). Adults know the language they are listening to in the sense of its phonemes, its words, and its grammar. They have subtly learned what phoneme sequences make up meaningful words and how the rules of grammar and semantics determine word order. The major effect of a hearing impairment is the loss of audibility for some or all of the important acoustic speech cues. Persons with hearing loss typically complain of an inability to understand speech. Conversation may be loud enough for them, but they cannot understand the words because the hearing loss distorts the acoustic signal and interferes with auditory processing.

Carney (1999) cautions audiologists against assuming linearity of a hearing loss. That is, hearing loss does not progress in an orderly fashion, and each 10 dB of additional hearing loss does not cause the same decrease in auditory function, regardless of the degree of hearing loss.

Skinner (1978) listed a number of detrimental "acoustic liabilities" to a child's language learning when a hearing loss exists:

• **Lack of Constancy of Auditory Clues When Acoustic Information Fluctuates.** When a child does not hear speech sounds in the same way from one time to another, there is confusion in abstracting the meanings of words due to inconsistent categorization of speech sounds.

- **Confusion of Acoustic Parameters in Rapid Speech.** Even the normal-hearing child suffers from variations of speech occurring among speakers and even in the same speaker. Frequency, duration, and intensity vary as a result of differences among speakers of different ages, genders, and personality types. The child with hearing loss will be confused in language learning as a result.

- **Confusion in Segmentation and Prosody.** The child with hearing loss may miss linguistic boundaries such as plurals, tenses, intonation, and stress patterns. These factors are requisite to meaningful interpretation of speech.

- **Masking of Ambient Noise.** As early as 1947, French and Steinberg noted that the normal-hearing child requires a signal-to-noise ratio of +30 dB (i.e., the speech signal must be 30 dB louder than the background noise) for speech learning to take place. Unfortunately, it is rare in our modern culture for such an easy listening ratio to be present. Public school classrooms typically have signal-to-noise ratio of +12 dB or less. Obviously, a child with even a minimal hearing loss is handicapped under such listening situations.

- **Breakdown of Early Ability to Perceive Speech Sounds.** The infant begins to learn to discriminate speech sounds almost immediately after birth. Studies have shown that between 1 and 4 months of age an infant can discriminate between most of the English speech sound pairs. By 6 months of age, the infant recognizes many of the speech sounds of language and is making ongoing cataloging of speech sounds (see Chapter 4). If the sounds of speech are not perceived early, due to the presence of a hearing loss, learning can be impeded.

- **Breakdown in Early Perceptions of Meanings.** During ordinary speech, the normal listener often misses some unstressed or elided words or sounds but is able to fill in by understanding the context of the message. However, when a hearing loss causes a young child to miss many of these soft or inaudible sounds, there is confusion in word naming, difficulty in developing classes of objects, and misunderstanding of multiple meanings.

- **Faulty Abstraction of Grammatical Rules.** When short words are soft or elided, as they often are, it becomes more difficult for a hearing-impaired child to identify the relationships between words and to understand word order.

- **Subtle Stress Patterns Missing.** Conductive hearing loss is usually worse in the low frequencies than in the higher frequencies. The emotional content of speech, its rhythm, and its intonation are communicated through the low frequencies. When these are lost, the emotional content of speech is confused—another condition that impairs the learning of speech and language.

DEGREES OF HEARING IMPAIRMENT

It is common practice to simplify hearing losses into terms such as mild, moderate, severe, and profound for ease of communication. However, this categorization by degree is potentially misleading and, perhaps, an unfortunate practice. Yet, these terms are in common use although there is no standard agreement as to the definitive criteria for each category. For example, a child labeled with "mild" hearing loss might be considered to have only minimal dysfunction—a descriptor that parents, teachers, and physicians may interpret to mean that no significant hearing problem exists. Yet, research by Wohlner (cited by Matkin, 1984) found that young children categorized with "mild" bilateral sensorineural hearing loss showed delay in development of at least 2 years in expressive oral language by the age of 7 years. Children in the study with "moderate'" hearing impairment at age 7 scored below the norms for normal-hearing 4-year-olds. Keeping in mind the limitations associated with such labels, the features commonly used to describe varying degrees of hearing loss are presented below and are summarized in Table 1-1.

Table 1-1.
Handicapping Effects of Hearing Loss in Children

Average Hearing Level (500–2000 Hz)	Description	Possible Condition	What Can Be Heard Without Amplification	Handicapping Effects (If Not Treated in First Year of Life)	Probable Needs
0–15 dB	Normal range	Conductive hearing losses	All speech sounds	None	None
15–25 dB	Slight hearing loss	Conductive hearing losses, some sensorineural hearing losses	Vowel sounds heard clearly; may miss unvoiced consonants sounds	Mild auditory dysfunction in language learning	Consideration of need for hearing aid; speech-reading, auditory training, speech therapy, preferential seating
25–30 dB	Mild hearing loss	Conductive or sensorineural hearing loss	Only some of speech sounds, the louder voiced sounds	Auditory learning dysfunction, mild language retardation, mild speech problems, inattention	Hearing aid, speechreading, auditory training, speech therapy
30–50 dB	Moderate hearing loss	Conductive hearing loss from chronic middle ear disorders; sensorineural hearing losses	Almost no speech sounds at normal conversational level	Speech problems, language retardation, learning dysfunction, inattention	All of the above plus consideration of special classroom situation
50–70 dB	Severe hearing loss	Sensorineural or mixed losses due to a combination of middle ear disease and sensorineural involvement	No speech sounds at normal conversational level	Severe speech problems, language retardation, learning dysfunction, inattention	All of the above plus probable assignment to special classes
70+ dB	Profound hearing loss	Sensorineural or mixed losses due to a combination of middle ear disease and sensorineural involvement	No speech or other sounds	Severe speech problems, language retardation, learning dysfunction, inattention	All of the above plus probable assignment to special classes

Mild Hearing Loss (15–30 dB HL). A 15- to 30-dB hearing loss will have a significant effect on communication and language learning and educational achievement. Vowel sounds are heard clearly, but voiceless consonants may be missed. In children with a 15- to 30-dB hearing loss, auditory learning dysfunction may result in inattention, mild language delay, and mild speech problems. This hearing-impaired child hears only the louder, voiced speech sounds. The short unstressed words and less intense speech sounds (such as voiceless stops and fricatives) are inaudible. The acoustic cues of speech that are audible may be perceived differently by someone with a 15- to 30-dB conductive loss than by someone with a 15- to 30-dB sensorineural hearing loss.

Moderate Hearing Loss (31–50 dB HL). These children miss most conversational speech sounds, but they typically respond well to language and educational activities with the help of hearing aid amplification. Children with moderate hearing loss may show inattention, language retardation, speech problems, and learning problems. These children will likely have difficulty learning abstraction in the meaning of words and the grammatical rules of language because they do not hear some of the speech sounds and they hear other speech sounds inaccurately. With this degree of hearing loss, vowels are heard better than consonants. Short, unstressed words such as prepositions and relational words, as well as word endings (-s, -ed), are particularly difficult to hear. This reduction of cues and information leads to confusion among speech sounds and word meanings, limited vocabulary, difficulty with multiple meanings of words, difficulty in developing object classes, confusion of grammatical rules, errors in word placement in sentences, and omission of articles, conjunctions, and prepositions. Omission and distortion of consonants typically characterize the speech articu-

lation of the individual with moderate hearing loss. Strangers may have difficulty understanding the speech of a child with moderate hearing loss.

Severe Hearing Loss (50–70 dB HL). Language and speech will not develop spontaneously in children with severe hearing loss. With early intervention, use of appropriately fit hearing aids, and special education, these children may eventually function very well. Without amplification, children with severe hearing loss cannot hear sounds or normal conversation. They can hear their own vocalizations, albeit distorted, some very loud environmental sounds, and only the most intense conversational speech when spoken loudly at close range. With the use of hearing aids, they can discern vowel sounds and differences in manner of consonant articulation. This degree of hearing loss generally results in severe language problems, speech problems, and associated educational problems.

Profound Hearing Loss (71 dB HL or Greater). Children with profound hearing loss can only learn language and speech with intensive special education. Their success in life is greatly improved with early identification and treatment of their hearing loss problem. Without amplification through hearing aids, children with profound hearing loss are generally unable to hear sounds. With appropriately fit amplification, they may hear the rhythm patterns of speech, their own vocalizations, and environmental sounds. Profound hearing loss results in severe language retardation, speech problems, and possible related learning dysfunction. Boothroyd (1993) suggested three additional categories to describe those children with more than profound hearing losses: (1) those children with considerable residual hearing with thresholds between 90 to 100 dB HL; (2) those with limited residual hearing between 101 dB and 120 dB HL; and (3) those children with no measurable hearing or auditory thresholds of 121 dB HL or greater.

The speech of children with profound hearing loss is characterized with voice, articulation, resonance, and prosody problems. Their vocal pitch is frequently higher than that of normal-hearing people, and the prosodic features of intonation and stress are missing, giving their voices a monotone quality. The speech of deaf children is characterized by (1) slow temporal patterning, (2) inefficient use of the breath stream, (3) prolongation of vowels, (4) distortion of vowels, (5) abnormal rhythm, (6) excessive nasality, and (7) addition of an undifferentiated neutral vowel between abutting consonants. The articulation of severely to profoundly hearing-impaired children has been observed to have excessive mandibular movement, lack of tongue movement, posterior tongue positioning, voiced-voiceless confusions for consonants, problems with coarticulation, substitution of visible sounds for those sounds that are difficult to see, better articulation for initial speech sounds than for medial or final speech sounds, stop/plosive confusion, and the intrusion of an undifferentiated neutral vowel between abutting consonants. Studies of speech intelligibility indicate that, at best, naive listeners understand 20–25% of the speech of children with profound deafness. Deaf children use concrete rather than abstract words and concepts with poor syntactic constructions limited by their lack of exposure to natural language.

DEFINING HEARING LOSS

The definition of a handicapping hearing loss in any given case lies in the entire diagnostic process, which includes not only hearing tests but requires measurements of a child's receptive and expressive language, vocalization and speech levels, and behavioral functioning evaluations. Such diagnostic evaluations are best conducted by enlisting professionals from other disciplines, such as a speech-language pathologist, to help determine if the child is sufficiently language-delayed to warrant educational intervention. The initial identification of these children generally occurs through the family practice physician or the pediatrician. As the sources of primary medical care, these professionals often serve as the gatekeepers for managed care organizations and therefore hold the keys to referrals to other specialists. The primary caregiver will also require support and help as to when to apply measures of language competence to determine whether a handicapping hearing loss is present in a young child.

The foregoing concepts can be used in proposing a realistic definition of hearing loss in children, namely: *A handicapping hearing loss in a child is any degree of hearing that reduces the intelligibility of a speech message to a degree inadequate for accurate interpretation of speech or as to interfere with learning.* Such a definition recognizes that it may not be possible to place specific measure on what precisely handicaps a child's ability to learn. Too many variables are present in the learning process of children: amount of parental stimulation, quality of parental stimulation, innate intelligence, age of onset of hearing loss, personality factors, health conditions, and socioeconomic status. These variables may so affect the learning abilities of children that a 15-dB loss may be a handicap to one child, whereas a 25-dB loss will not handicap another.

CHILDREN WITH UNILATERAL DEAFNESS

Unilateral hearing loss (involvement of one ear only) is a fairly common problem among children, with a prevalence of 3–13 in 1000 depending on the definition of the degree of hearing loss in the abnormal ear (Berg, 1972). Total unilateral deafness is most commonly due to mumps developed in very early childhood or as the sequel to a case of subclinical mumps with no obvious symptoms. In many instances, the child and family are unaware of the problem, and the parents do not discover the loss until some sequence of events suggests the presence of a hearing loss in one ear. Parents will finally realize that their child can only hear on the telephone with one particular ear, or the child cannot be awakened when the normal-hearing ear is pressed into a pillow.

When the unilateral hearing loss is confirmed by testing, the audiologist should take time to explain the ramifications of the problem. These patients, with only one hearing ear, have significant difficulties in localizing the source of a sound. They have pronounced difficulties in listening in backgrounds of noise, and they lose the binaural summation effect provided by two ears, creating overall and ongoing communication difficulties.

Children with unilateral deafness are educationally disabled. Studies by Bess and Tharpe (1984) and Bess, Klee, and Culbertson (1986) at Vanderbilt University have brought renewed attention to the child with only one normal-hearing ear. They identified 60 children with unilateral hearing loss who were enrolled in the Nashville Metropolitan School System and closely examined their educational records. They found that approximately one-third of this group had failed at least one grade during their school years and that nearly 50% of the group needed special resource assistance in the schools. In studies in which unilaterally hearing-impaired children were matched with normal-hearing children, Bess's group showed that the children with unilateral hearing loss performed much poorer on localization tasks and syllable recognition tasks. From these research efforts, it is clear that children with unilateral hearing loss experience considerably more difficulty in communication and in education than was previously supposed.

Oyler, Oyler, and Matkin (1987, 1988) challenged the Vanderbilt data on unilat-eral hearing loss by conducting a similar study in a large school district in Tucson, Arizona. They found a remarkably similar academic failure rate, proving again that children with unilateral hearing loss are at a risk factor approximately 10 times greater than that for the general school population for academic difficulties resulting in grade failure. In both the Nashville and Tucson studies, the recurring profile among the unilateral hearing loss students who experienced academic difficulties included (a) early age of onset, (b) severe to profound hearing impairment, and (c) right-ear impairment. Oyler et al. (1987) suggested several management recommendations for supporting the child with unilateral hearing loss. These recommendations are equally applicable for communicating with all children who have hearing loss:

- Gain the child's attention before beginning to speak
- Use familiar vocabulary and less complex sentence structure
- Rephrase statements that are misunderstood, rather than just repeating them verbatim
- Provide visual supplement to the communication to improve understanding
- Provide students preferential classroom seating to take advantage of the better hearing ear
- Minimize noise interference generated from within or outside the classroom
- Routinely monitor the child's speech and language development and academic progress
- Consider use of special hearing aid fitting systems such as cross routing of signals (CROS)
- Consider use of a personal FM or a classroom amplification system to enhance the signal-to-noise ratio
- Provide hearing conversation rules to protect the good ear:
  (a) Stay away from loud noises

(b) Get prompt medical care for any ear infection

(c) Avoid putting anything into the ear

(d) Avoid ototoxic drugs unless absolutely necessary

(e) Take special care of general health, especially during flu seasons

(f) Have an otologic and audiologic check once a year

(g) Do not get advice on treatment from anyone except qualified otolaryngologists and audiologists

THE MALINGERING CHILD

This section discusses the child who is malingering a feigned, functional, or nonorganic hearing loss for some consciously desired purpose. The pediatric audiologist will inevitably run into a child who responds as though a hearing loss is present when no problem really exists. The child who makes a pretense of having a hearing loss is quite different from the malingering adult. The child is typically much less sophisticated with the deception of poor hearing than the adult. More importantly, the underlying motives and the impelling factor are usually more obscure. The needs that drive the child to give an inaccurate hearing test are probably more honest, and certainly engender more sympathy, that those that drive the adult. Furthermore, it is often the last thought that some cute youngster is actually exaggerating an existing hearing loss or pretending to have a hearing loss in one or both ears.

Any child who presents with a functional hearing loss has a problem, whether it be a minor transient difficulty or a deep-seated permanent disorder, and has some sort of need. Malingering is a symptom of some other problem. It should never be disregarded or passed off as a temporary foible. It may represent a cry for attention, an apology for poor performance, or a rebuff to a hostile world.

Children who have some basic need that is unfulfilled may choose from a variety of symptoms that are available to them, ranging from the conscious to the psychosomatic. They may complain of stomachaches, headaches, poor vision, poor hearing, or specific pains. They may act out their needs in aggressive behavior or in withdrawal. Their symptoms may enter the psychosomatic realm, with disorders such as eczema or chronic stomach problems. Psychosis may even be present. When their behavior becomes outwardly aggressive and approaches delinquency, their disturbance becomes a threat to their families and to society.

The large majority of children who present with such problems are referred because of failure on the screening test in school. Johnny sees that Joe, who has failed the hearing test, is given special treatment—he is excused from school to have further examinations and is given special seating and attention in school. It is like having headaches or stomachaches—it gives an excuse for poor performance and a chance to bid for sympathy. Be aware that this discussion of feigned hearing loss does not include those children who simply did not understand the instructions given them during a previous test. However, this is also a primitive strategy used by the malingering, so care should be taken to ensure that the child has completely understood the directions.

The audiologist must learn to recognize the child with nonorganic hearing loss through exaggerated behaviors such as verbosity, brashness, overwithdrawal, lack of personal affect, exaggerated straining to hear the test tones, and inconsistent intratest results. The quickest and most obvious clue is poor agreement between the pure tone average of thresholds at 500, 1000, and 2000 Hz and speech reception threshold. The naiveté of young children in responding at normal levels with speech audiometry and exaggerated threshold levels with pure tones usually makes identification of the nonorganic hearing problem easy. Another common clue is wild audiometric threshold variation of 15–25 dB at the same test frequency.

In the final analysis, otoacoustic emission tests, acoustic immittance, audiometric techniques, and ABR measurement may be required to reveal the true state of hearing in the child with nonorganic hearing loss. Normal otoacoustic emissions and normal tympanograms and the presence of bilateral acoustic reflexes rule out any possible conductive hearing problem. The ABR threshold exploration procedure can be used to validate hearing thresholds. It is rare that any of the classic auditory tests for functional hearing loss used with adults need to be used on children. Occasionally, in the case of a monaural feigned hearing loss, the Stenger test can be used to estimate the level of hearing in the supposedly "bad" ear (Stach, 1998).

Once the inconsistencies have been identified, hostility and threats from the audiologist or the family toward the child tend to make matters worse. When the child realizes that the audiologist is suspicious of the responses, "saving face" is an important step toward resolution of the problem. The use of statements such as, "Perhaps you didn't understand my instructions clearly," or "The results of this hearing test are not coming out correctly, and I would like you to listen again as carefully as you can" can be helpful in such situations. The audiologist should take his or her time in the presentation of pure tones and be prepared to wait. If normal hearing levels can be established through traditional behavioral techniques, time and effort are streamlined. The task is to establish ear- and frequency-specific thresholds. The challenge of identifying the malingering child is only half the problem—the true hearing in each ear still needs to be determined.

In terms of general management of the child with nonorganic hearing loss, it is best to refer actual psychologic problems to the professionals best trained to deal with abnormal behavior. The continuum of severity of emotional causes of nonorganic medical problems runs a gamut from mild, transient behaviors to severe malingering. Transient, isolated instances describe most children's attempts to feign hearing loss and, when resolved, usually cause no additional concerns. As the nonorganicity of hearing loss appears to be somewhat more entrenched in the child's daily behavior, certainly the audiologist needs to talk frankly with the parents about the child's problem and to suggest professional counseling. Given truly bizarre behavior, including total noncooperation from the child in the hearing test situation, the main task of the audiologist is to establish the organic hearing levels of the youngster; and psychiatric counsel should urgently be advised with the agreement of the managing physician. The cry for help that is inherent in the presentation of nonorganic hearing loss in a child should not be taken lightly by the audiologist.

PARENT MANAGEMENT

Parents and families of children with special needs play a pivotal role in the successful development of the child. It has become increasingly clear that parents are the best advocates and facilitators for their child and must be actively involved in decision-making. Accordingly, the audiologist must be sensitive to the feelings and needs of families as the hearing loss in their youngster is revealed through the audiometric testing experience. In fact, it is often the audiologist who must inform the parents that their child has significant hearing impairment. This presents an important responsibility for the pediatric audiologist which requires the utmost in professionalism and genuine concern for the involved family.

If possible, it is beneficial to have the parents observe the child's responses in a free-field situation, so that they can see for themselves that the child does not hear normally presented sounds. This firsthand, controlled experience will help the parents realize what they have likely suspected as they note what their child can and cannot hear. Although in many instances the parents have a strong suspicion that their child has a hearing problem, confirmation of the handicap may still be an extremely traumatic situation for them. Whether the parents show grief openly or contain it within themselves, the audiologist can be sure that they will be deeply disturbed over the knowledge and he or she must find ways to help them over this initial shock.

Stein and Jabaley (1981) have published an excellent chapter on parent counseling in their textbook, "Deafness and Mental Health," in which they describe their conclusions based on 15 years of talking with parents of hearing-impaired children. They state that the two most common factors in the environment of deaf children that can account for their emotional or behavioral differences are (1) the lag in language development and its effect on family communication and socialization, and (2) the psychologic response of parents to the diagnosis of a hearing handicap in their child. Stein and Jabaley describe three stages of parental responses: (1) an initial expression of anger toward the professionals who diagnose the deafness in their child, (2) subsequent expressions of anger toward the child as they find it increasingly difficult to deny the existence of the hearing loss, and finally (3) the acceptance of the hearing-impaired child by the parents, which marks the transition from sadness and anger to the development of adaptation and coping behaviors. They urge the development of a working relationship with the involved parents to reduce the high prevalence of emotional and behavioral problems, while helping to establish the important parent-infant bond.

It is the usual tendency of parents to want to find out immediately everything that concerns the future of the child and his or her functioning. One must resist the temptation to go into great detail about the prognosis for the child's development. Whatever is said will be only half-absorbed and largely distorted on the first visit. One should limit the amount of information to the relative degree of loss that seems to be present—mild, moderate, severe, or profound—and concentrate on the implications of the loss and what is going to be done for the child. If the parents press the question as to whether the child will speak, what kind of school he or she will attend, or whether the child will ever communicate, they should be assured that their questions will be answered but only after a period of diagnostic therapy. No one can ever guarantee what a child will be able to do with training; only the results will demonstrate that.

There is perhaps no way to cushion the shock of finding out that a child is hearing-impaired. Any attempt to minimize the problem would be a disservice and would avoid the reality of the situation. Nevertheless, a sympathetic attitude and an understanding of the parents' feelings will help as much as possible. The audiologist could say things such as, "You probably feel pretty upset about this news," or "It's perfectly natural for you to feel badly about this." The parents should be allowed sufficient time to express their feelings and fears and to ask questions. The audiologist should offer to be available for any future questions and let the parents know that they will be closely involved in the process of discovering their child's capabilities. It should be emphasized that he or she is a child first, has a hearing loss only secondarily, and is just as lovable as any other child.

Whenever possible, parents' groups directed by qualified psychologic counselors should be organized to provide ongoing guidance. If further help seems indicated, psychiatric or psychologic counsel should be sought for individual parents. The audiologist should be aware of his or her limitations in providing psychotherapy for parents who cannot handle their problems.

In his or her relationship with the parents, the audiologist's responsibilities include the following:

- A complete explanation of what the audiogram means, and what the child can and cannot hear.

- A description of the type of loss, whether conductive or sensorineural, and what it means in terms of whether medical treatment may or may not be possible.

- A thorough explanation of the educational programs that are available for the child: auditory, oral, or total. The parents should be directed to visit each program so that they may participate in the decision as to which program will be chosen. With proper guidance, they should be able to make this decision themselves.

- Psychologic support to help the parents accept the situation of hearing impairment in their child. This may take the form of a one-to-one relationship, or the parents may require group programs or even individual psychiatric counseling. The audiologist should remember that in this difficult role, he or she can and should seek counseling both for oneself and for the parents if the parents are unable to cope adequately with the situation.

All students of audiology, as well as practicing clinicians, should read the excellent books written by David Luterman, PhD, "Counseling Parents of Hearing-Impaired Children" (1979) and "The Deaf Child" (Luterman, Kurtzer-White, & Seewald, 1999) for additional insight and understanding in managing parents.

ECONOMIC BURDEN OF DEAFNESS

A major concern that has a significant effect on parents when they learn that their child is hearing-impaired or deaf is the worry about potential financial stress. Although no specific amount of money can be identified that will apply to every hearing-impaired or deaf child, at least some consideration can be given to a number of possible factors that should be included to make the child's daily living optimal for communication and education purposes. This information may be used for parents' financial planning or for medical-legal purposes in establishing compensation awards for inadvertent hearing loss resulting from an accident or as the conclusion of an iatrogenic misadventure of medical treatment that is identified as the determinant of the child's hearing impairment.

It is a thought-provoking exercise to consider the economic burden created by childhood deafness. A number of general areas should be considered, including routine medical and audiologic expenses over the lifetime of the child as well as special educational and vocational expenses that are above and beyond those expenses incurred by parents of children with normal hearing. The deaf child will require a number of special living expenses for assistive listening devices and aids to meet ordinary daily life circumstances. Finally, there is the question of loss of income borne by every profoundly deaf individual over the course of his or her adult working life, which is due to the inability to obtain employment of full and equal status with the average, normal-hearing adult. In addition to specific expenditures that can be estimated, consideration must include a number of intangible costs of deafness that affect the deaf person in childhood and throughout adult life. Although statistics to determine the precise economic penalty of deafness are not available, our cursory overview reveals a potentially enormous financial obligation to be shared among the child's parents, state and federal social service agencies, and the hearing-impaired individual.

The amounts shown below are our estimates of approximate costs, based on 1999 dollar values, calculated for a child of 1 year of age with severe hearing impairment with a life expectancy, according to the National Center for Health Statistics, of 75 years:

Medical and Audiologic Expenses. $150,000

- Otolaryngology consultations twice annually until 16 years of age and then annual evaluations throughout adult life
- Audiologic services twice annually until age 18 and as necessary throughout adult life
- Hearing aids, batteries, maintenance, and insurance based on binaural amplification devices used daily and replaced every 4 years throughout life
- Cochlear implant surgeries and devices, follow-up rehabilitation, replacement, and upgrades

Education and Training Expenses. $1,000,000

- Parent-infant program training; speech, language, and auditory training therapy during preschool years; private school for the hearing-impaired, with special educational tutoring services as needed through age 18; computer-assisted learning systems; Gallaudet University, National Technical Institute for the Deaf, or regular college with interpreter services

Special Living Expenses. $150,000

- Baby-cry amplifier; personal FM auditory system; special signaling devices to include door bells, telephone TTY system, fire alarm, alarm clock, wristwatch, all with replacements as necessary and upgrades as needed through-

out life; special interpreter fees as needed for daily living; telecaption system for televisions; captioned films and videos for entertainment and recreational purposes; hearing dog services including provisions for food, shelter, transportation, and medical care

Loss of Income . . . . $500,000–$1,000,000

- Based on a work life expectancy of 50 years and a comparison of the average annual salary with the fact that employed deaf adults earn 30% less annually than normal-hearing persons (Schein & Delk, 1974); it can be further noted that unemployment of deaf adults is more than twice the United States national unemployment figure and (as reported by Internal Revenue Service statistics) more than 20% of deaf adults report no income

Intangible Costs of Deafness. The price of deafness is not limited to economic costs. One must also take into consideration the deep wounds of emotional trauma to the parents and family of the child found to be hearing-impaired. Many have compared the parent's realization of deafness in their child to an actual death, inasmuch as the parents have "lost" the normal child they thought they would have. Many parents go through a denial phase during which they may go from clinic to clinic, searching for a diagnosis and cure that will allow their child to be normal; an anger phase during which they may lash out at clinicians and doctors and try to place blame; a mourning phase during which they experience sadness and depression over the deafness; and finally an acceptance phase that allows them to become active participants in the child's habilitation process. Other intangibles comprise a never-ending recital of problems that only begin with the initial realization of deafness.

Breakdown of Normal Family Communications. Parents are denied the pleasure of being understood easily by their child and of hearing their child speak normally. Their child does not come when they call, does not obey their verbal commands, can neither be praised nor reprimanded orally, and cannot play the kinds of games the rest of the family plays—all these things present difficulties for the parents of a child with severe hearing loss.

Other children in the family are deprived of the attention of their parents, who must spend a great deal of time in coping with the needs of the deaf child. The extra time required to teach that child the basic elements of living, as well as communicating, is taken away from the other siblings who may suffer from this deprivation. The child with deafness suffers as well, for jealousy and anger can arise from siblings and cause family upheaval.

Problems in School. The child with profound hearing loss is isolated from peers in every educational system circumstance. As the mainstreamed child in normal-hearing classes, he or she stands aside while the other children play games involving verbal commands. In the classroom, he or she requires special attention and help that set him or her apart from peers. Studies have shown that although a deaf child may learn well in a mainstreamed environment, he or she may be scarred by the psychological feeling of inferiority and poor self-image (Davis, Elfenbein, Schum, & Bentler, 1986). In a special school for the deaf, he or she is among deaf peers but is only able to communicate fully with them if signing is the mode of communication.

Language learning is always impaired to some degree in the deaf child. The average language level of the young deaf adult has been shown to be often equivalent to the third- or fourth-grade level. This fact has accounted for the poorer earning power of the deaf. It also deprives them of one of the great joys of life: an appreciation of humor that relies on verbal play or on an understanding of some daily usages. For example, a deaf child takes expressions such as "put your best foot forward" absolutely literally unless additional explanation is provided.

Finally, speech defects associated with deafness seriously diminish the social relations of the deaf child with normal-hearing peers. Nothing makes a child an outcast more than "funny speech," and children are notoriously cruel to a child with any deviations from the norm. Unfortunately, few children with profound hearing losses have speech that approaches normal voice quality, so they will always be "different."

Problems in Adulthood. The lower income of the deaf necessitates a more modest lifestyle than is possible for their peers, consigning them to a lower level of living than their potential abilities would have allowed them. When it comes to marriage, the choices of the deaf are narrowed. If the deaf person has been led by his or her family and educational environment to expect to find a hearing mate, he or she may be doomed to disappointment.

One of the most devastating problems facing the deaf is dealing with the demands of the "hearing establishment." Society is organized around hearing people, and major adjustments have to be made for the deaf to confront everyday problems. When a person is deaf, how can he or she explain a tax problem to the Internal Revenue Service? How can he or she go to court and plead a case? Go to the doctor and explain a medical problem? Get out of a burning building in time without hearing the fire alarm? Mobilize the facilities to find a lost child in the mall?

Going through a college program for normal-hearing people requires a supreme effort by the deaf person. To profit from lectures, a note-taker and/or an interpreter to sign during the lectures may be necessary. Most colleges now have these special helps available for the deaf youth, but it requires constant concern and application to keep up with the college requirements. The hearing-impaired or deaf college student may depend on elaborate augmentative communication devices in lieu of helpful colleagues.

The choice of a career is limited for the deaf individual. He or she cannot become a physician without sufficient hearing to interpret heart beats and chest sounds, and he or she cannot become a trial lawyer unless speech is adequate for understanding in a courtroom. Many other occupations are closed to the deaf adult if they require verbal communication with hearing people. It is to the everlasting credit of the human spirit that deaf people are able to rise above these problems and lead the productive and happy lives that most of them have, for despite all the limitations described above, the deaf community is a cohesive, supportive group whose members are generally as contented as their normal-hearing peers.

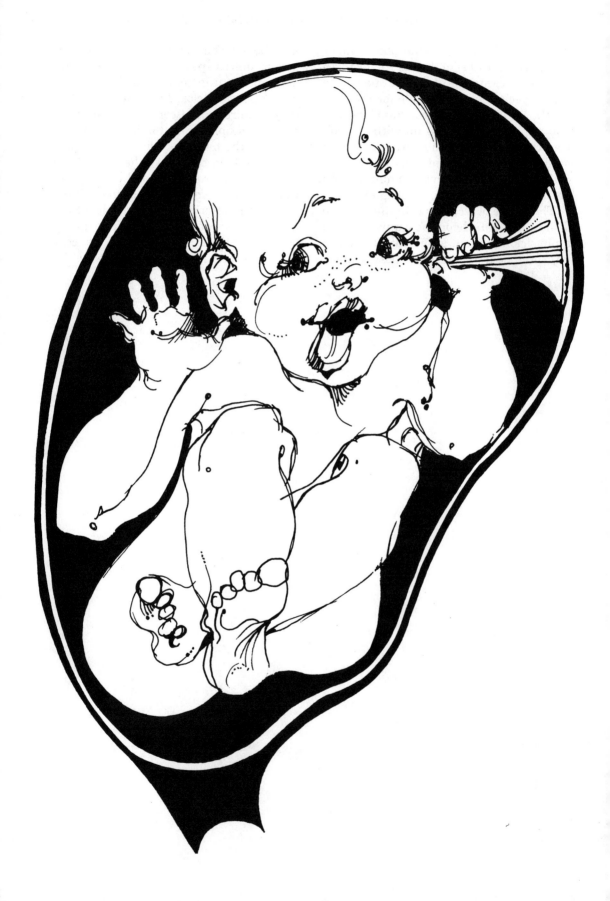

CHAPTER 2

The Auditory System

The mystery of the majesty of creation is abundantly evident in the structure and function of the human hearing mechanism. Originating as a simple extension of a pressure-sensing organ in primitive sea creatures, the human hearing mechanism is a product of evolution, resulting in the development of a highly complex sensory system (Lipscomb, 1996). Great strides have been made in recent years toward a more thorough understanding of how the auditory system translates physical acoustic energy into neural impulses that are interpreted by the brain. However, the truth is that many questions remain to be answered concerning the precise biologic, mechanical, neurochemical, and electrical mechanisms and relationships that operate at all levels within the auditory system.

This chapter presents a synopsis of the development of the major anatomic components of the ear and an overview of the anatomy and physiology of the hearing mechanism. Although many classic papers and textbooks are relied on for these topics, the interested reader is referred to more explicit references such as Glasscock, Shambaugh, and Johnson (1990), Schuknecht (1993), Hughes and Pensak (1997), and Lalwani and Grundfast (1998).

The embryologic development of the ear is of more than academic interest to the clinician. An understanding of embryologic relationships helps confirm a diagnosis and suggests the need for early hearing assessments. If one is aware of the timetable of prenatal development and the association of the various organs and structures with each other, the suspicion of deafness and its subsequent diagnosis and treatment become easier. The origination and major changes in the development of the ear and the hearing system take place in the mother's womb as the baby becomes a progressively more complex structure over time. Several processes occur concurrently to produce the final structure, including enlargements, constrictions, and foldings, which are further modified by evaginations and invaginations. However, development of the auditory structure does not cease, nor is it totally complete, at the time of birth.

Knowledge of the origins of auditory structures (known as *phylogeny*) can be of diagnostic significance to the clinician. For example, when an infant presents with a congenital skin disorder, the clinician considers the fact that the skin and the otocyst both originate from ectoderm. It may then be logical to suspect that anomalies of the cochlear structures may have occurred contiguously with the skin disorder and that a search for severe sensorineural deafness is in order.

Similarly, the timing of development of the various organ systems guides the clinician to suspect that a hearing loss may have occurred at the same time that other systems were affected. A noxious influence on the fetus at 2 months of gestation may result in a malformation of the pinna developing at that time. The pinna malformation, however, does not necessarily imply malformation of the ossicles of the middle ear. Although the ossicles of the middle ear share partially the same time clock as the pinna in embryologic development, the origins of the structures are different. On the other hand, an insult to one may well result in a related insult to the other.

Principles such as these allow clinicians to look for the occult symptom of hearing loss whenever an overt embryologic-related symptom becomes evident. The prognosis for auditory function can then be estimated from what is known of the origin and the expected pathology. A review of the embryologic development of the ear and its related structures will clarify some of these principles.

ORIGINS AND EVOLUTION OF THE HEARING MECHANISM

Unfortunately, "ears" and "hearing" are often synonyms to the naive student who may be unaware that the ability to hear is actually a secondary acquired characteristic of the ear. The primary responsibility of the auditory organ is maintaining equilibrium. The sense of hearing developed from the primordial structures developed for balance. Thus, there are many similarities between the cell structure and physiology of the vestibular and hearing systems in humans. The study of origins and evolution is known as *phylogeny*. The comparative anatomy of various animal auditory systems confirms that hearing is important only to higher forms of vertebrates, but the basic function of equilibrium remains essentially unchanged in the phylogenetic evolution between fish and humans.

In many fish, amphibians, and reptiles the paired internal ears are devoted primarily to functions related to equilibrium. In these creatures the membranous labyrinth of the inner ear is filled with endolymph, and two distinct sac-like structures are generally present, the utricle and saccule. An endolymphatic duct extends upward from these two sacs and terminates within the brain case as the endolymphatic sac. A structure known as the lagena, which is actually the forerunner of the cochlea, is formed as a depression pocket in the floor of the saccule. Even in these lower vertebrates, branches of the auditory nerve are associated in the sensory sacs with end organs known as macula.

The macula-type of sensory cell is found in all vestibular systems and is the basic means of transforming equilibrium information into neural codes. These sensory end organs, much like the human cochlear hair cells, have hair-like projections embedded in an overlying gelatinous material, the cupula. In the utricular and saccular maculae and often in the primitive lagena, this gelatinous material becomes a thickened structure in which crystals of calcium carbonate are deposited. Technically, the very small crystals in the human otolithic membrane are *otoconia* (Greek word meaning "ear dust"), whereas the somewhat larger concretions of some other vertebrates are *otoliths* (Greek word meaning "ear stones"). However, the two terms are often used interchangeably.

An interesting equilibrium system found in crayfish was described by Storer (1979). The crayfish has a small sac known as the statocyst that is located at the base of each antenna. The statocyst contains a ridge of sensory hairs to which sand grains are attached by mucus to form structures called statoliths. The action of gravity on the statoliths causes the sensory hairs to bend, informing the crayfish of its present orientation. Each time the crayfish molts, it loses the statolith lining and must acquire new grains of sand to deposit in the statocyst. The crayfish shows disorientation in an aquarium with no foreign debris particles after molting. When iron filings are placed in the aquarium, the crayfish will pick some up for use in its statocyst, and then its equilibrium may be controlled with a magnet held in various positions along the sides of the aquarium.

All vertebrates are dependent on information concerning turning movements provided by the semicircular canals. In every jawed vertebrate, three such canals arise from each utricle. The three canals are at right angles to each other and represent the three planes of space. Each canal has an enlargement at one end known as an ampulla. Within the ampulla is a sensory end organ, the crista. Displacement of the endolymph in the semicircular canal causes displacement of the cupula attached to the cristae, bending the sensory hairs and initiating neural impulses.

Some fish and amphibians have a peculiar sensory system termed the lateral line system. The receptor organ of the lateral line is the neuromast, a generalized name applied to nerve receptors that demonstrate a hair-like projection enclosed in a flexible mass of gelatinous material—the cupula. Neuromasts are generally located on the surface skin of the water-dwelling organism. Evidence of embryonic development of the sensory endings in the human cochlea, which closely resembles the externally placed neuromast organs, may indicate that the internal ear originated phylogenetically as a specialized, deeply sunk portion of the lateral line system.

As animals evolved to become land-dwelling creatures, adaptations in the hearing sense organ were necessitated to process airborne sound waves. Changes were in order to transmit sounds and amplify them to the inner ear, which was usually set deeply in the skull. A middle ear space with and ossicular bridge developed to overcome the energy loss as sound is transmitted by air. The middle ear of amphibians and reptiles is quite similar, in the sense that the hyomandibular bone seen in the fish has changed its function to become a rod-like stapes or columella. The columella crosses the middle ear between the tympanic membrane and the oval window of the inner ear. This columellar-type middle ear ossicle is of particular interest, because human middle ear malformations may show this type of deformity. It makes one wonder if this is a throwback to the primitive evolutionary forebears (Fig. 2-1). An abnormal structure reminiscent of normal structures in "lower" animals, such as a cervical fistula or a columella ossicle, is known as a reversion structure or *atavism*.

In mammals, the external ear becomes a prominent structure known as the pinna. A more fundamental change occurs in the middle ear where, instead of a single bone, an articulated series of three ossicles between the eardrum and oval window exists. The middle ear mechanism in humans is the result of a 400-million-year evolutionary process in which discarded parts from nearby structures, having lost their original function, became adapted for full use in the hearing apparatus. According to Romer (1986) the origin of this series of ossicles has long been debated. The question existed as to whether the three ossicles were really due to subdivisions of the columella. Careful study of paleontology and comparative anatomy, however, led to the conclusion that only the mammalian stapes is related to the lower vertebrate columella. Mammals have developed a new specialized jaw system, and the "older" jaw elements have been developed into the other two middle ear ossicles. The reptile eardrum lies close to a jaw joint known as the articular, which becomes the malleus in mammals. A second jaw bone, the quadrate, is attached to the articular in the reptile and to the hyomandibular bone (forerunner of the stapes) in the fish. The quadrate retains these primitive connections and becomes the incus in mammals. Thus, these bones, which were originally part of the gill structure in fish, developed into the jaw structure of reptiles and finally into ear structures in mammals. In Romer's words, the breathing aids of fish developed into feeding aids in reptiles and finally into "hearing aids" in mammals.

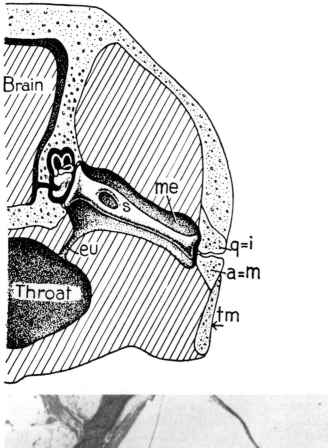

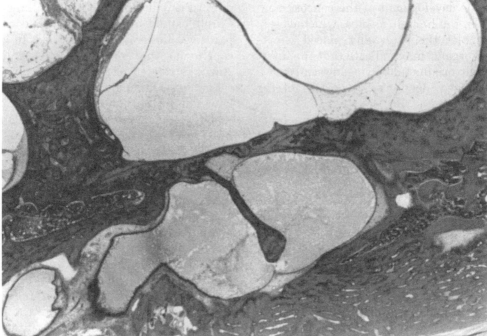

Figure 2-1. Example of an otic reversion structure. (Top) Ventricle cross-section of the normal reptile middle ear. *me,* middle ear; *s,* columella, which is the forerunner of the stapes; *q,* quadrate, which becomes the incus *(i); a,* articular, which becomes *m,* the malleus; *tm,* is to be the tympanic membrane; *eu* eustachian tube. (Reprinted with permission from Romer, A.S. (1986) *The vertebrate body* (5th ed.). Philadelphia: WB Saunders.) (Bottom) Horizontal cross-section of a human middle ear from a Treacher Collins patient showing congenital columella-type stapes with absence of malleus and incus. (Reprinted with permission from Sando, I., & Wood, R.P. (1971). Congenital middle ear anomalies. *Otolaryngology Clinics of North America (Symposium) 4,* 29–318.)

The inner ears of birds and mammals function from nearly identical physiologic mechanisms—auditory sensory structures vibrated by movements of a membrane located beneath them. Birds and mammals refined their hearing abilities with the advanced development of the cochlea. A hole exists through the bird's skull connecting both ears and permitting sound localization otherwise not available because of the bird's small head size. The number of coils present in the cochlea may vary among mammalian species. As indicated earlier in this phylogenetic discussion, the portions of the inner ear devoted to balance show little change in evolutionary development.

DEVELOPMENT OF THE EAR

Most audiologists have not had training or coursework in the field of embryology, so some basic background information is essential to appreciate fully the development of the ear. Only the general essentials of the development of the ear are presented here. The interested reader is referred to Zemlin (1998) for a thorough discussion of the embryonic development of the facial, head, and neck regions.

All growth is the result of cell division of preexisting cells. Through a process known as mitosis, changes take place in the nucleus of a cell that produce a specific number of double structures. The cell and nucleus then subdivide into two identical "daughter" cells. At the same time, "organizers" exist in the embryo which stimulate development of associated areas and create specific differentiation of cells in the developmental process.

One of the earliest organizational developments in the embryo is the differentiation of cells into three superimposed, cellular plates called germ layers. Initially, the cells of each layer are virtually indistinguishable, but chemical changes result in the distinct cell layers (ectoderm, mesoderm, and endoderm) even though all the cells are descendants of the same fertilized egg. *Ectoderm* is generally responsible for the development of the outer skin layers but also gives rise to the nervous system and the sense organs. *Mesoderm* is associated with skeletal and circulation structures, kidneys, and reproductive organs. *Endoderm* creates the digestive canal and respiratory organs. These germ layers are actually not quite as specific in their functions as outlined above; however, the outer and inner portions of the ear develop from ectodermal tissue, whereas the middle ear ossicles and the bone surrounding the inner ear originate from mesodermal tissue.

A developing baby is known as an *embryo* (from the Greek word meaning "to swell") during its first 8 weeks of gestation. At the end of the second week, a cellular disc exists that is composed of the three germ layers. By the end of the first month, the embryo is only about one-quarter of an inch long. The embryonic period terminates around the eighth week. At this time, the structure assumes a more human appearance and is known as a *fetus* (from the Latin word meaning "offspring") for the remainder of the gestation period.

The ear begins its development during the early life of the embryo, so some discussion of the detailed growth of the embryo itself is worthwhile. Very early in the developmental period, approximately 15 days after fertilization, the embryonic disc is split by a primitive streak. The primitive streak leads the way for development of the ectodermal-lined primitive groove and primitive fold (Fig. 2-2). The primitive groove deepens into a primitive pit, which in turn becomes the neural groove and neural fold (Fig. 2-3). An enlargement exists (the primitive knot) at the cephalic end of the primitive streak. This enlargement is destined to become the head of the organism. The ectodermal-lined neural folds come together to close off the neural groove, which is now known as the neural tube. It is during the

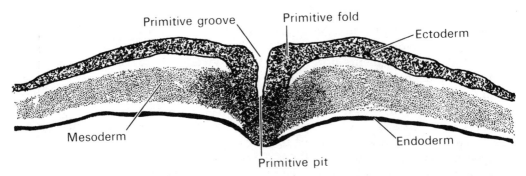

Figure 2-2. This drawing was made from a transverse cut through a chick embryo at approximately 25 hours after fertilization. (Modified with permission from Arey, L.B. (1940). *Developmental anatomy.* Philadelphia: WB Saunders.)

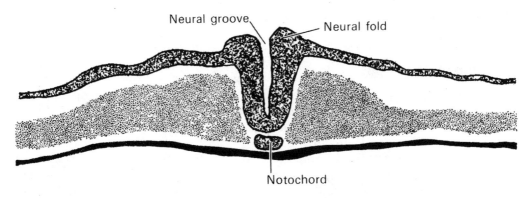

Figure 2-3. Cephalic transverse section through the fifth pair of somites in a seven-segment chick embryo. (Modified with permission from Arey, L.B. (1940). *Developmental anatomy.* Philadelphia: WB Saunders.)

stage of the neural tube that the earliest beginnings of the ear are seen.

Inner Ear. The earliest demarcations of the ear in the human embryo are seen early in the third week as thickenings in the superficial ectoderm on either side of the open neural plate. These thickenings are the auditory or otic placodes and are obvious by the middle of the third week (Fig. 2-4a). On approximately the 23rd day, the auditory placodes begin to invaginate into the surface ectoderm and are known as the auditory or otic pits. When the mouth of each auditory pit closes on or about the 30th day, it becomes the auditory vesicle or otocyst and appears as an ectodermal cavity lined with epithelium lateral to the now-closed neural tube, as shown in Figure 2-4c.

The auditory vesicle proceeds to differentiate through a series of folds, evaginations, and elongations and takes on an elongated shape divided into a utricular-saccule area and a tubular extension known as the endolymphatic duct. By 4.5 weeks, the portion of the auditory vesicle connected to the endolymphatic duct can be recognized as the future vestibular portion of the labyrinth, while the more slender portion of the vesicle begins to elongate from the saccular area as the future cochlea (Fig. 2-5a). At the end of the sixth week, three arch-like outpockets are visible and destined to become the semicircular canals. At this same time, the utricle and saccule become two definitive areas through a deepening construction of the vestibular portion of the auditory vesicle (Fig. 2-5b).

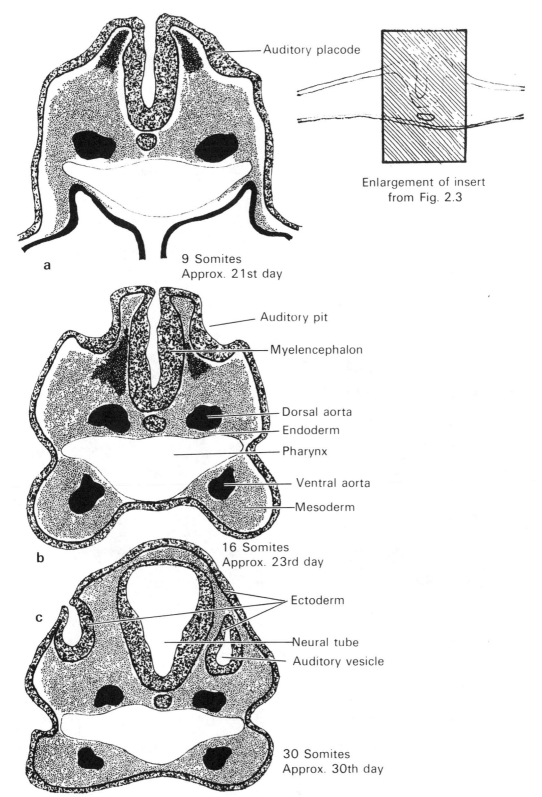

Auditory placode

Enlargement of insert
from Fig. 2.3

a   9 Somites
Approx. 21st day

Auditory pit

Myelencephalon

Dorsal aorta
Endoderm
Pharynx

Ventral aorta
Mesoderm

b   16 Somites
Approx. 23rd day

Ectoderm

c

Neural tube
Auditory vesicle

30 Somites
Approx. 30th day

Figure 2-4. Early development of the inner ear in a human embryo. (Modified with permission from Arey, L.B. (1940). *Developmental anatomy.* Philadelphia: WB Saunders.)

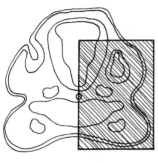

Enlargement of insert
From Fig. 2.4

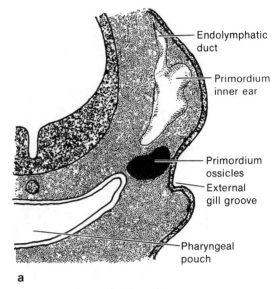

a

Approx. 4½ weeks

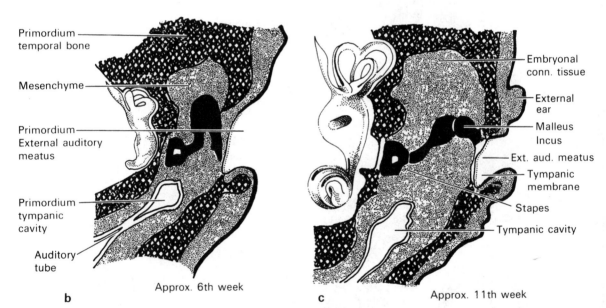

b   Approx. 6th week

c   Approx. 11th week

Figure 2-5. Schematic development of the inner and middle portions of the auditory mechanism from approximately 4.5–11 weeks. (Modified with permission from Patten, B.M. (1968). *Human embryology* (3rd ed.). New York: McGraw-Hill.)

By the end of the seventh week, the elongated outpocketing of the saccular portion of the auditory vesicle has completed one coil of the future cochlea. During the 8th through 11th week, the 2.5 coils of the cochlea are completed. The cochlear duct continues to be attached to the vestibular area by means of a narrow tube known as the ductus reuniens. The cochlear division of the eighth nerve follows the elongating and coiling of the cochlear duct, and fans its fibers out to be distributed along the duct's entire length.

During the seventh week, the complicated convolutions of the otic labyrinth continue to develop, and sensory end organs first appear as localized thickenings of epithelium in the utricle and saccule. Similar localized epithelial thickenings are found in the ampullated ends of the semicircular canals during the 8th week and in the floor of the cochlear duct at 12 weeks. These epithelial thickenings show differentiation into two types of cells including sensory cells with bristle-like hairs and supporting cells at one end. Complete maturation of the sensory and supporting cells in the cochlea does not occur until the fifth month, when the entire cochlear duct has shown considerable growth and expansion.

The membranous labyrinth of the inner ear reaches its full adult configuration by the early part of the third month. At this time the otic capsule, which has been encased in cartilage, begins to ossify (about the 16th week) through a complex system of 14 different endochondral ossification centers in the petrous portion of the temporal bone. The inner ear is the only sense organ to reach full adult size and differentiation by fetal midterm. However, the cochlear portion of the inner ear is the last inner ear end organ to differentiate and mature. Thus, the cochlea may be subject to more possible developmental deviations, malformations, and acquired disease than the vestibular end organs.

Middle Ear. While the sensory portion of the auditory system—the inner ear—is developing, the transmission portion of the auditory mechanism is developing as the middle ear. Unlike the inner ear, which originates from ectodermal tissue, the middle ear is an endodermal structure. The middle ear cavity begins its development during the third week while the auditory pit is sinking into the neural plate to become the auditory vesicle. The tympanic cavity and the auditory tube (later known as the eustachian tube) come from an elongation of the lateral-superior edge of the endodermal-lined first pharyngeal pouch. This elongation is called the tubotympanic recess (Fig. 2-5b).

By the time the human embryo is in its fourth week, a series of five branchial grooves or "gill slits" has appeared in the lower head and neck region on the lateral surfaces. On the inside of the embryo, a corresponding series of pharyngeal pouches develops, and the collective structures are identified as "arches." In fish, these grooves from the outside ultimately meet the corresponding pouches on the inside to form gills as part of its respiratory mechanism. In humans, most of the branchial grooves do not form slits with the pharyngeal pouches; however, the embryo's passing through this developmental stage is an example of human inheritance of embryonic structure from aquatic ancestors. It is of interest that in the human embryo one of the gill pouches does actually become perforated, forming a passageway from the pharynx to the outside of the head. This passageway becomes the external ear canal and eustachian tube. The eardrum forms a barrier between these two portions of the passageway, which otherwise would directly connect the pharynx and the exterior as does the gill slit of a fish. Occasionally, an additional opening will occur, forming a cervical fistula or branchial cyst that is an opening on the throat between the pharynx and the surface of the neck. The exact position of the fistula depends on which of the pouches is involved.

During the second month, the tubotympanic recess approaches the embryo surface between the first and second branchial arches, known as Meckel's (or mandibular) and Reichert's (or hyoid) cartilages, respectively. By the eighth week, the tympanic cavity is present in the lower half of the future middle ear, while the upper half is filled with cellular mesenchyme (Fig. 2-5b). The classic theory of ossicle origin holds that the malleus and incus arise from Meckel's cartilage and the stapes comes from Reichert's cartilage. Pearson et al. (1970) suggests a more complex and dual origin for the ossicles. Currently, the first branchial arch is credited for most of the body structure in the malleus and incus, whereas the second branchial arch gives rise to the lenticular process of the incus, the handle of the malleus, and the stapes. The middle ear cavity itself also has a dual origin, with the anterior area coming from the first arch and the posterior area coming from the second arch. It is noteworthy that the mandible also arises from the first arch.

By 8.5 weeks, the incus and the malleus have attained a complete cartilaginous form similar to that in an adult (Fig. 2-5c). The stapes continues to develop as a cartilaginous structure until the 15th week. By the 15th through 16th week, ossification begins to occur in the cartilaginous surface of the malleus and incus, which have nearly reached completion by the 32nd week. The stapes does not begin to ossify until the 18th week and continues to develop through life even after ossification is complete. Otologic surgeons recognize the stapes in a child to be more bulky and less delicate than the normal stapes seen in the adult.

As the ossicles begin to ossify, the surrounding mesenchymal tissue becomes loose and less cellular and is absorbed into the mucoperiosteal membrane of the middle ear cavity. When the ossicles are free from mesenchyma, mucous membrane connecting each ossicle to the walls of the middle ear cavity remains, eventually to become the ossicular supporting ligaments.

By the 30th week, development of the tympanum proper is almost complete. The middle ear cavity antrum is pneumatized by the 34th through 35th week, and the epitympanum is pneumatized during the last fetal month (36th to 38th week). The air cells of the temporal bone develop as outpouchings from the middle ear cavity during the 34th week. Air does not actually enter the middle ear cavity until the onset of respiration immediately after birth.

External Ear and Eardrum. The external ear (auricle) develops during the third or fourth week from the first and second branchial arches (Fig. 2-6a). Actually, the auricle is derived primarily from the second branchial arch, and only the tragus seems to originate from the first branchial arch. This is about the same time that the auditory vesicle is formed in the development of the inner ear.

During the sixth week, six hillocks or tissue thickenings form on both sides of the first branchial groove (Fig. 2-6b), arranged as three hillocks on each facing border. The ultimate shape and configuration of the adult auricle depend on the development of these six growth centers; thus, many divergent forms of the auricle are within the extremely wide range of normal (Fig. 2-6c). Darwin's tubercle forms in some people as an irregularity in the posterior margin of the helix or outer edge of the auricle, as shown in Figure 2-6d. At this time the mesenchymal folds of the auricle are beginning to become cartilage. From the 7th to 20th week, the auricle continues to develop, moving from its original ventromedial position to be slowly displaced laterally by the growth of the mandible and face. At the 20th week the auricle is in the adult shape (Fig. 2-6d) but continues to grow in size until the individual is 9 years old.

The external auditory meatus is derived from the first branchial groove during the fourth to fifth week. At this time, the ectodermal lining of the first branchial groove is in brief contact with the endodermal lining of the first pharyngeal pouch. Mesodermal tissue, however, soon grows between the two layers and separates the pharyngeal pouch from the branchial groove. In the eighth week, the primary auditory meatus sinks toward

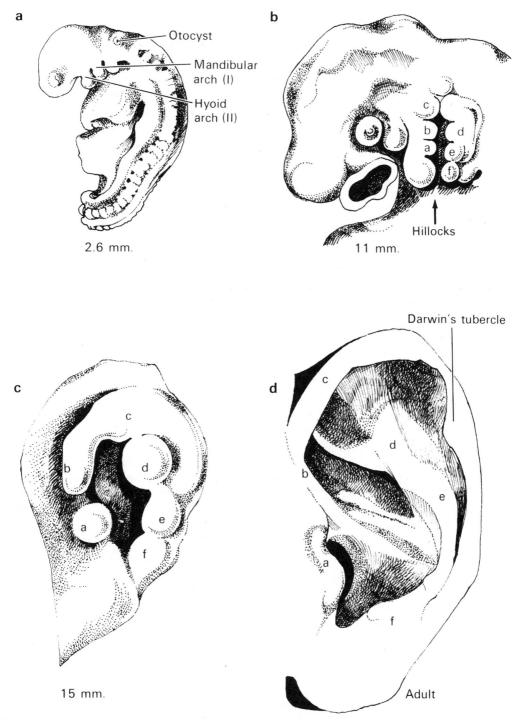

a

Otocyst

Mandibular arch (I)

Hyoid arch (II)

2.6 mm.

b

c

b

a

d

e

f

Hillocks

11 mm.

c

c

b

d

a

e

f

15 mm.

d

Darwin's tubercle

c

b

d

e

a

f

Adult

Figure 2-6. Schematic development of the auricle from the third to fourth week to adult stage. (Modified with permission from Anson, B.J. (1963). *An atlas of human anatomy* (2nd ed.). Philadelphia: WB Saunders.)

the middle ear cavity and becomes the outer one-third of the auditory canal, surrounded ultimately by cartilage.

The ectodermal groove continues to deepen toward the tympanic cavity from the external surface until it meets a thickening of epithelial cells known as the meatal plug, which has arisen from surface ectoderm. Mesenchyme grows between the meatal plug and the epithelial cells of the tympanic cavity. These three layers of tissue become the tympanic membrane, composed of inner circular fibers, the fibrous middle layer of tissue, and the outer radial fiber layer, before the ninth week. The solid meatal plug, however, keeps the external auditory canal closed until the 21st week. By this time the inner and middle ear structures are well formed and ossified. The meatal plug disintegrates and forms a canal, with the innermost layer of meatal plug epithelium becoming the squamous epithelial layer of the tympanic membrane. The external auditory canal continues to develop until the ninth year. At birth the floor of the external auditory canal has no bony portion. In the infant the external auditory canal is short and straight, whereas in the adult the canal is longer and curves. This suggests that the infant tympanic membrane might be easier to observe than the eardrum of the adult. That is not the case, however, because the infant tympanic membrane is in an oblique or almost a horizontal position and difficult to visualize. The bony portion of the external canal is not complete until about the seventh year. A summary of major embryologic features and their time sequence is presented in Table 2-1.

This discussion of the anatomy of the hearing mechanism is concluded with a brief case study to show the important relationship between disorder and function. A young patient with evidence of multiple congenital anomalies related to first and second branchial arch origins is shown in Figure. 2-7. This patient's condition was diagnosed as Moäbius' syndrome, also termed aplasia of the sixth and seventh cranial nerves. Her cranial deformities include obvious malformations of the external ear, bilateral facial weakness producing a consistent mask-like appearance, submucous cleft palate with a bifid uvula, and greatly exaggerated width of the mouth resulting from failure of proper union of the maxillary and mandibular processes. She is profoundly deaf with no measurable hearing responses and was a student in a residential school for the deaf. Radiographic studies revealed symmetric middle ear ossicular anomalies of the malleus and incus, the absence of the oval window bilaterally, and deformities of the mastoid. The cochlea and semicircular canal system appear normal on the radiographic study, but the internal auditory canals are abnormally narrow, measuring only 1.5 mm in diameter instead of the normal diameter of approximately 8.0 mm.

A general overview of human development is presented in Figure 2-8.

PHYSIOLOGY OF HEARING

To understand the nature of hearing impairments, one must understand the normal physiology of the hearing mechanism and the nature of hearing loss. These concepts are presented here only as background material, so that a discussion regarding the pathologies of hearing impairment can be developed in the following chapter. For a thorough description of the auditory pathways, the reader is referred to "The Human Brain" (Nolte, 1998).

Outer and Middle Ear. The phenomenon of hearing is the result of a complex series of events. Sound energy, originating as vibration and transmitted through an elastic medium such as air, is collected by the pinna and funneled into the ear canal. The sound vibrations impinge on the tympanic membrane causing it to vibrate. The vibrations are transmitted to the oval window of the otic capsule by the

Table 2-1.
Embryology Summary of the Ear

Fetal Week	Inner Ear	Middle Ear	External Ear
3rd	Auditory placode; auditory pit	Tubotympanic recess begins to develop	
4th	Auditory vesicle (otocyst); vestibular-cochlear division		Tissue thickenings begin to form
5th			Primary auditory meatus begins
6th	Utricle and saccule present; semicircular canals begin		Six hillocks evident; cartilage begins to form
7th	One cochlear coil present; sensory cells in utricle and saccule		Auricles move dorsolaterally
8th	Ductus reuniens present; sensory cells in semicircular canals	Incus and malleus present in cartilage; lower half of tympanic cavity formed	Outer cartilaginous one-third of external canal formed
9th		Three tissue layers at tympanic membrane are present	
11th	2.5 cochlear coils present; nerve VIII attaches to cochlear duct		
12th	Sensory cells in cochlea; membranous labyrinth complete; otic capsule begins to ossify		
15th		Cartilaginous stapes formed	
16th		Ossification of malleus and incus begins	
18th		Stapes begins to ossify	
20th	Maturation of inner ear; inner ear adult size		Auricle is adult shape but continues to grow until age 9
21st		Meatal plug disintegrates, exposing tympanic membrane	
30th		Pneumatization of tympanum	External auditory canal continues to mature until age 7
32nd		Malleus and incus complete ossification	
34th		Mastoid air cells develop	
35th		Antrum is pneumatized	
37th		Epitympanum is pneumatized; stapes continues to develop until adulthood; tympanic membrane changes relative position during first 2 years of life	

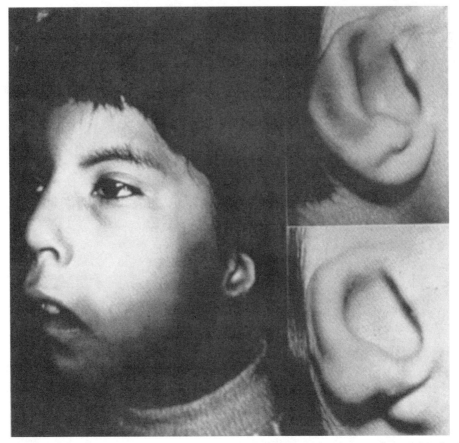

Figure 2-7. Patient with Möbius' syndrome, with first and second branchial arch anomalies as described in the text.

three middle ear ossicles. In addition to serving as a conductor for sound energy, the tympanic membrane and ossicles amplify the sound by two simple mechanical principles. First, there is a slight lever action created in the motion of the three middle ear ossicles. Second, the relationship between the relatively large surface area of the tympanic membrane that funnels sound energy onto the smaller surface area of the stapes footplate increases sound pressure. These two mechanisms provide middle ear amplification of the transmitted sound energy by approximately 30 dB. The 30 dB advantage may be lost when defects or pathologies inhibit either or both of the middle ear amplifying mechanisms (Lipscomb, 1996).

The mechanical vibration transmitted by the stapes to the oval window induces motion in the fluids of the cochlea, where traveling waves faithfully transmit the intensity and frequency of the vibrations. Perilymph fluid fills two ducts within the cochlea which are known as the scala vestibuli and the scala tympani. These parallel scalae communicate with each other at the helicotrema in the apical tip of the cochlear coils. When sound vibration displaces the stapes inward into the scala vestibuli, a simultaneous outward motion occurs in the scala tympani at the round window membrane; this movement is termed the round window reflex.

Inner Ear. The understanding of the anatomy and physiology of the fine structure of the inner ear has increased tremendously since use of the electron microscope began in the early 1950s. The

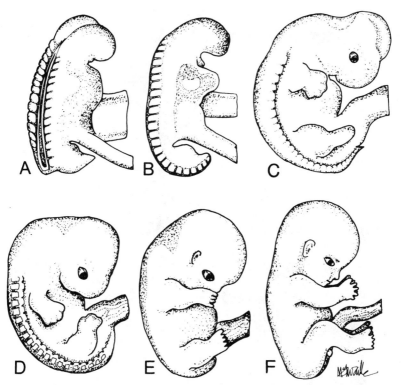

Figure 2-8. Human life and hearing develop together. **(A)** The neural tube, the heart, and the brain begin to develop at 3 weeks concurrently with the auditory pit and tubotympanic recess. **(B)** In the 4-week-old embryo, limbs begin to appear and the otocyst develops. **(C)** The embryo is only one-third inch in length at the fifth week when the auditory meatus starts to form. **(D)** At 6 weeks, eyes, semicircular canals, and external ear hillocks develop. **(E)** Embryonic seventh week includes initial formation of teeth, muscles, genitals, external ear, and cochlea. **(F)** Now nearly 1 inch long, at 8 weeks the embryo becomes a fetus, and the middle ear ossicles and tympanic membrane begin to form.

scanning electron microscope added a new dimension to the appreciation of inner ear structures. Unlike the conventional electron microscope, which transmits an electron beam through the specimen, the image in the scanning microscope is created by secondary electrons emitted from the excited surface of the specimen. The result is a picture similar to the image produced on a television screen. The depth of field obtained with the scanning microscope is approximately 500 times that of a light microscope. A photomicrograph of the organ of Corti taken with a scanning electron microscope is shown in Figure 2-9.

The vibrations of the stapes footplate displace fluids within the cochlea, resulting in traveling waves that stimulate the receptor cells within the cochlea. The receptor cells are present in orderly rows resting along the entire length of the basilar membrane. The basilar membrane moves in traveling wave patterns driven by the mechanical eddies in the cochlear fluids. The attached sensory cells follow the motion of the basilar membrane. Each sensory cell has a tuft of stiff cilia, or hairs, on its upper surface. For this reason the sensory cells are known as hair cells. The sensory cells occur in several rows of increasing length, with the tallest tufts of cilia on each cell embedded in the undersurface of the tectorial membrane, which is positioned directly over the hair cells. The basilar membrane, the sensory hair cells and their supporting cells, and the tecto-

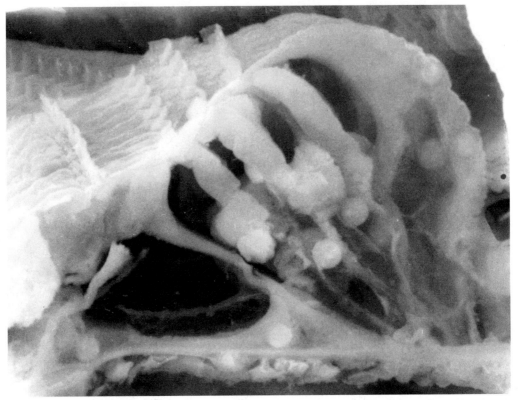

Figure 2-9. Scanning electron microscopic view of organ of Corti from a guinea pig. (Courtesy of David Asher, Ph.D.)

rial membrane comprise the organ of Corti.

Organ of Corti. The organ of Corti is a frequency analyzer, with the highest pitches monitored at the base of the coil of the cochlea and the intermediate and higher pitches tonotopically organized toward the apex. The organ of Corti is a papillary structure resting on the basilar membrane within the scala media (cochlear duct) and is composed of sensorineural receptors and supporting elements. The organ of Corti is designed to convert mechanical vibrations into electrical events that are then transmitted to the central nervous system. Technically, the hair cells convert the mechanical fluid vibration into electromechanical feedback, which amplifies the hydromechanical response of the cochlea, and electrochemical events, which in turn promote synaptic

transmission between the hair cells and the neurons of the auditory portion of the eighth nerve (Ryan & Dallos, 1996).

The vibratory fluid motion in the cochlea stimulates nerve impulses, with the cochlear neural epithelium acting as a mechanical transducer. The spiral-shaped organ of Corti contains two types of sensory cells, inner and outer hair cells, topped by several rows of stereocilia (Fig. 2-10). There are some 140 stereocilia extending from each of the 3500 inner hair cells and the 12,000 outer hair cells. The inner hair cells, which are shaped like a flask, are completely surrounded by specialized supporting cells except for their hair-bearing tops. The outer hair cells are arranged in three (at the base) to five (at the apex) parallel rows. The outer hair cells are rectangular, shaped like elongated cylinders, and in contact with supporting cells only at their very tops and

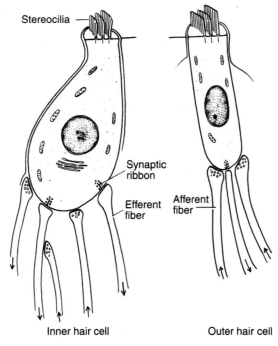

Figure 2-10. Diagrammatic representation of inner and outer hair cells found in the organ of Corti.

bottoms (Table 2-2). The total of approximately 15,500 hair cells rest on supporting cells that, in turn, rest on the basilar membrane and extend into a third cochlear duct filled with endolymph fluid which is known as the scala media or cochlear duct. This third duct is interposed between the scala vestibuli and scala tympani throughout the entire 2.5 turns of the cochlea. Hair cells have an orderly arrangement in the cochlea which is related to sound frequency. Hair cells that

respond to high frequencies above 2000 Hz are located in the basal turn of the cochlea, whereas hair cells that are tuned to stimulating frequencies below 2000 Hz are found in the middle and apical cochlear coils.

Thus, with the arrival of an auditory-vibratory stimulus to the cochlea, transduction of the mechanical traveling wave into a neural activity begins with the deflection of the outer hair cell's stereocilia rows. The tips of the tallest outer hair cell stereocilia are embedded within the tectorial membrane, where it appears that the inner hair cells do not touch the tectorial membrane. The stereocilia of the outer hair cells are displaced directly by the combined displacement of the tectorial and the basilar membranes. With the vibration of the basilar membrane, a shearing force is produced with an accompanying displacement of the stereocilia; this results because the tectorial membrane does not move to the same degree as the hair cells (Noback, Strominger, & Demarest 1996)

Table 2-2.
Comparison of Inner and Outer Hair Cells

Inner Hair Cells	Outer Hair Cells
3500	12,500
Flask shape	Cylinder shape
Single row	3–5 rows
"C"-shaped stereocilia	"V"-shaped stereocilia
Surrounded by support cells	Attached at top and bottom
Afferent innervation	Multiple innervation
One neuron—one cell	One neuron—multiple cells

Hair cells act both as transducers (converting mechanical energy into electrochemical energy) and biologic amplifiers (Noback et al., 1996). As early as 1948, a biophysicist named Thomas Gold hypothesized a "cochlear amplifier" system based on an "active" process originating within the cochlea. Nearly four decades were to pass before the predicted motility was observed in the organ of Corti. Brownell et al. (1985) demonstrated through dramatic single cell video recordings that the outer hair cells are mechanically active; that is, they shorten when depolarized and lengthen when hyperpolarized. This electromotility is extremely fast and occurs at frequencies up to the limit of human hearing. Obviously, this active process of length change of the outer hair cells, although miniscule in each hair cell, can be summed sufficiently to influence the mechanical responses within the organ of Corti. This finding is consistent with the cochlear amplifier concept and describes a mechanism for acoustic energy being generated from within the cochlea. This outer hair cell motility may be the source for otoacoustic emissions.

Ryan and Dallos (1996) demonstrated that the selective destruction of outer hair cells resulted in a loss of threshold sensitivity in the cochlea of approximately 40 dB. Van Tassel (1993) reviewed contemporary literature and concluded that hearing loss of cochlear origin, with air-conduction thresholds less than 60 dB HL, is consistent with damage to the outer hair cells, whereas hearing losses greater than 60 dB HL are likely to involve widespread destruction of inner hair cells and/or disruption of their afferent function in addition to the loss of outer hair cell function. This absolute loss in inner hair cell function, if extensive, can produce greatly degraded psychoacoustic abilities.

Bobbin (1996) offered an interesting description of both the active and passive cochlear mechanics involved in the hearing process. The passive mechanism is used during sound exposure greater than 40–60 dB SPL, where sound energy is powerful enough to move the cochlear partition directly and involves the outer hair cells as the key elements in the action. The active mechanism is used during low levels of sound exposure.

The peripheral neurons of the cochlear nerve are distributed to hair cells from beneath the basilar membrane and its supporting shelf, the osseous spiral lamina. The fluid motion of the scala tympani—due to its physical properties of width, length, thickness, mass, and elasticity—displaces the basilar membrane in a traveling wave pattern, producing torsion on the hair-like processes of the cell and creating a mechanical-chemical change resulting in peripheral nerve-ending stimulation (Ryan & Dallos, 1996). The resultant electrical potentials in the eight nerve dendrites initiate impulses that are transmitted to the central nervous system via the higher auditory neural pathways. Through this intricate and complex system, the external vibratory energy transmitted by the tympanic membrane is ultimately transformed into neural impulse code. Interested readers are referred to Yost and Nielsen (2000) for a more complete discussion of auditory physiology.

Bone Conduction. Humans also hear sounds by a bone conduction pathway that bypasses the external and middle ears. Bone-conducted sound stimulates the inner ear by mechanical vibrations of the bones of the skull. Bekesy (1960) researched the process of hearing via bone conduction through extensive experiments and concluded that the vibratory patterns of the basilar membrane for both air- and bone-conducted stimuli are exactly the same. The vibrations of the skull create the same current displacements within the cochlea as when the sounds are transmitted by the air-conduction pathway beginning in the ear canal and tympanic membrane. As the fluids within the cochlea are set into motion by the bone-conducted vibrations, the displacement of the basilar membrane initiates the hydroelectromechanical processes that stimulate neural impulses to the brainstem and the temporal cortex. The perception of sound at the brain is exactly the same whether the activity is stimulated by air conduction or bone transmission of the vibrations.

Auditory Nerve. The nerve fibers that innervate the hair cells have their cell bodies in the bipolar spiral ganglion located in Rosenthal's canal. Axons from the spiral ganglion cells join in the modiolus and collect as the auditory, or cochlear, branch of the eighth nerve. Just outside the cochlea, the vestibular portion of the eighth nerve coming from the semicircular canals, utricle, and saccule joins the cochlear portion. The two portions of the eighth nerve come together like a rope and pass through the internal auditory meatus toward the medulla. The structure of the auditory nerve is orderly, with fibers from the apical quarter of the cochlea forming the core of the nerve. Around the core, nerve fibers from the apex of the cochlea twist one way, while the fibers from the middle turn of the cochlea twist the opposite way. Fifty percent of the nerve fibers from the cochlea come from the basal coil and represent sensory elements that respond to frequencies higher than 2000 Hz.

Research by Spoendlin (1967, 1969) has shown that the vast majority (90%) of the afferent neurons innervates the inner hair cells, whereas only some 10% of the fibers come from the outer hair cells. Each outer hair cell is innervated by several different neurons, and each neuron innervates a large number of outer hair cells. The inner hair cells are innervated by a large number of different neurons, but each neuron innervates only one inner hair cell. Most of the information transmitted to the brain originates from the inner hair cells, not the outer hair

cells (Ryan & Dallos, 1996). Although the cochlea is stimulated by hydromechanical pressures, the neural impulses leave the cochlea via the afferent neurons which join together to form the acoustic division of the eight cranial nerve.

The eight nerve divides into acoustic and vestibular branches before it reaches the brainstem. The acoustic nerve enters the brainstem at the level of the pons. The auditory portion divides into dorsal and ventral branches that go to corresponding nuclei in the brainstem wherein the second-order afferent auditory neuron cell bodies are located.

The fibers in the eighth nerve are "tuned" to certain frequencies. That is, certain fibers are more responsive to certain stimulating frequencies. This fact is shown by inserting microelectrodes into single nerve fibers, determining the threshold for the action potential "spike" of that nerve fiber for a variety of frequencies, and then plotting the response area for that particular fiber. The threshold sensitivity of a fiber increases gradually and is most sensitive at its "tuned" frequency. The tuned frequency is used to name the fiber (e.g., 7000 Hz fiber). Most of the auditory fibers are high-frequency units, usually above 1000 Hz. Recent observations indicate that individual inner hair cells also maintain characteristic responses to tuned frequencies and may actually be more finely tuned than the nerve fibers (Evans, 1975). It is remarkable that only a few fibers of the eighth nerve are required to preserve "good" hearing. The auditory nerve must be sectioned more than halfway to have any measurable effect on auditory thresholds, and then, if indeed any hearing remains, it is predominantly low-frequency hearing (Neff, 1947; Wever & Neff, 1947). The individual nerve responses, tuned to different frequencies, fire in close synchrony to click stimuli, so that the amplitude of the action potential is representative of the number of fibers that respond (Davis, 1961).

Brainstem Pathways. Much of the brainstem auditory pathway can be seen in Figures 2-11 and 2-12. The higher auditory pathways are complex and often escape significance with students who tend only to memorize the names of the relay stations and major neuronal paths. It is important to realize that although first-order neurons from the cochlea reach the brainstem in the cochlear nuclei, most of the activity that ultimately reaches the cortex is by way of fourth-order neurons. This seemingly too complex system seldom breaks down because of alternate paths to the cerebral cortex (Thompson, 1983).

Two pairs of cochlear nuclei exist, a dorsal and a ventral cochlear nucleus on each side of the medulla; they are referred to collectively as the cochlear nuclei of the medulla. Although some of the neurons of the cochlear nuclei ascend to higher nuclei on the same side of the system, most cross over to the opposite side in the trapezoid body. Auditory units in the cochlear nuclei are also sensitive to specific frequencies as noted previously with the auditory nerve fibers. Inhibitory units have also been reported in the cochlear nuclei, which under certain circumstances actually inhibit response rather than excite the unit under examination. Thus, a

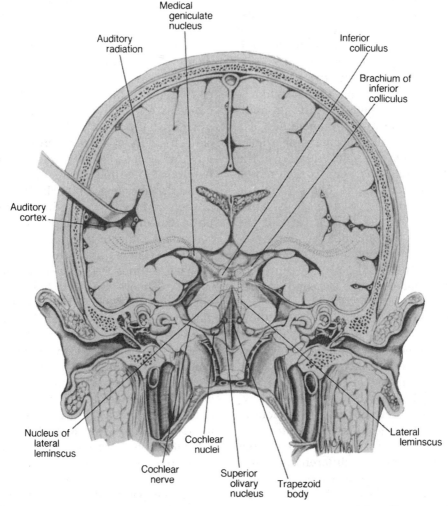

Figure 2-11. Ascending auditory pathway. (Reprinted with permission from Nolte, J. (1988). *The human brain: An introduction to its functional anatomy* (4th ed.). St. Louis: CV Mosby.)

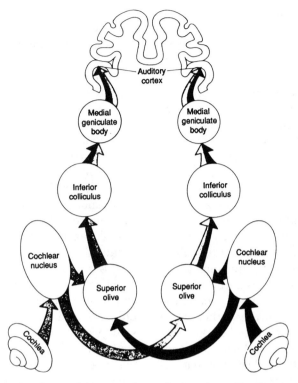

Figure 2-12. A diagrammatic scheme of the ascending auditory pathway. (Reprinted with permission from Yost, W.A. (2000). *Fundamentals of hearing: An introduction* (4th ed.). San Diego: Academic Press.)

particular frequency stimulus may excite certain neurons of the auditory system while inhibiting other units from firing. What starts out in the cochlea as the excitation of the relatively large group of hair cells is narrowed down to a smaller group of neurons through this process of inhibition. In addition, the cochlear nuclei, like the cochlea, exhibit tonotopic organization, or an orderly arrangement of responsiveness to different frequencies. In fact, Rose, Galambos, and Hughes (1959) reported one unrolling of the cochlear frequency distribution in the dorsal cochlear nucleus and two separate complete frequency patterns in the ventral nuclei. The number of discharges from a single cochlear nucleus unit is related to the intensity of the acoustic stimulus.

The principal terminations of second-order afferent auditory neurons are in the nuclei of the trapezoid body and superior olivary body. The superior olive is the first

structure in the medulla that receives fibers from both ears, and it may play a role in the localization of sound. From here, neurons originate that course upward in the loosely compacted neurons of the lateral lemniscus to another principal relay station, the inferior colliculus. Collaterals of second- and third-order neurons are given off to the reticular formation that provides an indirect, diffuse, sensory pathway to the cerebral cortex. The reticular formation is closely related to arousal and attention during sleep and may be responsible for the fact that a crying baby may wake only the mother but no one else in the family, or that a person may sleep soundly through a barrage of noise but wake suddenly on hearing a soft familiar voice.

Most of the fibers in the lateral lemniscus pathway terminate in the inferior colliculus, but some may bypass and end in the next relay station, the medial geniculate body. So far as is known, all direct projections to the auditory cortex are relayed in the medial geniculate body. The auditory cortex is, of course, responsible for the fine discrimination necessary in the understanding of speech. The "tuning" function of the higher auditory centers including the inferior colliculus, the medial geniculate body, and the auditory cortex has been summarized by Ryan and Dallos (1996): some units at higher levels in the auditory system are frequency specific, and some are not; many units respond only to clicks with a complex spectrum and are unresponsive to pure tone signals; many units show spontaneous firing that can sometimes be inhibited by acoustic stimuli; and of the units that are frequency-specific, the response areas of the units higher up in the auditory system tend to be narrower than those units found in lower auditory centers. An estimated cell count of each of the levels in the afferent auditory pathway is presented in Table 2-3.

Attempts to map the cortical responses to auditory stimuli have identified the temporal lobe as the responsive area, sometimes further localized as Brodmann's areas 41 and 42. The primary cortex (area 41) area in the temporal lobe has at least five tonotopic frequency projections that are the reverse of each other. Kryter and Ades (1943) established a very important fact with significant clinical implication. They showed that under appropriate conditions, cortical lesions have no appreciable effect on the absolute

thresholds of pure tone stimuli. This is true even when extensive bilateral cortical lesions are made. Thus, the ability to respond to tones is not dependent on the cerebral cortex. These same investigators reported that removal of the inferior colliculi created an approximate 15-dB loss in pure tone sensitivity; destruction of the entire auditory system from the midbrain to the cortex created a pure tone hearing loss of about 40 dB. It may be concluded that the most important aspect of auditory sensitivity to pure tones is due to intact neurons below the inferior colliculi, and a nearly normal audiogram may be obtained with a loss of 75% of the neurons of the auditory nerve. Unilateral lesions of the ascending auditory pathways above the level of the cochlear nuclei produce only minor impairments because of the strong bilaterality of the pathway. Bilateral lesions of the central auditory pathways are relatively uncommon because tracts and nuclei of the system are widely separated.

In addition to the afferent (ascending) auditory pathways to the cortex, a separate system of neurons provides an efferent (descending) pathway from the cortex to the cochlea. Of particular interest is the olivocochlear bundle, which consists of (1) lateral olivocochlear neurons that project ipsilaterally and terminate on the peripheral processes of afferent fibers beneath the inner hair cells, and (2) medial olivocochlear neurons that project contralaterally and terminate primarily beneath the outer hair cells. The medial olivocochlear pathway is associated with interaction between the two ears at the level of the brainstem and most likely has a role in suppression of otoacoustic emissions (Hood & Berlin, 1996). The inhibitory influences conveyed by these efferent fibers act to suppress the activity of the afferent fibers of the cochlear nerve and fine-tune the basilar membrane through the outer hair cells (Noback et al., 1996).

Table 2-3.
Afferent Auditory Pathways and Estimated Cell Count at Each Level

Cochlear nuclei	8800
Superior olivary complex	34,000
Nuclei of lateral lemniscus	38,000
Inferior colliculus	392,000
Medial geniculate body	364,000
Auditory cortex	10,000,000

ANATOMY OF THE EAR THROUGH TEMPORAL BONE STUDY

Knowledge concerning the anatomy of the temporal bone is increasingly important to the audiologist. More and more journal articles and presentations at meetings include histologic temporal bone sections to demonstrate some aspect of deafness. Many significant advances in knowledge about the etiology of deafness have come from careful study of temporal bone histologic sections. Yet many questions remained unanswered. Why do people develop sensorineural hearing loss? Which otologic diseases produce hearing losses, and what can be learned to facilitate improved diagnosis and treatments? What are the processes of progressive sensorineural hearing losses? The answers to such questions may lie in the study and understanding of pathology of the otic capsule and temporal bone. This scientific information will likely lead to improved patient treatment outcomes in many areas of clinical services, including hearing aid fittings, educational recommendations and referrals, genetic counseling, and patient prognosis.

Most speech and hearing training programs have infrequent access to normal or pathologic temporal bone sections. In fact, only a handful of nonmedical clinicians are experienced enough with this technical discipline to teach through the use of histologic sections. Yet this method of instruction enables the student to achieve an understanding of the anatomy of the structures of the ear and vestibular system as well as an appreciation for the complexity of the hearing mechanism. An understanding of the anatomy of the normal temporal bone will provide the audiologist with new insight into the etiology and pathology of deafness.

The paucity of temporal bone anatomic sections available for the benefit of hearing and speech students has prompted the authors to include this section of his-tology samples from a normal temporal bone. The authors' understanding of deafness has been enhanced greatly by careful study of temporal bone anatomy and pathology. Thus, it is the authors' belief that it is important for students to examine fully the normal temporal bone sections presented in this chapter. These normal histologic samples may be used as a comparative reference for pathologic temporal bone sections shown in other chapters of this book. The clinician can extrapolate from what is known about the pathology of a given ear disease or genetic entity to other similar cases or patients. As an example, knowledge of the temporal bone pathology of meningitis deafness can suggest that when little or no hearing can be detected in a child who has had meningitis, the probability of destruction of cochlear structures is quite high. Temporal bone studies of rubella deafness may demonstrate sections of nearly normal tissues that suggest the possibility of residual hearing despite clinical failures in obtaining measurable audiometric responses.

The National Temporal Bone, Hearing and Balance Pathology Resource Registry was established in 1992 by the National Institutes of Health to promote temporal bone donations for research purposes. The Registry, based in Boston, Massachusetts, coordinates a national network of 26 temporal bone laboratories and contains a library of more than 12,000 well-documented human temporal bone specimens that have been catalogued for research purposes. The scientific value of temporal bones is enhanced when a premortem hearing test was conducted, so that the postmortem analysis can identify the number and position of health sensory cells. A graph can then be created to relate the physical location of the healthy hair cells to the premortem auditory thresholds to create a "cytococheogram." Although much has been learned through the study of temporal bones, there is still a strong need for donations from individuals with hearing-impairment representing many ear diseases and treatments that do not exist in the National Temporal Bone Registry.

Temporal Bone. The temporal bone forms part of the lateral wall and base of the skull, as shown in Figure 2-13. It articulates with other bones of the skull, including the sphenoid, parietal, and occipital bones. The petrous part of the temporal bone is the densest bone of the body and contains, among other things, most of the structures of the ear. The temporal bone is generally divided into four sections: the squamous, mastoid, petrous, and tympanic areas. In general terms, the squamous portion of the temporal bone is superior to the external auditory meatus; the mastoid area is posterior, while the tympanic portion forms the anterior, inferior, and part of the posterior walls of the external auditory meatus.

The petrous portion of the temporal bone extends medially from the external auditory canal, and its middle third contains the structures of the middle and inner ear. In the petrous bone it is noteworthy that the cochlear portion of the inner ear is situated anteriorly and medially to the internal auditory meatus and the vestibular portion of the inner ear. The internal auditory meatus houses the facial nerve (seventh), which lies superior to the auditory portion of the acoustic nerve (eighth) and anterior to

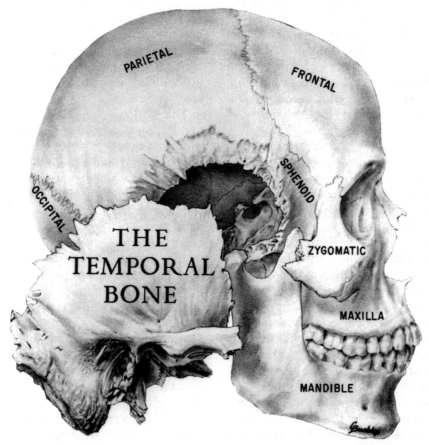

Figure 2-13. Temporal bone section of the human skull. (Reprinted with permission from Anson, B.J., & Donaldson, J.A. (1967). *The surgical anatomy of the temporal bone and ear.* Philadelphia: WB Saunders.)

the superior vestibular branch of the eighth cranial nerve. The petrous bone is shown in Figure 2-14 as part of the base of the skull as seen from above.

Preparation of Temporal Bone Histologic Sections. Examination of the stained sections of the temporal bone under high-powered magnification takes expert skills and knowledge gained only through experience and thorough study. The procedure involved in preparation of a single temporal bone is expensive and complex and requires numerous labora-

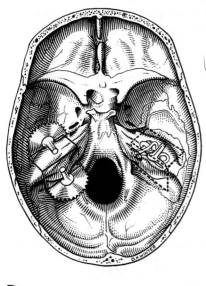

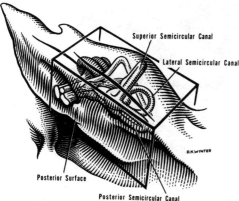

Superior Semicircular Canal

Lateral Semicircular Canal

D.K.WINTER

Posterior Surface

Posterior Semicircular Canal

Figure 2-14. Petrous portion of temporal bone shown as part of the skull viewed from above. (Reprinted with permission from Gallagher, J.C. (1967). *Histology of the human temporal bone.* Washington, DC: Armed Forces Institute of Pathology.)

tory personnel processing the tissue for 9 months. The scientific value of temporal bone studies depends, in great part, on the accuracy with which the clinical manifestations can be correlated with pathologic findings. The validity of such interpretation is strongly influenced by (1) the completeness of the relevant medical history, 2) the timeliness of the auditory and vestibular laboratory test data, (3) the quality of the histologic preparations, and (4) the experience of the otopathologist making the interpretations (Schuknecht, 1993).

The density of the temporal bone and the intricacy of the inner ear structures make preparation of suitable histology slides from the gross bone specimen very difficult. The processing of a temporal bone into slides is a difficult, demanding, precise, time-consuming, and expensive procedure. Initially, the temporal bone must be removed from the skull of the donor within 24 hours of death, or the inner ear structures undergo autolysis. The bone is immediately submerged in formalin for 2 or 3 weeks for fixation of structures. An extensive decalcification process follows for some 5 weeks in an adult bone to remove the dense calcium from the temporal bone. Infant temporal bones that are hours or days old may not show the presence of calcium after the first or second week in the decalcification solutions. Excess bone is then pared from the gross structure, the decalcification chemicals are neutralized, and the bone is carefully washed.

The temporal bone is then dehydrated with ethyl alcohol solutions, infiltrated, and embedded into varying solutions of celloidin for nearly 3 months. The celloidin provides support for the bone tissues to permit sectioning with a microtome. The temporal bone is sliced into sections 20 μm thick, forming some 400 sections from each temporal bone. Only every 10th section is initially stained with dyes, generally hematoxylin and eosin, to give the various tissues color for ease in identification. The dyed sections are mounted on microscope slides and are ready for study.

Anatomy of a Normal Temporal Bone. An understanding of normal temporal bone structures is necessary before one can appreciate the abnormalities found in temporal bone from patients with various kinds of deafness. Temporal bone study is usually reserved for residents in otolaryngology or physiologists interested in studying mechanisms of hearing, but there seems to be sufficient reason for all students of hearing disorders to have some familiarity with anatomy as demonstrated by horizontally cut, temporal bone histopathologic sections.

One must keep in mind the general level of the section under study as it was taken from the inner ear or temporal bone block. Figure 2-15 shows the gross structure of the inner ear. If one imagines a horizontal line drawn through the most superior portion of the inner ear, one will see that the only structure represented might be the arch of the superior semicircular canal. As the microtome blade cuts off horizontal sections from a temporal bone block, the superior semicircular canal will be the initial structure to be sectioned. One must then imagine how a horizontal slice of temporal bone tissue will appear when placed on a microscope slide and viewed from above. The student of temporal bone anatomy must have a draftsperson's ability to imagine three-dimensional structures from a two-dimensional picture.

Sample sections from a horizontally sectioned petrous portion of a temporal

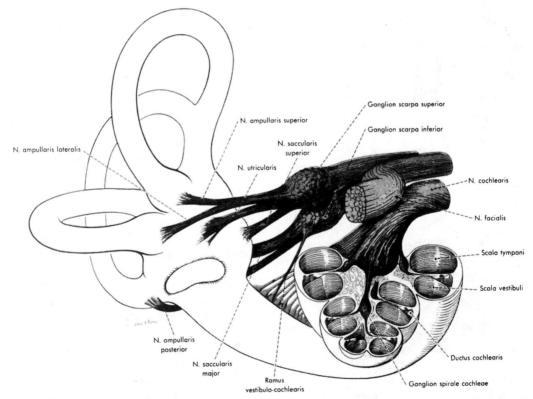

Figure 2-15. Inner ear. Note the position of the facial nerve to the cochlear nerve and to the superior and inferior vestibular nerve. The cochlea is open to illustrate the midmodiolar view as observed in temporal bone sections. (Reprinted with permission from Melloni, B.J. (1957). *Some pathological conditions of the eye, ear, and throat: An atlas.* Chicago: Abbott Laboratories.)

bone are shown in the next few pages. The sections have been selected because they show specific portions of the inner ear that are of interest to audiologists. Photographs of the midmodiolar section of the cochlea and a single coil, turn of the cochlea and a single coil, and turn of the cochlea have been included at higher magnifications so readers can appreciate these interesting structures.

A well-pneumatized mastoid can be seen in the posterior (or left) area of the section shown in Figure 2-16. The ampulla of the superior semicircular canal is shown as a nearly round structure enclosing the membranous labyrinth. The crista is noticeable on the anterior edge of the superior semicircular canal ampulla. The facial nerve and its genu are very clearly shown in this slide, which has been cut across the superior portion of the internal auditory canal. Immediately anterior to the genu of the facial nerve is the dense

bone of the otic capsule, which contains the cochlea. The lateral semicircular canal and its membranous labyrinth are also present at the peripheral edges of the structure.

The section shown in Figure 2-17 is approximately 1 mm below the section in Figure 2-16. The middle ear cavity is obvious in this section, which contains a cross-sectional view of the malleus and incus joined by the malleoincudal joint. The facial nerve is encased in the facial canal. The upper portion of the basal turn of the cochlea is present anteriorly and medially to the facial nerve. The superior branch of the vestibular nerve is visible in the internal auditory meatus and is shown passing to the macula of the utricle. The endolymphatic duct is also present.

Figure 2-18's section is approximately 1 mm below the section shown in Figure 2-17. The middle ear cavity shows the malleus and incus with its short process

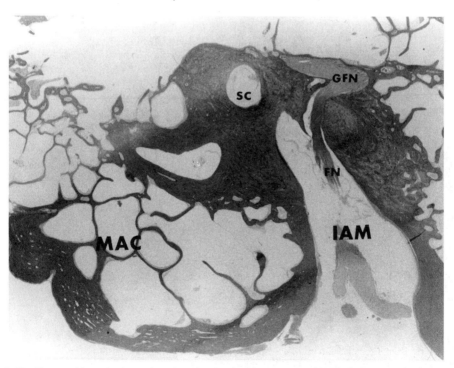

Figure 2-16. Temporal bone horizontal section showing facial nerve genu (GFN), facial nerve (FN), internal auditory meatus (IAM), ampulla of superior semicircular canal (SC), and mastoid air cells (MAC). (Courtesy of I. Sando, M.D.)

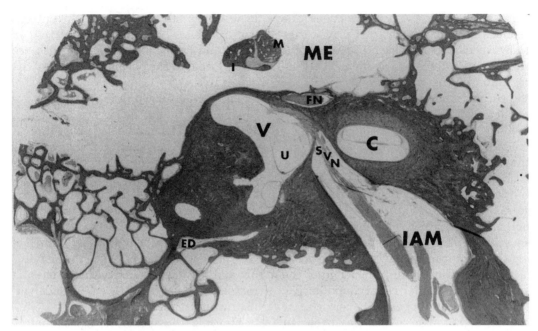

Figure 2-17. Horizontal section of normal temporal bone showing malleus (M) and incus (I) in the attic of the middle ear (ME), utricle (U), basal turn of the cochlea (C), and superior vestibular nerve (SVN), feeding into vestibule (V) from the internal auditory meatus (IAM). The endolymphatic duct (ED) is seen at lower left corner. (Courtesy of I. Sando, M.D.)

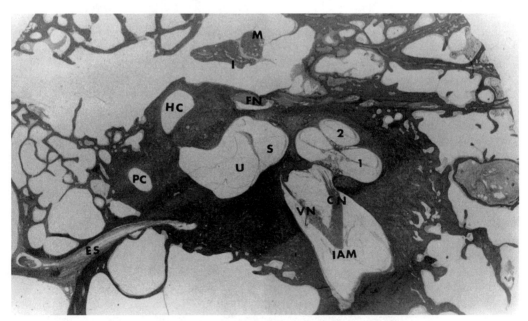

Figure 2-18. Horizontal section from normal temporal bone showing two cochlear turns, basal (1) and middle (2); vestibular (VN) and cochlear (CN) portions of the eighth nerve in the internal auditory meatus (IAM), and the endolymphatic sac (ES) is shown at lower left. The utricle (U) and the saccule (S) can be seen in the vestibule. The horizontal (HC) and posterior (PC) semicircular canals are also identified. *M,* malleus; *I,* incus; *FN,* facial nerve. (Courtesy of I. Sando, M.D.)

pointing posteriorly toward the aditus and antrum into the mastoid air spaces. The anterior mallear ligament can also be seen. The large space immediately medial to the facial nerve and canal contains the utricle. This section passes through the basal and middle turns of the cochlea that extend laterally. Reissner's membrane, the basilar membrane, and spiral ligament are obvious, even at this magnification. The modiolus is evident in the center of the basal turn of the cochlea. The inferior division of the vestibular nerve and the cochlear branch of the auditory nerve are shown in the internal auditory meatus. The endolymphatic sac is apparent in the posteromedial portion of the photograph.

The section shown in Figure 2-19 is 1 mm lower than the section shown in Figure 2-18. This section passes through the bony modiolus of the basal and middle turns of the cochlea and now includes the final cochlear turn, the apical coil. In the middle ear, the malleus and incus are no longer touching. The large tensor tympani muscle in its canal is obvious immediately adjacent to the cochlea and running anteroposterior. This section shows the processus cochleariformis extending posteriorly into the middle ear cavity from which the small tensor tympani tendon can be seen attaching to the anterior surface of the malleus. Part of the stapedial crura can be seen with the stapes footplate in the oval window niche. (An enlargement of the stapes in the oval window with the attachment of the stapedial tendon is shown in Fig. 2-20.) The saccule and its innervation can be seen clearly in the vestibule along with the lateral semicircular canal and utricle. The large circular structure at the anterior edge of the section is the internal carotid artery. All three ossicles are difficult to demonstrate on one temporal bone section because they are not lined up equally on a single horizontal plane level.

Figure 2-21 shows an enlargement of the cochlea as seen in Figure 2-19. It may be useful to the reader to review the gross view of the inner ear in Figure 2-15 to see how this exposure of the cochlea is obtained. This is a midmodiolar section of the cochlea showing the basal, middle, and apical turns. The nerve fibers are easily seen in the internal auditory meatus, and the ganglion cells of the spiral

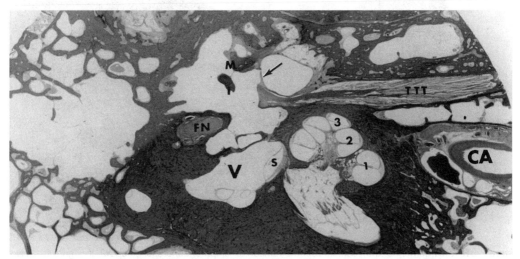

Figure 2-19. Cochlear midmodiolar horizontal section of normal temporal bone. All three coils of cochlea (1, 2, and 3) are evident; the malleus (M) is attached to tympanic membrane; the tensor tympani muscle (TTT) extends through the processus cochleariformis with tensor tendon (identified by the arrow) to malleus. *FN,* facial nerve; *V,* vestibule; *CA,* internal carotid artery; *I,* incus; *S,* saccule. (Courtesy of I. Sando, M.D.)

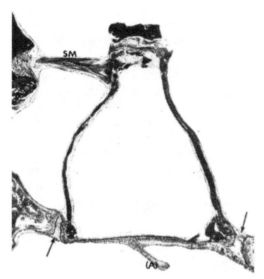

Figure 2-20. Enlargement of the stapes in the oval window and stapedial tendon (SM). Note normal attachment of stapes footplate in oval window by annular ligament (arrows). (Courtesy of E.L. Grandon, M.D.)

ganglion may be seen in Rosenthal's canal. The osseous spiral lamina extends radially from the modiolus in each turn. The basilar membrane can be seen extending from the osseous spiral lamina to the spiral ligament and stria vascularis. Reissner's membrane is seen in each coil of the cochlea, separating the scala vestibuli from the scala media. The basilar membrane supports the organ of Corti, which can just barely be seen at this magnification.

Figure 2-22 shows a classic view of a cochlear turn and emphasizes the structures of the scala media. These structures can be observed on a human temporal bone section by increasing the magnification on a single cochlear turn. The cochlear nerve fibers are shown under the spiral osseous lamina at the left of the photograph. The limbus supports one end of the tectorial membrane, which in its natural position should extend over the outer hair cells. The tectorial membrane, however, is very often seen in distorted position as an artifact of the temporal bone preparation procedure. Reissner's membrane extends from the limbus (crista spiralis) to the edge of the spiral ligament and stria vascularis. The curve between the limbus and the organ of Corti is the internal sulcus. The lower

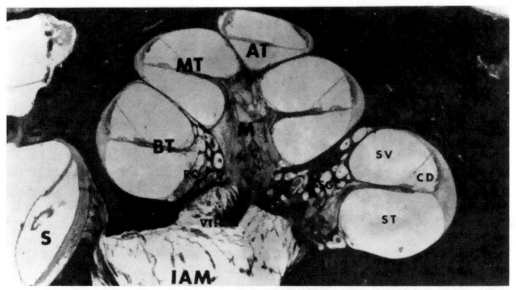

Figure 2-21. Enlargement of the cochlea from the horizontal temporal bone section shown in Figure 2.15. Note the auditory nerve (VIII N) in the internal auditory meatus (IAM) with ganglion cells (SGC) in Rosenthal's canal (RC). The cochlear basal turn (BT), the middle turn (MT), and apical turn (AT) are clearly shown. Three ducts are seen in each turn: the scala vestibuli (SV), the cochlear duct (CD), and the scala tympani (ST). The saccule (S) with its innervation is also obvious in this view. *M*, modiolus. (Courtesy of I. Sando, M.D.)

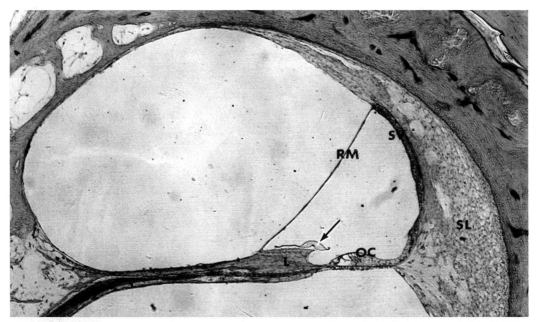

Figure 2-22. Higher magnification of one cochlear duct, showing organ of Corti (OC), spiral ligament (SL), stria vascularis (SV), Reissner's membrane (RM), tectorial membrane (arrow), and limbus (L). (Courtesy of I. Sando, M.D., and L. Bergstrom, M.D.)

edge of the limbus, pointing and extending toward the organ of Corti, is known as the tympanic lip, which has numerous holes, termed the habenula perforata. The habenula perforata permits cochlear nerve fibers to enter the organ of Corti from below the osseous spiral lamina. The basilar membrane supports the organ of Corti, which includes inner hair cells, outer hair cells, and the tunnel of Corti. Inner and outer pillar cells form the tunnel of Corti. Various supporting cells are seen next to the hair cells. Hensen's and Claudius' supporting cells are found between the outer hair cells and the external sulcus formed by the lower curve of the stria vascularis. Nuel's space is between the outer pillar and the first row of outer hair cells. The outer hair cells are supported by outer phalangeal cells (Deiter's cells). Thus, the outer hair cell rests on a Deiter's cell and extends hairs from its upper surface toward the tectorial membrane. The lower portion of the stria vascularis contains a bulge known as the spiral prominence.

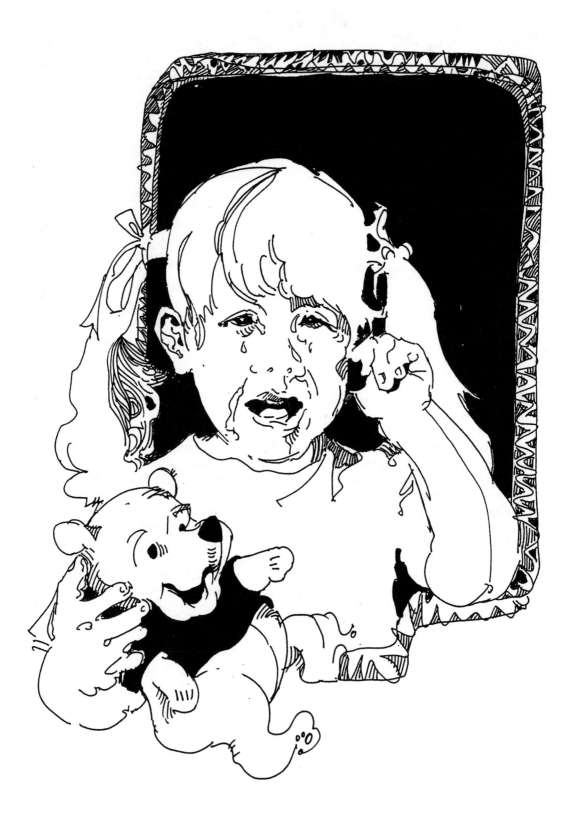

CHAPTER 3

Otitis Media

Ear infection can be very distressing in a child, and prompt, effective evaluation and treatment are required. Otitis media, or infection of the middle ("media") ear ("oto") is the most common childhood diseases and one of the most frequent reasons for concerned parents to take their child for medical services. According to the National Center for Health Statistics, visits to the doctor for diagnosis of otitis media increased from 10 million in 1975 to more than 25 million in 1990 (Schappert, 1992). Children younger than 2 years of age have the highest rate of visits to physicians' offices for otitis media and showed the highest rate of increase in visits between 1975 and 1990. Although improved accuracy in diagnosis accounts for some of this increase in reported cases, there is widespread recognition that the prevalence and incidence of otitis media has indeed grown over the years.

Parental concern is foremost because otitis media is usually a disease of infants, toddlers, and young children. The disorder is particularly difficult for parents to deal with because the symptoms can be so variable. Preverbal children are especially problematic because they are unable to localize and describe the sources of their pain. It has been estimated that 25 to 40% of all upper respiratory infections (URIs) in children younger than 3 years of age are associated with acute otitis media (Karver, 1998). Unfortunately, many parents have come to believe that ear pulling is a reliable sign of an ear infection. Baker (1992) has shown that ear pulling, in the absence of other symptoms, is not usually related to ear infections.

By technical definition, otitis media is an inflammation of the middle ear. The disorder is characterized by the presence of negative middle ear pressure and possible fluid (effusion), and may exist without obvious clinical signs or symptoms of infection. Otitis media creates a mild to moderate degree of conductive hearing loss by compromising the traditional air-conduction sound pathway. A current hypothesis about the natural history of the pathology is that the clinical variations of otitis media form a continuum of the disease process and are dynamically interrelated—that is, the simple beginning forms of otitis media, if untreated, may lead to more complex and severe disease processes.

The underlying cause of otitis media is nearly always the result of poor eustachian tube function, which leads to the production of sterile fluid by the mucosal lining of the middle ear. The eustachian tube has three general purposes: (1) protection of the middle ear from invading microbes, (2) clearance of middle ear secretions, and (3) equalization of pressure between the middle ear space and the nasopharynx. The child's eustachian tube is short, horizontal, and composed of relatively flaccid cartilage, whereas the adult eustachian tube lies in a more vertical position (Fig. 3-1). The adult vertical position provides more effective protection for the middle ear. The nearly horizontal position of the child's eustachian tube more

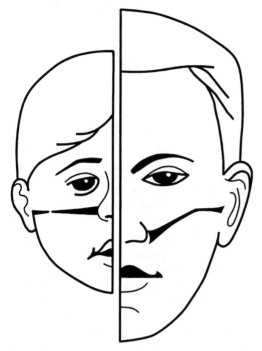

Figure 3-1. A comparison of the anatomic orientation the eustachian tube in a young child and an adult.

easily permits retrograde reflux of bacteria from the nasopharynx into the middle ear.

Nearly every aspect of childhood otitis media, from diagnosis to treatment to sequela, raises controversy and debate among professionals. Whereas recurrent otitis media is a well-recognized medical problem in children, the treatment and the management of this common disorder have been the focus of numerous research efforts. Questions regarding the short-term and long-term effects of the otitis media continuum, and the effect of the accompanying mild to moderate conductive hearing loss, on child development continue to raise unresolved questions. Pediatric patients and their parents are often caught in the middle between policies of cost-oriented health care management and the recommendations for treatment provided by patient-oriented physicians (Gates, 1998). It is surprising that so little substantive data are available to chart natural course and developmental effects of this problem. Numerous unresolved questions surround the relative efficacy and risks of medical and surgical treatments. Also debatable are the outcome results of the speech and language delays considered by many to be the direct result of the transient and recurrent mild conductive hearing loss. Excellent summaries of multidisciplinary workshops concerned with otitis media identification and management have been published by Bluestone, Klein, and Paradise (1983) and Bluestone, Fria, and Arjona (1986).

The hearing acuity of children with otitis media with effusion (fluid) in the middle ear has been reported by Fria, Cantekin, and Eichler (1985). Average air conduction thresholds, based on careful audiometric examination of 762 children with documented middle ear effusion (MEE), were 27 dB HL at 500, 1000, and 4000 Hz, with a better average hearing threshold of 20 dB HL at 2000 Hz. Hearing sensitivity in this study was approximately 10 dB worse in children with bilateral effusion than in children with unilateral effusion.

In general terms, the hearing loss associated with otitis media is either flat or slightly rising from the low frequencies, with the best hearing at 2000 Hz (Fig. 3-2). However, hearing loss due to otitis media can vary from nearly normal hearing to as much as 50 dB of hearing loss. Bone-conduction thresholds are usually not affected by the presence of MEE. Gravel and Ellis (1995) point out that the hearing of children with otitis media can differ substantially both by degree and symmetry between the two ears. Otoscopic observation of an air-fluid level or air bubbles within the middle ear fluid is generally associated with less hearing impairment. Studies of extended high-frequency hearing showed that children with a history of chronic or recurrent otitis media had significantly impaired

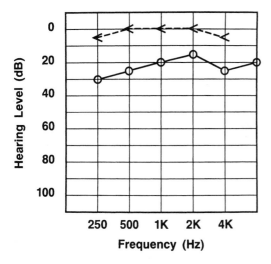

Figure 3-2. Typical audiometric results showing conductive-type hearing loss from the right ear of a child with otitis media. Note the normal hearing bone-conduction threshold responses (open arrows) with diminished air-conduction thresholds (open circles).

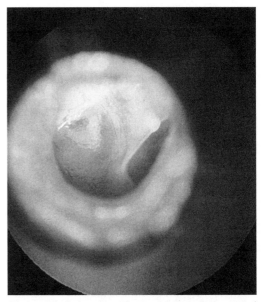

Figure 3-3. A view through an operating microscope of a normal tympanic membrane. Viewed posteriorly through the translucent eardrum, the incus and stapedius tendon can be noted.

hearing in the 12–20 kHz range in light of normal hearing in the conventional audiometric frequency test range (Trine, Hirsch, & Margolis, 1993; Margolis, Rykken, Hunter, et al., 1993).

The general definitive and descriptive categories of otitis media are (1) otitis media without effusion, (2) acute otitis media, (3) otitis media with effusion, and (4) otitis media with tympanic membrane perforation. Each of these categories may be classified by duration into acute (0–21 days), subacute (22 days–8 weeks), and chronic (more than 8 weeks). In otitis media with effusion, with or without tympanic membrane perforation, the fluid or discharge may be characterized as serous (thin, watery liquid), purulent (pus-like liquid), or mucoid (thick, viscid, mucus-like liquid). An otoscopic view of a normal tympanic membrane is shown in Figure 3-3 with normal landmarks clearly visible. The otoscopic photomicrograph shown in Figure 3-4 was taken from an ear with serous otitis media characterized by the absence of all normal landmarks.

ECONOMIC CONSIDERATIONS

The economic considerations of otitis media have a tremendous influence on national health expenditures. Otitis media

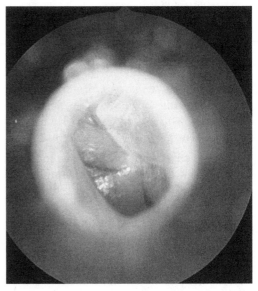

Figure 3-4. An otoscopic view of serous otitis media. The eardrum is retracted, with the short process of the malleus prominent and the long process foreshortened in appearance. Inferiorly, the eardrum is sucked inward from effusion in the middle ear space.

represents huge financial considerations for numerous health-care professionals, pharmaceutical companies, and hospitals as detailed in "Ear Infections in Your Child" by Grundfast and Carney (1987):

- The total cost related to the management of otitis media in the United States is estimated to be $5 billion per year. This figure includes physician fees and surgery, prescribed medications, and speech-language and audiology examinations.

- Nearly 30 million visits to physicians per year are estimated to take place for the diagnosis and treatment of otitis media. This includes emergency visits, follow-up visits, consultations with ear, nose, and throat (ENT) medical specialists, hearing tests by audiologists, and evaluations of speech and language.

- It has been estimated that on any winter day in the United States, up to 30% of children are suffering an ear infection or have an abnormal middle ear condition. This means that up to 900,000 children a day may suffer an ear-related condition.

- Before the age of 6, approximately 85 to 90% of all U.S. children will have had at least one ear infection. Half the children who have one ear infection before age 1 will have six or more episodes in the following 2 years. Nearly 20% of children who suffer ear infections will require surgery to correct the problem.

- Otitis media is one of the most common indicators for outpatient antimicrobial use in the United States, with the number of prescriptions doubling from 12 million in 1980 to 24 million in 1992.

Otitis media is most common during the first 2 years of a child's life and then decreases in incidence as the child grows older. As the young child ages, the inclination of the eustachian tube increases to about a 45° angle, thereby decreasing the incidence of ear infections. The incidence of otitis media has been studied by many investigators and has been found to be a function of age, gender (more otitis media in boys), race (native Americans, Eskimos, and whites have higher incidences than blacks), genetic factors, socioeconomic status, season, and climate.

A number of research studies have identified risk factors that may make certain children more likely to have recurrent otitis media. Children living in households with many members have more episodes of otitis media than children living in households with fewer members. Children with siblings or parents who have a history of otitis media show a higher incidence of otitis media than children with family members without a history of the disease. Other risk factors include certain socioeconomic factors such as overcrowding with poor sanitation, inadequate diet, and the absence of routine health care; secondary cigarette smoke exposure; and possibly sleep position. Breast-feeding and group day care also play roles in URIs in general, including otitis media (Duncan et al., 1993; Aniansson, Alm, & Anderson, 1994; Paradise Elster, & Tan, 1994). Infants who are bottle-fed in the supine position are more at risk for otitis media than infants who are fed while being held upright. Children in day care have more otitis media than do children who are cared for at home, because of endemic URIs passed among children (Teele, Klein, & Rosner, 1980b; Bluestone, 1998).

The statistical implication of otitis media in the general population is impressive. In a study of preschool children in Pittsburgh, Pennsylvania, Casselbrant, Brostoff, Cantekin, et al. (1985) confirmed that nearly 60% of children aged 2–6 years who were examined monthly for 24 months had documented otitis media with effusion episodes that averaged 2 months in duration. Approximately 80% of 103 young children diagnosed as having otitis media with effusion experienced a spontaneous recovery within 2 months without medical treatment. In a larger cohort study of 1439 Dutch children, approximately 60% of children recovered from otitis media with effusion without intervention within 3 months (Zielhuis, Straatman, Rach, & van den Broek, 1990). Although otitis media may resolve spontaneously without treatment in most children, the disorder may return with a high recurrence rate in some children.

The prevalence of otitis media among children shows strong seasonal variation associated with the presence of URIs. Otitis media is common among patients with allergies. Inflammation of the eustachian tube, along with allergic rhinitis, is a common cause of MEE. Klein (1979) suggests that children can be divided into three groups with regard to otitis media: one-third of children have no episodes, one-third may have an occasional episode, and one-third have frequent episodes of otitis media. The problem, of course, is how to identify in advance the children who belong to the group with frequent and recurring otitis media.

Of particular importance is the concept of the "otitis-prone" child described initially by Howie, Ploussard, and Sloyer (1975). An otitis-prone child is the youngster who has the condition 6 or more times before the age of 6 years, or whose initial episode of otitis media was due to bacteria and occurred before the age of 1 year. The otitis-prone child is destined to have continued and recurrent bouts of otitis media throughout childhood and requires careful monitoring and management. Other special populations with a predisposition for MEE and otitis media include children with Down, Turner, Apert, or Crouzon syndromes; cleft palate (overt or submucous); or any craniofacial malformation. Craniofacial malformations, including dentofacial abnormalities, may have an associated congenital anatomic or physiologic abnormality that results in eustachian tube dysfunction.

EAR DISEASE IN NATIVE POPULATIONS

Otitis media was one of the most serious health problems among the native American Indian and Eskimo populations of North America. Much effort and money were expended during the 1970s and 1980s to gain control over the widespread problems of alcoholism and tuberculosis among American Indians. The success in reducing these health problems brought to light a new health problem challenge—otologic disease and hearing impairment.

Health problems existed among native American populations because of poor living conditions, harsh physical and psychological environment, inadequate water facilities, crowded living conditions, unsanitary waste disposal, inadequate refrigeration, nonexistent insect control, and poor nutrition. With federal financial support, great strides in the health care for American Indians and Eskimos have been accomplished. However, cultural barriers, poverty, poor transportation, and lack of education about health issues make solutions to health problems difficult. The success of well-planned and implemented health programs with native American children provides a clear blueprint for other at-risk populations. The widespread health problems associated with otitis media are not uncommon in many of the developing countries around the world.

Hearing Impairment in Eskimos. During the early 1950s, ear disease in native Eskimo children was such a common occurrence that parents did not consider otorrhea (drainage from the ear) to be a serious problem. Brody (1964) and Brody, Overfield, & McAlister (1965) reported that 31% of an Eskimo village population had at least one episode of draining ears within the evaluation year, with two-thirds of the ear disease group indicating more than one episode of otorrhea. It was shown that ear pathology in Eskimos is established by the age of 2 years, and those children who by age 2 did not have draining ears were unlikely to develop ear pathology. Several additional studies on Eskimo populations were published, confirming the extraordinarily high incidence of middle ear disease. Reed, Struve, and Maynard (1967) followed 378 Eskimo children during their first 4 years of life. They reported that the *frequency* of episodes had more influence on the degree of hearing impairment than did the age of onset of the initial otorrhea episode. Reed and Dunn (1970) found that 43% of 641 Eskimo children experienced 532 episodes of otitis media, with the highest incidence occurring in children less than 2 years of age. Kaplan, Goddard, Van Kleeck, et al. (1973) reported that 38% of a group of Eskimo children had one or more bouts of otorrhea before age 1 and that 76% of these children commonly experienced otorrhea when they were subsequently evaluated at 7–10 years of age.

Ear Disease in American Indians. American Indian populations also show a high percentage of middle ear disorders. In 1967, Johnson reported the incidence of chronic otitis media in the Navajo population to be 12–15 times higher than that found in white Americans. Jaffe (1968b) studied the incidence of ear diseases of all types in the Navajo. Aural atresia was found in 58 of 60,000 persons. Chronic suppurative otitis media was the most common Navajo otologic disease, with 4.2% central perforations in 2000 patients. Jaffe cites the closed genetic pool among the Navajos as a major cause of frequently seen bifid uvula and aural atresia. One hundred years ago there were only 5000 Navajos; the current Navajo population is estimated to be at least 170,000. Other reports have been published on various American Indian tribes (Johnson & Watrous, 1978; Fischler, Todd, & Feldman, 1985).

Moore (1999) examined the risk of conductive hearing loss in native Inuit patients who live in the western Canadian Arctic area. The study showed an increase in conductive hearing losses throughout childhood. The identification and treatment of otitis media in this native group is especially important due to the negative impact that hearing loss is likely to have on the children's abilities to learn both their native language and English.

PATHOPHYSIOLOGY OF OTITIS MEDIA

Eustachian tube dysfunction has long been recognized to be a significant factor in the development of otitis media. The most important function of the eustachian tube is ventilation of the middle ear space. When the eustachian tube malfunctions, from either a mechanical or a functional cause, the air trapped in the middle ear cavity is absorbed by the mucosal lining of the middle ear, creating negative middle ear pressure and, ultimately, transudation of fluid into the cavity. As stated previously, otitis media with effusion is characterized by fluid in the middle ear without evidence of infection. A long litany of synonyms is used to describe this condition including serous otitis, secretory otitis, allergic otitis, catarrhal otitis, nonsuppurative otitis, mucoid otitis, glue ear, fluid ear, and MEE.

The tonsils and adenoids have traditionally been implicated in the pathophysiology of otitis media, although current medical research questions this assumption. Tonsils and adenoids are part of a ring of glandular tissue encircling the back of the throat. The adenoids are located high in the throat behind the soft palate and are not visible through the mouth without special instruments. The tonsils are the two masses of tissue on either side of the back of the throat. These structures are strategically located to "sample" incoming bacteria and viruses, and they often become infected themselves. It is thought that they help form antibodies to those "germs" as part of the body's immune system to resist and fight future infections. Chronic infections in the tonsils and adenoids can affect nearby structures, and their swelling may create blockage around the base, or opening, of the eustachian tubes. This situation may lead to mechanical blockage or interference in the function of the eustachian tube. Eustachian tube dysfunction leads to ineffective aeration of the middle ear spaces, thereby ear infections and subsequent hearing loss.

Eustachian tube dysfunction is often treated indirectly by surgical insertion of tiny, hollow, plastic tympanostomy tubes into the tympanic membranes (Fig. 3-5). Treatment of otitis media with tympanostomy tubes is the most common surgical operation performed in children. The tubes, inserted into the tympanic membrane, serve to aerate the middle ear space until the eustachian tube recovers and functions normally. The tubes are left in place for several months until they naturally extrude, in hopes that the eustachian tube dysfunction, which initially caused the otitis media, has resolved naturally. There is a wide variety of tubes available to surgeons which differ by lumen size, tube length, and retention time. In general, short tubes extrude sooner than longer "T"-shaped tubes. The larger-bore tube may aerate the middle ear better and stay in place longer, but it

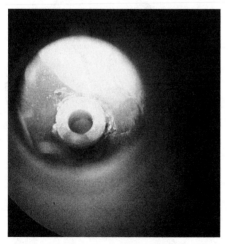

Figure 3-5. A view of a tympanic membrane with a tympanostomy tube in place. The tube is patent to aerate the middle ear space and will gradually be pushed out by the regrowth of the tympanic membrane behind it.

is more likely to leave a persistent perforation of the tympanic membrane (Gates, 1998).

TREATMENT OF OTITIS MEDIA

The diagnosis of otitis media is based on clinical manifestations, physical examination of the tympanic membrane, as well as acoustic immittance testing, otoacoustic emissions, and routine audiometry. The mainstay of the diagnosis of otitis media is pneumatic otoscopy—a procedure in which a hermetically sealed otoscope is used to visualize the tympanic membrane with magnification while the air pressure in the external ear canal is varied. This permits evaluation of tympanic membrane mobility that is not possible by simple inspection through a simple otoscope. Although hearing loss is the most prevalent complication associated with otitis media, possibly characterized by fluctuating hearing levels, the hearing loss usually returns to normal following resolution of the effusion. The symptoms of otitis media can be classified as either specific or systemic. Specific symptoms include earache, rubbing or tugging at the ears, otorrhea (drainage), hearing impairment, and balance disturbance. Of these, only earache and otorrhea are generally associated with active infection. The systemic symptoms include fever, temperament disorders and restless sleep, irritability, or low-grade discomfort. Effective treatment is important to provide rapid symptomatic relief but also to reduce the likelihood of long-term sequelae such as hearing loss, permanent middle ear damage, and development and learning dysfunction.

The most common infective pathogens causing otitis media are *Streptococcus pneumoniae, Haemophilus influenzae,* and *Moraxella catarrhalis. S. pneumoniae* has become resistant to a variety of antibiotics. This has emerged as one of the most serious problems affecting antibiotic treatment in the 1990s. In addition, about 30% of *H. influenzae* and up to 75% of *M. catarrhalis* strains are now resistant to common antibiotics. No single antimicrobial agent appears to be suitable for all patients with otitis media. There is growing concern that prescribing antibiotics without due consideration of factors such as changing resistance patterns and individual patient variables is leading to a greater level of treatment failures. Difficult cases of otitis media require aspiration of the fluid, which is then cultured to identify the specific organism responsible for the infection (Fig. 3-6). Evidence exists that antimicrobial use may have little or no effect on the long-term course of otitis media (Culpepper & Froom, 1995). Paradise (1995, 1997) cites the increasing prevalence of multiple resistant pneumococcal infection and the heightened risks associated with antimicrobial usage to recommend restricting antimicrobial treatment of otitis media in children as much as possible. It has been shown that up to 85% of cases of acute otitis media clear up without antimicrobial treatment, compared with improvement in 95% of patients treated with antimicrobial therapy (Rosenfeld, 1996).

Considerable research is underway in the areas of microbiology and immunology as the necessary steps toward the development of a vaccine to prevent otitis media (Lim, Bluestone, & Casselbrant, 1998). Although much remains to be learned about the pathophysiology of otitis media and the most effective means to combat the major infective agents, the basic evidence presented at this time suggests that it will be feasible to develop bacterial vaccines in the future which will prevent otitis media. Clearly, this protective strategy for children at risk for otitis media will be beneficial in reducing this enormous health problem from the points of view of human suffering and economic consequences.

Recurrent tonsillitis and enlarged adenoids were once thought to be the major cause of otitis media. The number of tonsillectomies and/or adenoidectomies performed yearly in the United States has steadily decreased each year since 1965

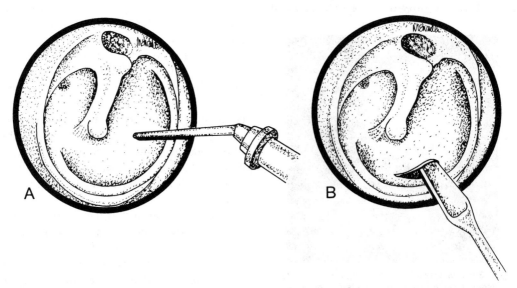

Figure 3-6. A. (A) Tympanotomy, or surgical puncture of the tympanic membrane, is used to aspirate fluid by suction for culture. **(B)** Myringotomy, or surgical incision of tympanic membrane, is performed in the lower half of the tympanic membrane to avoid damage to middle ear ossicles. Myringotomy is conducted to provide instant relief from pain, to drain fluid from the middle ear space, and thus to help initiate rapid recovery from middle ear disease.

(Grundfast & Carney, 1987). The tonsillectomy and adenoidectomy ("T&A") operation, once the most common surgical procedure for children, is now only performed occasionally. Experts agree that tonsillectomy alone is not recommended as treatment for otitis media, although the role of adenoidectomy in treating otitis media is somewhat more controversial.

The goal of surgery is to correct the underlying pathophysiologic condition when possible. Gates (1998) points out that surgical treatment is recommended only when medical treatment fails. Thus, medical and surgical therapies for otitis media are sequential, not alternative, treatments. If otitis media is likely due to inadequate ventilation of the middle ear, then insertion of tympanostomy tubes, also known as pressure equalization (PE) tubes, is the recommended surgical treatment. If infection of the middle ear from reflux of nasopharyngeal organisms is the problem, adenoidectomy is the treatment of choice. In most cases of chronic otitis media, both pathophysiologic conditions exist concurrently; thus, the combined operation of tympanostomy tubes with adenoidectomy is indicated.

According to Rosenfeld (1997) children with middle ear problems tend to fall into two treatment groups: those who get better no matter what treatment they receive, and those who get better only with surgery and placement of ventilation tubes. Rosenfeld dispels several common myths about tympanostomy tubes:

- Tympanostomy tubes do not cause significant scarring of the eardrum, and the small mark that may form when the tube falls out does not affect hearing.

- A properly placed tympanostomy tube cannot fall into the middle ear. Instead, the tube is naturally pushed into the external ear canal after 6–18 months.

- Water precautions are typically unnecessary for most children with tympanostomy tubes. Research and clinical experience have shown no benefit from the routine use of earplugs, bathing caps, or custom fitted swim molds during normal bathing or swimming. Water precautions may be necessary for those children who swim in lake water or a spend a substantial amount of time totally immersed underwater.

- The tympanostomy tube does not cure the ear infection; it simply controls the infection by temporarily ventilating the middle ear. By the time the tube falls out naturally, approximately 80% of children will have outgrown their tendency for middle ear problems.

Opposing points of view regarding the use of tympanostomy tubes for treatment of otitis media with effusion cite the lack of convincing evidence linking otitis media early in life to either otologic or developmental difficulties later in life. That is, if the majority of patients with otitis media spontaneously recover, why is surgical intervention necessary? Other considerations to be weighed before surgical intervention include the cost and risk of surgery as well as the potential complications resulting from tympanostomy tube insertion. Comparison of preoperative threshold audiometry with thresholds measured after tympanostomy tube placement is important to document improved hearing.

Controversy, confusion, and misunderstanding surround the various philosophies for treatment and the standard of care required in patients with otitis media. Tremendous benefits would be gained for patients and rising health-care costs if otitis media could be prevented or substantially reduced in frequency. Accordingly, the Agency for Health Care Policy and Research (AHCPR) of the U.S. Department of Health and Human Services convened a panel of experts to summarize current scientific knowledge and develop a clinical practice guideline for otitis media. Their findings and recommendations were published as "Otitis Media With Effusion in Young Children" (Stool, Berg, Carney, et al., 1994) to codify the diagnosis and treatment and to recommend management guidelines for this growing problem in health care. The panel made recommendations for the diagnosis and treatment of otitis media with effusion in children between the ages of 1 year and 3 years, based on extensive literature review, expert testimony, and consensus of the primary physician panel members.

AHCPR RECOMMENDATIONS

Diagnosis of Otitis Media

- Pneumatic Otoscopy. The diagnosis of suspected otitis media with effusion should include pneumatic otoscopy. Otoscopy alone (without the use of pneumatic otoscopy to test tympanic membrane mobility) is not recommended.

- Tympanometry. This may be used as a confirmatory test for otitis media with effusion.

- Hearing Evaluation. This is recommended for a child who has bilateral otitis media with effusion for 3 months. As an optional recommendation, hearing evaluation may be performed before otitis media with effusion has been present for 3 months. The panel members apparently believed that insufficient scientific evidence was available to substantiate the use of hearing tests as a necessary procedure in the diagnosis of otitis media.

- Tuning Forks and Acoustic Reflectometry. No recommendations were made regarding acoustic reflectometry as a technique for screening or diagnostic evaluation of otitis media. Tuning fork tests were noted to be inappropriate for young children.

The AHCPR panel made numerous recommendations concerning treatment and management of otitis media with effusion in otherwise healthy youngsters

from 1–3 years of age. In each category presented below, the panel included a recommendation that parents should be encouraged to follow to control environmental risk factors (i.e., infant feeding practices, passive cigarette smoke exposure, and child care situations).

Initial Management of Otitis Media

- Observation or antibiotic therapy may be chosen for management of otitis media with effusion in an otherwise healthy child.

- Myringotomy with or without tubes should not be performed for initial management of otitis media.

Treatment of Otitis Media After 3 Months

- Observation or antibiotic therapy may be chosen if the child has normal hearing, as indicated by hearing threshold levels better than 20 dB HL in the better hearing ear.

- If the child has bilateral hearing deficits of 20 dB HL or worse, antibiotic therapy or myringotomy tubes may be chosen to manage otitis media.

Treatment of Otitis Media After 4–6 Months

- Myringotomy with tubes is recommended to manage otitis media with effusion that has lasted for 4–6 months.

Not Recommended for Treatment at Any Age

- Management procedures that are not recommended at any time for otitis media with effusion are steroid medications, antihistamine/decongestant medications, adenoidectomy, and tonsillectomy.

In a study designed to evaluate the AHCPR otitis media treatment guidelines, Griffith, Levine, and Giebink (1998) found generally poor compliance with the recommended treatment protocols. Their review of patient medical records revealed low utilization of pneumatic otoscopy, audiometry, and tympanometry. Nearly 34% of patients treated by pediatricians had delayed referral to otolaryngologists, with some patients having ear disease for 7 years before referral. The average length of MEE present in the cohort children before referral was 5.2 months. In the study, flat tympanograms were found in 70% of all ears, and hearing loss was present in 92% of patients. Nearly 50% of children had complications or sequelae from otitis media at the time of referral, the most common being speech and language delay. The records showed that as many as seven different antibiotic agents had been prescribed for some patients. The authors called for better education of primary care physicians about otitis media so that the use of diagnostic tools and the time to specialist referral could be improved.

COMPLICATIONS ASSOCIATED WITH OTITIS MEDIA

Complications of untreated otitis media with effusion include hearing loss, perforation of the tympanic membrane (with or without effusion), tympanic membrane retraction, cholesteatoma, mastoiditis, adhesive otitis media, tympanosclerosis, ossicular discontinuity, facial paralysis, and labyrinthitis. Intracranial complications may include meningitis, encephalitis, brain abscess, and sinus thrombophlebitis. The most prevalent adverse sequel to tympanostomy tubes is purulent otorrhea (infected drainage from the tube itself). Treatment of otorrhea consists of a topical steroid and oral antibiotic that is usually sufficient to clean up the discharge. In 1–15% of patients, the tympanic membrane fails to heal following extrusion of the tympanostomy tube, leaving a small perforation in the eardrum. The perforation rate has been shown to be significantly higher

when the tympanostomy tubes are retained longer than 36 months (Nichols, Ramadan, Wax, & Santrock, 1998). The treatment of the persistent perforation generally requires a minor surgical procedure, known as a myringoplasty, to seal the perforation. Finally, persistent and recurrent otitis media in early life may impair the development of children's cognitive abilities and detrimentally influence behavior (see Speech and Language Development below).

An enlightening and extremely important finding was reported by Teele, Klein, and Rosner (1980a) concerning persistence of MEE following medical treatment. After the first episode of otitis media, 70% of children in the study still had effusion at 2 weeks, 40% at 1 month, 20% at 2 months, and 10% at 3 months. Pelton, Shurin, and Klein (1977) also found that approximately one-third of unselected children with acute otitis media had persistent fluid in the middle ear for 4 or more weeks. These statistics confirm the importance of careful and thorough medical and audiologic follow-up for all children with otitis media with effusion.

Acute Otitis Media. Acute otitis media presents with sudden onset accompanied by severe ear pain, redness of the tympanic membrane, and fever. Acute otitis media is an inflammatory disorder caused by microorganisms in the middle ear, usually as a sequel to a URI. Otitis media without effusion is usually present in the early stages of acute otitis media. The diagnosis of acute otitis media is usually made with otoscopy based on the color, decreased mobility, and outward bulging contour of the tympanic membrane. It is not uncommon for an episode of acute otitis media to be associated with a spontaneous perforation of the tympanic membrane, which results in otorrhea. At the time of the spontaneous rupture of the tympanic membrane, the acute pain typically ceases. Although generally an easy diagnosis, sometimes acute otitis media presents without a red tympanic membrane, without fever, and without pain. Treatment is usually dependent on eliminating the infecting organism through adequately prescribed antibiotic treatment. When the diagnosis of acute otitis media is in doubt, or when determination of the causative agent is in question, aspiration of the middle ear fluid is performed with tympanocentesis or myringotomy. In patients with unusually severe earache and pain, myringotomy may be performed to provide immediate pain relief.

Bullous Myringitis. Blisters occasionally form on the tympanic membrane in association with a coincident URI. The blisters, or bullae, represent an accumulation of fluid between the layers of the tympanic membrane and may appear to the untrained observer to represent acute otitis media. This disorder is extremely painful and accompanied by a feeling of pressure in the ear. Hearing levels may be within normal limits. According to Bluestone (1998), bullous myringitis is not a separate clinical entity but is merely acute otitis media with blisters on the eardrum.

Serous Otitis Media. This is the most common form of otitis media and may be recalcitrant to medical treatment. The tympanic membrane is usually opaque, and there may be relatively normal mobility to applied heavy positive and negative pressure from the pneumatic otoscope. The effusion is usually asymptomatic in most children. However, if pain is present in this disorder, it is usually intermittent and mild. Following an episode of acute otitis media, an effusion may persist despite antibiotic treatment of the condition. Persistent MEE that follows an attack of acute otitis media usually clears without further treatment. About 50% of pediatric cases of serous otitis media show no significant hearing loss (Cohen & Sade, 1972).

Adhesive Otitis Media. This form of otitis media is a thickening of the fibrous tissue of the tympanic membrane that may be accompanied by severe retraction and negative pressure in the middle ear space (Fig. 3-7). When a retraction pocket forms in the superior portion of the pars tensa of the tympanic membrane, the development of cholesteatoma (see below for definition) is probable.

Chronic Suppurative Otitis Media. This is a late stage of ear disease in which there is infection of the middle ear and mastoid as well as a "central" perforation of the tympanic membrane and discharge. This condition most often has its onset in childhood, between the ages of 5 and 10 years. Mastoiditis is invariably a part of the pathologic process. Recurrent otitis media may halt or reverse the process of mastoid pneumatization or cause mastoid sclerosis. Severe forms of chronic otitis media may damage the middle ear ossicles, depending on the severity and duration of the disease (Fig. 3-8). Severe otitis media may produce areas of os-

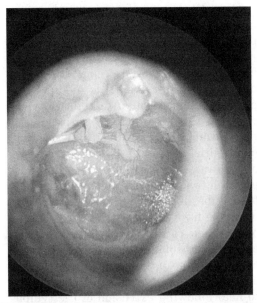

Figure 3-7. Adhesive otitis media with severe retraction of the tympanic membrane. The eardrum is draped around the incus posteriorly, and the stapedius tendon is clearly seen.

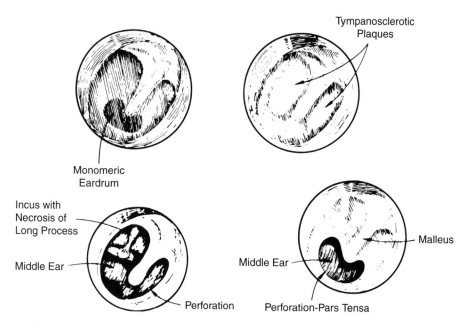

Tympanosclerotic
Plaques

Monomeric
Eardrum

Incus with
Necrosis of
Long Process

Middle Ear

Malleus

Middle Ear

Perforation

Perforation-Pars Tensa

Figure 3-8. Otoscopic drawings of the tympanic membrane showing sequelae of chronic otitis media. (Courtesy of Gerald M. English, MD, Denver, Colorado.)

teitis in the mastoid septae, resulting in a continuous foul discharge in the ear canal (Bluestone, 1998).

Cholesteatoma. Cholesteatoma is a growth of skin from the external ear canal which invades the middle ear space by pressing into a retraction pocket in the tympanic membrane. Repeated infection and persistent negative middle ear pressure typically cause the retraction pocket (also known as a pouch or sac). The continuing growth of the squamous epithelium (skin) into this retraction pocket takes the form of a cyst formed by new layers of skin growing over older layers of skin. Over time, cholesteatoma can increase in size and destroy the surrounding tissues and structures of the middle ear. In otitis media with perforation, the tissues of the middle ear intermittently undergo destruction, healing, and scarring during the recurrent infection process.

Initially, the symptoms of cholesteatoma include drainage (sometimes accompanied by a foul odor), conductive hearing loss, fullness or pressure in or behind the ear, dizziness, and facial weakness. Usually, although not always, cholesteatoma is a unilateral problem. This is a very serious ear condition that must be examined and evaluated by an otolaryngologist. Cholesteatomas that are undiscovered or untreated can be dangerous, with resultant bone erosion leading to deafness, brain abscess, and meningitis; death can sometimes occur. Because of the seriousness of this disorder, audiologists must be extremely careful in the evaluation and referral of children with unilateral conductive hearing losses that do not respond to traditional medical treatment.

The cross-section shown in Figure 3-9 shows an attic and a middle ear cholesteatoma. Moisture and bacteria may gain access to the cholesteatoma, creating infection and drainage. Initial treatment may consist of careful cleaning of the debris, topical eardrops, and antibiotics to clear up the infection process. Large or complicated cholesteatomas usually re-

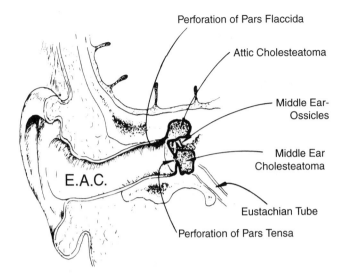

Perforation of Pars Flaccida

Attic Cholesteatoma

Middle Ear-Ossicles

Middle Ear Cholesteatoma

E.A.C.

Eustachian Tube

Perforation of Pars Tensa

Figure 3-9. Cross-section of the external and middle ear showing an attic cholesteatoma through a perforation of the pars flaccida portion of the tympanic membrane. A perforation of the pars tensa portion of the tympanic membrane may lead to development of a middle ear cholesteatoma. (Reprinted with permission from English, G.M., Northern, J.L., & Fria, T.J. (1973). Chronic otitis media as a cause of sensorineural hearing loss. *Archives of Otolaryngology, 98,* 17–22.)

quire surgical removal to protect the patient from more serious complications. The purpose of the surgery is twofold: to remove the cholesteatoma and infection as well as to preserve or improve hearing. In some cases, these goals are accomplished through two separate operations. Tos (1983) reviewed surgical results from 122 children operated on for removal of cholesteatoma. He found recurrent cholesteatoma in 12% of patients and remarked that recurrent growth of cholesteatoma is more common in children than in adults and develops faster in young people. Following surgical removal of the cholesteatoma, routine visits are scheduled to examine the ear for possible recurrence of the skin tumor. In some patients, an open mastoid cavity is surgically created, and office visits every few months (perhaps for life) are necessary to clean out the cavity and prevent new infections.

Mastoiditis. Mastoiditis is categorized into either acute or chronic stages. The terms represent the degree of involvement of the infected mastoid air cell system. The anatomic continuity between the middle ear and the mucosal lining of the mastoid antrum allows for the coexisting inflammatory process associated with these structures. With the onset of edema or in-

sufficient drainage of the mastoid mucosa, pressure is created within the air cells, causing localized discomfort. Some of the clinical manifestations of mastoiditis are fullness, pain, otitis media, tenderness, edema, and conductive hearing loss. Other clinical findings may consist of tympanic membrane and middle ear ossicular destruction.

Acute mastoiditis is an inflammation of the ciliated mucosa of the antrum. Until the 1940s, acute mastoiditis was a complication of acute otitis media in 25–50% of cases. With the advent of antibiotics such as penicillin, the incidence of acute mastoiditis has been lowered considerably. However, antibiotic therapy has been said to "mask" the presence of mastoiditis, whereby the disease is suppressed enough to reduce the symptoms but not enough to resolve the ongoing destructive process.

Chronic mastoiditis occurs with chronic inflammation of the membrane lining the mastoid antrum and ciliated cells. The bone structure is often involved in the infection. Generally, chronic mastoiditis is associated with a history of otitis media, which may be active or inactive, depending on whether purulent discharge is present. The symptoms of chronic mastoiditis are similar to those of acute mastoiditis, with the exception of the hearing loss, which often takes on a sensorineural component.

During the preantibiotic era, some of the most life-threatening complications of mastoiditis were meningitis, brain abscess, and cerebellar abscess. Current complications still include facial nerve paralysis, labyrinthitis, meningitis, and cholesteatoma. Intracranial complications have decreased since the 1930s and 1940s, along with a significant decrease in patient mortality rates. In cases in which antibiotics have been ineffective in treating acute mastoiditis, a simple mastoidectomy is performed with surgical drainage of the mastoid air cells. Patients with chronic mastoiditis are initially treated nonsurgically to dry the ear and prevent factors that would complicate surgical treatment. When medical management fails, a surgical modified or radical mastoidectomy is performed.

Tympanosclerosis. Following recurrent episodes of otitis media, the middle ear and tympanic membrane may develop *tympanosclerosis,* which is hyalinized and calcified scar tissue. Tympanosclerosis deposits may cause stiffening of the tympanic membrane or fusion and fixation of the middle ear ossicles. Middle ear granulation tissue, polyps, and monomeric membrane formation are also associated with various types of chronic otitis media, as shown in Figure 3-6.

Paparella and Brady (1970) reviewed more than 200 patients with chronic suppurative otitis media and mastoiditis. They found a definite increase in the incidence of sensorineural hearing loss that they suggested was due to a cochlear biochemical change created by toxic materials passed into the inner ear through the round window, resulting in gradual destruction of the organ of Corti. English, Northern, and Fria (1973) evaluated 404 patients with various forms of otitis media and reached similar conclusions. The authors found that bone conduction

thresholds worsened with the severity and duration of chronic otitis media. These studies confirm that sensorineural hearing loss can be a sequelae of chronic otitis media.

MIDDLE EAR EFFUSION (MEE) IN NEONATES

The diagnosis of MEE in neonates and infants presents special problems. A number of investigators in the early 1970s showed that MEE occurs commonly in neonates, both in the outpatient population and in the intensive care nursery. However, otoscopy is not routinely performed on neonates because the infant tympanic membrane is difficult to visualize (Fig. 3-10). In an infant, the external ear canal is flexible and often collapsed, and the tympanic membrane lies in a nearly horizontal plane. Balkany, Berman, Simmons, & Jafek (1978) reported results from examining 125 consecutive infants from the neonatal intensive care unit (ICU) and found MEE to be present in 30%. They believed that this finding was especially important because unrecognized middle ear fluid may act as a focus for the dissemination of bacteria into the circulation and/or central nervous system. They also found that nasotracheal intubation of longer than 7 days is

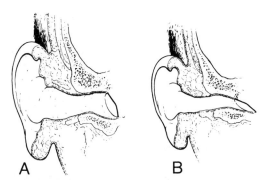

A   **B**

Figure 3-10. Orientation of the tympanic membrane in the adult **(A)** and in the infant **(B)**. Note the horizontal plane of the infant eardrum, which makes visualization of the tympanic membrane difficult. (Reprinted with permission from Balkany, T.J., Berman, S.A., Simmons, M.A., & Jafek, B.J. (1978). MEE in neonates. *The Laryngoscope, 88,* 399.)

highly associated with suppurative MEE. Technological advances in the objective identification of MEE by acoustic immittance measures and otoacoustic emissions tests will help greatly in identifying MEE in neonates (see Chapter 7). The age at which tympanometry becomes reliable for detecting MEE in infants is not fully agreed on, but many clinicians believe that it is probably not until the infant is 4–6 months of age.

The relationship of early otitis media to subsequent language and learning difficulties is of special importance to audiologists. Wallace et al. (1988) conducted a prospective study of neonates from birth until 1 year of age. Their results demonstrated language deficits in children who had otitis media in the first year of life. These researchers concluded that infants who suffer repeated episodes of bilateral otitis media during the first year of life are more likely to have reduced auditory sensitivity and to be at risk for expressive language difficulties.

SPEECH AND LANGUAGE DEVELOPMENT

The role of otitis media relative to the development of cognitive and linguistic function has divided professionals into two opposing camps. Menyuk (1986) described these two opposing positions concerning the relationship of persistent otitis media and speech and language disorders. One viewpoint is that otitis media has no effect on speech and language development in children, because the hearing loss is only slight and short-term and the child's hearing returns to normal between the recurring episodes of MEE. The other viewpoint is that persistent otitis media does have a detrimental effect on speech and language development, because of the fluctuating hearing loss during the early years of life and that this inconsistent auditory-receptive status creates problems for some children with mild to moderate hearing loss. A plethora of research studies have been conducted over the past decade to sub-

stantiate one or the other viewpoint. Unfortunately, the research designs in a large number of these projects have been less than adequate to reach significant conclusions (Paradise 1981, Ventry, 1983; Roberts & Wallace, 1997; Roberts et al, 1998). Thus, there remains a confusing array of statistics that leaves questions concerning the impact of otitis media on linguistic development as an unresolved issue.

A complete review of the literature pertaining to the developmental sequelae thought to be associated with otitis media is beyond the scope of this book. In recent years, a number of excellent publications have summarized the overwhelming accumulation of such studies, and interested readers are referred to Kavanagh (1986), Hasenstab (1987), Haggard and Hughes (1988), and Chalmers, Stewart, Silva, and Mulvena (1989). Brief descriptions of seminal research publications on otitis media and developmental sequelae are presented below to provide the reader with a sense of the history of this research body and an overview of various efforts to study this perplexing problem. Despite the acknowledged shortcomings of these research studies, the overall picture is that linguistic, cognitive, and behavioral effects can be documented as real sequelae of otitis media. The important factors seem to be the onset of the recurrent problem in the first few months of life and the duration of time the child has MEE (and thus conductive hearing loss) during the initial 2 years. Roberts et al. (1998) suggests that the child with otitis media often experiences a mild to moderate fluctuating hearing loss and thus receives partial or inconsistent auditory input, making speech more difficult to detect. This may impair the discrimination and central processing of speech and thus cause the child to encode information inefficiently, incompletely, or inaccurately into the database from which language develops.

One of the earliest reports on the developmental effect of ear disease was made by a psychologist working with language learning problems (Eisen, 1962). He described a child with auditory learning difficulties who had had a history of otitis media in early childhood, starting in infancy. Although this child now had normal hearing, Eisen blamed the early otitis media for causing irreversible auditory language learning problems. He believed that a new syndrome had been identified and called it the "quondam hard-of-hearing" ("at one-time hard-of-hearing") syndrome.

In a classic study reported by Holm and Kunze (1969), an experimental group of children 5.5–9 years of age was identified who had had no other medical problems except middle ear disease that had had its onset before the age of 2. Hearing levels had fluctuated from normal to greater than 25 dB. A well-matched control group of children with no history of ear disease was used for comparison. Each group was given a battery of tests, including the Illinois Test of Psycholinguistic Abilities (ITPA), the Peabody Picture Vocabulary Test, the Templin-Darley Tests of Articulation, and the Mecham Verbal Language Development Scale. The otitis media group showed significantly lower scores in all tests requiring the receiving or processing of auditory stimuli or the production of a verbal response. No differences between the groups were found in tests requiring visual skills, but all language skills were lower in the experimental group.

Howie, a pediatrician with a long-time interest in problems presented by young children with otitis media, studied the whole of his private practice caseload and noted that one group of children could be identified as "otitis-prone" (Howie et al., 1975). These children had had six or more recurrent bouts of otitis media before the age of 6 years. With additional analysis of the children who fell into this otitis-prone category, Howie et al. noted that the majority had had their first episode of otitis media during the first 18 months of life.

This finding has been replicated in numerous other subsequent studies that verify that if a child has an initial bout of otitis media very early in life, the chances of recurrent episodes of MEE are high. On the other hand, the research shows that if a child's first bout of otitis media occurs after 18 months of age, the child is likely to have only a singular, or a few isolated, occasions of MEE during childhood.

Howie (1975) also identified two matched groups of paired children from his private practice: one group having had no otitis media during the first 12 months of life, and the other group having had at least three documented episodes of otitis media during this period. He applied the Wechsler Adult Intelligence Scale (WISC) IQ test to the two groups of matched children at the age of 7 years to determine that the mean IQ scores of the otitis media group were significantly lower than the mean IQ scores obtained by the non-otitis group. A similar finding was reported by Paradise (1976b), who compared the IQs of a group of 32 children with cleft palate, two-thirds of whom underwent aggressive otologic management of their otitis media with repeated myringotomy and ventilation tube placement, and one-third of whom received "poor" otologic management of their otitis media. The mean IQ of the children in the aggressive care group was 110 compared with 98 in the poor-care group.

Needleman (1977) identified 20 children aged 3–8 years who had recurrent serous otitis media that initially occurred between birth and 18 months of age and continued for at least 2 years. She compared this group with a matched group of otitis-free children, studying the comprehension and production of aspects of the phonologic system as measured by various tests. She found the otitis media group to score significantly lower than the non-otitis group in production of phonemes and words, in production of phonemes in connected speech, in the use of combinations of phonemes and word endings, and in varying morphologic contexts. She pointed out that the phonologic skills that were deficient were necessary for reading skills and that this fact may account for the educational retardation of the children who have had early otitis media.

An important research effort was conducted by Teele, Klein, Rosner, and the Greater Boston Otitis Media Study Group (1984) on approximately 2500 Boston children, all of whom were evaluated in a prospective manner. The children were examined before 3 months of age and routinely until age 3 years for the presence of middle ear disease. The children had generally normal developmental histories and were stratified for study purposes by the estimated daily presence of MEE, gender, type of health care, and socioeconomic status. The project, known as the Boston Cohort Study, found a significant correlation between estimated time spent with MEE (unilateral or bilateral) and low test scores on vocabulary, comprehension, and verbal ability. The Boston Cohort Study data showed that it is the history of otitis media in the first 6 months of life that accounts for the significant differences in cognitive abilities.

An extremely well designed, prospective study known as the Dallas Cooperative Project followed a cohort of more than 450 middle-class, normally developing children with concurrent and repeated measures of hearing, MEE, and language development (Friel-Patti & Finitzo, 1990). Measurements on the cohort children were collected in a variety of settings, including a pediatrician's office, a community hearing-speech-language center, and home/day care settings. Among other findings, the Dallas Cooperative Project reported significant correlations for hearing and days with effusion over the same period. These measures were then related to emerging language patterns at 12, 18, and 24 months of age and were found to show significant negative correlations beginning with receptive language at 12 months; by 18 and 24 months, both ex-pressive and receptive scores were significantly related to hearing thresholds. Receptive language scores were significantly higher for children who had hearing better than 20 dB HL as early as 12 months of age. By 2 years of age, both receptive and expressive language performance were higher for children who had better hearing between 6 and 18 months of age. Thus, these findings confirm that there is a definite causal relationship between otitis media and language performance based on hearing levels—not the number of bouts of otitis media with effusion.

Question has always existed relative to the fact that perceptual deficits associated with otitis media are subtle and may not persist through school age. Mody, Schwartz, Gravel, and Ruben (1999) examined some of the long-term consequences of otitis media on phonologic processing skills in 9-year-olds with and without early histories of otitis media. In their study, children with strong first-year histories of otitis media tended to have long-lasting but subtle deficits in speech perception that may be linked to their early, transient, mild conductive hearing losses. The authors hypothesized that weak phonologic coding abilities may result in poor lexical organization, which might later be manifested in difficulties with word retrieval and semantic processing. These findings support earlier studies by Gravel and Wallace (1995) and Roberts and Wallace (1997), which showed that the effects of early hearing deficits, even if they are transient, might have far-reaching perceptual and academic consequences.

The majority of studies of otitis media with effusion in children younger than 4 years of age have shown a mild association between its presence and speech and language development (Teele, 1994). Even after the age of 4 years, there is continued association between otitis media with effusion, expressive language development, behavior, and cognitive function (Haggard, Birkin, Browning, et al., 1994).

Although one can be critical of small-sample retrospective studies, recent, well-planned, large-sample prospective studies such as the Boston Cohort Study and the Dallas Cooperative Project confirm the suspected association between frequency occurrence of otitis media during early childhood and impaired speech and delayed language development. To this point, we cite a well-controlled study of 394 Finnish children younger than 4 years of age with concurrent otitis media episodes. Five years later, these Finnish children were reexamined and found to perform poorer than control subjects in reading and tests of comprehension (Luotonen, Uhari, Aitola, et al., 1996). Critics claim it is premature to reach conclusions about the impact of otitis media on children's development, but to wait for a definitive answer while the suspicion remains is an untenable position for those who advocate for optimal child development.

In conclusions reached following a long-term prospective study, Roberts et al. (1998) evaluated language and cognitive development in control and study groups of young children at 1 and 2 years of age. Although the proportion of time spent with otitis media or with hearing loss was modestly correlated with lower scores of language and cognitive skills, of special interest was the finding that the children with more otitis media tended to live in less-responsive caregiving environments. The question remains whether these results suggest that children in less-responsive caregiving environments experience conditions that make them more likely to experience otitis media—or is it more difficult for caregivers to be responsive and stimulating to children with more otitis media?

Downs (1985) proposed a high-risk model for susceptibility to recurrent otitis media with effusion. She reviewed more than 140 research studies to develop a risk profile to identify those children who may develop language delays after suffering recurrent otitis media in infancy. Downs acknowledged that it may be impossible to resolve the controversy over the extent of language delay caused by recurrent otitis media because of the influence of family predisposition to language disorder and the inability of any test to determine the maximal potential function of any child at a point in time that is not corrupted by other influences. Nonetheless, factors to be given emphasis in a high-risk model should include the following: (1) hearing loss greater than 20 dB HL due to otitis media, (2) infants with three or more episodes of otitis media during the first year of life, (3) middle socioeconomic living status, (4) quality of home environment, (5) maternal caregiving, and (6) quality and environment of day care when applicable.

In summary, there is a growing consensus among researchers and clinicians that the relationship between otitis media and language is mediated by hearing and hearing loss. Many children with otitis media have mild to moderate hearing losses for prolonged periods that may affect speech perception. The transient hearing loss associated with otitis media may result in an incomplete or an inconsistent auditory signal leading to weak encoding of auditory-based phonemic distinctions (Gravel & Nozza, 1997). A fluctuating speech signal to an infant with otitis media may impede accurate perceptions of sounds, making it difficult to discriminate between the phonetic characteristics of sounds. It appears that the emerging relationships between communicative disorders and otitis media with MEE during the early stages of language development create new opportunities and new challenges for audiologists and educators.

Screening tests for speech and language delay have been developed that are well validated and cost-effective for use in primary care physicians' offices (Coplan, Gleason, Ryan, Burke, & Williams, 1982; Capute, Palmer, Shapiro, et al., 1986;

Walker, Downs, Gugenheim, & Northern, 1989). In as much as speech and language delays are recognized sequelae of otitis media, it is appropriate to recommend that these tests be incorporated into well-child care and in particular for those children who have experienced recurrent or persistent otitis media with effusion. Language screening tests should be performed on all children starting at 6 months and every 6 months thereafter until 3 years of age. Ruben (1991) suggests that such screening would detect children who have or have had hearing losses that could result in language delays. There should also be a hearing screening of every child at well-baby visits and especially for every child younger than 3 years of age who has had 3 months of otitis media and/or 3 bouts of otitis media in 6 months.

MANAGEMENT OF THE CHILD WITH OTITIS MEDIA

When a child presents with otitis media and there is an indication that it may be a recurrent problem, a speech and language screening or evaluation must be recommended. Whether or not the child turns out to be otitis-prone, the evaluation will serve as a baseline for future reference. It is particularly urgent to be zealous about applying these evaluations in the first 2 years of life, because during this period of language learning 3 months of poor hearing is an eternity in the development of language skills. A recommended sequence of management and intervention with these children is discussed below.

Medical Intervention. Medical treatment is the first line of defense in otitis media. The choice of treatment depends on the specialty training of the responsible physician, and the treatment regimen may vary considerably among physicians. The American Academy of Pediatrics published a policy statement in 1984 concerning the medical management of otitis media with a special caution regarding the relationship between middle ear disease and language development (italics added by the authors):

There is growing evidence demonstrating a correlation between middle ear disease with hearing impairment and delays in the development of speech, language and cognitive skills. A parent or other caretaker may be the first person to detect such early symptoms as irritability, decreased responsiveness and disturbed sleep. Middle ear disease may be so subtle that a full evaluation for this condition should combine pneumatic otoscopy, and possibly tympanometry, with a direct view of the tympanic membrane. This statement is not meant to be a recommendation for specific treatment methods. *When a child has frequently recurring acute otitis media and/or middle ear effusion persisting for longer than 3 months, hearing should be assessed and the development of communicative skills must be monitored.*

The Committee feels it is important that the physician inform the parent that a child with middle ear disease may not hear normally. Although the child may withdraw socially and diminish experimentation with verbal communication, the parent should be encouraged to continue communicating by touching and seeking eye contact with the child when loudly and clearly speaking. Such measures, along with prompt restoration of hearing whenever possible, may help to diminish the likelihood that a child with middle ear disease will develop a communicative disorder. Middle ear disease can occur in the presence of sensory neural hearing loss. *Any child whose parent expresses concern about whether the child hears should be considered for referral for behavioral audiometry without delay.*

Ruben (1986) points out that treatment for otitis media is directed at the return to "normal," and he outlines two forms of medical intervention. The initial choice of treatment is the administration of antibiotics for chronic and/or recurrent otitis media. This medical treatment appears to be efficacious for approximately half of patients, with the other half continuing to harbor MEE with accompanying hearing loss.

Those patients who do not respond by returning to normal are candidates for the second treatment approach, which consists of surgical placement of a tympanostomy tube (also known as ventilation tubes) through the tympanic membrane to permit aeration of the middle ear space and, it is hoped, to improve hearing. Ruben points out that the insertion of a tympanostomy tube does not ensure that the threshold of hearing will return to normal. Further, the drawback to this treatment is that as a surgical procedure, certain risks and complications may be expected in a small percentage of cases.

Language and Speech Screening. Delayed early language milestones are often the keystone for identifying possible developmental delay in children and may indicate slow cognitive development or the presence of hearing loss. Further, many studies have noted that children who are experiencing otitis media with effusion may score poorer on tests of articulation than those children who are otitis-free. From a retrospective point of view, speech-language pathologists often comment that children with a significant history of otitis media have phonologic or articulation deficiencies. Children who have significant communication deficiencies should be referred for diagnostic language evaluation and possible remediation through speech therapy.

Our suggested guideline is that if MEE exists for 3 months despite vigorous medical or surgical treatment or if the hearing impairment persists after 3 months, a language screening test should be applied. Coplan et al. (1982) developed a useful screening test for language development known as the Early Language Milestone (ELM) Scale with which we have had good success in young children between 12 and 26 months of age (Walker et al., 1989). Coplan's ELM Scale has been well normed for the presence of 41

language milestones during the first 36 months of life in normal children. It is a brief language assessment tool with both receptive and expressive items that are specifically age-related, and it reportedly yields 97% sensitivity and 93% specificity as a detector of developmentally delayed children.

Because language delay can be a significant factor in the identification of young children with mild to moderate hearing impairment or history of otitis media with effusion, it behooves the audiologist to develop competency in the observation of normal speech-language milestones as well as skill in administering language screening tests. Naturally, when a child is noted to be functioning at a level significantly less than normal for his or her age, referral should be made for a comprehensive language evaluation and a thorough hearing evaluation.

Educational Intervention. If a child fails the language screening test at his or her age level, an initial program that encourages home language stimulation may be recommended. During the past decade, the areas of early development, education, and especially infant intervention have become ever-expanding fields for study and research. Since the 1960s there has been an increase in awareness of the value of early intervention for young children in general, particularly for infants and toddlers who have handicaps or who are at risk for developing handicaps. Research suggests that early intervention with infants, in whom problems are identified and treated as early as possible, can make significant differences in their later physical, cognitive, and social abilities and can minimize the effects of present or potential handicaps (Weiner & Koppelman, 1987).

Traditionally, the approach to delivering services to very young children has focused on identifying strengths and weaknesses, then remediating deficits and "teaching" the child the needed skills. In recent years, however, the focus in many early intervention programs offers a more positive approach for children, their families, and the professionals who work with them. This approach, often referred to as prevention-intervention, recognizes that not all problems or deficits can be "fixed" through many of the medical or educational therapies available and that parents and professionals cannot change the long-term problems that occur at birth, such as brain damage or severe hearing loss. Parents and professionals can, however, minimize or prevent impairments from causing secondary handicaps, such as emotional problems or problems with thinking or communicating. They can work through a child's strengths to help the child develop alternative or compensatory learning strategies (Campbell & Wilcox, 1986).

Whereas many programs focus on parents being given advice and educational and therapeutic tasks to do at home, others are beginning to develop systems that recognize parents and professionals as equal partners. In such programs, professionals serve as consultants to families, helping them determine the goals and activities they want for their child. The changes in the approaches taken and attitudes adopted by professionals working with parents reflect a focus on family needs, with an emphasis on enhancing the child's growth, development, and sense of well-being, rather than a singular focus on correcting a problem. Parents need to be regarded as full partners in this effort and valued as prime contributors in decisions made about their child's program and progress.

We believe that the child at risk for any developmental delay, whether from auditory deprivation or neurologic condition, requires a stepped-up language enrichment program such as those offered in child developmental centers under the direction of a qualified speech-language pathologist. However, the initial step may be the instigation of a simple program designed to improve parent-infant interaction and communication. Matkin (1984) developed the following as a useful list of suggestions for parents of children with middle ear problems:

- **The Importance of Talking.** Talking to a child is necessary for his or her language development. Because children usually imitate what they hear, how much parents talk to their child, what they say, and how they say it will affect how much and how well the child talks.

- **Look.** Parents should look directly at the child's face and wait until they have his or her attention before they begin talking.

- **Control Distance.** Parents should be sure to be close to the child when they talk (no farther than 5 feet). The younger the child, the more important it is to be close.

- **Loudness.** Parents should talk slightly louder than normal. The radio, TV, dishwasher, etc. should be turned off to remove background noise.

- **Parents Should Be Good Speech Models.** Describe daily activities as they occur. Expand on what the child says. For example, if the child points and says "Car," the parent should say, "Oh, I see, you want the car."

  Add new information. A parent might add, "That car is little."

  Build vocabulary. Make teaching new words and concepts a natural part of everyday activities. Use new words while shopping, taking a walk, washing dishes, etc.

  Repeat the childs's words using adult pronunciation.

- **Play and Talk.** Every day, some time should be set aside for "play time" for just the parent and child. Play can be looking at books, exploring toys, singing songs, coloring, etc. The parent should talk to the child during these activities, keeping the conversation at his or her level.

- **Read.** Parents should begin reading to their child at a young age (before 12 months). Librarians can provide books that are appropriate for a child's age. Reading can be a calming activity that promotes closeness between parent and child. It provides another opportunity to teach and review words and ideas. Some children enjoy looking at pictures in magazines and catalogs.

- **Don't Wait.** A child should have the following skills by the ages listed below:

  18 months: 3-word vocabulary.
  2 years: 25- to 30-word vocabulary and several 2-word sentences.
  2.5 years: at least a 50-word vocabulary and 2-word sentences consistently.

- **If a Child Does Not Have These Skills, Tell the Doctor.** A referral to an audiologist and speech-language pathologist may be indicated. Hearing, speech, and language testing may lead to a better understanding of a child's language development.

Hearing Aid Placement. A mild ear-level hearing aid, with appropriate limitations on maximum saturation and gain, may be considered in extreme cases of persistent conductive hearing loss. The obvious drawbacks are that it is difficult to convince parents of the necessity for such an extreme antidote, and there are problems in keeping such an instrument on an infant or toddler. Hearing aid placement is a feasible procedure only if (1) the parents are highly motivated; (2) continual guidance by an audiologist or speech therapist is obtained; (3) a total support system by physician, parent, and therapist is in effect; and (4) a period of diagnostic therapy with a loaner hearing aid is initiated to judge the effectiveness of the aid.

Multidisciplinary Otitis Media Team. By the time a child with recurrent otitis media reaches age 2, his or her parents may be purchasing services from a variety of professionals: pediatrician, otologist, audiologist, and speech/language pathologist. Although decisions made by these various individuals may be in the best interest of the child, the outcomes may not be consistent with each other, therefore disrupting the continuity of the child's care and creating a financial burden for the family. The otitis media clinic is similar to other multidisciplinary clinics in that at one appointment various professionals evaluate a child's medical and developmental status relative to otitis media, share results at a staff meeting, and make recommendations for further care. The clinic, therefore, performs as a body of professionals who provide a consensus of recommendations for the child's primary caregivers.

The disciplines involved include otology, pediatrics, speech/language pathology, and audiology. The role of the otologist is to assess middle ear status and the health of the child as it may relate to middle ear problems. This is accomplished through use of pneumatic otoscopy and microscopic examination. Evaluation of tonsils, adenoids, allergies, constant congestion, and eustachian tube dysfunction are some additional areas of assessment. The pediatrician is responsible for overall evaluation of the child's health, including developmental concerns. In addition, the pediatrician conducts a review of the patient's medical chart before each clinic visit and identifies pertinent information relative to otitis media. Routine speech/language screenings are administered by the speech/language pathologist, who also provides information on language stimulation techniques to be used by the parents at home. The audiologist performs tympanometry and audiometry.

Consideration for entry into an otitis media clinic is determined by any one or a combination of the following factors: (1) 3 episodes of otitis media within 3–6 months, (2) 3 months of effusion, and (3) 1 or more episodes of otitis media before 6 months of age. During the otitis media clinic visit, children and their parents rotate between four stations: otology, pediatrics, speech/language pathology, and audiology. A staff meeting follows the clinic visit, at which each of the professionals describes their findings, and suggestions for management are agreed on and discussed with the parents.

RECOMMENDED AUDIOLOGIC GUIDELINES

It must be recognized that there are children who do not function to their full communicative and developmental potential because of hearing loss associated with early, recurrent episodes of otitis media with effusion. Accordingly, the American Academy of Audiology issued a position statement in 1992 recommending audiologic guidelines as an effort to decrease substantially the number of children who will be burdened with persistent communicative and learning deficits related to undetected and/or untreated otitis media:

1. The *identification process* should include screening of hearing, middle ear function, and communication development, particularly in "at risk" populations. Such groups would include infants who develop otitis media at or before the age of 6 months, infants and young children cared for in multi-child day care settings, and infants and children with known risk factors such as those with cleft lip or palate, native Americans, or those with Down syndrome.

   Children who have had MEE that persists for 3 months despite medical treatment should undergo monitoring hearing screenings, routine tympanometry, and language and speech screening. Those children who fail any of these screening procedures should be referred for complete assessment with in-depth testing. Those children

for whom communication skills are found to be delayed or abnormal may need more assertive medical attention from a certified/licensed speech-language pathologist.

2. The *assessment process* should include complete audiologic evaluation to characterize the audiometric profile including the configuration and degree of hearing loss for each ear independently using air- and bone-conduction testing. In addition, it would be appropriate to include speech audiometry tests of speech thresholds and word recognition abilities (including higher-order auditory processing capabilities when indicated), acoustic immittance assessment, and a formal language screening of the child's receptive and expressive language abilities. Children failing this screen should be referred to a certified/licensed speech-language pathologist for a formal comprehensive evaluation and for the determination of the need for therapeutic intervention.

3. Audiometric monitoring of hearing sensitivity should be a routine component of the *management process*. Children having documented histories of otitis media and accompanying hearing loss should receive periodic hearing evaluations by a certified/licensed audiologist even when they appear to be symptom free. In particular, hearing assessment should be completed at the onset of the school year in preschool and elementary students and at least once during the winter months. The management of infants and young children with otitis media must further include parent/caregiver and teacher awareness of the implications of hearing loss on the communication process.

Additional management considerations include (1) providing information optimizing auditory-based communication strategies during bouts of otitis media when hearing sensitivity might be compromised, (2) monitoring auditory behaviors that might signal subsequent episodes of otitis media, and (3) providing suggestions for optimizing the classroom environment for all children who might experience "minimal fluctuant hearing loss" through the reduction of classroom noise and/or the provision of sound field amplification systems. A comprehensive discussion of the audiologic management of children with otitis media has been published by Gravel and Wallace (1998).

Additional guidelines for management of hearing loss in school-aged children have been developed by ASHA (1993) and the American Academy of Audiology (1997). These guideline documents are very useful in developing comprehensive programs so that children with undetected hearing loss and/or persistent middle ear disease will be identified and appropriate treatment and management interventions can be provided.

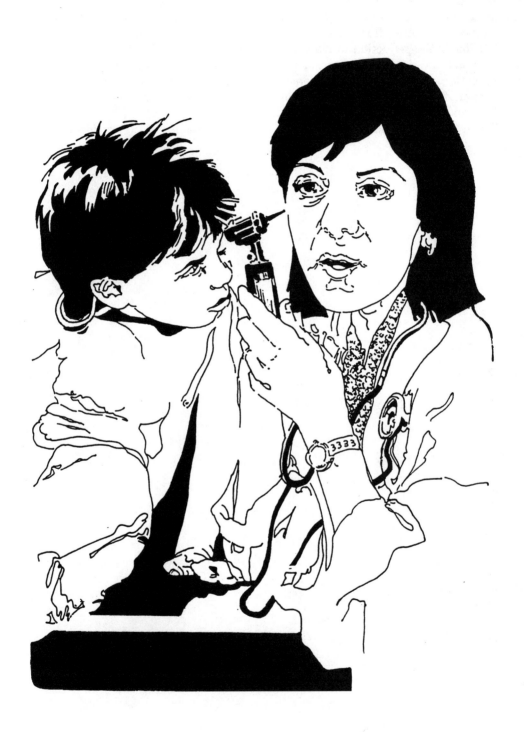

CHAPTER 4

Medical Aspects of Hearing Loss

It is the audiologist's responsibility to insist that regular medical examinations be performed for the hearing-impaired child. Until the child is at least 10 years of age, an otolaryngologic examination should be insisted on at least annually or more frequently as warranted. An erroneous assumption is that after a child has sustained a hearing loss, nothing more can happen to his or her ears. Not only is this belief incorrect, but there may be progressive sensorineural hearing impairment accompanied by increased susceptibility to other ear diseases, to noise-induced loss, or to ototoxicity. Therefore, it is imperative that the auditory thresholds of the hearing-impaired child be monitored frequently. The importance of every decibel of residual hearing that the child possesses may be in exponential ratio to each decibel of hearing loss. Routine audiologic monitoring of the degree of loss pays dividends in information on changes in hearing that are pertinent for the habilitation program. A more extensive otologic and physical examination may be suggested when deterioration of the auditory threshold or the speech discrimination is found.

Detailed medical descriptions of disorders associated with hearing loss in children are presented in textbooks such as "Pediatric Otolaryngology" by Bluestone and Stool (1990) and "Pediatric Otology and Neurotology" by Lalwani and Grundfast (1998). Audiology textbooks may offer material on hearing pathology, but it is usually offered in a nonmedical manner, so that insufficient information is available to audiologists who work in medical settings. The material presented below is not as complete as that found in otolaryngology textbooks, but it is our hope it is more pertinent to childhood disorders than that commonly found in basic audiology textbooks. A thorough presentation on medical problems associated with hearing loss in infants has been published by Hayes and Northern (1996). For the child with hearing loss, the audiologist must advocate prompt medical referral to evaluate all new complaints including reports of changes in hearing, onset of tinnitus, dizziness, or changes in the quality of sound.

DISORDERS ASSOCIATED WITH HEARING LOSS

Conditions of the External Ear and Ear Canal. The audiologist will likely confront various medical conditions involving the pinna and external auditory canal. The making of earmolds and swimmolds, as well as the insertion of acoustic immittance and otoadmittance probe tips during diagnostic and hearing screening testing, make it imperative for the clinician to recognize disorders of the external ear.

To recognize the presence of a diseased state, one must appreciate the normal anatomy of the external ear. The pinna or auricle is an appendage attached to the side of the head, level with the middle third of the face. It is composed of a piece of elastic cartilage with numerous convolutions, covered with thin skin, and fixed in position at the lateral aspect of the external auditory canal by its direct continuity with the cartilaginous canal, auricular muscles, and auricular ligaments. Its major convolutions include the helix, anthelix, tragus, antitragus, and concha. The lobule is unique in that it contains no cartilage and, therefore, has been designated by various cultures as the appropriate place through which and on which to hang ornaments for decoration.

An opening, the external auditory meatus, is cartilaginous in the lateral third and bony in the medial two thirds. The cartilage of the external auditory canal is generally continuous with that of the pinna. Present in the cartilaginous canal wall are several fissures to permit flexibility. Hence, the curved path of the ear canal can be partially straightened to facilitate inspection by gently pulling back and up on the pinna. Squamous epithelium lines the external canal and covers the tympanic membrane. This skin is thicker laterally with hair follicles, sebaceous glands, and earwax-producing glands, but it is quite thin over the more medial bony portion of the canal with fewer skin structures present. This skin is unusual because it does not flake, as does other squamous epithelium, but migrates laterally toward the external meatus, providing a self-cleaning mechanism unique to the ear canal.

At the onset of every clinical evaluation or testing procedure, the audiologist should take note of the location, size, and shape of the pinnae and their relationship to the remainder of the structures of the head and face. Normally, the superior border of the helix is located at the outer canthus of the eye, and the tragus is roughly level with the infraorbital rim (Fig. 4-1). Low-set pinnae are frequently associated with other anomalies of the first and second branchial cleft. Although the pinna may have no abnormality in its location or basic shape, the alert clinician should be aware of any lump, ulcer, or lesion on the pinna.

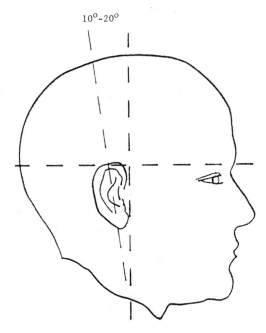

Figure 4-1. Position of the pinna in relationship to the face.

The child with ears that stick out from his or her head in a prominent fashion faces possible social problems from the ridicule of classmates. Successful surgical treatment of a patient with this deformity before the patient's entering school may save a great deal of emotional anguish. Correction of these deformities is easily accomplished through an operation known as otoplasty, which consists of an incision of the back of the pinna, cinched with stitches, to hold the ear in its new position closer to the head.

Aural Discharge. The presence of fluid running from the external auditory meatus should give the clinician concern. Fluid from the external auditory canal may be divided in three categories: (1) clear; (2) cloudy, whitish, or yellow; and (3) bloody. Presence of these fluids in the ear canal requires immediate medical referral.

Clear Fluid. Clear fluid may represent cerebral spinal fluid leaking from a temporal bone fracture, which offers a ready route for access for infection into the cranial cavity. This condition requires prompt otologic consultation by physical examination, radiographic studies, and perhaps surgical exploration of the ear to confirm and repair the leakage.

Cloudy Fluid. Cloudy fluid usually represents inflammation of the external auditory canal, a condition known as external otitis (see below). Less often, cloudy discharge may result from an inflamed middle ear space with existing perforation of the tympanic membrane.

Blood. Blood coming from the external auditory canal frequently results from self-instrumentation of the ear canal to relieve itching or remove earwax. Blood coming from the ear canal requires immediate medical consultation.

Cerumen and Foreign Bodies. Cerumen, or earwax, is a combined product of the apocrine and sebaceous glands located in the skin of the ear canal. Cerumen comes in two varieties: wet and dry. Wet earwax varies from yellowish to dark brown and, at times, even resembles blood. Dry earwax tends to be whitish scales or powdery feathery-like material. Most people's ear canals are self-cleaning of cerumen because of the migratory pattern of the epithelium toward the external auditory meatus. The cerumen may easily be wiped away with a washcloth. People with excessive production of cerumen or inadequate self-cleaning mechanism may accumulate wax in the external auditory canal, which can cause hearing loss. These individuals should have the wax removed by a physician who will frequently utilize magnification for improved visibility. The use of a Waterpik or the use of the infamous Q-tip applicator is to be condemned. Cotton tip applicators, in the hands of an aggressive parent, are a major source of lacerated ear canals, perforated eardrums, and occasional sensorineural hearing loss.

Children are the leading candidates to appear with a foreign object in their ear canal. Objects may include broken crayons, food, small toys, or pieces of jewelry. Hearing loss is usually not a major concern in such cases unless the foreign object has ruptured the tympanic membrane. Referral to a medical specialist for removal of the object is, of course, mandatory.

Bony Growths. Occasionally, bony outgrowths in the external auditory canal may create problems. These come in two forms: (1) multiple growths termed exostoses, and (2) single growths termed osteomas. These appear as smooth, hard, round nodules in the external ear canal covered with normal skin. Exostoses do not require removal unless they cause cerumen accumulation, impair hearing, or create canal obstruction. Osteomas usually continue to grow and, hence, require surgical removal.

Inflammatory Conditions. Occasionally, just touching the pinna will cause the patient to wince or react with noticeable discomfort. Conditions most frequently responsible for this phenomenon are (1) external otitis, (2) perichondritis, and/or (3) furunculosis of the external auditory canal. Each of these conditions is usually quite painful, and the patient needs prompt medical attention.

Otitis Externa. Otitis externa is an inflammation of the skin of the external auditory canal, most frequently due to bacterial infection or fungal infection. The presence of water in the ear canal against the tympanic membrane provides ideal circumstances for bacterial growth. The skin of the canal on acute external otitis is usually red and quite tender, with some form of drainage present. External otitis is not uncommon in persons who wear hearing aids. The presence of an occlusive earmold traps moisture in the ear canal and may contribute to external otitis. The otolaryngologist may suggest that the patient either switch the hearing aid to the opposite ear or, in certain instances, go without the hearing aid until the condition clears. The use of open-type earmolds helps prevent this condition.

Perichondritis. Perichondritis is an inflammation of the covering of the cartilage of the ear or ear canal. It is usually secondary to trauma to the cartilage, either accidental or surgical. The pinna is usually red and tender with generalized swelling. Repeated episodes may lead to cartilage deformities of the pinna known as "cauliflower ears."

Furuncle. A furuncle of the external canal is a boil or pimple. It is exquisitely tender because the skin of the ear canal is tightly applied to the cartilage.

Perforations of the Tympanic Membrane. Perforations may occur from some sort of trauma (such as a blow to the side of the head, a water-skiing fall, diving, or sudden changes in air pressure) or from middle ear infections leading to acute otitis media (Fig. 4-2). The tympanic membrane is about 8 mm in diameter, and perforations from acute otitis media are usually much smaller, 1–2 mm in diameter. Because the outer layer of the tympanic membrane is squamous epithelium, small traumatic perforations will often heal spontaneously within a matter of days.

Conductive hearing loss occurs as a consequence of poor vibration of the tympanic membrane. The degree of loss, however, is variable and dependent on the size of the perforation and its location on the tympanic membrane. Small perforations may be obvious with hearing levels within normal limits. Complications from perforations may be serious, and all such children should be immediately referred to a medical specialist. Parents should be advised to practice aural hygiene by keeping water out of the ear when the child is swimming or bathing until proper medical care of the ear has been given.

CLEFT PALATE

Deformities of the lip and palate are among the most common major congenital malformations, occurring once in 900 newborns. The incidence of hearing problems in children with cleft lip and/or palate is very high and requires special attention in the audiology clinic. A substantial number of articles have been published concerning the otologic and audiologic problems of children with overt cleft palate. The incidence of recurrent otitis media in such children is quite high and has been reported to be from 50–90% by various investigators.

Paradise and Bluestone (1974) reported the "universality" of otitis media findings in 50 infants with cleft palate. Hearing loss as a secondary problem to the middle ear disorder related to cleft palate is so common that it may exist in nearly all such patients. Sterile inflammatory effusions that vary in viscosity are commonly found in the ears of these infants. Paradise (1980) recommended that infants with cleft palate receive

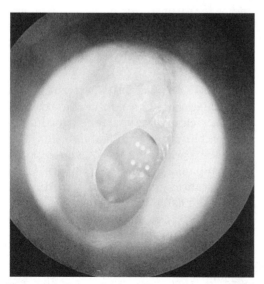

Figure 4-2. Otoscopic view of a tympanic membrane with a chronic perforation.

myringotomy and tympanostomy tube insertion at a relatively early age, within the first 6 months of life if possible, especially if hearing loss seems to be present or discomfort or infection is present. Repeat myringotomy and tubes may be necessary to keep the infant's ears clear and hearing normally. Complications such as cholesteatoma and adhesive otitis may accompany repeated middle ear effusion in children with a cleft palate. The incidence and severity of middle ear problems related to cleft palate decrease as the patient grows older.

Otologic and hearing problems may also be associated with submucous cleft palate. Although overt cleft palate is diagnosed at birth, submucous cleft palate may not be diagnosed until years later. The submucous cleft palate is an imperfect union of muscle across the soft palate that tends to "tent" when the patient phonates. The area may appear bluish because it is covered by only nasal and oral mucosa. The dehiscence of muscle and bone may be obvious with palpation and is often accompanied by a bifid uvula. Most clinicians agree that the deficiency of palate musculature is the probable cause of poor eustachian tube function. This results in inadequate middle ear ventilation, effusion of fluid, tympanic membrane retraction, and hearing loss.

Hearing loss related to cleft palate is most common between 3 and 8 years of age, which also corresponds to the increased exposure and susceptibility to upper respiratory infections found in this age group (Bluestone & Klein, 1988). Audiologists must be aware of this increased incidence of hearing difficulty and recurrent middle ear disease in children with cleft palate. The hearing of such patients must be monitored on a regular basis with close medical follow-up. Our experiences with these children have identified numerous youngsters with recurrent episodes of otitis media accompanied by hearing loss who undoubtedly miss auditory information at school and home.

Medical and surgical treatment is often necessary for these children who may qualify for repeated myringotomy and ventilation tubes. Mild- to moderate-power hearing instruments may be in order for children who do not respond well to medical treatment, especially during the school years.

It is important that the audiologist be included on the cleft palate team because routine hearing evaluations contribute substantially to the total management of these children. Acoustic immittance audiometry is an especially valuable clinical procedure in children with cleft palate. Immittance audiometry may identify conductive impairments in even very young infants (Bess, Lewsi, & Cieliczka, 1975; Bess, Schwartz, & Redfield, 1976).

DOWN SYNDROME

Down syndrome, also known as trisomy 21, is one of the most commonly seen clinical conditions, occurring in 1 in 800 live births. These special needs children have a high incidence of hearing loss that may further hinder their developmental delay. The child with Down syndrome often has a narrow external auditory canal, making otoscopic examination difficult. Their developmental delay and retardation make them difficult patients from which to obtain valid hearing test results without careful testing protocols. External ear abnormalities such as small and/or deformed pinnae are frequently noted in Down syndrome. These children have a high incidence of otitis media with complications causing conductive hearing loss. The degree of hearing loss is usually mild to moderate and may also have a sensorineural component. The child with Down syndrome may be more susceptible to upper respiratory infection than is the normal child because of abnormal nasopharynx and eustachian tube development that adversely affects proper drainage of the sinuses and middle ear spaces.

Downs (1980) published a comprehensive study of hearing impairment in children with Down syndrome. She noted that the child with Down syndrome is usually treated medically for persistent middle ear effusion; however, her clinical experience showed that conductive hearing loss often persisted after medical treatment. She conducted a comprehensive study of 107 noninstitutionalized children with Down syndrome and found 78% to have hearing loss in one or both ears. Fifty-four percent of children had conductive loss, 16% had sensorineural loss, and 8% had mixed-type hearing loss. Otologic examinations were conducted on each of the 107 children. According to Balkany, Berman, Simmons, et al. (1978), middle ear effusion or chronic otitis media could not explain approximately 40% of the children with conductive hearing loss. On microscopic pneumatic otoscopy, the patients had normal-appearing tympanic membranes suggesting the presence of middle ear anomalies as the etiology for the conductive hearing loss. Seventeen operative procedures on carefully selected patients with Down syndrome revealed congenital ossicular malformations and ossicular destruction caused by inflammation due to chronic infection. These findings lead us to recommend that children with Down syndrome and persistent conductive hearing loss be treated aggressively to normalize their hearing, break the cycle, and prevent recurrent and chronic ear disease.

Roizen, Walters, Nicol, and Blondis (1993) recommend that auditory brainstem response (ABR) audiometry be performed routinely during the initial 6 months of life, as their evaluation of 47 unselected young children with Down syndrome resulted in finding 66% with significant hearing loss. The high incidence of conductive hearing loss in the Down syndrome population makes acoustic immittance audiometry and/or otoacoustic emissions an imperative part of each hearing evaluation (Northern, 1980a). Every hearing test on a child with Down syndrome should utilize insert earphones or sound field testing (without traditional earphones) to rule out erroneous "conductive losses" due to collapsed ear canals. Down syndrome children require vigorous hearing screening and monitoring of middle ear problems. Some children with Down syndrome who have persistent hearing loss may do well with mild hearing aid amplification. In addition, a total team approach including an ear, nose, and throat specialist, pediatrician, audiologist, and speech-language pathologist is recommended for the child with Down syndrome to provide optimal opportunities for advancement.

AUTISM

Autism is classified as one of the pervasive developmental disorders (PDD) because of three major characteristics of the disorder: (1) impairment in social interaction, (2) impairment in verbal and nonverbal behavior, and (3) insistence on sameness—described as repetitive movements, abnormal preoccupations, ritualistic behaviors, and resistance to change. Autism is a severely debilitating disorder that has an occurrence rate of 5 in 10,000 and affects boys 3 times more often than girls (Rutter, 1978). The disorder is diagnosed by observation of a cluster of behaviors associated in some manner with central nervous system pathology. Autism may be defined through the following criteria: early onset (before 30 months of age), disturbances of social relationships, disturbances of speech and language, and extremely deviant behavior characterized by preoccupation with particular objects and/or self-destructive activities. Autistic patients show a pervasive lack of responsiveness to other people and gross deficits in language development. When speech is present, it is characterized by peculiarities such as immediate and delayed echolalia, metaphorical language, and pronoun reversal

(Wing, 1993). Autistic individuals may exhibit bizarre responses to various aspects of the environment and failure to use or comprehend verbal and nonverbal messages, with illogical and inconsistent responses to sensory, especially auditory, stimuli. For example, autistic children may be easily distracted, enraged, or frightened by normal background noises. These children may present serious challenging behaviors during the audiologic evaluation. It is not unusual for the autistic child to refuse to cooperate or follow instructions. They are likely not to respond consistently to auditory stimuli, and they may demonstrate non-stop repetitive behavior such as banging their head against the sound room wall or throwing themselves on the floor. These problems make autistic children among the most difficult to assess for hearing function.

Several auditory evaluation studies on autistic individuals have been reported in the literature. In general terms, auditory evoked brainstem response is the test of choice, and considerable effort has been conducted to identify differences in ABR patterns between autistic and normal children (Gillberg, Rosenhall, & Johansson, 1983; Rosenblum et al., 1980; Tanguay & Edwards, 1982a; Tanguay, Edwards, Buchwald, Schwafel, & Allen, 1982b). Many believe the basis of autism to be a neurodevelopment disorder with abnormalities of the limbic system, thalamus, basal ganglia, and cerebellum. Although minor differences in ABR patterns have been reported between normal and autistic patients, the differences are not consistent across studies, and the reports are difficult to compare because control conditions and experimental variables are often not well described. Some authors have attempted to use central auditory tests to speculate about the specific loci of dysfunction in autistic children (Wetherby, Koegal, & Mendel, 1981). Although it is probable that the organic dysfunction is clearly implicated in autism, no precise etiologic mechanisms have been identified.

ACQUIRED HEARING LOSS IN CHILDREN

Ototoxic Hearing Loss. Unfortunately, almost every available drug effective for treatment of disease has the potential to compromise the human system through possible side effects. Hearing loss due to the administration of certain drugs is not an uncommon side effect. Drugs that damage the cochlea and/or vestibular portion of the inner ear are known as ototoxic. Ototoxic drugs may cause permanent sensorineural hearing loss that may be accompanied by vertigo, nausea, and gait instability. Considerable individual susceptibility to ototoxic drugs exists and is generally unpredictable. The resultant hearing loss is usually, but not always, sensorineural, bilateral symmetrical impairment of varying degree, audiometric configuration, and severity. The physician's management of illness with drugs and chemotherapy becomes a fine-line judgment, weighing the potential benefit to the patient against the potential risk of adverse side effects.

The drug family of antibiotic aminoglycosides, such as kanamycin, neomycin, and gentamicin, are the most commonly used ototoxic drugs. Other ototoxic aminoglycosides, including vancomycin, amikacin, and tobramycin, have also been documented to cause hearing loss. Streptomycin, long the front runner for the treatment of tuberculosis, is well known to be destructive to the cochlea and vestibular system. Because aminoglycosides are cleared more slowly from the fluids of the inner ear than from the bloodstream, the high concentration of the drug in the perilymph of the inner ear may result in ototoxic effects long after the drug has been discontinued (Fausti, Henry, & Frey, 1996). Physicians monitor drug dosages by determining serum drug peak and trough concentrations routinely to achieve and maintain serum levels within a therapeutic range.

Aminoglycosides are commonly used in the treatment of infection in newborns. The evaluation of aminoglycoside ototoxicity in infants presents a problem, because these babies are usually receiving medical therapy for severe life-threatening problems. Infants with low birthweight who contract systemic infection may also experience jaundice or other health disorders that are of themselves associated with deafness. Salamy, Eldredge, and Tooley (1989) examined very-low-birthweight infants and found a significant association between the long-term administration of the diuretic, furosemide, and aminoglycosides with sensorineural hearing loss. Infants receiving such drugs require extensive audiologic follow-up, otoacoustic emission tests, and ABR measurements to confirm or rule out mild to moderate hearing loss.

Other drugs are known to be ototoxic and may lead to hearing loss. Several cancer chemotherapeutic agents are also damaging to hearing. They include cisplatin, carboplatin, caroplatin, nitrogen mustard and alpha-difluoromelthylornithine (DFMO). Cisplatin is used commonly in cancer treatment for both children and adults, and irreversible ototoxicity is well documented.

Aspirin, quinine, and some diuretics produce temporary hearing loss, which may be fully or partially reversed when the medication is stopped.

Impaired kidney function may result in increased serum levels for drugs that are poorly metabolized; thus, the potential for ototoxicity is increased. Renal failure, concomitant use of loop diuretics such as ethacrynic acid and furosemide, and a prolonged course of drug therapy are the most important factors in the development of ototoxicity. Other important factors include mode of drug administration, dose per treatment, length of administration, and cumulative dosage. Ingestion of ototoxic drugs by pregnant women can result in a multitude of congenital abnormalities, including hearing loss, because of passage of the drugs across the placenta (Siegel & McCracken, 1981).

The ototoxic pathology in the cochlea begins with cell damage in the innermost row of the outer hair cells at the basal turn. As the damage progresses toward the apex of the cochlea, it also involves the outer rows of hair cells. This cell damage is consistent with the onset of high-frequency sensorineural hearing loss. Genetically predisposed susceptibility to aminoglycoside ototoxicity has been identified as a risk factor by Prezant, Shohat, Jaber, et al. (1992). Thorough information on ototoxic drugs and hearing loss was prepared for audiologists and published by Fausti et al. (1996). In addition, the American Speech-Language-Hearing Association has published guidelines for the audiologic management of individuals receiving ototoxic drugs (1994).

Perilymph Fistula. A perilymph fistula (PLF) is a leak of inner ear fluid through a tear or hole in either the round window membrane or the oval window annular ligament. This defect permits an open communication between the middle ear and the fluids of the inner ear. The perilymph leak is associated with certain cases of stapes footplate defect or may occur through the otic capsule bone from trauma or cholesteatoma erosion. PLF was not implicated as a cause of sensorineural hearing loss in children until the late 1970s. It is now estimated that 6–11% of unexplained pediatric sensorineural hearing loss is the result of PLF (Reilly, 1989). In data for children with progressive sensorineural hearing loss, estimates of PLF increase to nearly 25% (Pappas et al., 1998). It is believed by some that the perilymph leak can occur spontaneously, but it more typically occurs as the result of trauma to the head or from heavy lifting. The diagnosis of PLF is often tenuous and difficult in children, and may be a diagnosis of last resort when other possible etiologies are systematically eliminated (Balkany & Pashley, 1986).

Because sensorineural hearing loss results from PLF, many otologic surgeons perform exploratory operations to seek evidence of fluid leakage that can be repaired by patching the defect. Petroff, Simmons, and Winzelberg (1986) summarize several facts about PLF, including the following: (1) the relationship between fistulas and hearing loss is not completely understood, (2) PLF may occur in normal-hearing ears, and (3) surgical repair of PLF does not usually restore or improve hearing, although a successful repair may stabilize progressive sensorineural hearing loss. Some physicians believe that PLF may self-heal without surgery and with sufficient bedrest.

Diagnosis of PLF is difficult at best, because it is a condition with a wide variety of signs and symptoms. There is no consistent pattern of diagnostic findings, but "typical" symptoms may be as subtle as fluctuation in speech recognition scores, aural fullness, dysequilibrium, positive fistula test, or fluctuating severe hearing loss, which may be unilateral or bilateral. Factors that suggest PLF include precedent history of head trauma, hearing loss in the presence of craniofacial anomalies, radiographic evidence of inner ear dysplasia, signs of enlarged vestibular aqueduct, unexplained vestibular or balance abnormalities, progressive or fluctuating hearing loss, and/or history of previous meningitis or labyrinthitis (Marple & Meyerhoff, 1998). Caution must be exercised to separate fluctuating hearing loss from test-retest normal variations noted during testing in children (Myer, Farrer, Drake, & Cotton, 1989). PLF should be considered in any child with a progressive sensorineural hearing loss and intermittent dizziness, because total hearing loss can result if the condition is left untreated (Parnes & McCabe, 1987; McCabe, 1989).

Temporal Bone Fracture. Amnesia and loss of consciousness usually accompany a blow to the head that is severe enough to cause a temporal bone fracture. Skull fractures of the occipital or squamous portion of the temporal bone may extend into the petrous portion of the temporal bone and involve the otic capsule. Temporal bone fractures are classified as longitudinal and transverse. The longitudinal fracture often results in mild to moderate sensorineural hearing loss that exhibits the audiometric pattern of acoustic trauma. Should the fracture line cross the external auditory canal, laceration of the skin and bleeding of the external canal may occur with no loss of hearing. More medial fractures may produce bleeding in the middle ear or disruption of the ossicular chain. When the middle ear ossicles have been dislocated, severe conductive hearing loss will be present, requiring correction by reconstructive middle ear surgery.

The transverse temporal bone fracture typically passes through the vestibule of the inner ear, causing extensive destruction of the membranous labyrinth accompanied by complete loss of cochlear and vestibular function (Schuknecht, 1993). Severe vertigo and facial nerve palsy may exist for a few weeks following the traumatic event.

Relatively moderate trauma to the occiput of the skull can cause a permanent sensorineural hearing loss. Trauma to the head may produce temporary and/or permanent sensorineural high-frequency hearing loss. A sharp blow to the head creates a pressure wave in the skull that is transmitted through bone to the cochlea, often causing hearing loss on the contralateral side. Meningitis may occur as a late complication of temporal bone fracture months or years later, usually associated with upper respiratory infection (Schuknecht, 1993).

Noise and Hearing Loss. A sound of sufficient intensity and duration can cause injury to the cochlea, producing a temporary or permanent hearing loss. Such injuries often occur accidentally from a single exposure to very high sound pressure levels (noise trauma) or as a result of gradual, long-term exposure to loud sounds (noise-induced hearing loss). Different ears vary in their resistance to noise-related hearing loss. The extent of noise-induced or traumatic noise-inflicted hearing loss in children is difficult to ascertain, but its presence is relatively common. Mills (1975) published a thorough review of the early literature concerning noise and children. Noise-related hearing loss can be both cumulative and progressive over time.

A number of toys used by children produce sound levels capable of producing acoustic injury (Axelsson & Jerson, 1985). Toys and devices with sufficiently high sound levels include firecrackers, model airplane engines, toy firearms, and fireworks. Examples of noisy toys include certain rattles and squeaky toys (110 dBA), some musical toys (120 dBA), toy telephones (125 dBA), and toy firearms (150 dBA). For noise-emitting toys to conform to the safety requirements of the American Society of Testing Materials, they should not produce impulsive noises with sound pressure levels exceeding 138 dBA—this is as loud as a jackhammer or a jet airplane at takeoff. If a toy produces a sound that seems too loud, it probably is too loud. Parents should pay attention to noise exposure in children's recreational activities, encouraging children to lower the volume on stereos and noisy computer games, remember to take hearing defenders to loud movies and rock concerts, and monitor the volume of personal stereo systems.

Literally thousands of children have permanent hearing losses caused by the acoustic impulses of excessively loud toys. Weber, McGovern, and Zink (1967) evaluated 1000 children from Colorado with hearing loss and found 249 boys and 51 girls with noise-exposure–characteristic audiograms. These authors suggest that noise-induced losses are first identified in junior–senior high school boys who have a history of experience with firearms and farm machinery. Litke (1971) evaluated higher frequency hearing among 1516 South Dakota school children. He found high-frequency hearing loss in 6% of the population, with 5 times more boys involved than girls. The hearing loss due to noise exposure typically consists of sensorineural impairment at 4000 Hz in the affected ear, regardless of the type or frequency spectrum of the noise exposure.

Concerned parents often ask if listening to or playing loud rock and roll music can damage the hearing of their children. Although research in the issue of hearing loss and rock music is somewhat conflicting, there is little doubt that exposure to loud music can produce temporary threshold shift. Rintlemann and Borus (1968) studied rock musicians and found that only 5% of them incurred noise-induced hearing losses. Jerger and Jerger (1970) reported that eight of nine rock and roll musicians, aged 14–23 years, showed temporary threshold shift in excess of 15 dB on at least 1 frequency between 2000 and 8000 Hz. A study by Danenberg, Loos-Cosgrove, and LoVerde (1987) showed that hearing threshold shift can be measured in persons attending a typical school dance with loud, live rock music.

A thorough history may identify unrecognized situations of excessive noise exposure. Those youngsters routinely exposed to high noise situations must be counseled carefully regarding the potential hazards of additional noise exposure and fitted with ear defenders as soon as possible. Hearing protection, worn correctly, can reduce the noise reaching the cochlea to safe levels. A very successful program to protect teenagers from loud music has been developed by the nonprofit group Hearing Education and Awareness for Rockers (HEAR).

Noise Levels in the Intensive Care Unit. Any visitor to the newborn intensive care unit (ICU) is immediately aware of the high noise levels. Originally, hospital nurseries were small rooms with four to eight infants in incubators or cribs with virtually no life-support equipment. However, modern technology has created a much noisier nursery environment with the use of machines for life support, diagnosis, and monitoring of activity. The modern day ICU is a multitude of sound sources, respirators, and monitors that generate both background sound and alarm signals.

Noise levels in the ICU may be 20 dB higher than in the well-baby nursery, day and night, causing staff aggravation, fatigue, and stresses, possibly leading to potential patient care errors. Ambient noise levels in ICU have been reported to range between 56 and 77 dBA. This noise is generally low frequency (most energy lower than 250 Hz), persistent, and continuous (Falk & Woods, 1973; Redding, Hargest, & Minsky, 1977). Although prolonged exposure to the noise levels characteristic of intensive care equipment and infant incubators may be harmful to the developing neonate, direct evidence for such insult has not been reported. In 1974, the American Academy of Pediatrics Committee on Environmental Hazards recommended that manufacturers of incubators reduce noise levels below 58 dBA.

A number of concerned investigators have measured the ambient sound level generated within infant incubators. In general, the SPLs of incubators have been reported to be greater than 60 dBA (League et al., 1972; Falk & Farmer, 1973; Blennow, Svenningsen, & Almquist, 1974; Douek, Dodson, Banister, et al., 1976). Although these sound levels are not in excess of acceptable damage risk criteria, it must be remembered that infants in such incubators are usually in poor health, may be undergoing treatment with potentially ototoxic drugs, and are exposed to the noise continuously for several weeks to months (Falk, 1972). Long, Lucy, and Philip (1980) recorded polygraphic tracings from infants' heart rates, respiratory rates, transcutaneous oxygen tensions, and intracranial pressures during the routine ICU schedule. They found that sudden loud noises usually caused agitation and crying in the infants, which led to decreases in transcutaneous oxygen tensions and increases in intracranial pressures, as well as increases in heart and respiratory rates.

Bess, Peek, and Chapman (1979) measured incubator noise with different types of life-support equipment when impulse noise was created by health professionals striking the side of the incubator or by opening and closing the doors of the storage unit. The life-support equipment increased the overall noise levels of the incubators by as much as 20 dBA with a predominance of high-frequency energy. The impulse signals created by striking the side of the incubator (a common practice of physicians and nurses to forcefully stimulate breathing in apneic infants) ranged from 130 to 140 dBA SPL. Opening and closing the storage unit doors created peak amplitudes of 114 dBA SPL.

CHILDHOOD INFECTIONS ASSOCIATED WITH HEARING LOSS

Prenatal and postnatal bacterial and viral infections have long been recognized as causes of hearing loss and deafness. Widespread vaccine programs in the modernized nations have done much to decrease common childhood infectious diseases such as measles, mumps, diphtheria, tetanus, hepatitis B, meningitis, pertussis, and polio. However, the Centers for Disease Control (CDC) has reported that less than 80% of U.S. children are adequately protected by immunization by the time they reach 2 years of age. Vaccination programs have also practically eradicated maternal rubella infections in the United States. Stein and Boyer (1994) described medical advances in the treatment and prevention of bacterial meningitis due to *Haemophilus influenzae* type b through universal immunization programs and the introduction of cephalosporin antibiotics and corticosteroid treatment of congenital toxoplasmosis. These public health programs represent important progress in the prevention of childhood deafness. Unfortunately, without widespread vaccination programs in developing countries, children with these diseases continue to show a high incidence of significant hearing loss due to infectious diseases.

Common childhood viruses known to cause deafness, sometimes with vestibular symptoms, include mumps (perhaps the most common cause of unilateral sensorineural hearing loss), measles, chickenpox, influenza, and even the viruses of the common cold. Deafness occurs when the inner ear is damaged as a result of direct infiltration from the bloodstream or meninges via the internal auditory meatus. Viral infections may cause any degree of hearing loss from mild hearing impairment to profound deafness. Residuals of postnatal viral infections can also include optic nerve atrophy, cerebral palsy, mental retardation, disturbances of respiration, muscular atrophy or paralysis, convulsions, disturbances of autonomic system, and disturbances of metabolism.

Maternal infections during pregnancy have been demonstrated as the cause of a host of other congenital malformations and abnormalities (Hayes & Northern, 1996). However, congenital infections often cause fetal death and miscarriage. Damage to the fetus attributed to congenital viral infections has included congenital malformations such as clubfoot, intrauterine growth retardation, serious damage to the nervous system (including spina bifida), congenital heart disease, and disease of other organs (such as the liver, pancreas, and adrenals). Additional information about childhood infections of premature and newborns is presented in Chapter 8 in the discussion of neonatal and infant hearing screening. The reader is also referred to specific disorders in the appendix.

Meningitis. Sensorineural hearing impairment is the most common complication of bacterial meningitis in infants and young children. The microorganisms associated with hearing loss include *H. influenzae, Neisseria meningitidis*, and *Streptococcus pneumoniae*. Infectious meningitis causes deafness as the result of bacterial labyrinthitis due to an extension of the infection from the meninges. The infecting virus has been traced from the meninges to the inner ear through the cochlear aqueduct and along vessels and nerves of the internal auditory meatus. Serous or purulent labyrinthitis may follow with partial or complete destruction of sensory receptors in the cochlea and eighth nerve elements. Subsequent replacement of the membranous labyrinth in the cochlea and vestibular divisions of the inner ear with fibrous tissue and bone ossification is common.

The severity of the sensorineural hearing loss configuration ranges between mild and profound hearing loss, and the audiometric pattern is typically bilateral, symmetrical, and irreversible. Conductive hearing loss due to acute otitis media and upper respiratory infection are commonly associated with bacterial meningitis. Estimates of the frequency of hearing loss following bacterial meningitis, based almost entirely on retrospective studies, have been reported in the range of 4–29% of children who survive this illness (Kaplan, Catlin, Weaver, Feigin, 1984). Arditti et al. (1998) reported an incidence of 32% of sensorineural hearing loss in patients with pneumococcal meningitis. The number of children who suffer hearing loss due to bacterial meningitis from *H. influenzae* type b has decreased sharply with the development and widespread application of a protective vaccine. The vaccine is recommended for all children.

In earlier years, clinicians noted partial hearing recovery in some patients following bacterial meningitis infections. However, research based on prospective auditory evaluations of meningitic infants with ABR techniques confirm that documented hearing improvement occurs in only isolated cases, primarily those from *H influenzae*. Previous "improved" hearing levels following meningitis may have been related to inaccurate behavioral hearing tests obtained during the acute illness stage of the disease or to resolution of the conductive element of the hearing loss. On the other hand, certain sequelae of meningitis, such as elevated intercranial pressure or neuritis of the eighth nerve, may explain temporarily reduced hearing that improves with time and treatment. When improvement in hearing is noted, the increase is more common at frequencies lower than 3000 Hz and associated with moderate to severe hearing losses. Roeser, Campbell, and Daly (1975) and Ozdamar, Kraus, and Stein (1982) reported documented cases of hearing improvement following meningitis.

Vienny et al. (1984) of Switzerland examined 51 children with bacterial meningitis hearing loss with serial ABR recordings beginning with the earliest phase of the disease. They found that 35 children (68%) always showed normal ABR recordings, 11 children (21%) had transient ABR tracing abnormalities, and 5 children (10%) had persistent pathologic ABR tracings with permanent sensorineural hearing impairment. This study showed the early occurrence of deafness in the course of meningitis, with a crucial phase of possible recovery (or worsening) happening during the initial 2 weeks. In this cohort of patients, there were no incidences of "late" deafness or "late" hearing recovery, based on thorough audiometric follow-up studies 3 months after discharge from the hospital.

In a prospective evaluation of acute bacterial meningitis in children, Dodge, Davis, Feigin, et al. (1984) tested the hearing of 185 infants and young children older than 1 month of age. Of this population, 19 children (10.3%) showed permanent sensorineural hearing loss. Tran-

sient conductive hearing loss was identified in 16% of the sample of patients, but in no case was there improvement of the sensorineural hearing loss with time. Based on their analyses of the data, the authors concluded that the presence of hearing impairment in children who had meningitis does not correlate with the number of days of illness (symptoms) before hospitalization or with the number of days before the initiation of antibacterial treatment.

Although the ABR technique has significant prognostic value in estimating hearing levels in infants with meningitis, clinicians are cautioned that the ABR tests only the higher frequencies and is therefore insufficient as a singular hearing test. Clinical audiologic surveillance with behavioral testing is the only means by which to determine hearing levels with certainty at all frequencies in infants and young children who had meningitis. Because hearing deficits are so common in patients with bacterial meningitis, a hearing evaluation by ABR is recommended as a routine practice as close as possible to hospital discharge. Follow-up audiometric evaluation to obtain frequency-specific thresholds for each ear must be conducted when initial findings suggest the presence of hearing loss.

Congenital Syphilis. In many parts of the world, congenital syphilis is one of the most important contributors to perinatal mortality and morbidity. In Western countries, the disease is now relatively rare, but recent increases in sexually transmitted diseases (STD) suggest that congenital syphilis may again become a threat to neonates. Detection of syphilis is typically the result of a positive finding with the fluorescent treponemal antibody-absorption test, commonly known as the FTA-ABS test.

The most severe form of the disease manifests before 2 years of age. However, the majority of cases of syphilis manifest during the second or third decades of life.

Early signs include nasal discharge (snuffles), rash, anemia, jaundice, and osteochondritis. Later manifestations include saddle nose, saber skin, Hutchinson teeth, mulberry molars, and other dental anomalies. Congenital syphilis may demonstrate a multitude of central nervous system abnormalities including vestibular dysfunction, sensorineural hearing loss, and, occasionally, aortic valvulitis. Possible accompanying mental retardation depends on the severity of the neurologic damage.

Auditory impairment may not be present at birth. Onset of hearing loss may appear in early childhood with sudden onset, bilaterally symmetrical hearing loss causing severe to profound impairment. Poor hearing function and limited use of the hearing aid can be expected as a result of neural atrophy. The general treatment of congenital syphilis consists of prompt treatment of the infant with strong antibiotics. Chan, Adams, and Kerr (1995) demonstrated that proper drug treatment may be effective in treating the syphilitic effects on both the auditory and the vestibular system and may be performed in utero when an infected mother is identified.

Cytomegalovirus. Cytomegalovirus (CMV) is a member of the herpes family of viruses which includes herpes simplex, Epstein–Barr, and varicella (chickenpox) viruses and is endemic throughout the world (Hayes & Northern, 1996). CMV is now recognized as the most common infective virus with an incidence of 0.3–3% of all live births (Irving & Ruben, 1998). Fortunately, CMV is not highly contagious and is harmless to most people who experience a CMV infection with no symptomatology. Although antibodies are established, the virus remains in body cells in an inactive state, making future infection possible for the remainder of the person's life. This inactive virus can be reactivated under certain circumstances, including pregnancy. When the virus is reactivated, it is excreted in body fluids such as urine, saliva, feces, blood, semen, and cervical secretions. Unlike rubella, infection by CMV in any stage of gestation may result in damage to the fetus. CMV accounts for 6000 cases of sensorineural hearing loss annually (McCollister, Simpson, Dahle, et al., 1996). The hearing loss varies in severity from mild to profound and may be unilateral

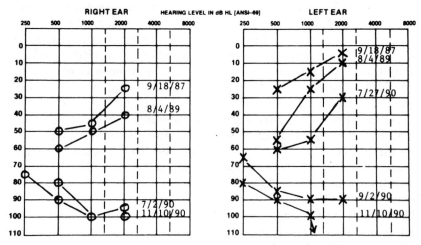

Figure 4-3. Audiogram of a patient with documented progressive bilateral sensorineural hearing loss. This child had normal hearing by observation of responses from birth to age 2.5 years.

or bilateral (Fig. 4-3). It is also known to be progressive, and routine audiometric evaluations are required.

CMV causes cytomegalic inclusion disease that is a generalized "herpes-like" viral infection of infants caused by intrauterine or postnatal contraction from the mother. The infection may be contracted during the perinatal period with passage down the birth canal (Peterson, 1977). The viral infection shows little pathogenicity in the mother, who may be totally asymptomatic. An infant may acquire the infection during the postnatal period from breast milk, blood transfusions, or older children and adults. CMV infection acquired postnatally is not associated with hearing loss.

One in 100 infants born in the United States has active CMV infection but appears normal at birth. Of these infants, 10–15% will develop central nervous system disabilities including hearing loss, developmental delay, psychomotor retardation, and intellectual problems. Approximately 1 infant in 1000 live births in the United States will show severe forms of cytomegalic inclusion disease (Stagno et al., 1982). Most infants with mild CMV infections remain asymptotic with no permanent sequelae and will develop within normal limits. However, infants with the most severe form of CMV usually die during the newborn period. Pappas (1983) concludes that the majority of congenital asymptotic CMV infections of the inner ear are undetected at birth and the deafness is subsequently incorrectly attributed to genetic etiologies.

If CMV disease is clinically detectable at birth, some 80% of infants have sequelae related to the central nervous system. CMV, when transmitted in utero, may be associated with a spectrum of problems including varying degrees of mental retardation, spasticity, hyperactivity, microcephaly, optic atrophy, congenital cataracts, and convulsive seizures. Associated complications may include facial weakness, cleft of the hard or soft palate, and a fairly high incidence of sensorineural hearing loss. Strauss (1985) stated that 20–65% of infants with symptomatic CMV infection have sensorineural hearing loss severe enough to be handicapping. Unfortunately, there is no treatment for congenital CMV. Although congenital CMV infection can be detected at birth through laboratory studies, screening for congenital CMV is not routinely performed in U.S. hospitals.

Harris, Ahlfors, Ivarsson, Lemmark, & Svanberg (1984) reported data from a large-scale prospective study conducted in Sweden. Some 10,328 infants were followed for a 5-year period in which it was shown that 50 (0.5%) had a congenital CMV infection. Of this group, five children had sensorineural hearing loss (four with total deafness and one with mild hearing loss). Hicks et al. (1993) reported the rate of sensorineural hearing loss resulting from congenital CMV infection to be 1.1 per 1000 live births. Fowler et al. (1997) found that 70% of children with asymptomatic congenital CMV infection also had sensorineural hearing loss characterized by delayed onset and threshold fluctuation. Fowler et al. (1992) found that the risk of acquiring hearing loss from CMV increases substantially if the infection is acquired during pregnancy. Further, the presence of antibodies to CMV in the mother before conception may improve the infant's protection against hearing loss.

PERSISTENT PULMONARY HYPERTENSION OF THE NEWBORN

Infants with persistent fetal circulation (PFC), also known as persistent pulmonary hypertension (PPHN), present with progressive hypoxemia (despite ventilatory support) and cardiac failure. This cardiac abnormality, previously known as patent ductus arteriosus, is relatively common in newborns. The defect occurs as an isolated abnormality as the persistence of the normal fetal vessel that joins the pulmonary artery to the aorta. Surgical correction is usually the treatment of choice and is performed between 2 and 5 years of age.

Naulty, Weiss, and Herer (1986) followed 11 patients with PPHN for 36 months with behavioral audiometry and auditory brainstem evaluations. Three babies (27%) had bilateral, progressive hearing loss with language delays 4–12 months below age level. Sell et al. (1985) pointed out that PFC babies are potentially at risk for long-term neurologic problems because of their history of severe hypoxemia. Hendricks-Munoz and Walton (1988) reported sensorineural hearing loss in 21 of 40 PFC infants, 14 of whom required hearing aids. In their study, the authors reported a high association of delayed onset and progressive sensorineural hearing loss. Nield, Ramos, and Warburton (1989) routinely refer all infants who have been mechanically ventilated because of PFC for 20 days or more for audiologic evaluation. PFC babies are at higher risk for sensorineural hearing loss than others in the ICU. Fujikawa, Yang, Waffarn, and Lerner (1997) reported treatment of 28 PPHN infants with inhaled nitric oxide; none of these infants had significant sensorineural hearing losses.

RH INCOMPATIBILITY

Exposure to high levels of circulating unconjugated bilirubin can result in hearing loss in the newborn. Due to Rh incompatibility, this condition involves the destruction of Rh-positive blood cells of the fetus by maternal antibodies. Owing to improved technology in perinatal care, newborns with access to modern medical treatment of Rh incompatibility are unlikely to have hearing loss, even with complete blood transfusions at birth. Clinical symptoms, when they occur, develop during the immediate neonatal period and include elevated bilirubin, jaundice, and possible brain damage.

Kernicterus is a condition with severe neural symptoms, associated with high levels of bilirubin in the blood (sometimes called bilirubin encephalopathy). Infants with severe kernicterus may die during the first week of life, with 80% of those surviving having complete or partial deafness. Other common residuals reported included cerebral palsy, mental retardation, epilepsy, aphasia, and behavioral disorders. Audiometric findings may show mild to profound sensorineural hearing loss. Hearing loss is usually sensorineural and bilaterally symmetrical. Central auditory pathways are also affected in kernicterus encephalopathy.

DIABETES MELLITUS

Diabetes mellitus is a chronic hormonal disorder of carbohydrate metabolism that is believed to result from insulin deficiency. There are two types of diabetes mellitus: juvenile onset and maturity onset. Juvenile onset is the more severe of the two and usually appears suddenly in childhood or in the teen-age years. Daily insulin injections are required to compensate for a lack of native insulin. The young untreated diabetic is often quite thin and experiences excessive hunger, thirst, need to urinate, weakness, and weight loss. Diabetics are more susceptible to infection. Long-term complications of this disorder include blindness, kidney dysfunction, and gangrene of extremities. Deafness is not an invariable accompaniment, but when it occurs it is usually a mild to moderate, progressive, bilaterally symmetrical sensorineural hearing loss. The incidence of hearing loss is higher in diabetics than in nondiabetics of the same age (Axelssen & Fagerberg, 1968; Friedman, Schulman, & Weiss, 1975).

AUTOIMMUNE DISEASE

There are reports in the literature of children with nonsyndromic hearing loss and serum abnormalities compatible with an autoimmune process (Irving & Ruben, 1998). In children, this problem may be seen as rapidly progressive bilateral sensorineural hearing loss leading toward deafness. Although hearing aids may provide an immediate resolution to alleviate parents' worries, the instability of these ears may lead to a continual decline in function. If in fact the disorder can be identified as related to an autoimmune problem, the condition is potentially treatable. Of paramount importance is the ability of the physician to diagnose the condition and institute prompt and effective treatment (Harris, 1998). Fortunately, autoimmune disease in children is rare.

ACOUSTIC NEUROMA

Tumors arising from the eighth nerve and extending into the cerebellar-pontine angle have been reported in children. According to Angeli and Brackmann (1998), the most common pediatric tumor of the posterior fossa is the acoustic neuroma in the context of neurofibromatosis II, formerly known as von Recklinghausen's disease. Neurofibromatosis type 2 is a genetic progressive neurodegenerative disease associated specifically with sensorineural hearing loss, but often includes other cranial nerve problems. Acoustic tumors should be expected in all children with von Recklinghausen's disease or who have a family history of neurofibromatosis. The hearing loss is unilateral in 95% of cases (bilateral in patients with neurofibromatosis type 2), progressive, and sensorineural. It appears slowly and may be difficult to identify in children. Children with bilateral acoustic neuromas may experience profound bilateral deafness that cannot be treated by conventional cochlear implants. The acoustic tumor diagnosis is generally made from ABR wave morphology abnormalities as well as specialized radiographic techniques and positive family history. Treatment requires careful monitoring and ul-

timately surgical removal of the tumor. After surgery, children often must live with neurologic and cognitive deficits that greatly affect their quality of life. Acoustic neuromas are uncommon in children.

HEREDITARY DEAFNESS

Hereditary deafness is a fairly common disease entity, occurring in 1–3 children in 1000 live births. The term "hereditary deafness" is used rather than "congenital deafness" to describe children with profound, irreversible, bilateral sensorineural hearing loss present at birth and related to any condition including anatomic malformation, in utero infection, birth trauma, and genetic causes. Congenital deafness would include those children with hearing loss due to osseous malformation in the middle ear. In studying a child with apparent congenital severe deafness, the clinician must be aware of possible exogenous, or outside, factors that can cause childhood deafness, as summarized in Table 4-1. Fraser published a classic contribution to the study of etiologic factors in deafness, "The Causes of Profound Deafness in Childhood" (1976).

A high percentage of congenital deafness is hereditary, according to Konigsmark (1972) and Fraser (1976). About 40% of profound childhood deafness is autosomal recessive in origin; 10% dominant transmission; and some 3% due to a sex-linked gene. Because deaf persons tend to marry other deaf persons, statistics regarding their potential for producing deaf offspring are of interest. The marriage of two deaf persons gives only a slightly increased risk of deafness in their children because there is small chance that two such persons would be affected by the same exact genetic deafness. Should the same recessive gene be carried by two normal-hearing parents, theoretically one-fourth of their offspring would be affected and one-half of their

Table 4.1.
**Summary of Known Exogenous Causes
of Prelingual Deafness**

Preconception and prenatal causes
  Rubella
  CMV
  Ototoxic and other drugs, maternal alcoholism
  Hypoxia (and its possible causes: high altitude,
    general anesthetic, severe hemorrhage)
  Syphilis
  Toxemia, diabetes, other severe systemic maternal
    illness
  Parental irradiation
  Toxoplasmosis

Perinatal causes
  Hypoxia
  Traumatic delivery
  Maternal infection
  Ototoxic drugs
  Premature delivery

Neonatal and postnatal causes
  Hypoxia
  Infection
  Ototoxic drugs
  Erythroblastosis fetalis
  Infantile measles or mumps
  Otitis media (acute, chronic, serous)
  Noise-induced
  Meningitis
  Encephalitis

children would be carriers. However, if the same recessive type of hereditary deafness overtly affects both parents, they are homozygous for the trait; therefore, all their children will be affected and will also be capable of passing the trait on to some of their offspring.

A means of identifying the causes of deafness has been accomplished by interviewing large samples of adult deaf persons. Deaf adults, however, are often poorly informed regarding the cause of their hearing problems. Such analyses are usually obtained through a written questionnaire or personal interview, but in this type of population in which language and communication are problems, such information-gathering techniques suggest caution in data interpretation. A summary of results from two studies of deaf adults who were asked the cause of their hearing loss (Schein, 1965; Northern et al., 1971) is shown in Table 4-2.

Gorlin, Toriello and Cohen (1995) describe more than 150 syndromes associated with deafness. The alert clinician is soon aware that malformations and anomalies often "run together." Congenital defects may be caused by prenatal misfortunes that influence the development of specific body systems or create generalized malformations of all the structures undergoing growth at that time. On the other hand, when multiple congenital malformations appear together frequently, the patient is described in terms of a "syndrome." The term syndrome is often overused and misapplied. The difficulties of syndrome classification lie in terminology problems, the broad spectra of signs and symptoms, and differences in the basis of diagnosis. Experts often disagree on the identification of a syndrome, or young patients present such a variety of symptomatic signs that clear-cut diagnosis is not possible. The definition of a syndrome depends on the level of acuity of observation and becomes easier as the demonstrative features are more pronounced.

As an example of a syndrome involving deafness, consider CHARGE—an acronym for several genetic complications including *c*olobomas (clefts in the iris or retina of they eye), *h*eart defects, *a*tresia

Table 4-2.
Etiology of Hearing Loss as Expressed by Manually Communicating Deaf Adults

Etiology	Northern et al. (1971)	(1965)
Unknown	35.8%	32.2%
Congenital	25.5%	10.5%
Meningitis	13.1%	12.7%
Scarlet fever	9.5%	4.6%
Result of a fall	8.1%	7.7%
Whooping cough	3.6%	2.3%
Measles	2.2%	3.4%
Pneumonia	—	2.3%
Mastoiditis	—	1.9%
Other	2.2%	16.7%
Total	137	1132

of the choanae (blockages of passages from the throat to the back of the nose that interfere with breathing), *retardation* of growth and development, *genital* and urinary abnormalities, and external *ear* abnormalities and hearing loss (Harvey, 1991). These patients have a characteristic abnormality of the pinnae in which the concha bowls are triangular with narrow ear canals (Fig. 4-4). These children present with abnormalities of the middle ear ossicles and inner ear dysplasias, creating sensorineural, conductive, and mixed-type hearing losses. These children have chronic ear infections throughout childhood and must be aggressively treated for recurrent and persistent otitis media. Although not common (reported to be 1 in 12,000 live births), it is advantageous for the audiologist to be well aware of this cluster of symptoms forming the CHARGE syndrome, as these children present with very difficult hearing problems to evaluate and manage (Toriello, 1995).

Some syndromic disorders may manifest progressive-type hearing loss, so that although normal hearing is noted on the initial visit, these children require regular reevaluation. The verification of hearing loss is the realm of the audiologist who can substantiate accurately hearing levels in such children. Siegel-Sadewitz and Shprintzen (1982) published a summary of communication disorders found in various syndromes. A concise system of classifying deafness was prepared by Bergstrom, Hemenway, and Downs (1971), ordered around types of hearing loss and body systems as shown in Table 4-3.

Hearing loss is often associated with congenital craniofacial anomalies such as malformations of the external ear and canal, cleft lip and palate, ear tags, and other dysmorphic features. Hayes (1994) described results of auditory evaluation of 145 infants with craniofacial anomalies and found that 50% evidenced hearing loss. The presence and degree of hearing loss varied by the specific craniofacial anomaly. In 92% of infants identified with hearing loss, results of ABR testing were consistent with conductive hearing problems.

Malformations of the External Ear and Canal. The auricle develops around the first branchial groove as six knob-like protrusions early in embryonic life. These six hillocks soon lose their identity as they coalesce to form the pinna. With six separate growth centers developing at differing rates, it is not surprising that a wide variation exists in final ear configurations that are within normal limits. The shape of the auricle is so different among individuals that European police forces utilize the configuration of the ear much like American police use fingerprints.

Supernumerary hillocks, known as "tags" or preauricular appendages, may remain with an otherwise normal-appearing pinna (Fig. 4-5). However, the presence of tags may suggest anomalies of the external and middle ear systems. A Swedish study established an incidence

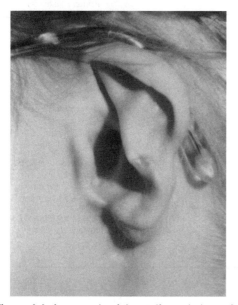

Figure 4-4. An example of the malformed pinna of a child with CHARGE syndrome.

Table 4-3.
Classification of Hereditary Deafness

Congenital Sensorineural Hearing Loss Disorders	Congenital Conductive Hearing Loss Disorders	Disorders of Congenital Sensorineural and/or Conductive Hearing Loss	Progressive Hearing Loss Disorders
Craniofacial and skeletal disorders Absence of tibia Cleidocranial dysostosis Diastrophic dwarfism Hand-hearing syndrome Klippel-Feil Saddle nose and myopia Split-hand and foot	**Craniofacial and skeletal disorders** Apert's syndrome Fanconi's anemia syndrome Goldenhar's syndrome Madelung's deformity Malformed, low-set ears Mohr's syndrome Otopalatodigital Preauricular appendages Proximal symphalangism Thickened ears Treacher Collins	**Craniofacial and skeletal disorders** Achondroplasia Crouzon's syndrome Marfan's syndrome Pierre Robin Pyle's disease	*Sensorineural progressive hearing loss of later onset* **Craniofacial and skeletal disorders** Roaf's syndrome Van Buchems syndrome
Integumentary and pigmentary disorders Albinism with blue irides Congenital atopic dermatitis Ectodermal dysplasia Keratopachyderma Lentigines Onychodystrophy Partial albinism Piebaldness Pili torti Waardenburg's syndrome	**Integumentary and pigmentary disorders** Forney's syndrome **Eye disorders** Cryptophthalmos Duane's syndrome **Renal disorders** Nephrosis, urinary tract malformations Renal-genital syndrome Taylor's syndrome	**Integumentary and pigmentary disorders** Knuckle pads and leukonychia **Eye disorders** Möbius' syndrome **Miscellaneous somatic disorders** Turner's syndrome	**Eye disorders** Alström's syndrome Cockayne's syndrome Fehr's corneal dystrophy Flynn-Aird Norrie's syndrome Optic atrophy and diabetes mellitus Refsum's syndrome
Eye disorders Hallgren's Laurence-Moon-Biedl-Bardet			**Nervous system disorders** Acoustic neuromas Friedreich's ataxia Herrmann's syndrome Myoclonic seizures Sensory radicular neuropathy Severe infantile muscular dystrophy
Nervous system disorders Cerebral palsy Muscular dystrophy Myoclonic epilepsy Opticocochleodentate degeneration Richards-Rundel			**Endocrine and metabolic disorders** Alport's syndrome Amyloidosis, nephritis, and urticaria Hyperprolinemia II Hyperuricemia Primary testicular insufficiency
Cardiovascular system disorders Jervell and Lange-Nielsen			*Sensorineural or conductive progressive hearing loss* **Craniofacial and skeletal disorders** Albers-Schönberg disease Engelmann's syndrome Osteogenesis imperfecta Paget's disease
Endocrine and metabolic disorders Goiter Hyperprolinemia I Iminoglycinuria Pendred's			**Endocrine and metabolic disorders** Hunter's syndrome Hurler's syndrome
Miscellaneous somatic disorders Trisomy 13-15 Trisomy 18			*Progressive conductive or mixed hearing loss* Otosclerosis

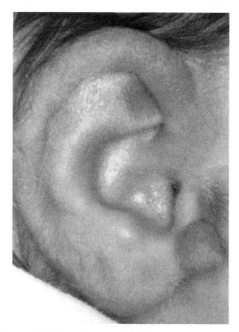

Figure 4-5. View of a preauricular tag.

figure for preauricular tags of 5.4 in 1000 live births. Kankkunen and Thuringer (1987) studied 188 Swedish babies with preauricular tags and noted that when the tag was the only facial defect, mild to moderate sensorineural hearing loss was found in 23% of patients. However, in 10 patients with preauricular tags and associated facial anomalies (facial paralysis, mandibular anomalies), 8 patients had conductive hearing loss, 1 patient had a mixed-type hearing loss, and 1 patient showed sensorineural hearing loss.

Atresia or Stenosis of the Canal. Atresia is the complete closing off of the ear canal. Stenosis is a narrowing of the canal. Atresia or stenosis of the external ear canal may accompany microtia (congenital malformation of the auricle, see below) or occur in conjunction with a normal auricle (Fig. 4-6). Stenosis of the external canal may be congenital or acquired following trauma. In congenital stenosis, the embryonic atresia plate may be solid bone or membranous; radiographic examination distinguishes between these two possibilities. The inci-

dence of aural atresia (with or without abnormalities of the pinnae) is estimated to be between 1 and 5 per 20,000 live births (Cooper & Jabs, 1987). Atresia is frequently observed with cranial, facial, mandibular, or acrofacial dysostoses such as Crouzon's disease or Treacher Collins syndrome. Aural atresia may also be associated with facial, labial, and/or palatal clefts. Abnormalities of the skeletal system and visceral organs or chromosomal aberrations may also accompany atresia. Children with these defects usually suffer conductive-type hearing losses and may do well with bone conduction hearing aids if medical or surgical treatment is not in order. Jahrsdoerfer and Hall (1986) reviewed surgical results and complications from operating on 202 patients with congenital malformations of the external ear.

Defects of the external ear and canal may be apparent without damage to the middle or inner ear structures. However, severe middle ear anomalies or aplasia of the middle ear may be associated. External ear and canal anomalies may be visible at birth, but they are often overlooked, and the defect is not noted until hearing loss is suspected or discovered. Sometimes the auricle and the opening to the external auditory meatus appear normal, but the meatus may funnel down to complete closure lateral to the tympanic

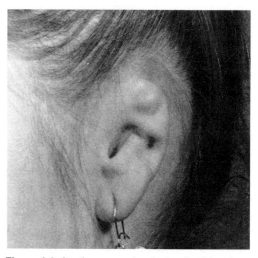

Figure 4-6. Atretic ear canal and microtia of the pinna.

membrane. If the atresia is bilateral, the child should be fitted with a bone-conduction hearing aid as soon as possible. If the atresia is unilateral and normal hearing can be established in the opposite ear, treatment or habilitation is generally deferred. Aural atresias may accompany other defects of the cranium, face, skeleton, or mandible. The etiology of aural atresia may be a chromosomal aberration, heredity, maternal thalidomide use, or maternal rubella. In cases of an atretic ear canal, surgery occasionally reveals thick soft tissue where the tympanic membrane should be; more often, a bony atresia plate of varying degrees of thickness is present.

Microtic Ear. Microtia or "small ear" is an abnormally formed, or absent, pinna. Fortunately, this occurs only once in 20,000 births (Holmes, 1949). Nevertheless, the authors see a number of such cases each year. The congenitally microtic ear varies from the mildly deformed ear to total absence of pinna with no external auditory meatus or to complete atresia of the canal. Unilateral microtia is about 6 times more frequent than bilateral microtia (Dupertius & Musgrave, 1959), is more common in males than females, and is found predominantly on the right side (Brown, Fryer, & Morgan, 1969).

When a patient has one normal-hearing ear, obviously the problem of unilateral microtia is not so bad. When hairstyles are long, the deformity of the auricle is easily covered. Patients who wish to do something about the microtia have a choice between attempted surgical improvement or the use of a prosthetic-type pinna that is attached to the side of the head by special adhesive material. Regardless of the surgical techniques used, parents should be aware that the reconstructed ear seldom has the appearance of a normally developed pinna, and the result is not totally inconspicuous. For improved hearing benefit, however, as in the patient who has bilaterally stenosed ear canals, surgical intervention may be successful. Bone-conduction hearing aids work very well for patients with bilateral atresia.

Congenital Middle Ear Malformations. Interest in middle ear anomalies has increased with the advent of microscopic surgical techniques and improved diagnostic capabilities of clinicians. Many patients with abnormal middle ears can have the deformity corrected by surgery. Since the middle ear is largely formed during the first trimester of fetal life, gross developmental anomalies of the middle ear are often related to factors that influence the fetus during that time.

Malformation of the middle ear may be due to hereditary factors or to disturbances during embryonic development. Failure in the proper development of the first and second branchial arches may result in the absence of the ossicles or a fusion of the ossicles. A malformation of the stapes footplate, however, is related to the development of the otic capsule. A disturbance in the fetal growth of the first branchial pouch may affect the eustachian tube, middle ear cavity, and the ultimate pneumatization of the mastoid air spaces.

Isolated anomalies of the middle ear ossicles are not particularly rare. Malleus anomalies include fixation or deformation of the malleus head and bony fusion of the incudomalleolar joint or absence of the malleus. Incus deficiencies may exist in isolation or in conjunction with other middle ear ossicular problems and range from total absence to a deficiency of the lenticular process. The incus may have only a fibrous connection to the malleus or be fused to the lateral semicircular canal wall. Stapes anomalies may involve fusion of the stapes head to the promontory, absence of the head and/or crura, absence of the entire stapes itself, or presence of a columellar ossicle. Congenital absence of the oval window or the round window may also exist as a unilateral or bilateral defect.

Middle ear anomalies should be suspected whenever other branchial arch anomalies are observed and are often noted as part of congenital syndromes. Branchial arch disorders include atresia of the external auditory canal, cleft palate, micrognathia, Pierre Robin syndrome, Treacher Collins syndrome, and low-set auricles. Disorders that feature other skeletal defects may also include middle ear anomalies such as Apert's syndrome, Klippel-Feil syndrome, and Crouzon's, Paget's, and van der Hoeve's diseases. Middle ear anomalies have been reported in disorders of connective tissue such as gargoylism or Hunter-Hurler syndromes, Möbius' syndrome, and dwarfism.

Congenital Inner Ear Malformations.
Aplasia of the inner ear implies failure of the ear to reach full development. Accordingly, inner ear aplasia is always a congenital malformation. Of course, the embryonic time of developmental failure determines the ultimate structure and appearance of the deformity. An individual may possess different degrees of aplasia in the two ears. Aplasia of the inner ear is a relatively uncommon aberration. Although wide variety exists in anatomic abnormalities of the inner ear, three classic types exist. These include Michel (complete failure of development of the inner ear), Mondini (incomplete development and malformation of the inner ear), and Scheibe (membranous cochleosaccular degeneration of the inner ear).

Knowledge of these inner ear anomalies is important for accurate diagnosis, proper treatment, and genetic counseling for the parents of the handicapped child, as well as for the child when he or she is old enough to become a parent. Therefore, differentiation and specific diagnosis of the inner ear problem is crucial in the determination of whether the hearing loss in question is of a genetic or an acquired origin. The degree of abnormal development that is actually involved in any specific patient may vary considerably from other patients with similar inner ear malformations. Diagnostic considerations

must include petrous pyramid polytomography of the inner ear and a complete evaluation of the hearing impairment. Malformations in the bone of the otic capsule can be detected by radiology so that differential diagnosis of the Michel and Mondini aplasias is now possible.

Michel Aplasia of the Inner Ear.
Michel first described the macroscopic description of this temporal bone anomaly in 1863. This type of anomaly is represented by a complete absence of the inner ear and auditory nerve. The outer ear may be completely normal with a narrow middle ear cavity. The malleus and incus may be present, but the stapes and stapedius muscle may be absent or abnormal. Maternal thalidomide use during pregnancy has been associated with this anomaly, and it has been observed in at least one case of Klippel-Feil deformity (McLay & Maran, 1969).

Mondini Aplasia of the Inner Ear.
Mondini described a temporal bone in 1791 that showed incomplete development of a flattened cochlea that consisted of only a single basal coil. In 1904, Alexander added more detail to this type of anomaly, indicating involvement of the auditory nerve and the vestibular canals. Characteristic of this anomaly is that it involves both the bony capsule and the membranous labyrinth. This anomaly is associated with Klippel-Feil and Wildervanck syndromes. Middle ear anomalies may be present in these cases, and atresia of the external canal has also been reported. Many temporal bone studies have described this deformity, which varies considerably from one case to another and may be unilateral or bilateral (Fig. 4-7).

Scheibe Aplasia of the Inner Ear.
The Scheibe abnormality of the inner ear, originally described in 1892, is characterized by involvement of only the membranous portion of the cochlea and saccule. This type of dysplasia is the most com-

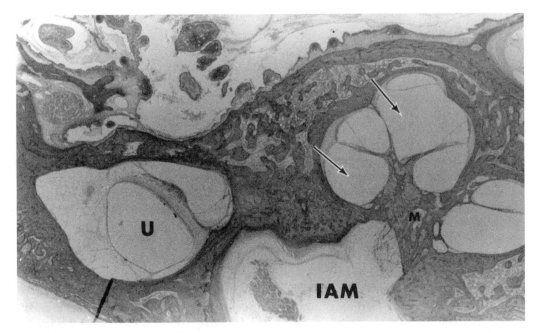

Figure 4-7. Mondini type of incomplete development with malformation of the inner ear from a patient with trisomy 13-15 syndrome. Note the incompletely developed cochlea with absence of the interscalar osseous septum (arrows) and poorly developed modiolus (M). *U,* utricle; *IAM,* internal auditory meatus. (Reprinted with permission from Sando, I., Baker, B., Black, F.O. & Hemenway, W.G. (1972). Persistence of stapedial artery in trisomy 13-15 syndrome. *Archives of Otolaryngology 96,* 441–447.)

mon of the inner ear aplasias. Histopathology of these inner ears shows atrophy of the stria vascularis, degeneration of the organ of Corti, and rolling up of the tectorial membrane, especially in the basal turn of the cochlea. This anomaly has been identified in cases of Waardenburg's syndrome, the cardioauditory syndrome of Jervell and Lange-Nielsen, Usher's syndrome, Refsum's syndrome, and maternal rubella.

Knowledge regarding the residual hearing in children with inner ear anomalies may be of great value in the habilitation of the child so deafened. Audiometric patterns in the Michel ear should show no hearing, because no true inner ear exists. True hearing is impossible, and a hearing aid for such a patient is of limited, if any, value. It is possible for the Mondini malformed inner ear to have some hearing, since the basal coil of the cochlea may be present; thus, a cochlear implant may be a consideration. The

Mondini ear is often a candidate for cochlear implantation (see Chapter 8). The Scheibe ear may show residual hearing in the low frequencies, since in this ear the major damage is in the basal coil of the cochlea. The Scheibe and Mondini malformations may be unilateral. Black, Bergstrom, Downs, et al. (1971) report that asymmetry of malformation is not uncommon and the patient may demonstrate one type of inner ear anomaly on one side and another type of inner ear anomaly on the other side. In such cases, radiographic findings and the degree or pattern of the hearing loss may be quite unlike each other.

More information is needed regarding the presence of these inner ear malformations. As of now, the risk of occurrence and the ratio of male-female incidence have not yet been securely determined. The bony inner ear dysplasias may be diagnosed soon after birth by polytomography and other radiology techniques, but the soft tissue malformations of the membranous labyrinth cannot be seen on radiographs and therefore must be inferred.

GENETICS

Humans take great pride in identifying distinguishing traits from one generation to the next. We enjoy speculating on the resemblance of children to their parents and question which child has, for example, the father's eyebrows or the mother's chin. With such observations begins the study of genetics and the submicroscopic structures known as genes. The audiologist concerned with hearing disorders should have some basic knowledge of genetics. There is probably some genetic component in almost all disease processes, but the extent of this component varies. Some diseases, such as Down syndrome, are entirely determined by a person's genetic constitution.

Genes are found in the nuclei of the many cells that compose the body. Genes are concerned with the determination of what a person's characteristics shall be, and they form the hereditary link between one generation and the next. The characteristics of an offspring are, to a large degree, determined by the genes he or she receives from parents—from the mother through the ovum or egg and from the father through the sperm cell that fertilized that ovum at the time of conception. Genetic factors present at conception are largely unaltered throughout life. The genes are contained in chromosomes that occur in pairs. One member of each chromosome pair is inherited from the father, the other chromosome member is inherited from the mother.

Nearly 3000 genetic disorders have been identified. Of the 4,000,000 babies born in the United States each year, 2–3% have a major genetic or congenital disease. The average person has 4–8 potentially harmful genes out of a total of 50,000–100,000 genes that determine his

or her neonatal and physical traits. A number of important technologic advances will help reduce these statistics. Amniocentesis (and a related procedure known as chorionic villus sampling) is a procedure in which physicians withdraw amniotic fluid from the mother's uterus for laboratory examination to search for abnormal cells that indicate the condition of the fetus. Ultrasound techniques bounce sound waves off the fetus to produce pictures. Fetoscopy permits the physician to examine the fetus directly with a lighted lens inserted into the uterus.

Of course, the problem of identifying an abnormal fetus may be simpler than the decision regarding abortion. The problem of deciding whether to abort a fetus is complicated by the fact that many genetic disorders present with a wide spectrum of severity. For example, some children born with cystic fibrosis have only minor symptoms throughout their lives, while others die a slow death from respiratory failure. Some children with mild Down syndrome may lead useful, productive lives, while others with the same chromosome picture but more severe retardation will be more severely disabled.

The following presentation will include basic information concerning chromosomes, chromosome defects, patterns of inheritance, the genetics of deafness, and genetic counseling. The goal is to acquaint the audiologist who has had little or no formal course work in genetics with the fundamentals of this important aspect of life that contributes to many of the cases of deafness commonly seen in the patient population.

Chromosomes and Chromosomal Defects. All hereditary material, in the form of deoxyribonucleic acid (DNA), is carried as genes on the chromosomes. All human body cells contain 23 pairs of chromosomes or 46 total chromosomes. Twenty-two of these pairs are known as autosomes; the remaining two chromosomes are called the sex chromosomes, two X-chromosomes constituting a female (written as 46,XX in genetic nomenclature), and one X and Y constituting a male (46,XY). The reproduction process of the body (or somite) cells is known as mitosis, whereas the reproduction of the germ (or sex) cells is called meiosis. Mitosis results in the development of genetically identical cells; meiosis results in the development of genetically unique cells.

During the process of mitosis, each chromosome becomes shortened and thickened and splits longitudinally into two chromatids joined at the point called the centromere. This is the form in which most chromosomes are pictured. They are then aligned and split longitudinally through the centromere, separating the two chromatids that then migrate to opposite ends of the cell. Cleavage then occurs in the cell to produce two genetically similar cells (Fig. 4-8).

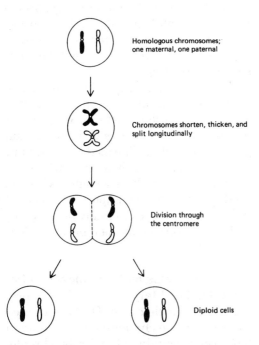

Homologous chromosomes; one maternal, one paternal

Chromosomes shorten, thicken, and split longitudinally

Division through the centromere

Diploid cells

Figure 4-8. Process of mitotic cell division. (Reprinted with permission from Stewart, J.M. (1973). Genetic counseling. In J. Clausen et al. (Eds.), *Maternity Nursing Today.* New York: McGraw-Hill.)

An essential factor in the reproductive process is the formation of additional sperm and eggs by a special type of cell division (meiosis) that involves only the germ cells, as shown in Figure 4-9. In this process, the chromosomes again shorten and thicken and split into two chromatids joined at the centromere as described in mitosis. Matching pairs are arranged together, and at this time material may be exchanged between paired chromosomes (known as *crossing over*). Crossing over, or the exchange of genetic material between chromosome pairs, results in unique genetic combinations. The paired chromosomes then separate (known as dysjunction) and move to opposite poles of the cell, forming two cells now with 23 chromosomes each (known as the haploid number). Each cell contains two chromosomes—X chromosomes, Y-chromosomes, or a combination of each. The next step in the process is simple mitotic division in which there is a longitudinal split at the centromere and migration of the chromatids to opposite poles. In this manner new ova and new sperm are formed, each with 23 chromosomes. At some future time of fertilization, one ovum and one sperm will unite to form a cell, known as the zygote, with a full 46-chromosome constitution.

Abnormalities may occur during meiotic or mitotic division, producing an individual with a chromosomal defect. These abnormalities may involve one of the autosomes or one of the sex chromosomes and consist of either too much or too little total chromosome material. In certain types of tissue and under certain conditions, chromosomes are readily visible under high magnification. A photographic record of chromosomal constitution of a cell is called a karyotype (Figs. 4-10 and 4-11). The human karyotype is often described in terms of the "Denver system," so-called because it was formulated at the meeting of cytologists in Denver, Colorado. In the human karyotype the pairs of somatic chromosomes (autosomes) are identified

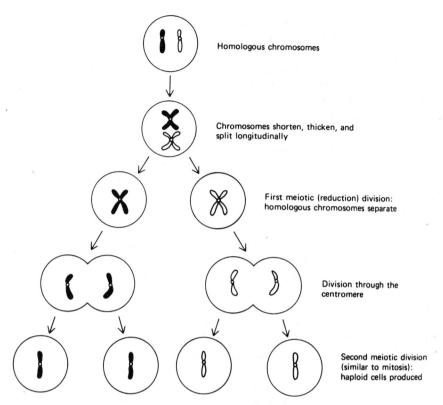

Figure 4-9. Germ cell division or meiosis. (Reprinted with permission from Stewart, J.M. (1973). Genetic counseling. In J. Clausen et al. (Eds.): *Maternity Nursing Today.* New York: McGraw-Hill.)

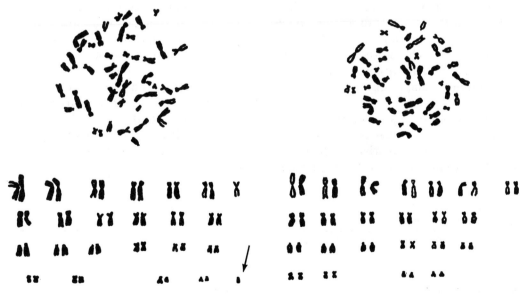

Figure 4-10. Human male karyotype with normal chromosomes. (Courtesy of A. Robinson, MD, Cytogenetics Laboratory, University of Colorado Medical Center.)

Figure 4-11. Human female karyotype with normal chromosomes. (Courtesy of A. Robinson, MD, Cytogenetics Laboratory, University of Colorado Medical Center.)

by number (1–22) as nearly as possible in descending order of length and are divided into seven groups (usually designated as group A through group G). Each group is composed of chromosome pairs with similar morphologic features. The symbols X and Y identify the sex chromosomes.

The most common autosomal defect is known as Down syndrome, or mongolism. The affected individual has an extra number 21 chromosome (trisomy 21) for a total of 47 chromosomes. The clinical features of Down syndrome are described in the appendix. Down syndrome can also occur in another form. An occasional child with Down syndrome will have only 46 chromosomes, including one large abnormal chromosome that consists of the translocation of the extra 21 to another chromosome. Clinically, the child with the translocation type of Down syndrome is indistinguishable from the child with the more common form, trisomy 21.

Hearing loss may also occur with trisomy 13 and trisomy 18, as described more fully in the appendix. These children usually have many severe abnormalities and rarely live beyond a few months of age. The total absence of an autosome is believed to be incompatible with life, although a few exceptions have been reported. For example, a deletion of the short arm of chromosome 5 results in severe mental retardation and a cat-like cry in infancy, comprising the cri du chat syndrome.

Unlike the loss of autosomal material, an individual may lose one of the sex chromosomes with surprisingly little defect. Sex chromosome defects cause disorders usually less severe than autosomal defects, such as Turner's syndrome and Klinefelter's syndrome. About 1% of residents of institutions for the retarded have sex chromosome anomalies (Robinson, 1972).

Patterns of Inheritance. The chromosomal defects that have been described above are all grossly obvious in a standard karyotype. Defects involving single genes, however, are much more discrete. Genes occur in pairs and are located on homologous chromosomes. One gene is maternal in origin, and the other paternal. If the two genes have the same effect, the person is said to be *homozygous* for the gene. If the effect is different, the person is said to be *heterozygous* for the gene. The expression of each gene factor depends on its interaction with other genes and the environment. Genetic defects can be inherited in three well-known ways and in a fourth less well understood, but commonly occurring, manner. A summary of the patterns of inheritance is presented in Table 4-4.

Autosomal Dominant. A condition or trait is dominantly inherited if it is manifest in the heterozygous state. This is a type of inheritance with an affected person having a 50% chance of passing the gene on to each of his or her offspring. Every afflicted person will have a similarly afflicted parent. An unaffected person in most cases does not carry the abnormal gene, and all of his or her offspring will be normal. Dominantly inherited traits have several distinguishing characteristics. They are usually milder

Table 4-4
Patterns of Inheritance

Characteristic	Dominant	Recessive	X-linked
Parental genetic status	Homozygous	Heterozygous	Mother heterozygous
Disorder in parents	Present	Absent	Mother = carrier
Chance of inheritance	50%	25% affected 50% Carriers	50% daughters carriers 50% sons affected

because the affected individual, who is capable of reproduction, passes on the gene. There is much variation in the clinical manifestations of a dominant gene, which is known as *variation in expressively*. In other words, a few persons are so very severely affected, while those at the other end of the spectrum may be so mildly affected, that they have no obvious clinical manifestation of the gene problem. If this occurs, a gene is said to have *decreased penetrance*. On occasion, a dominant trait will seem to appear as a spontaneous gene mutation. The parents of such a child are not at an increased risk for future pregnancies, although the affected person would have a 50% chance of passing the trait on to his or her offspring.

Autosomal Recessive. A condition is said to be recessively inherited if it is manifest only when the person is homozygous for the defective gene. This is a type of inheritance in which the carrier parents are asymptomatic with a 25% chance of producing an affected child. Fifty percent of their children will be carriers, like themselves, and 25% will be genetically normal. In many cases, recessive conditions are more severe than dominant conditions, as the asymptomatic carrier passes on the abnormality and the affected person need not reproduce. If a particular recessive condition is rare, there is an increased incidence of consanguinity in the parents. Consanguinity, which refers to a marriage of parents with recent common ancestors, such as cousin to cousin or uncle to niece, has genetic significance in that there is a greatly increased chance that two parents who have a recent common ancestor may each have the same recessive gene inherited from that common ancestor. Each partner, then, could give a child this gene, so that the child would possess two such genes and be homozygous for the abnormal gene. The pattern of this type of inheritance shows a cluster of affected persons among brothers and sisters, with normal parents. It is not possible to identify such families in the general population until they have produced affected children. An example of an autosomal recessive disorder is Pendred's syndrome, a condition characterized by hearing loss and a goiter, which appears in adolescence. Both parents in some circumstances might have normal hearing with no other family history of deafness.

Sex-Linked. If the gene for a particular trait or abnormality is located on the X chromosome, the condition is inherited in an X-linked or sex-linked manner. The condition then is X-linked recessive if it is manifest only in the male who is homozygous (i.e., the abnormal gene on the single X chromosome is genetically unopposed). The female who has a normal gene on one X chromosome and an abnormal gene on the other is a carrier and usually asymptomatic. The carrier female passes the gene on to 50% of her sons, who then manifest the abnormality, and to 50% of her daughters, who are also carriers but who will not manifest the abnormality. The cardinal feature of an X-linked trait is the lack of male-to-male transmission, since the male may pass on his Y chromosome only to his sons. The pattern of father-daughter alternation is characteristic because affected fathers have only one X chromosome, so they must pass the gene to their daughters, and none of their sons, who get the father's Y chromosome and the mother's X chromosome. Sex-linked inheritance patterns have been familiar since biblical times when it was noted that hemophilia, as well as color blindness, seemed to be passed from unaffected females to males.

Polygenic. Many of the more common congenital abnormalities, such as cleft lip, cleft palate, and spina bifida, are not inherited in one of the manners described above, and yet it is well known that these defects cluster in families. It has been postulated that multiple genes contribute to these defects and that each individual has a threshold above which the abnormality will be manifest. This condition is known as polygenic inheritance. The more severe the defect, the more the predisposing genes must present. Unlike single-gene defects, the recurrence risk varies with the number of affected persons in the family.

Genetic Counseling. Genetic counseling is often given to parents who have had one abnormal child and who are interested in knowing the potential for having additional children with the same defect. Genetic counseling may also be offered to siblings of an abnormal person and to the affected person as he or she approaches marriage age and possible parenthood. Genetic evaluation and counseling may be done in any of some 400 genetic counseling centers in the United States today.

The steps of genetic counseling vary with the complexity of the problem but include a careful family, pregnancy, birth, and infancy history to find factors that might explain the abnormality; careful physical examination of the affected individual and other family members; and necessary laboratory work as required. When the evaluation has been completed and the diagnosis reached, the parents return for the actual counseling sessions. Both parents are generally required to attend, and the counseling is done in an unhurried and relaxed atmosphere. They are given the final diagnosis and the risk figures for future pregnancies. When possible, an attempt is made by the genetic counselors to minimize guilt; however, in situations in which one parent is obviously the carrier of the gene causing the defect, it may be better to acknowledge the guilt and help the parent deal with it. In many instances, more than one counseling session is necessary. There is good evidence that parents who seek genetic advice will usually make appropriate and expected decisions about future children.

According to Keats (1996) comprehensive medical histories for all family members are essential to determine the etiology of a disorder, especially if genetic factors are likely to play a role. Family history may demonstrate a clear pattern of inheritance on which recurrence risk calculations for family members can be based. Single genes mutations probably account for at least 60% of all congenital deafness. These calculations become more definitive when the location of the gene causing the disorder is known. The transmission from parents to offspring of DNA markers that are very close to the gene can be determined by laboratory analysis, and this information predicts with high probability (usually greater than 98%) whether or not a family member has the defective gene. Identification of the gene allows direct mutational analysis to be performed on an individual's DNA without the need for DNA samples from other family members.

The diagrammatic construction of a family pedigree, which is a representation of the family medical history used to determine if the etiology of a disease is indeed familial, is helpful to indicate modes of inheritance. The pedigree may provide evidence to establish whether a trait carried by a single gene is dominant, recessive, or sex-linked. Simple pedigrees showing classic types of single-gene inheritance are presented in Figure 4-12.

The field of genetics is old, yet it is filled with new discoveries. In 1956, human chromosomes were first accurately counted, and in 1959 the first chromosomal abnormality—the trisomy 21 associated with Down syndrome—was accurately described. Progress has been rapid, however, in the past 40 years, and considerable research effort is now being directed toward the identification of specific genes responsible for familial deafness. As many as 100 genes may be involved in orchestrating sound acquisition and vestibular function on many levels, including neuronal and structural integrity and electricalmechano transduc-

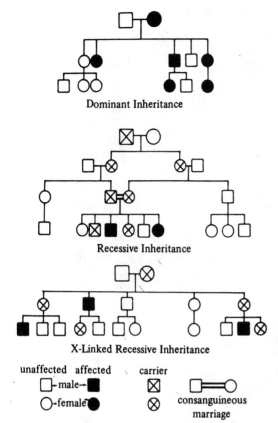

Dominant Inheritance

Recessive Inheritance

X-Linked Recessive Inheritance

unaffected	affected	carrier
□-male-■	⊠	□▬○
○-female●	⊗	consanguineous marriage

Figure 4-12. Family pedigrees showing simple inheritance patterns of single-gene factors.

role of the audiologist in decisions concerning diagnosis and management is a vital one. The audiologist contributes essential information on the degree of loss, auditory behavior and development, and auditory functioning of the child. He or she also provides familiarity with training methods in decisions on the placement of the hearing-impaired child. The clinical insight and observation of the experienced pediatric audiologist contribute a much-needed element to the decisions that will be made. How does the child relate to the clinician? Is eye contact good? Is the behavior even minimally distractible? Does there seem to be perseveration of auditory behavior? What is the vocal quality and how does the child use his or her voice? How do parent and child relate to each other? These are the questions that can be answered more through the audiologist's observations than through calibrated measurements.

Once the audiologist has specified the degree of hearing loss that exists and has delineated the status of the auditory development of the child, a standard protocol of examinations is indicated. Any of these studies, if made in isolation, will furnish only a fragment of the total picture of the child and his or her needs. When these fragments are brought together in a team conference, the picture becomes a whole. The team together makes a diagnosis of the etiology, extent, and degree of the problem and decides on the proper management for the child. A summary of the recommended medical workup for the child with hereditary deafness is shown in Table 4-5.

After the initial thorough evaluation, it is customary to follow the young child every 3–6 months to observe his or her progress and to pick up any loose ends of diagnosis. Not until all facets are put together and the child has stabilized satisfactorily in his or her program will the child be seen only once a year. Such stabilization does not occur until the child is 5 or 6 years of age. From then until adoles-

tion; however, only a small number of genes have been identified that cause nonsyndromic hearing loss (Vahava, Morell, Lynch, Weiss, Kagan, et al., 1998). Defining the molecular events leading to deafness may form the basis for new ways to help the hearing-impaired population in the future.

TEAM MANAGEMENT OF CHILDREN WITH HEARING IMPAIRMENT

The complex nature of hearing losses in children, and the fact that the hearing function is not an isolated phenomenon, makes it imperative that a team of professionals work together to diagnose and manage each case (Fig. 4-13). Emphasizing the team approach in no way minimizes the audiologist's contribution. The

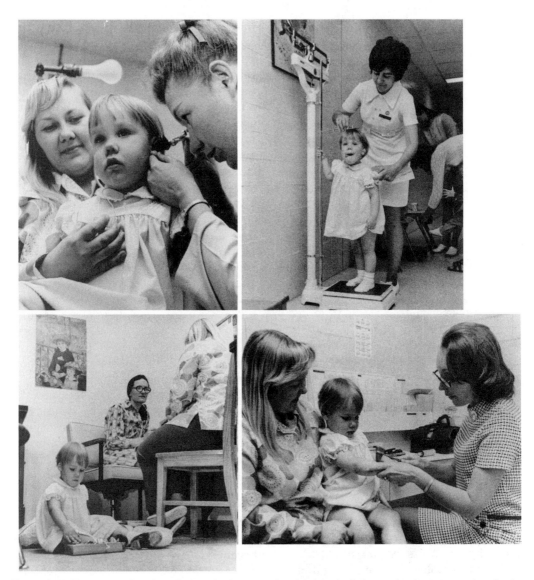

Figure 4-13. The nature of modern-day hearing losses makes it increasingly imperative that a team of profession-als work together in the management of a child with hearing loss. In addition to the audiologist's services, the reg-ularly scheduled checkup should include otologic examination (top left), physical examination (top right), social work interview (bottom left), and pediatric evaluation (bottom right). (Courtesy of The National Foundation-March of Dimes.)

cence the child should be evaluated once a year and, after that, whenever indicated.

Diagnosis. Diagnosis is a cooperative effort of all the specialists involved, but the pediatrician or family practitioner is the primary manager of the child's care. The physician can determine the etiology,

identify other associated anomalies, and suggest myriad laboratory tests that will contribute to the diagnosis. The physician also assesses the overall development of the child and provides for genetic coun-seling once the etiology is determined.

The audiologist contributes baseline audiometry, evaluates possible vestibular

Table 4-5.
Diagnostic Medical Workup of the Child With Hereditary Deafness

History
    Detailed family pedigree   Perinatal and neonatal history
    Maternal prenatal history   Subsequent medical history

General physical examination

    Generalized congenital bone disorders   Pigmentary disorders
    Congenital absence or sparseness of hair and/or nails   Congenital heart disease
    Congenital neurologic deficits   Hand anomalies
    Ataxia of gait

Concomitant head and neck physical findings
    Atresia of the external auditory canals   Retinitis pigmentosa
    Malformed external ears   Rubella retinopathy
    Facial anomalies, especially of mandible   Congenital cataracts
    Congenital facial nerve paralysis   Dental anomalies
    Branchial anomalies   Short neck; neck anomalies
    Heterochromia of the irises   Goiter
    Increased intercanthal distance   Quality of voice and speech
    White forelock in scalp hair

Routine laboratory tests
    Family audiometry   Urinalysis
    Complete blood count

Special laboratory tests (when appropriate)
    Age 1 year and under
        Rubella titer
        CMV   Immunoglobulin M
        Other viral titers   Viral cultures of urine, throat, and nasopharynx
                                          for rubella and CMV

    Any age
        Electrocardiogram   Dermatoglyphics
        Protein-bound iodine   Karyotype, buccal smear
        Syphilis serology   Radiographs as necessary
        Serum pyrophosphate and uric acid   Petrous pyramid polytomography
        Urine mucopolysaccharide screening   Electroretinography
                                            Vestibular testing

Courtesy of LaVonne Bergstrom, MD.

involvement when appropriate, and evaluates the relationship of the child's functioning to the degree of hearing loss. The speech-language pathologist provides a baseline speech and language evaluation that will be used to compare later functioning. During the diagnostic workup, the social worker becomes involved in helping determine where parents are in their process of accepting the problems of the deaf child. Are they in the denial, anger, or mourning stage? How can they be helped to an acceptance of the problem, which will allow them to best nurture the child? It may be necessary, at any given point, to bring in a psychologist for counseling.

The ophthalmologist evaluates associated eye abnormalities. All hearing-impaired children should have routine vision testing, and those children without a clear syndrome should be checked for retinitis pigmentosa with electroretinography to rule out Usher's syndrome. A renal consultant should be involved in cases such as hereditary chronic nephritis or Alport's syndrome. Cardiologists and neurologists are called in as indicated, and it is found that in such complex cases as Hunter-Hurler syndrome that the entire roster of a hospital's specialists may be involved.

Placement Counseling. The decision regarding placement of the child in an educational program must be the parents' prerogative. Unless the parents have made the decision, there will be second thoughts and possibly recriminations at a later date. The parents' decision is based on the following contributions from the child's deafness team: (1) information as to the degree of loss; (2) results of the speech and language evaluations, if relevant; (3) an introduction to the types of education available in the community (this would include visits to each of the facilities that are offering programs for hearing-impaired children); and (4) encouragement to choose freely and to feel comfortable with making a change at a later date if at any time it appears that another program will better benefit the child.

Routine Monitoring. During the first year or two, the hearing-impaired child should be seen every 3–6 months for periodic reassessment of the hearing impairment and progress in rehabilitation for the reasons listed below:

- Repeat audiometry may reveal progression of loss or unsuspected opposite ear involvement.

- Case history review may reveal overlooked historical items such as early history of disease.

- Physical examination may reveal overlooked physical findings or newly developed symptoms, such as thyroid problems, renal problems, and night blindness.

- Repeat family history may show suppressed information or false-positive items.

- An incorrect initial diagnosis may be corrected by reevaluation.

- Progressive concomitant disease may be identified by follow-up evaluations.

- New information, new scientific knowledge, and new technology may become available.

- Aided thresholds may reveal the need to adjust amplification.

Speech and language evaluations are given to monitor the performance of the child in the particular program in which he or she has been entered. If at any point it is obvious that the child is not making reasonable progress in the system, consideration can be given to looking at a change of program.

Psychosocial reevaluation and monitoring is extremely useful to determine whether any help should be given to the family in psychologic or social matters. It may be necessary to solicit public funds to help the family's finances in supporting the child in the particular program in which he or she is functioning.

In the hearing team's function as an objective advocate for the child (apart from the methodology of the program the child is in), it may be necessary to arbitrate between the family and the system. If the parents believe that the school system has mismanaged the child's placement, it may be necessary for the team to represent the family at a hearing called to evaluate the disagreement. Federal law mandates hearings that the parents can request whenever they believe a change is indicated (see Chapter 10). When college age is reached, the team may be called on to support the special interests of the student in obtaining a specific type of education.

It should be evident that the work of a child's hearing team may be never-ending. It will continue until the patient is fully achieving and completely comfortable in the environment that has been chosen.

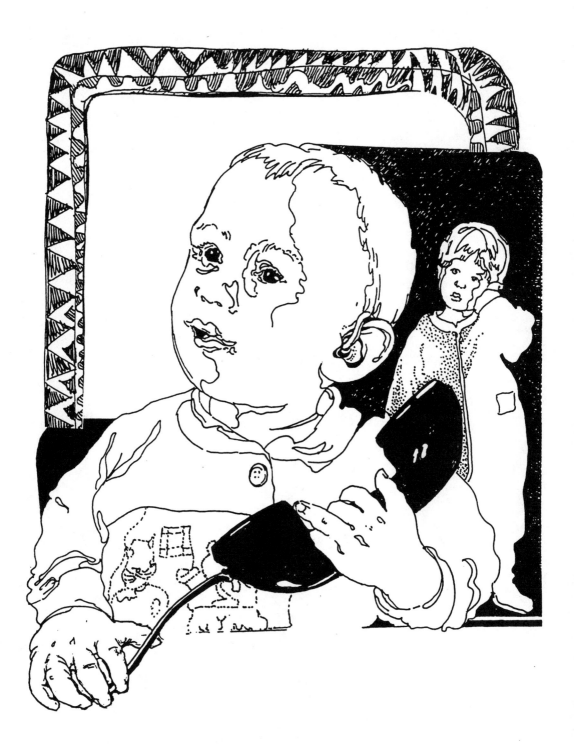

CHAPTER 5

Auditory Development and Early Intervention

Perhaps the most important aspects in any child's development are the acquisition and production of spoken language. Spoken language is the doorway to successful communication and the social interaction that is so important to daily life. Language is the key to the doors by which we express our thoughts, needs, and feelings and by which we receive and comprehend the thoughts, needs, and feelings of others (McConnell & Liff, 1975). Although it is language in a child that opens the door to education, the successful acquisition of language is highly dependent on an adequately functioning auditory system.

As adults, we give little thought to the development of speech and language because it comes so naturally and easily to most children. We listen with awe, however, as the child's sounds develop into phonemes, then into words, and finally into sentences complete with appropriate expression and speech patterns. As audiologists we know that the child with hearing loss does not automatically develop speech. The child with hearing loss may be confronted with a life of language difficulties and educational struggles. Language develops so rapidly in the first few months of life that the longer an infant's hearing loss goes undetected, the worse the outcome is likely to be; thus, we realize the importance of early intervention.

The audiologist has a unique contribution to make to the understanding of how language develops in infants—one that linguists and psychologists cannot offer. That is, the study of the degree to which the acoustic parameters of language learning in the infant are innate, preprogrammed processes and how acoustic factors influence language learning. There is research evidence that there are special biologic predetermined processes of perception for the various acoustic dimensions of speech. For example, we know that the newborn infant responds selectively to the dimensionality of human speech within hours after birth and is especially tuned to the voice of its mother (DeCasper & Fifer, 1980). It appears that the perception of speech signals by infants is mediated in some manner by central neural events, because although infants have had little listening experience by 2 months of age, they can differentiate between voiced stops /b/ and /g/ (Lieberman, 1975).

According to Stark (1996), Jacobson, a well-known linguist of the 1940s, made the claim that the vocal sounds made by infants during their first year of life are completely at random. Jacobson believed that these early infant sounds are made only for "practice" in the manipulation of the oral articulators, because their vocal productions do not resemble the sounds of any known language. Stark, an expert in child language development, pointed out that the International Phonetic Alphabet cannot be used to transcribe the unique sounds made by very young infants. However, in contrast to Jacobson's beliefs of the 1940s, other researchers documented that infants produce similar sounds across all languages. By the early 1970s, scientists noted that the patterns of vocal development in all infants, regardless of nationality, are universal. The milestones of cooing, vocal play, and replicated babbling appear in that general order in all normally developing infants. There is, furthermore, a lawful relationship between sounds that babies make in babbling at the end of the first year of life and those they make in their first attempts at words during the second year (Stark, 1996).

It is important for us to know that the auditory development and maturation of a normal-hearing baby follows a standard sequence of behaviors from birth to 12 months that is as regular as clockwork. It is the experiences of sounds and exposure to speech that shape the auditory system of infants during their first year of life. Although infants are unable to produce recognizable words until about 12 months of age, they quickly develop a remarkable ability to distinguish auditorily among speech sounds. Newborns quickly learn to recognize words, phrases, vocal intent, rhythm, and names and to perform sophisticated auditory functions long before they produce their own speech.

This chapter discusses the intricate pattern of auditory development in normal-hearing infants and contrasts their auditory, speech, and language development with infants who have significant hearing impairment. The classic studies that established the basics of prenatal and neonatal hearing development, the plasticity of the auditory system and central nervous system (CNS), and normal speech and language development are reviewed. The case is made for early intervention for children with hearing loss. It is critical that the pediatric audiologist completely understands the normal development of auditory behavior in normal-hearing infants to be able to recognize the similarities and differences in infants with congenital and acquired hearing impairments.

NEUROPLASTICITY

During the past decade, researchers have gained new insights into the early development of the brain and nervous system. Sophisticated technologies, such as elaborate brain scans and brain mapping, have helped illuminate the developing brain in greater detail than ever before. One of the most important conclusions from such studies is that the brain development that takes place during the first 12 months of life is more rapid and more extensive than previously realized. Since the late 1950s, one of the major themes in neuroscience is that the brain is not a "rigid" structure but a malleable, "plastic" organ with the capability of reorganizing itself based on sensory and motor input, a phenomenon known as "neuroplasticity." The neurons in the cortex mature during the first 3 years of life, and after that the brain's general organization does not change significantly. Knowledge of these facts demands that more attention be focused on the importance of early childhood intervention.

From the beginning of life brain cells proliferate rapidly, making connections that will shape a lifetime of experiences. The growing brain of an embryo, by 6 weeks nearly as big as its entire body, is richly irrigated by a vast system of blood vessels. At this embryo stage, the brain produces many more neurons (or nerve cells) than it actually needs. As the neurons carry electrical signals along the nervous system, systematic pathways are established through coordinated routes that are used over and over again. The stimulated neurons develop long axons that spin out multiple branches that connect with a vast number of different neurons. Current theory suggests that spontaneous bursts of electrical activity strengthen some of these pathway connections, while other neurons that are not reinforced by electrical activity begin to atrophy and finally disappear. The brain, during the early years of life, eliminates the excess neurons and connections that are seldom or never used. During early life, the number of neuronal connections explodes, and each of the brain's billions of neurons will forge links to thousands of other neurons. The resultant increase in cortical and brainstem electrical activity, triggered by the new flood of sensory experiences, fine tunes the brain's circuitry and determines which connections will be retained and which will be pruned (Chugani, 1993).

Brain mapping studies show that the biochemical patterns noted in a 1-year-old's brain qualitatively resembles those patterns found in the brain of a normal young adult. Brain cell formation is virtually complete before birth, but brain maturation is far from over. The next challenge is the formation of connections among the neurons to form the brain's physical "maps" that allow learning to take place. It is estimated that there are up to 15,000 connections, or synapses, per neuron. In the months after birth, this process proceeds with astounding rapidity, growing the number of synapses 20-fold, from 50 trillion to 1000 trillion (Chugani, Phelps, & Mazziotta, 1987; Kolb, 1989).

Among the first systematic circuits laid down by the brain are those that govern the emotions such as contentment, distress, and anger. Although the newborn can indeed feel, see, hear, and smell, these senses operate somewhat dimly and reflexively. Over the first few days, weeks, and months of life, sensory activity stimulates the neuronal connections from the brainstem to the appropriate areas of the cortex. The results of these early sensory experiences are those actions we have come to expect as normal infant development: by 2 months the baby is able to grasp objects, by 4 months the complex actions required to locate a sound in

space are initiated, by 6 months a baby can recognize and mimic the vowel sounds that are the precursors to speech formation, and by 12 months, we begin to see the results of neural pathways formed to produce the first words that mark the beginning of language expression.

Scientific study has shown that early brain development is much more vulnerable to environmental influence than previously suspected. The influence of environment on early development may be long lasting. The prenatal environment and conditions affect not only the number of brain cells and the number of connections among them, but also the way that these connections are "wired." For example, we know that inadequate nutrition before birth and during the first years of life can seriously interfere with brain development. Poor early nutrition may lead to a host of neurologic and behavioral disorders, including learning disabilities and mental retardation. Other detrimental changes in the environment of the embryo, such as drug abuse or viral infection, can wreck the clockwork precision of neural development, resulting in epilepsy or perhaps autism. Thus, one can understand and appreciate the increased focus that society has given to the importance of proper prenatal care (Carnegie Corporation, 1994).

Sininger, Doyle, and Moore (1999) reviewed the experimental evidence to support the notion of auditory system plasticity. Animal experiments show that the developing auditory nerve, brainstem nuclei, and auditory cortex have the capacity to change during normal development and during times of interrupted sensory input. There is also experimental evidence that reintroduction of sensory input after auditory deprivation induces further plastic changes, and deleterious effects may be reversed only during early stages of development. This important research evidence obtained in animal anatomic studies supports the view that critical periods may exist for intervention to ameliorate the experimentally created deficits.

The brain's growth spurts begin to slow down around 10 years of age. By the end of adolescence, around age 18, the brain has declined in plasticity but increased in power. These physiologic findings, confirmed by modern neuroscience, show the importance of early intervention. Although the adult nervous system continues to lay down new synaptic connections as we learn new ideas and skills, never again will the brain be able to assimilate and master new information so readily as during the first 3 years of life.

PRENATAL HEARING

Elliot and Elliot (1964) confirmed that the human cochlea has normal adult function after the 20th week of gestation. Johansson, Wedenberg, and Westin (1964) were among the first to attempt to test hearing function in the fetus. Using high-frequency pure tones presented through a microphone placed on the mother's abdomen, fetal heart rate increase response to the tones was recorded after the 20th week of gestation. The demonstration of fetal hearing has value in contradicting the theory that the child is born a *tabula rasa* insofar as hearing is concerned. At the time of birth, the infant has actually been hearing sounds for at least 4 months—fluid-borne sounds, to be sure—but nonetheless, true hearing.

Knowing that the fetus is physiologically prepared to respond to sound is important, but the difficult task is determining how to elicit a response and measure it. Birnholz and Benacerraf (1983) observed the auropalpebral reflex in 236 human fetuses in a study of screening for gross deafness. Stimuli were presented via vibroacoustic stimuli applied to the maternal abdominal wall directly over the fetal ear, and fetal eye clenching was observed with ultrasonic imaging. Their results, confirmed by Kuczwara, Birnholz, and Klodd (1984), indicated that auropalpebral reflexes consistently occur at approximately 24–25 weeks gestational age in normal fetuses.

How early does the infant perceive speech and act on the acoustic environment? To be sure, the developmental response to sound in the fetus is primarily reflexive, including startle, generalized body movement, possible cessation of activity, and the auropalpebral reflex (involuntary eye-blink). Nevertheless, there is also research evidence for the existence of preadaptive processes of perception of the acoustic dimensions of speech.

At birth the infant is able to discriminate his or her mother's voice and will behave in such a way as to elicit the mother's voice in preference to the voice of another female. DeCasper and Fifer (1980) used a sucking stimulus-response paradigm to demonstrate these capacities with infants shortly after delivery. Earphones were placed over the ears of the supine infant, and a nonnutritive nipple was placed in his or her mouth. The nipple was connected by way of a pressure transducer to recording equipment that produced either another non-maternal voice or the mother's voice. For five randomly selected infants, sucking bursts first produced only the mother's voice on the tape for a predetermined interval and then the voice of another infant's mother. For another five infants the conditions were reversed. A preference for the maternal voice was indicated if the infant produced the sucking response more often to his or her own mother's voice than to the nonmaternal voice. The infants soon learned to gain access to their own mother's voice, because specific temporal properties of sucking could be used to produce the recorded maternal voice.

Is there sufficient acoustic exposure in the uterus to permit such a precocious development? Bench (1968) reported that for a 72 dB SPL signal there is the least attenuation of sound going into the uterus at 200 Hz (19 dB), slightly more at 500 Hz (24 dB), more at 1000 Hz (38 dB), and the most at 2000 and 4000 Hz (48 dB). The frequencies below 1000 Hz contained the frequency response of the maternal voice that may be heard from the fourth month of gestation.

A later study by Armitage, Baldwin, and Vince (1980) measured the actual sound level inside the amniotic sac of pregnant ewes by means of hydrophones inside the sac, within the normal fluid environment of the fetus. These investigators found that although sounds from the maternal cardiovascular system were not perceived, the sounds of the mother's eating, drinking, ruminating, breathing, and muscular movements were discernible, as were sounds from outside the mother. They found that the attenuation of sounds measured reached a maximum of 37 dB below 1000 Hz, but it was reduced below and above this frequency. The higher frequencies were attenuated about 20 dB up to 5000 Hz. Human conversations at normal levels outside the sheep could be understood and raised voices were heard distinctly. If the leap is made from this animal model to the case of the human fetus, then it is likely that the mother's and even the father's voices can be heard by a fetus.

Querleu, Renard, and Crepin (1981) performed intrauterine measures on humans and demonstrated that the fetus could indeed hear the mother's voice and other voices, which were perfectly audible but lacking in tone because the high frequencies were absorbed. When there is no fetal distress the fetus reacts to the sound stimulus by a change in heart rate, often associated with movement. In 1981 Querleu et al. made more careful observations of seven patients during term labor after amniotomy, implanting hydrophones and microphones in the uterine cavity. When external speech was recorded through the uterus, two observers could recognize 64% of the mother's phonemes and 57% of a male's speech.

Apparently a great deal of auditory experience is necessary to produce the abilities of the newborn to prefer the mother's voice to other voices. Before such early discriminations can be made, the infant auditory system has to be preadapted to various acoustic discriminations. Such discriminations have been shown to be present in the newborn and, assuming a normal hearing system and normal CNS, the same capabilities are present in the 4-month-old fetus. The innate discriminations that subserve the preference for the mother's voice require the auditory competencies of discriminating rhythm, intonation, frequency variation, stress (suprasegmental aspects of speech), and phonetic components of speech (linguistic aspects).

NEONATAL HEARING DEVELOPMENT

It has long been established that normal-hearing infants and neonates between the ages of 4 and 16 months undergo an orderly maturation and development of predictable auditory response behaviors. These responses are easily observable and can be elicited with soft acoustic signals or simple noise-makers. In the hands of an experienced audiologist, knowledge of the normal auditory behavioral responses may be used as a hearing screening procedure. The normal-hearing, alert infant will respond in the predictable manner in accordance with his or her mental age. In fact, the kinds of responses one looks for are very age-specific, depending on the maturation of the infant, as shown in Figure 5-1.

The pediatric audiologist should be aware that the easiest response to elicit and observe is the startle, or Moro's, response. All normal-hearing infants and babies younger than 36 months will show an easily observable startle response to a sudden onset stimulus of 65 dB SPL or louder. We have found that an easy way to observe this response is to present a sudden speech stimulus through the sound

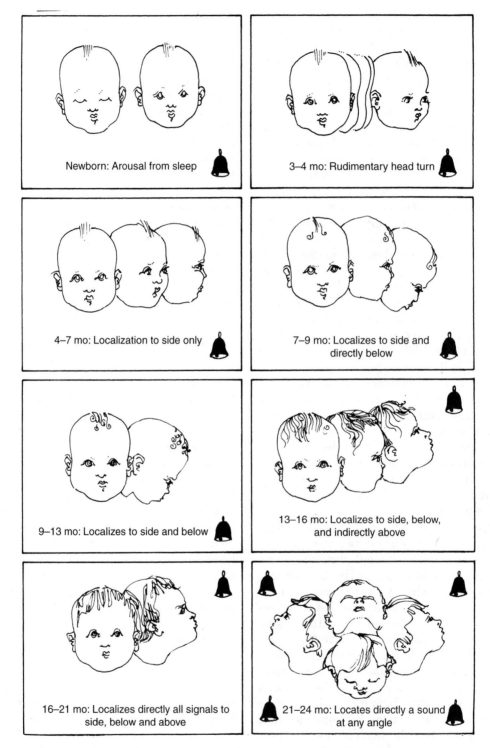

Newborn: Arousal from sleep

3–4 mo: Rudimentary head turn

4–7 mo: Localization to side only

7–9 mo: Localizes to side and directly below

9–13 mo: Localizes to side and below

13–16 mo: Localizes to side, below, and indirectly above

16–21 mo: Localizes directly all signals to side, below and above

21–24 mo: Locates directly a sound at any angle

Figure 5-1. Normal maturation of the auditory localization response.

field speakers, with the baby seated quietly on the parent's knees as far forward as possible with minimal support. When a sudden and loud auditory stimulus is presented—such as an intensity controlled speech signal—the normal infant will likely provide a brisk, reflexive, whole-body response coincident with the presentation of the signal. We reserve observation of this startle response as our final presentation of the screening procedure, because the loud stimulus may actually frighten the baby into crying. The parent should be warned beforehand about the presentation of the sudden loud sound as to not jump and startle the child. We recommend that infants and babies who do not demonstrate the appropriate startle response to intense auditory signals should be scheduled for an immediate complete audiologic evaluation.

Other normal developmental auditory maturation milestones can be used in hearing screening protocols. It has been our experience that at least 95% of normal-hearing babies will demonstrate the following auditory maturation responses when properly administered by an audiologist in a quiet setting with minimal visual distractions. Babies with severe to profound hearing loss, or developmental delay problems, are unlikely to show age-appropriate auditory maturation responses. It behooves the pediatric audiologist to observe these normal-hearing responses from a large sample of normal-hearing infants before using the techniques with more babies who are more difficult to test.

Birth to 4 Months. At this early age, auditory responses are limited and largely reflexive. In a very quiet environment one may see an eye-blink or eye-widening response to soft sounds from noise-makers or other subtle auditory signals, but the tester must be aware that these responses are highly variable. The only reliable auditory response is the Moro startle response or the "surprise"

eye-blink to louder sounds. At 3 or 4 months of age, the infant may begin to show a slow head turn toward a sound, but this response is also not yet consistent and quite variable.

4–7 Months. By 4 months the infant begins to turn his or her head toward the sound source in a more consistent, but still wobbly, manner. By 7 months, the infant's neck muscles will be strong enough to permit a direct turn toward the side from which the sound is presented. The head turn may not be a direct localization to a sound presented at a lower level beneath the eyes. For this preliminary localization response, the infant initially turns toward the side but only on a lateral plane.

7–9 Months. Between 7 and 9 months the infant begins to identify the precise location of the sound source with a direct head turn. By this age the localization response is brisk and firm. However, it is likely that the infant will not yet look directly at a sound on a higher plane (i.e., above eye level) as the ability to localize sound above the head is not demonstrated for another month or two.

9–13 Months. By the end of 13 months of age, the infant is able to localize sounds briskly and directly in any plane above or below eye level. By 12 months of age, the curiosity of the child is full blown and quick localization to an appropriately presented auditory stimulus will be noted by children with bilaterally normal hearing. Full maturation of the child's auditory development has been attained.

13 Months and Older. Although it is generally easy for the trained audiologist to elicit and observe these nonconditioned localizing auditory responses in this older age group, other factors influence expected behaviors up to 36 months of age and must be taken into consideration. For example, a 2- or 3-year-old may hear the auditory stimulus sound, but one can actually see the child willfully inhibiting the orienting response, because the child may suspect that the examiner is making the sound. Skill and experience of the audiologist must prevail with these younger children to be sure any responses noted are specific only to the presentation of the auditory stimulus. Of course, for this older age group, reinforced response techniques such as visual response audiometry or conditioned orientation response audiometry are preferred testing methods (see Chapter 6).

Condon and Sander (1974) and Demany, McKenzie, and Vurpillot (1977) demonstrated that neonates move in precise and sustained segments of movements that are synchronous with the articulated structure of speech. Spring and Dale (1977) showed that 1- to 4-month-old babies could discriminate linguistic stress as well as location, fundamental frequency, intensity, and duration. Thus, the entire gamut of *suprasegmental* aspects of speech is available and understandable to the infant at birth.

Rhythm, intonation, duration, and stress are extremely important to understanding multiple meanings of words as well as the meanings of homophones. Many words and phrases contain multiple meanings that are made clear only by intonation, rhythm, duration, and stress. This fact explains a part of the problem of a deaf child in understanding some of the subtle parameters of irony, satire, scorn, implied anger, or humor that convey the sense of multimeaning words or phrases. "You're tired." and "You're tired?" are two different sentences depending on the intonation of the rising or falling fundamental frequency. Sentences such as, "You drive me up the wall," and "I can't bear it," make for humorous misconceptions, but it is the kind of thing that is difficult for the concrete-minded deaf child who has not heard the stress and intonations that made the phrases meaningful.

Eimas et al. (1972, 1975, 1979) documented evidence that the very young child is also able to discriminate the *segmental* aspects of speech in a categorical and presumably linguistic manner. In an experiment with 26 1-month-old infants, Eimas used the classic sucking paradigm in discriminating the differences between the voiced stop /b/ and the voiceless stop /p/ combined with the vowel /a/. His results indicated that infants as young as 1 month of age are not only responsive to speech, but are able to make fine distinctions between similar speech sounds.

Eisenberg (1970, 1976) demonstrated that newborns, including those with known CNS abnormalities, can discriminate sound on the basis of frequency, intensity, and stimulus-dimensionality. Thus, neuronal mechanisms for processing and discriminating between SPLs are fully mature at birth. She found that the low frequencies tend to have a soothing or inhibiting effect on the infant, while sounds with higher frequencies have the property of occasioning distress rather than inhibiting it. However, signals in the range below 4000 Hz are 2 or 3 times more response provoking than those in the very high frequency ranges. It is intriguing to speculate whether speech dimensional signals are more attention-getting because of some preadaptive auditory reactivity or whether the known frequency-dependent sensitivity of the human ear is operating here. That dependency in itself is intriguing; one wonders which came first, the human ear's greater sensitivity to frequencies in the speech range or the peculiar properties of the human larynx and resonators to produce speech in that particular range of frequencies.

Kearsley, Snider, Richie, et al. (1962) found that if an unexpected noise of 70 dB SPL reaches maximum intensity within a few milliseconds, a newborn infant closes his or her eyes, startles, and shows an increase in heart rate. If the same sound reaches its maximal intensity in 2 seconds, the infant opens his or her eyes, looks around, and is likely to show a decrease in heart rate. The first reaction is a defensive one; the latter displays interest in the changing environment. Later studies by Morse (1972) confirmed that infants respond in a linguistically relevant manner, showing that categorical perception is present in infants before the onset of speech production.

The theoretical considerations of the infant's ability to process a segmental unit of speech have occasioned a great deal of speculation. The arguments revolve around the fact that speech is a very complex code; transformation of the acoustic energy signaling speech to the perceptual event may not be a simple conversion mediated by an auditory decoder. Lieberman (1975) states: "The acoustic cues for successive phonemes are intermixed in the sound stream to such an extent that definable segments of sound do not correspond to segments at the phoneme level." So all theories lead to the inescapable conclusion that the infant enters this world with considerable knowledge of the phonologic component of language.

That the infant is able to discriminate the acoustic features of speech means that the infant can segment an almost continuous acoustic input into discrete elements. This ability to process language into discrete elements is a basis for development of full language competence. The infant's ability to do this at the very beginning of language acquisition means that he or she does not have to learn that language is formed by discrete elements. The result is a facilitation of the language acquisition process, and indeed, the ability to break down discrete elementary language may even be requisite to its formation.

Bench (1971) described the relationship between the infant's activity or sleep state and auditory response in terms of the law of initial value: the magnitude of response change is influenced by the state of the infant before stimulation. The lower the initial or prestimulus state, the greater the increase in level of activity on stimulation; the higher the initial state, the greater the decrease in level of activity. Bench measured the heart rate of 10 normal newborn babies for 10 seconds before and after stimulation by a 95 dB SPL broadband noise. The results indicated that the heart rate change to auditory stimulation was dependent on the prestimulus heart rate. The implication of this work for infant audiometry is that any given baby may show an increase or decrease in behavioral activity, or no change at all, depending entirely on the prestimulus state. Exploring the responsiveness of 0- to 6-month-old infants to various stimuli, Bench, Collyer, Mentz, et al. (1977) found that infants up to 6 months of age were notably unresponsive to pure tone and narrow-band auditory stimuli. However, broad-spectrum noise elicited better responses in the younger infants (1 week and 6 weeks), and the 6-month-olds responded well to recorded voice stimuli. Moderate-intensity signals were not effective for the 6-month-olds. The younger infants were mostly in sleep states when studied, so stimuli of 90 dB SPL were necessary for response.

In addition to responding differently in a passive way to stimulus patterns and intensity, newborns can be active in regulating auditory events in their environment. Butterfield (1968) reported that babies made bursts of contingent sucking responses that controlled the onset and offset of tape-recorded music: classical, popular, and vocal. An instrumental pacifier nipple operated the musical selections. Four 1-day-old infants were used in his study, and all responded consistently over several tests. This study leaves no doubt but that newborn infants are not passive in their hearing function. Their feedback loop operates actively at as early an age as study is possible. The availability of such an auditory function strengthens the idea of early application of hearing aids to hearing-impaired infants who have sufficient residual hearing to benefit from them.

Eisenberg's (1976) observations on the responses of newborns give substance to the description of responses to auditory stimuli. She included as possible overt newborn reactions a listing that included arousal, gross body movements, orienting behavior, turning of head, wide-eyed "what-is-it" look, pupillary dilation, motor reflexes, facial grimaces, displacement of a hand or single digit, crying, or cessation of crying. Eisenberg's studies have important significance to those interested in early auditory behavior of infants. It was she who first described differences in habituation to sound as an index of CNS integrity. Newborn infants with known CNS involvement failed to extinguish their responses to repeated acoustic signals. Normal infants habituated to the repeated stimuli in a short time, a behavior known as *response decrement*. Neonates' sensory habituation to a pure tone was shown by Bridger (1961) using heart rate measures to indicate a startle response to pure tones. All babies who were tested showed a cessation of marked startle to successive stimuli presentations, provided the interval between the stimuli was less than 5 seconds. Bridger also showed that changing the frequency of the pure tone would renew the startle response after habituation to one tone, showing that babies do discriminate between frequencies.

What do these studies mean in terms of differential development in children? An early study by Irwin (1947) described the early effects of different kinds of auditory input given to infants. He applied both quantitative and qualitative measures to two groups of infants from the time of birth to the age of 1 year. One group was composed of infants of highly verbal, "white-collar" and professional people; the other group was composed of infants of low-verbal, "blue-collar" workers and laborers. The variable was that the first talked a great deal directly to the infant and in its presence; the second group of parents was less communicative both to each other and to the child. The quantity and quality of their vocalizations showed that at about 3 months, something changed the vocalizations of the two groups. The infants of the highly verbal parents began to increase the number of their vocalizations and the quality of the phonemes used more rapidly than the infants of the low-verbal group. It can be inferred that by 3 months, the amount and the quality of the auditory input to these infants was already being transformed into commensurate output. The more highly stimulated infants had greater opportunity to select acoustic information and to apply it to their own auditory feedback loop. Active participation and expression resulted, but differentially in the two groups. What more pragmatic proof can there be that infants are active, not passive, in their utilization of incoming acoustic stimuli?

Carney (1996) noted that the presence of adequate audition is critical to the development of long-term oral communication competency. Carney, however, raises legitimate questions and seeks hard data answers about how much audition is needed, how best are auditory skills developed, and when are auditory skills manifested in oral communication competency. It is unfortunate that the paucity of hard data complicates finding the answers to these questions without considerable additional research.

DEVELOPMENT OF ORAL COMMUNICATION

Concurrent with the maturation of the auditory function is the development of speech and language and other developmental skills. The beginnings of language learning occur at birth and possibly before birth. Condon and Sander's (1974) studies showing that the human neonate moves in segments of movements synchronous with the articulated structure of adult speech demonstrate that the infant is a participant in the rhythm of many repetitious speech structures long before use in communication. These rhythms comprise a prelinguistic activity of the human infant even at birth.

It is difficult to state with certainty the absolute age of onset and cessation of various stages of speech development during the first year of life. However, there is agreement about the general order of succession of speech development—the onset of cooing, laughter, and reduplicated babbling follows the onset of vocal play and ultimately leads to single-word production.

The infant's first use of sounds in a repetitive manner indicates the time at which the auditory feedback loop has become effective. By 2 months the baby is beginning to make certain sounds more than others. The selection of which sounds to repeat seems to depend on the nature of the sound. From 2 to 4 months these sounds are vowel-like. The sequence of use of vowels is presumably from middle (the "schwa" sound /ə/) to front and back vowels (Menyuk, 1972). By 5 months the consonant-vowel (CV) sequences begin. Irwin (1947) states that back consonants (velars and glottals) predominant at 5–6 months of age, with some of the labial (front) consonants entering in. At 9–10 months, the glottal sounds decrease and the alveolar sounds (middle) are frequently used.

Although the infant is able to differentiate various speech sounds in the first few months of life, production of the sounds does not develop at the same rate. Berko and Brown (1969) described the lag between the perception of differences in speech signals and the production of those speech sounds. In the newborn period the infant does not produce phonated sounds, only cries and physiologic sounds.

Lieberman (1975) identified the range of format frequencies that are necessary to human speech. The well-developed pharynx, with the posterior one-third or so of the tongue forming its anterior wall, is the structural arrangement required for a wide range of formant frequencies. In the newborn and in the nonhuman primate, the hyoid bone is high in the throat, so that the tongue lies completely within the oral cavity. There is little or no pharynx. As the larynx and tongue descend, a pharynx is formed and speech sound production becomes possible.

Mother's feedback of the child's sounds lays the groundwork for the first production of a word. The mother imitates the sounds the child makes, and she may add additional speech improvisations. Soon the child imitates the mother's imitations, and speech control is under way. Sometimes, the comprehension of the sound sequence precedes the imitation; sometimes, imitation precedes understanding of the meaning of the sound sequence. Films of babies as young as 2 months reveal a kind of "prespeech" activity by movements of lips and tongue, with or without sounds (Trevarthen, 1975). Even in the second month the baby may imitate a mouth movement of the mother or a protrusion of her tongue, but this kind of behavior is most often seen after 6 months of age and only after the act is pointedly repeated in a teacher-like way. For Trevarthen, such embryonic speaking confirmed the psycholinguistic theory that language is embedded in an innate context of nonverbal communication.

Developmental Speech Milestones. Any introductory textbook in normal childhood development or human communication will have extensive information on the development of speech in newborns, infants, and young children. Pediatric audiologists must have a firm understanding of the development of speech production and perception in children with normal hearing. The following is a basic framework to aid pediatric audiologists in understanding the general milestones of speech development in the normal child so that they can contrast the typical delays in speech production demonstrated by young children with hearing disabilities. Table 5-1 provides a quick checklist to mark the expected age-specific characteristics of speech, language, and hearing development in normal children.

The Newborn. The most common sounds made by the newborn are cries and vowels. By the end of the first month, the cries take on meaning and mothers can differentiate anger and pain from tiredness. The noncrying sounds include normal phonation but lack resonance. Near the end of the first month the infant begins to initiate sounds characterized as "coos" and "gurgles." The newborn can discriminate between different phonemes and different intonational and stress patterns, but this auditory discrimination does not involve sound-meaning relationships.

2–3 Months of Age. By 2 months of age the infant has developed muscle control to stop and start oral movements and vocalizations. The infant seems to focus on the production of vowel-like sounds such as "ooh" and "aah." By 3 months, babbling and laughter are likely to begin.

4–6 Months. At this stage, the infant is into strings of sound known as *true babbling* and begins to respond to noise-making toys. There is definitely more control of the tongue. The infant may spend long periods experimenting and listening to his or her own vocalizations. At about 5 months of age, the infant vocal emissions include consonant-vowel combinations. Glottal and labial sounds are heard from the infant by the age of 6 months.

Table 5.1.
Quick Checklist for Speech-Language-Hearing Milestones

Birth–3 Months
✔ Startles to loud noises
✔ Calms to familiar voices
✔ Makes vowel sounds"ooh" and "ahh"

3–6 Months
✔ Makes a variety of sounds"ba-ba" and "ga-ba"
✔ Enjoys babbling
✔ Likes sound-making toys
✔ Changes voice pitch at will
✔ Turns eyes and head toward sound

6–9 Months
✔ Responds to own name
✔ Imitates speech with nonspeech sounds
✔ Plays with voice repetition, "la-la-la-la"
✔ Understands "no" and "bye-bye"
✔ Says "da-da" or "ma-ma"
✔ Listens attentively to music and singing

9–12 Months
✔ Responds differently to happy or angry talking
✔ Turns head quickly toward loud or soft sounds

✔ Jabbers in response to human voice
✔ Uses two or three simple words correctly
✔ Gives up toys when asked
✔ Stops in response to "no"
✔ Follows simple directions

12–18 Months
✔ Identifies people, body parts, and toys on request
✔ Turns head briskly to source of sound in all directions
✔ Can tell you what he or she wants
✔ Talks in what sounds like sentences
✔ Gestures with speech appropriately
✔ Bounces in rhythm with music
✔ Repeats some words that you say

18–24 Months
✔ Follows simple commands
✔ Speaks in understandable two-word phrases
✔ Recognizes sounds in the environment
✔ Has a vocabulary of 20 words or more

6–10 Months. Babbling ceases at approximately 6 months of age. During the next few months there is undistinguished progress in vocalizing speech sounds. The speech unit becomes the consonant-vowel. During this period, the mother's feedback of the child's sounds provides the groundwork for the first production of words—yet some 6 months in the future. As the infant gains increasing control of oral movements and vocalizations, speech production progresses to repetitive syllables such as "bababa" and "dadada." Recall that Menyuk (1972) showed that the frequency of consonant appearance in babbling is reflected in the order of speech-sound acquisition. With increasing age and vocal experience, the baby's babbling increasingly reflects adult speech in syllable structure and intonation. As mother (or father) imitates the sounds of the infant, and in turn begins to add additional speech improvising, the baby soon begins to imitate the parent's improvisations; the shaping of the infant's speech patterns is underway. Comprehension of the sound sequence may precede the imitation; sometimes imitation precedes understanding of the meaning of the sound sequence which the parents learn to associate with specific facial expressions or emotions. By now the infant responds to its own name, plays with voice repetition, understands "no" and "bye-bye," may be able to repeat "ma-ma" or "da-da," and listens attentively to music or singing.

11–18 Months. The child's first meaningful word is usually uttered around the first birthday and is dependent on a full year of attentive listening activities. Soon after utterance of the initial word, the child begins to rapidly build a vocabulary. By 12–14 months the child can follow simple directions; use two to three words in a meaningful phrase; may correctly identify people, body parts, and toys by name; bounce in rhythm to music; and attempt to imitate words. By 18 months the child should have at least a 6- to 10-word vocabulary.

Questionnaires for Parents. It is useful to get some idea from the parents as to how the child is functioning in terms of communication. The parent can be questioned either by written questionnaire or by oral query, depending on what suits the needs of the population served. A detailed developmental questionnaire for parents is presented in Table 5-2. Use of these questions may bring out facts that do not present themselves during the routine hearing test. The questions presented in Table 5-2 cover auditory behavior, communication skills, and developmental milestones of the child. If any category indicates developmental delay, the child may benefit from referral for additional evaluation.. The questionnaire includes information on developmental status and communication abilities in addition to the questions concerning hearing status. It is recommended that this kind of questionnaire be used as a screening device to identify other problems that might benefit from treatment at an early age. The hearing questions are separated from the developmental questions because most of the commonly used developmental milestones are present in otherwise-normal deaf babies and, therefore, would not identify a hearing loss.

Some knowledge of the attributes of the deaf is necessary for the questioner to understand why the questions in Table 5-2 are worded as they are. For example, a deaf child will look around or will wake up when a door slams, when someone stamps a foot on the floor, when a large truck rolls by on the street, or when a loud airplane flies low overhead. Therefore, if the parent states that the child awakens to a loud sound, the parent must be asked to specify the type of sound, because clearly the perception of vibration may actually be the stimulus involved. Another characteristic of the deaf infant is that he or she may be unusually visu-

Table 5.2.
Child Development Questionnaire for Parents

2 Months of Age

Hearing

Have you had any worry about your child's hearing?	❏ Yes	❏ No
When your child is sleeping, does he[a] move and begin to wake up to a loud sound?	❏ Yes	❏ No

Development and communication

	❏ Yes	❏ No
Does he lift up his head when he is lying on his stomach?	❏ Yes	❏ No
Does your child smile at you when you are looking face to face?	❏ Yes	❏ No
Does he move both hands together in the same way?	❏ Yes	❏ No
Does he look at your face without you making gestures to him?	❏ Yes	❏ No

4 Months of Age

Hearing

Have you had any worry about your child's hearing?	❏ Yes	❏ No
When your child is sleeping, does he move and begin to wake up to a loud sound?	❏ Yes	❏ No
Does he try to turn his head toward an interesting sound or when his name is called?	❏ Yes	❏ No

Development and communication

	❏ Yes	❏ No
Does he lift his head up to 90° and look straight ahead?	❏ Yes	❏ No
Does your child touch his hands together and play with them?	❏ Yes	❏ No
Does he laugh and giggle without being tickled or touched?	❏ Yes	❏ No
Does he coo to himself and make noises when he is alone?	❏ Yes	❏ No

6 Months of Age

Hearing

Have you had any worry about your child's hearing?	❏ Yes	❏ No
When your child is sleeping, does he move and begin to wake up to a loud sound?	❏ Yes	❏ No
Does he try to turn his head toward an interesting sound or when his name is called?	❏ Yes	❏ No

Development and communication

Does he lift his head and chest with his arms?	❏ Yes	❏ No
Does he keep his head steady when sitting?	❏ Yes	❏ No
Does he roll over in his crib?	❏ Yes	❏ No
Does he reach for objects within his reach and hold them?	❏ Yes	❏ No
Does he see small objects like peas or raisins?	❏ Yes	❏ No

8 Months of Age

Hearing

Have you had any worry about your child's hearing?	❏ Yes	❏ No
When your child is sleeping, does he move and begin to wake up to a loud sound?	❏ Yes	❏ No
Does he try to turn his head toward an interesting sound or when his name is called?	❏ Yes	❏ No
Does he enjoy ringing a bell, playing with a noisy toy, or shaking a rattle?	❏ Yes	❏ No

Development and communication

Does he support most of his weight on his legs?	❏ Yes	❏ No
Can he sit alone without help for 5 minutes?	❏ Yes	❏ No
Can he sit and look for objects that have fallen out of sight?	❏ Yes	❏ No
Can he pick up two objects, one in each hand?	❏ Yes	❏ No
Can he transfer an object from one hand to the other?	❏ Yes	❏ No
Can he feed himself a cracker?	❏ Yes	❏ No
Does he make a number of different sounds and change their pitch?	❏ Yes	❏ No
Does he clap his hands in imitation and make noises at the same time?	❏ Yes	❏ No

10 Months of Age

Hearing

Have you had any worry about your child's hearing?	❏ Yes	❏ No
When your child is sleeping, does he move and begin to wake up to a loud sound?	❏ Yes	❏ No
Does he turn his head toward an interesting sound or when his name is called?	❏ Yes	❏ No
Does he try to imitate you if you make his own sounds?	❏ Yes	❏ No

Development and communication

Does he play peek-a-boo with you?	❏ Yes	❏ No
Can he stand for at least 5 seconds, holding on to a crib or chair?	❏ Yes	❏ No
Does he try to hold a toy when it is pulled away?	❏ Yes	❏ No
Is he shy or afraid of strangers?	❏ Yes	❏ No
Can he pull himself to a standing position alone?	❏ Yes	❏ No

(continued)

Table 5.2.
Child Development Questionnaire for Parents (Continued)

12 Months of Age

Hearing

Have you had any worry about your child's hearing?	❏ Yes	❏ No
When your child is sleeping, does he move and begin to wake up to a loud sound?	❏ Yes	❏ No
Does he turn his head toward an interesting sound or when his name is called?	❏ Yes	❏ No
Is he beginning to repeat some of the sounds you make?	❏ Yes	❏ No

Development and communication

Can he pick up tiny objects with his fingers such as a raisin or candy?	❏ Yes	❏ No
Can he get to a sitting position without help?	❏ Yes	❏ No
Does he wave bye-bye or play pat-a-cake when you encourage him?	❏ Yes	❏ No
Can he say "mamma" or "dada" appropriately?	❏ Yes	❏ No

ªThe pronouns "he" and "his" are used throughout in the generic sense and are intended solely to avoid the redundancy and awkwardness created by using "he or she" and "his or her."

ally alert and attends to movement in peripheral vision. Therefore, if the parent reports that the child turns around to an interesting sound or name, the parent must be asked if the sound is out of the child's peripheral visual field.

Until the age of 6 months the deaf infant sounds to the uninitiated person much like the normal-hearing infant. The deaf infant vocalizes when the parent appears and coos just as the normal-hearing child does. Only an expert phonetician can identify the subtle qualitative differences in the babbling sounds that the deaf child makes.

A common misleading indication is a parent's report that the baby says "mamma" at around the age of 1 year and that, therefore, the baby must be hearing at that point. Oddly enough, the parents of most deaf children make just such a report, and it is universally true that a profoundly deaf infant appears to be saying "mamma" at around 1 year of age. Actually, what the baby is saying is "amah," which is the most primitive sound that can be made, involving as it does the almost animal-like "ah" vocalization plus the coming together of the lips. It has been postulated that one of the reasons for the "amah" development is that in infancy the baby is carried close to the mother, feels the vibrations or hears low frequencies of the mother's voice, and thus is stimulated to perpetuate the

sounds. At any rate, the sounds soon drop off, and nothing remains except the "ah" vocalization in a strident voice.

To be sure, it is recognized that speech develops at different rates in children depending on a wide variety of factors. Often it is the pediatric audiologist, listening to a child's speech patterns for the first time, who is in a position to recognize speech delay or inappropriate speech for the child's age. Generally, when speech problems are identified, the audiologist should be prepared to recommend that a full evaluation be performed by a qualified speech-language pathologist. Matkin (1984) organized some general guidelines as presented in Table 5-3 to assist in knowing when the child's speech patterns require referral for further evaluation.

STUDIES OF SPEECH DEVELOPMENT

Menyuk (1972) suggests that experimental results comparing primate vocalizations with those of human infants and adults "indicate that speaking is not simply a learned overlaid function on the muscles and structures of breathing and eating, but that man is preprogrammed to develop a vocal mechanism that is specifically adapted to produce speech." Studies of the development of infant vocalization show a logical, orderly sequence of utterances between the initial sounds made by the baby until the first words are achieved. As the infant's one-word vocabulary grows beginning at about 12 months, the frequency of babbling declines until it is entirely omitted between 18 and 20 months of age. Measurements of the fundamental frequency of the baby's voice (*f*o) were made by Kent (1976). He showed that during the first 3 weeks of life *f*o is around 400 Hz; then it increases to around 480 Hz by the fourth month, where it stabilizes for 5 months. At 1 year it begins to decrease sharply and levels off at 300 Hz at 3 years.

Regardless of the linguistic community in which they are raised, babies begin by cooing, then producing reduplicated CV syllables, and finally "variegated" babbling with sentence-like intonational patterns (Oller, 1978, 1980). By 1 month, typical cooing and gurgling sounds are made in addition to the crying; by 3 months, true babbling begins. True babbling consists of the pleasurable repetition of sounds. Babbling is not easily defined in terms of phonetic or acoustic characteristics. Babbling is defined by Kent, Osberger, Netsell, and Hustedde (1987) as "an infant's vocal behavior excepting the

so-called vegetative sounds associated with respiratory and gastric events and sounds of obvious distress or discomfort (such as cry or fuss sounds)." Stoel-Gammon and Otomo (1986) define babbling as "relative speech-like utterances." The sounds produced by infants include reduplicated syllables, sustained fricatives and trills, prolonged vocalic phonations, prolonged nasal murmurs, grunt-like short vowels, and complex sequences in which variations can be heard in manner, place, voicing, or any combinations of these (Kent et al., 1987).

The last stage of progress in the vocal capabilities required for the production of speech-like syllables is called the *canonical stage*. Canonical babble is the well-defined mature syllables, a clear vocalic sound with consonant margins that appears between 5 and 8 months of age. The canonical stage is followed typically by strings of syllables that are so speech-like that parents often assert that the infant is talking. These canonical syllables are not used in association with word meaning, but they are certainly the precursors to spoken language (Oller & Eilers, 1988). The differences between the vocalizations of hearing infants and deaf infants are important to note, and considerable new evidence supports the need for early auditory experiences critical to the development of canonical babbling and ultimately speech.

In a convincing study of infant vocalizations from 94 babies with normal hearing and 37 infants with severe to profound hearing impairment, Eilers and Oller (1994) showed that the vocal differences between the two groups was not subtle, but rather salient and striking. The onset of the canonical stage virtually always occurs by 11 months of age (range, 3–10 months) in normally developing, hearing infants. In deaf infants, however, careful studies of the onset of canonical babbling showed significantly delayed development in this speech stage until 11 months or older, often well into the third year of life (range, 11–49

Table 5.3.
Referral Guidelines for Children With Speech Delay

By 12 months
   No differentiated babbling or vocal imitation

By 18 months
   No use of single words

By 24 months
   Less than 10 single words

By 30 months
   Fewer than 100 words
   No 2-word combinations
   Unintelligible speech

By 36 months
   Fewer than 200 words
   No telegraphic sentences
   Clarity of speech less than 50%

By 48 months
   Fewer than 600 words
   No use of simple sentences
   Clarity of speech less than 80%

From Matkin, N. (1984). Early recognition and referral of hearing-impaired children. *Pediatrics in Review, 6*(5), 153.

months, with a mode onset at 24 months). In their study, no deaf infant ever reached the canonical stage before 11 months of age. The fact that there was no overlap in the distribution of the onset of canonical babbling between infants with normal hearing and infants with hearing impairment led to the suggestion that the failure of otherwise healthy infants to produce canonical syllables before the age of 11 months should be considered a serious risk factor for the presence of hearing impairment. Eilers and Oller noted that as the infants with hearing impairment were fitted with amplification, there was significant correlation between the onset of canonical babbling and the age at which hearing aids were fit.

Up to 5 or 6 months of age, the sounds made by the infant do not seem to be related to the speech sounds heard. The infant's productive capacity for speech lags significantly behind his or her demonstrated ability to perceive differences. From our observations of otherwise normal deaf infants, their vocalizations are identical to those of normal infants until 5 or 6 months. Furthermore, deaf infants increase their vocalizations when parents speak to them, just as normal infants do. It is obvious that the reason for this increase in vocalizations is not the baby's hearing the parent's voice. We postulate that it is a preadaptive, reflexive response stimulated by the presence of the parent's face, much as is the smile response that appears at the same age. The phenomenon of increased vocalization may indeed be a milestone that is predictive of eventual communication skills. Certainly the established fact that the auditory feedback loop is present at birth indicates that the elementary babbling sounds have a significant prelinguistic function. The lack of auditory feedback in the deaf child deprives him or her of early prelinguistic experiences.

An important research project was conducted by Stoel-Gammon and Otomo (1986) during which they produced phonetic transcriptions of babbling samples from 11 normal-hearing babies aged 4–18 months and compared their findings with phonetic transcriptions that they obtained from 11 hearing-impaired infants aged 4–28 months. The normal-hearing babies showed an increase in size of their consonantal repertoires with age in contrast to the hearing-impaired babies, who had smaller repertoires that decreased over time. A comparison of multisyllabic utterances showed a general tendency for the hearing-impaired infants to produce fewer multisyllabic utterances containing true consonants and for some of the hearing-impaired babies to produce a high proportion of vocalizations with glides or glottal stops. This study confirmed both qualitative and quantitative differences in the babbling development of normal-hearing and hearing-impaired infants.

Because their study included infants with varying degrees of hearing loss, Stoel-Gammon and Otomo noted that although all the hearing-impaired babies' babbling development was different from that of the normal-hearing infants, the magnitude of difference appeared to be smaller for those with moderate hearing loss compared with those with severe to profound hearing loss. The parental histories obtained in this study suggested not only that normal prelinguistic and early linguistic development (i.e., onset of babbling and meaningful vocal play) was arrested as a result of sudden onset of deafness, but also that the developing speech patterns reverted to behaviors resembling those predominating at earlier stages of development.

This study and others showed the important link between random articulatory movements and the resulting acoustic outcomes to the presence of self-monitoring through the auditory sense. The inability of hearing-impaired babies to hear their own vocalizations prevents them from the acoustic self-stimulation that encourages additional babbling and the consequential expansion of new speech sounds. The results obtained by Stoel-Gammon and Otomo suggest that significant hearing loss affects prelinguistic vocalizations by 8 month of age and possibly earlier. In their analysis of consonantal utterances, the point of divergence between their two groups of subjects was around 6–8 months, implying that at that age hearing loss began to influence the development of the consonantal repertoire.

By 5 months, Chinese children produce the intonation of the Chinese language. Also, by 5 months Polish infants' babbling can be distinguished from the babbling of English infants (Weir, 1966). The later skills of linguistic organization are undoubtedly dependent on these early activities. Reddy and Rao (1977) found that infants between 12 and 21 days of age could imitate both facial and manual gestures. Even sequential finger movement (opening and closing the hand by serially moving the fingers) was imitated. The infant, indeed, enters the world equipped with skills that appear innate to humans. Even facial expressions can be discriminated, according to Field, Woodson, Greenberg, et al. (1982). They exposed 74 neonates (average, 36 hours) to 3 facial expressions (happy, sad, and surprised) and observed diminished visual fixation on each face over trials. The fixations were renewed on presentation of a different expression. What was surprising was that the babies made imitative facial movements that clued observers to the expressions of the model, at greater than chance accuracy.

A most intriguing opportunity for research presented itself to Kent et al. (1987) when they identified two identical twin boys, one of whom had a severe to profound, bilateral hearing loss and one of whom had normal hearing. The etiology of the hearing loss was undetermined, although the infant was first suspected to be hearing-impaired when he failed a routine hospital-screening test. Auditory brainstem (evoked) response and behavioral testing confirmed his

hearing loss, and he was fitted with binaural ear-level hearing aids and enrolled in habilitative services at the age of 3 months. These twin boys offered a rare opportunity to study the effects of hearing loss on vocal development with reasonable control over environmental and genetic factors. The primary objectives of the study conducted by Kent et al. were to obtain longitudinal information on (1) fundamental frequency levels and contours, (2) formant frequencies of vocalic utterances, and (3) spectral characteristics of fricatives and trills. The acoustic data were collected via video and audio while the twins interacted with each other and with an adult (parent or investigator). The twins were evaluated at approximately 3-month intervals, beginning at the age of 8 months, again at 12 months, and again at 15 months.

The results of this unique investigation are presented for syllable shapes, formant patterns, and phonetic inventories obtained from transcriptions of the audiotapes of the twins between 8 and 15 months of age. Histograms of peak fundamental frequencies of syllable productions of the normal-hearing child (called Ned) and the hearing-impaired child (called Hal) at the age of 8 months are shown in Figure 5-2. According to the research team, Hal often showed a phona-

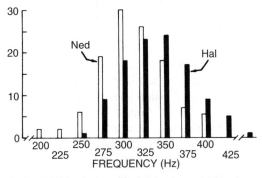

Figure 5-2. Histograms of peak fundamental frequencies of syllable productions of Ned and Hal at 8 months. (Reproduced with permission from Kent, K.D., Osberger, M.J., Netsell, R., Hustedde, C.G. (1987). Phonetic development in identical twins differing in auditory function. *Journal of Speech and Hearing Research, 52,* 66.)

tory pattern in his utterances that was highly variable, and this hearing-impaired twin had a larger range of peak fundamental frequency values and a higher model value as shown in the histograms. The composite data for vocalic formant frequencies F1 and F2 were determined from spectrograms and plotted as shown in Figures 5-3 and 5-4. The composite F1-F2 results for Ned, the normal-hearing twin (Fig. 5-4), show a configuration of the vowel region over the developmental period. A very different pattern is shown for Hal in Figure 5-4, where the developmental pattern is one of marked constriction such that by the age of 15 months the F1-F2 region is contained within the low-frequency portion of the pattern exhibited at 8 months.

As would be expected from the syllable structure data, Hal and Ned differed significantly in their consonant productions. Of special interest is the fact that unlike the normal-hearing twin—who produced fricatives at several places of articulation, including labiodental, alveolar, palatal, and pharyngeal—Hal was not heard to make even a single fricative sound. Table 5-4 shows the frequency of occurrence

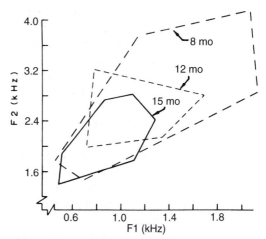

Figure 5-4. Composite F1-F2 data for Hal's vocalic segments at 8, 12, and 15 months. (Reproduced with permission from Kent, K.D., Osberger, M.J., Netsell, R., Hustedde, C.G. [1987]. Phonetic development in identical twins differing in auditory function. *Journal of Speech and Hearing Research, 52,* 68.)

data for place of consonant production in the spontaneous vocalizations of Hal and Ned at 24 months. Although Hal's syllable production was greatly diversified at 24 months compared with 8 months, his vocalizations continued to be narrower in range than those of Ned.

In their summary, Kent et al. indicate that the spontaneous vocalizations of the twin boys were clearly different as early as 8 months of age. The hearing-impaired twin's vocal productions were much less

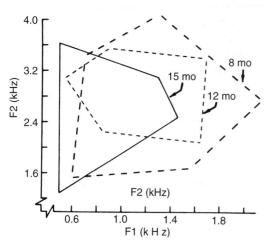

Figure 5-3. Composite F1-F2 data for Ned's vocalic segments at 8, 12, and 15 months. (Reproduced with permission from Kent, K.D., Osberger, M.J., Netsell, R., Hustedde, C.G. [1987]. Phonetic development in identical twins differing in auditory function. *Journal of Speech and Hearing Research, 52,* 67.)

Table 5.4.
Frequency of Occurrence Data for Place of Consonant Production in the Spontaneous Vocalizations of Hal and Ned at 24 Months of Age

Place	Hal	Ned
Bilabial	12 (15%)	29 (43%)
Dental	1 (1%)	9 (13%)
Alveolar	60 (77%)	15 (22%)
Palatal	4 (5%)	5 (7%)
Velar	0 (0%)	5 (7%)
Glottal	1 (1%)	6 (9%)
Total	78	67

With permission from Kent, K.D., Osberger, M.J., Netsell, R., & Hustedde, C.G. (1987). Phonetic development in identical twins differing in auditory function. *Journal of Speech and Hearing Research 52,* 69.

variable than the normal-hearing twin, with a fundamental frequency variability that had a wide range extending from a glottal roll to a shriek. The hearing-impaired twin had a restricted range of vowel production and few consonants as late as 15 months of age. This incredible research study has provided the basis of quantitative speech science differences in a unique study sample (identical twins) in which genetic and environmental differences can be assumed to be minimal.

Research has shown that babies learn the basics of their native language by the age of 6 months, long before they utter their first words. Newborns are "language universalists" in that they can learn any sound in any language and distinguish among all the sounds that adults utter. Continued exposure to their native language, however, reduces babies' ability to perceive sounds that are not in that language set. Kuhl, Williams, Iacerda, Stebens, and Lindblom (1992) used computerized speech to generate identical English and Swedish sounds that were presented to 64 6-month-old babies in a double-blind experiment conducted in both the United States and Sweden. The infants showed a significantly stronger preference for and accuracy in identifying the sounds from their own language. This important study demonstrates again that linguistic experience during the first 6 months of life affects an infant's perception of speech sounds.

More amazing than imitation is the *auditory localization* (finding a sound in space) of very young infants (Bower, 1975). Young babies observed their mother through a soundproof glass screen, with the voice of the mother coming at various positions of a loudspeaker. So long as the sound came from where the mother was, the baby was quite happy. But when the voice came from a speaker in another position, the infants manifested surprise and upset, indicating not only auditory localization but also an expectation that voices will come from mouths. Clifton (1998) demonstrated experimentally in newborns that normal-hearing infants show dramatic improvement in precision of localization ability within the first year of life, when the minimum audible angle detectable decreases from more than 20° to approximately 8°. Infants must make constant adjustments between timing and localization based on visual feedback to be able to improve performance over time. Sininger et al. (1999) states that localization ability is a clear example of the way in which human newborns integrate auditory experience (in this case with visual experience) to rapidly develop near-normal function in the first year of life. Adults seem to have lost such localization, being unaware for example that voices in movies come from a place other than the screen.

The long period of reception of auditory language symbols is the prerequisite to later language formulation. By the time speech and language emerge, there have been 12–18 months of receiving complex adult spoken language and distilling it into the matrix of the child language structure. This act of refining out of a complex language structure the basic one- and two-word sentences that are the baby's first speech language utterances must rank as creation's noblest day. Listening to language for a long period is essential to the ultimate usage of language. From the studies described above, it is evident that this listening is not a passive process but one in which the infant participates by acting on the incoming signals. By the time the child's first meaningful word is uttered, miraculously full-blown at around 1 year, a whole world of listening activity has taken place. Nothing the infant will ever achieve is as intellectually complex as what preceded that first speech utterance.

OPTIMAL PERIODS

How early is it necessary for the hearing-deprived child to receive language input to avoid language retardation? The answer to this question is based on whether there exist critical, or optimal, periods for the development of various functions. The theory of critical periods states that there are certain periods in development when the organism is programmed to receive and utilize particular types of stimuli, and that subsequently the stimuli will have gradually diminishing potency in affecting the organism's development in the function represented. In the case of audition, it means that at a certain developmental stage auditory signals will be optimally received and utilized for important prelinguistic activities, but that once this stage has passed, the effective utilization of these signals gradually declines. An analogous theory for language development holds that language input must be experienced at a certain stage, or it becomes decreasingly effective for utilization in emergent language skills.

The most vociferous opponent of this theory was Bench (1971), who claimed that the concept has no more than heuristic value and that its importance in the field of diagnostic audiology has been greatly overemphasized. Bench's argument requires the critical period theory demand an irreversibility of the effects. That is to say, if a method can be found to change the effects back to normal (reversing the apparently irreversible), then the so-called critical period is not critical after all. Although Bench's logic holds true, recent experiments have revealed promising retraining possibilities, beyond critical periods of time, which are thought to be due to the plasticity of the brain.

The modern theory of neuroplasticity is based on beliefs in optimal periods. A flood of scientific research in recent years has substantiated the fact that the neuronal pathways are laid down in the brain during the first 3 years of life, and after that time it is very difficult to rewire the pathways. This is probably the basis of the proverb, "You can't teach an old dog

new tricks." However, knowledge of the plasticity of the brain has opened new doors for various therapies, including sports training, wherein repetition exploits the neuroplasticity of the brain to retrain the cortex and form new pathways.

Lenneberg (1967) is of the opinion that puberty marks the last milestone for acquisition of language. With regard to the effects of early deprivation, he cites the difference between the congenitally deaf child and the child who acquires deafness through meningitis after a brief exposure to language. He states that those who lose hearing after having been exposed to the experience of speech, even for as short a period as 1 year, can be trained much more easily in all language arts, even if formal training begins some years after they had become deaf. According to Lenneberg, "It seems as if even a short exposure to language, a brief moment during which the curtain has been lifted and oral communication established, is sufficient to give a child some foundation on which much later language may be based."

In a well-designed study, Templin (1966) compared the language skills of deaf children with the skills of matched groups of normal-hearing children. In some of the language areas the deaf showed no systematic improvement in their performance beyond 11 years. At that point such skills as understanding of word meanings, sentence construction, and analogies reached a plateau and remained there without further insights or improvements. The normal-hearing children went on to achieve to the 14-year language level that was the upper limits of the study. It should be emphasized that there was no substantial difference in intellectual abilities between the deaf and the normal-hearing group and that the deaf had had intensive language training in their schools. Their rate of learning up to 11 years was comparable with that of the normal-hearing group. But an irreversible language deficit appeared at this age level and precluded further development. The complexity of language forms and of abstract language symbols takes a great leap around this age and leaves the deaf helplessly behind. The blame was ascribed to early language deprivation covering many periods optimal for language learning.

Yoshinaga-Itano and Apuzzo (1995) compared the language abilities of 46 hearing-impaired children identified before 6 months of age with 63 similar children identified after 6 months of age. All the children had bilateral hearing losses ranging from mild to profound. In longitudinal evaluations of both groups, a consistent advantage existed for the group identified before 6 months of age. The language skills advantage for the early identified children became more pronounced as the children aged. For children assessed between 13 and 18 months, there was only a slight advantage for the early group compared with the late group. For children in the 19- to 24-month-old category, the early group showed a 3-month developmental advantage; for children in the 25- to 30-month category, the early children showed a 4-month advantage. By the age of 31–36 months, the children identified early had a 10-month language advantage over the late identified group. Although these studies speak volumes for support of early intervention, they also reflect results that may be interpreted in favor of optimal period theory.

The reports of animal research supporting optimal period theory of development are numerous. Reisen (1947) reported that a chimpanzee raised in total darkness for the first 3 months of life never developed adequate vision. However, if chimpanzees are raised in light for the first 3 months and subjected to total darkness for the next 6 months, they quickly regain perfect vision when exposed to light. The analogous situation in humans is found in the child born with strabismus of one eye (thrown to a side focus). Ophthalmologists report that unless that eye is forced to be used, through patching the other eye, by the age of 4 no useful perceptions can ever be developed in it despite the fact that organically it is a perfect organ of vision. It is the central perception of vision that, untrained during critical periods, can never regain function. There seems to be no demonstrated reason why auditory perceptions do not fall into the same category as the visual modality.

According to Sininger et al. (1999), mice raised in a regular sound environment have, as expected, normal development in the neurons of the auditory nervous system, whereas mice exposed to noxious stimuli throughout development showed nonnormal neurons in the auditory pathway. Other animal studies have shown that the type of acoustic stimulation to which the auditory nervous system is exposed determines its mature response pattern. Reisen (1960) reported that chimpanzees showed a reduction in the efficiency of auditory learning following early sensory deprivation of hearing. In addition, he found that in cats deprived of visual sensation, three concomitant manifestations were present: hyperexcitability, increased susceptibility to convulsive disorder, and localized motor dysfunction.

These animal experiments have profound implications for the student of human deafness development. What is the effect of language deprivation on the deaf infant? If biologic theories of language acquisition are correct, then the human infant is just as preprogrammed to develop language skills as to develop motor skills. The effect of early sensory deprivation could then be expected to have far-reaching consequences on CNS functioning in integrative areas of the brain. The concept of language as a biologically predetermined function thus extends the speculation of early sensory deprivation in humans to another plane where animal research cannot apply. What are the effects of early learning deprivation on the CNS? Many clinicians have described symbolic language disorder, minimal cerebral dysfunction, or other kinds of central involvement in the deaf. Can these disorders be a direct result of auditory deprivation?

Edwards (1968) described the educator's attitude toward optimal periods in words that still ring true today:

The supremely difficult feat of building language recognition and response which takes place during the first years of life can occur because there is a built-in neurological mechanism for language learning present in every normal human organism. But like the image on the sensitized negative, this potential will not appear as reality unless the proper circumstances develop it. Experience—the right experience—is essential.

Heredity and environment interact. Hereditary possibilities are shaped by the influence that only human culture can provide; they are potentialities that must be developed while the young neurological organism is still rapidly growing, malleable, open to stimulus. If the "critical periods in learning" hypothesis applies to human beings...then the right experience must come at the right time, or the potential must remain forever unrealized.

We are going to have to make educational stimulation available from babyhood on for the children whose families cannot provide it for them. Whether tutors should go into the homes, whether children should be brought into carefully planned, well staffed *educational* (as distinct from baby-sitting day-care) programs, we do not now know. Experiments going on in several places in the country should help us decide. But however we do it, intervention by the age of 18 months should be the rule for the children of deprived inner-city or poor rural families. [Reprinted with permission from Edwards, E.P. (1968). Kindergarten is too late. *Saturday Review,* 70–77.]

Considered from the physiologic point of view, the infant's auditory system is plastic (i.e., it can be modified not only by anatomic alteration but also by variations of acoustic stimuli). Absent or faulty sound stimuli will result in deviant auditory function. According to Ruben and Rapin (1980), the central and peripheral auditory systems exert reciprocal control over each other. As the inner ear matures, its input is necessary to the development of at least part of the auditory nervous system. By the time the peripheral auditory system is fully developed, its input seems to be necessary for the maturation and innervations of portions of the central auditory system (Webster & Webster, 1977, 1979, 1980; Clopton & Silverman, 1977). Therefore, environmental sounds have the greatest effect in shaping auditory ability from the time the inner ear and eighth cranial nerve first become functional to the time when maturation of the CNS is achieved, roughly from the fifth month of gestation to between 18 and 28 months. The consequences of these findings for intervention programs for the hearing-impaired are strikingly apparent. The time for action is early in the first year of life, as demonstrated by numerous studies described in this chapter.

Consider the results of a study conducted at the Lexington School for the Deaf (Greenstein, Greenstein, McConville, et al., 1976). Thirty severely hearing-impaired children who had been admitted to the school before their second birthdays were studied. Two groups were identified: those who had been admitted before 16 months of age and those admitted between 16 and 24 months of age. The children were given standardized tests that revealed that the children admitted before 16 months of age were consistently superior to the later-admitted children in all aspects and at all age levels. Regardless of what caused the differences, its occurrence before 16 months was the variable responsible for the improved speech and language. Here is evidence relating learning ability in the hearing-impaired to time of identification of the hearing loss.

We have looked to studies of children who have been socially and sensorally deprived since infancy to shed light on the periods necessary for acquisition of language. The 1797 "wild boy of Aveyron" remained mute and incapable of even subtle communication even after Dr. Itard attempted to teach and socialize him in his preteen years (Lane, 1977). The description of Genie (Fromkin, Krashen, Curtiss, et al., 1974), who was isolated in a closet for 11 years of her life, states that this is "a case of language acquisition beyond the 'critical period.'" However, Genie's history shows that she was exposed to family life for her first 20 months before being placed in isolation until age 13 years, 9 months. The reported language abilities that she acquired after being rescued from a pitiful situation are actually what one could predict for anyone having had 20 months of normal language input. The really critical periods for language during which Genie had exposure laid the matrix from which her language skills could develop.

EARLY INTERVENTION

Early intervention is a broad term that describes the need to begin habilitation services as soon as a disability is confirmed. In children with hearing loss, early intervention means providing and fitting of hearing aids as well as providing counseling and supportive services to parents and primary caregivers to help them accept and understand the child's diagnosis. Early intervention is the course of action taken to achieve the proper steps to obtain the services needed by the child. The pediatric audiologist may be the first informant to the parents that their child has a hearing loss. Following confirmation of the hearing loss through a medical specialist's evaluations, the audiologist may again be the first professional to discuss intervention steps with the parents. As pointed out by Luterman (1996), this may present a challenge because the ability to impart knowledge and expertise to parents, without imposing personal opinions, is a delicate art. It takes time and confidence to build a trusting relationship with parents so that all parties are comfortable shar-

ing and disagreeing about strongly held beliefs. Intervention planning requires ongoing sharing of information in interactive sessions that allows the audiologist and parents to respect, react, and respond to each other.

Scientists have thoroughly documented the importance of early developmental years for the well-being and normal development of each individual. The goal for deaf and hearing-impaired children is the development of language skills commensurate with their normal-hearing peers, regardless of the degree of hearing loss, the mode of communication, socioeconomic status, cultural ethnicity, or gender. Pediatric audiologists strive to achieve language development that is commensurate with the child's cognitive potential. Rather than focusing energy on closing the developmental delay, Yoshinage-Itano (1999) believes that the focus should be on prevention of developmental delay though early identification and appropriate early intervention services. The manner in which individuals are able to function in preschool, adolescence, and even adulthood often depends on their experiences before the age of 30 months of age.

The basic components related to early hearing intervention include the following: (1) immediate counseling to support the parent's adaptation to the diagnosis and provide a forum in which they can express and work through their feelings, (2) the infant's impaired auditory system should be attended to and supplemented as quickly as possible through the appropriate fitting of hearing aids, and (3) encouragement should be given to the early development of a rich symbolic communication system between family members and the infant (Greenberg, Calderon, & Kusche, 1984). Early identification and intervention allow the family members to feel that they are doing all they can to assist the child and to bolster the child's sense of being. Such a program provides direct intervention with the child and a psychotherapeutic counseling experience for the parents to help them achieve satisfactory emotional adjustment to the birth of an infant with hearing impairment (First & Palfrey, 1994).

Many attempts have been made over the years to prove the efficacy of early intervention for hearing loss. The early research was limited by the fact that few children with hearing loss were identified before the age of 2 or 3 years. The early studies were also flawed because nearly all of them were retrospective rather than prospective. Fortunately, the past few years have been especially profitable in terms of prospective research in the area of early intervention, and a great many valuable insights have been established.

A number of development improvements have influenced the efficacy of studies of early intervention and hearing loss (Yoshinaga-Itano, 1995): These developments include the following points: (1) the age of identification has steadily decreased since the 1960s as assessment technologies have improved; (2) pediatric hearing aid strategies and fittings have improved dramatically; (3) advances in computer technology have influenced nearly every aspect of pediatric audiology; (4) changes have occurred in the modes of communication used in the education of children with hearing loss; (5) the widespread provision of parent-infant intervention and preschool education changed from the private sector to the public sector; (6) assessment tools for hearing, speech, and language development have improved; (7) the type of school placement and service delivery systems have improved; (8) the educational philosophies of parent-infant and preschool intervention have shifted to the family; (9) the basic etiologies of pediatric hearing loss have changed; and (10) the incidence of multiple handicapping conditions has increased.

An extremely important issue that affects the outcomes of early identification and intervention is the time interval, or delay pattern, between age of detection of the hearing loss and the age at which the initiation of services occurs. Fortunately, this time interval has decreased dramatically during the past 25 years. In 1984, Bergstrom called the situation "disgraceful." She reported data showing that although the average age of parental suspicion of deafness in a group of children was 10 months of age, it took until the children reached an average age of 21 months before a medical diagnosis of the hearing loss was determined. Further delay was noted because amplification and other intervention services were not initiated in these families until the children reached an average age of 27 months. The pattern of delays in these earlier years seemed to be due to three factors: (1) initial parental disbelief or denial of the fact that their child was hearing impaired, (2) delays due to physician scheduling and referrals to other specialists, and (3) many babies had multiple handicaps in which hearing was only part of the total concern of the parents. By the mid-1970s, statistics from our infant hearing-screening program at the University of Colorado Medical Center (Downs, 1986) showed that the average time between confirmation of the hearing loss and initiation of habilitation procedures was 6.5 months. In 1994, Strong, Clark, and Walden reported an average interval of 12 months from the time of diagnosis to intervention. Therefore, because their average age of identification was 2.5 years of age, the average age of intervention was 3.5 years of age—still too late. The 1994 and the 2000 Joint Committee on Infant Hearing statements called for infant hearing screening programs that will identify infants with hearing loss by 3 months of age so that intervention services can be instigated before 6 months of age.

Clearly, infants who are identified at birth with hearing loss have an important advantage over their later identified peers. Optimal intervention should begin as soon as the hearing loss in an infant is confirmed. Those infants identified early must receive intervention services so that they will have the opportunity to be exposed to a more abundant language environment that will enable them to achieve maximal language skills. The current universal infant-hearing screening programs are helping to identify infants with hearing loss at birth so that their hearing losses may be confirmed and diagnosed by the age of 2 months, and intervention begun immediately. Early identification of hearing loss can only be efficacious if quality early intervention is provided at the earliest possible time, certainly within the first year of life.

Federal law provides funds for states to participate in early intervention services for infants with hearing loss through Public Law 105-17. When hearing loss is identified, evaluation and early intervention services should be provided in accordance with the Individuals with Disabilities Educational Act (IDEA), Part H, Public Law 102-119 (formerly PL 99-457). Components of an early intervention program for children with hearing loss and their families should include the following:

- Family support and information regarding hearing loss and the range of available communication and educational intervention options. Such information must be provided in an objective, nonbiased way to support family choice. It is recommended to use consumer organizations and persons who are deaf or hard-of-hearing to provide such information. Professional, consumer, state, and community-based organizations should be accessed to provide ongoing information regarding legal rights, educational materials, support groups and networks, and other relevant resources for children and families.

- Implementation of learning environments and services designed with attention to the family's preferences. Such services should be family-centered and should be consistent with the needs of the child, the family, and their culture.

- Early intervention activities that promote the child's development in all areas, with particular attention to language acquisition and communication skills.

- Early intervention services that provide ongoing monitoring of the child's medical and hearing status, amplification needs, and development of communication skills.

The classic study by Levitt, McGarr, and Geffner (1987) reported measures on the development of speech and language in 120 children in the 10- to 14-year age bracket over a 4-year period. The children's hearing losses ranged from moderate 40 dB HL levels to profound hearing losses in excess of 80 dB HL. All the children in the study cohort were identified after 30 months of age. Following numerous longitudinal testing procedures, it was clear that the highest language skills were found in the children with the earliest intervention. A surprising finding in this research, however, was that the degree of hearing loss did not constitute a significant factor in later language skills and educational performance. The children with milder hearing losses showed the same reduced language skills as those children with profound hearing loss. The answer to this paradoxical finding is, of course, that none of these children had been identified at an age young enough to take advantage of the optimal periods for language learning. The equivalence of the language scores represented only the intense educational training that the children received, and did not reflect any benefit from a truly early intervention course of action. Speech intelligibility skills, as would be expected, were indeed directly proportional to the children's degree of hearing loss. Those children with the mildest hearing losses had the best speech; the children with the most severe hearing losses had the poorest speech. This finding is related to the fact that speech is an overlaid function, derived from a number of organs and structures that were developed for other uses, and dependent on accurate auditory reception for its production. The pathway to normalized speech and language patterns for the hearing-impaired child is a long journey (Fig. 5-5).

In another study of "earlier versus later," Watkins (1987) studied three groups of children with hearing impairment who received intervention services at different times in their developing years. Group 1 children received 9 months of home intervention before 30 months of age; group 2 children attended preschool beginning at 36 months of age; group 3 children did not receive any intervention services until they began school at 60 months of age. When all three groups of children were 10 years old, the results of a number of evaluations showed that for all variables assessed, the children who received the earliest and therefore the most intervention performed the best. The average child in this study who received early intervention performed better than 75–92% of the children in the groups that received later or no intervention.

In England, Robinshaw (1995) described a group of 5 young children whose deafness had been confirmed between 3 and 5 months of age, and who received intervention with hearing aids before the age of 7 months. He compared these deaf children with 5 normally hearing children and 12 similarly deaf children whose average age of identification was later than 24 months. His results showed that by 5 years of age, the earlier-identified group of children developed speech and language skills similar to the normal-hearing control group of children. These results buttress the argument for early intervention.

The Colorado Projects in Early Intervention. Under the direction of Christine Yoshinaga-Itana, a professor at the University of Colorado, the last half of the 1990s produced a number of important research studies that have had a profound effect on the acceptance of early identification of children with hearing loss and the concomitant value of early intervention. These research projects were largely made possible by the fact that several newborn hearing screening programs had been in effect in Colorado for nearly 20 years, making a large sample of children with hearing impairment of varying degrees available for studies. These now classic studies provide an impressive framework in which to develop additional studies as more is learned about the importance of early intervention in the lives of special needs children.

Yoshinaga-Itano, Sedey, Coulter, and Mehl (1998) reported on a selected group of children with hearing losses gleaned from a database of nearly 500 Colorado children with hearing impairment who had been carefully monitored for 10 years. From this series of subjects, 150 children with varying degrees of hearing losses and varying ages of identification and intervention were enlisted for her preliminary study. Approximately 50% of the group were identified and entered intervention activities before the age of 6 months; the remaining 50% were identified, and of course intervened with, at

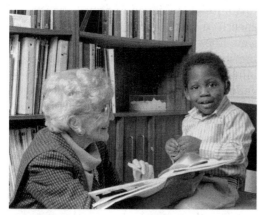

Figure 5-5. Language and speech development is a life-long task for the child with hearing impairment.

later ages. The children in both groups all had bilateral, congenital hearing losses ranging from a 27 dB HL average to hearing losses greater than 110 dB HL. Particular attention was given to matching the two groups of subjects as closely as possible to be sure that all of the children had received intervention immediately as soon as they were identified to have significant hearing loss.

All study children were given the Minnesota Child Development Inventory (MCDI) when they were between 13 and 36 months of age (Ireton & Thwing, 1974). The MCDI is a 320-item questionnaire that is filled out by the child's primary caregiver. It is composed of eight subtests that evaluate different areas of development including general development, gross motor skills, fine motor skills, expressive language, comprehensive-conceptual (language understanding), personal-social, comprehensive-situational (nonverbal understanding), and self-help scales. Children are considered to be functioning within normal developmental limits if their developmental age is greater than 75% of their chronologic age. The MCDI identifies children as "borderline delayed" (delay between 25 and 30% of chronologic age) and "delayed" (developmental age lower than 70% of chronologic age). Yoshinaga-Itano used the MCDI to compare the developmental scores of the children who were earlier-identified versus later-identified by a number of variables that included cognitive ability, age at time of testing, communication mode, minority status, gender, degree of hearing loss, socioeconomic status, and presence or absence of other disabilities in addition to hearing impairment.

The positive effects of early identification and early intervention showed consistently across all the variables analyzed by the Yoshinaga-Itano group. The group of children with hearing losses identified between birth and 6 months of age had significantly higher developmental functioning at 40 months of age than the group of later-identified children. Both

the receptive language and expressive language scores reflected a significant difference between the two groups in favor of the early identified-early intervened children. In addition, those children with normal cognitive abilities who were identified and received intervention before the age of 6 months achieved language skills well within the normal range of functioning for their age. Even children with lower cognitive quotients showed positive benefit from early identification and intervention. Somewhat surprisingly, when the early-identified children with mild hearing losses (26–40 dB HL) were compared with children in their cohort with profound hearing losses (greater than 90 dB HL), there was no appreciable difference in language skills. Personal-social quotients were significantly lower in the mild hearing loss group than for the profound hearing loss group, suggesting a greater need for attention to those children with milder hearing losses than previously thought necessary.

Finally, analysis of speech intelligibility concurred almost exactly with the earlier Levitt et al. (1987) findings. Speech intelligibility of the Colorado study children was directly proportional to the degree of hearing loss, regardless of the age of identification or the age at which intervention services were initiated. However, the early-identified children with all degrees of hearing loss (except the profoundly deaf) ultimately achieved normal range of speech intelligibility, albeit on different time lines. The children with milder hearing losses acquired good speech intelligibility by 31–36 months of age, whereas the children with moderate and severe hearing loss took 37–61 months to achieve optimal speech intelligibility. The effects of other demographic variables such as ethnicity, maternal education level, and communication mode were generally nonsignificant except for gender. Males in the study yielded a higher total intelligence quotient than females.

The findings of the important studies from Colorado demonstrate that early identification of infants with hearing problems, when followed by immediate and appropriate intervention, does indeed improve the outcomes for these children by resulting in significantly better performances in language, speech, and educational progress. Although mean language scores for early-identified children were within the low normal range, their developmental quotients were lower than those reported for normal-hearing children. Most of the children identified early in the Colorado programs are performing better than traditionally expected. Their performance is remarkably close to age level as measured in the children who were identified by 2 months of age. Regardless of the degree of hearing loss present, the trend for significant improvement in the children of the study cohort is related to early identification and early intervention (Yoshinaga-Itano & Apuzzo, 1995; Yoshinaga-Itano, 1999).

There is a growing body of research demonstrating that intensive early intervention can alter positively the cognitive and developmental outcomes of young infants with disabilities and reduce the levels of family stress reactions, as cited in a valuable tutorial review prepared by Carney and Moeller (1998). They concluded that enriched intervention programs provide some children with hearing loss with the ability to overcome developmental lags in language and academic skills. There has been considerable evidence that the natural give-and-take of communication that typically occurs with parents and infants can be disrupted when deafness occurs. In contrast, deaf parents of deaf infants appear to be effective interventionists for their children because of their understanding of deafness, their ability to communicate with sign, and their lack of conflict with deafness as a disability (Meadows-Orlans, 1987).

Optimal early intervention strategies provide appropriate services for the child with hearing loss and assure that families receive a full complement of consumer-oriented information. Families should be informed of organizations that enhance informed decision-making such as peer models, persons who are hearing-impaired or deaf, and consumer and professional associations. The 2000 Joint Committee on Infant Hearing Position Statement cites six principles of effective early intervention:

1. Developmental timing, referring to the age at which intervention services are initiated with the knowledge that programs that enroll infants at younger ages and continue longer are found to produce the greatest intervention benefits.
2. Program intensity, referring to the amount of intervention provided. This is measured by multiple factors such as the number of home visits or individual contacts per week.
3. Direct learning, implying that learning experiences are more effective when center-based educational activities are provided by trained professionals in addition to indirect home-based training.
4. Program breadth and flexibility, referring to the fact that successful intervention programs offer a broad spectrum of services and are flexible and multifaceted to meet the unique needs of the infant and family.
5. Recognition of individual differences, referring to the basic principle of education that states that individual progress and benefits from programs are functions of infant and family differences (i.e., not everyone progresses or benefits at the same rate).
6. Environmental support and family involvement, referring to the fact that the benefits of early intervention continue over time depending on the effectiveness of existing family and other environmental support (i.e., home, school, health, and peer).

FAMILY-CENTERED COUNSELING

Parents are their children's first teachers. Accordingly, the role of parental and family involvement with the child with hearing impairment is absolutely crucial. Although early intervention based on this premise has been suggested since the early 1950s, PL 94-142 mandated the shift to family-centered practices. Families can play a critical role in fostering language development. Children need to be immersed in a language-rich environment, and the family or the primary caregivers play an optimal role in accomplishing this. In the family-centered paradigm the basic concept is that parents, or the primary caregivers, will be able to make appropriate decisions if they have sufficient information and understand the factors involved in reaching these decisions. The audiologist performs the role of guide as an educator and facilitator in the provision of resources and in answering questions. Because of the enormous learning potential of infants, early parent intervention training programs have received considerable attention in recent years (Laughton, 1994).

When parents learn that their child has a disability or chronic illness, they begin a journey often filled with emotion, difficult choices, and interactions with many different professionals with an ongoing need for information and services. Parents react in ways that are entirely predictable and often documented. As summarized by Luterman (1996), parents are likely to go through periods of denial, grief, fear, and guilt followed by confusion, helplessness, disappointment, and even rejection. Not all parents go through each of these emotions, but it is important for parents to know that they are neither alone nor unique in all of these troublesome feelings. Table 5-5 provides suggestions for constructive actions that may help parents or primary caregivers through their rampant emotional reactions to learning that their child has a hearing loss.

Parents can easily become overloaded by the onslaught of information that is communicated when they learn that their child has a disability. The process is part

Table 5.5.
Constructive Suggestions and Actions for Parents

Seek assistance from another parent

Talk with your mate, family, or significant other

Rely on positive sources in your life

Take one day at a time

Learn the terminology

Seek information

Do not be intimidated

Show emotion

Learn to deal with natural feelings and emotions

Maintain a positive outlook

Keep in touch with reality

Remember that time is on your side

Find programs for your child

Take care of yourself

Avoid pity

Decide how to deal with others

Keep daily routines as normal as possible

Remember to love your child

Recognize that you are not alone

Adapted from Smith, P.M. (1997, February). *National parent network on disabilities, news digest* (2nd ed.). Washington, DC.

of the effort to initiate early intervention services and must be handled with confidence and skill. The parents or primary caregivers are suddenly immersed in information regarding management of their hearing impaired child, application of personal amplification devices, recommended changes in their daily living, concerns for the social interactions and communications within the family structure, as well as decisions that must be made regarding educational approaches and placements. The role of the audiologist is an important one in this context, and a thorough understanding of the many complexities, potential diversions, and personal conflicts that may arise among family members must be taken into account in each counseling session.

Lucker (2000) describes two cognitive modes used by people to reach decisions. The first is the holistic approach in which information is best understood when it is presented in whole stories. Holistic thinkers tend to gather information from the totality of the situation and then break it down into its parts. The second method is the analytic approach demonstrated by thinkers who need the pieces broken down first, and then they put the pieces back together to understand the information. Audiologists can be more successful in the roles of educators and facilitators if they first identify which type of approach would better convey information to parents, families, and caregivers. The efficacy of audiology services largely depends on whether patients thoroughly understand the counseling and advice given them. Being aware of how they communicate with patients can indeed have a significant impact on the success of audiologists' services.

An interesting discussion presented by Rushmer (1994) helps one understand the family constellation. The pediatric audiologist must develop a keen sense of appropriate timing and respect for the family's role in determining future directions for their child newly identified as having a hearing loss. Families are a collection of unique individuals, usually related but not always, who represent certain cultural and social histories. Most importantly, successful families alter their life styles to accommodate a child with special needs. Unfortunately, not all families can be considered successful in this ability to adjust to the needs of the hearing-impaired child. The audiologist needs to understand the complexities of a specific family unit, such as its size, health, interaction patterns, and socioeconomic factors, to assist effectively in developing a habilitation program that best fits its members. Added to these complexities presented by the traditional family are the special problems faced by working parents, the single parent, and various other nontraditional families.

The changing roles of the parents and the professional reflect the important fact that the child must always be considered an extension of the family. Typically, hearing-impaired children are born to parents who have little knowledge of the child's disability. In the past, the professional acted as an outside expert who imparted selected information to the uninformed parents and then made critical decisions on behalf of the child. However, in the 1980s a new awareness developed for the importance of the family in the successful habilitation of the child with special needs. The professional's role changed to being involved in a collaborative process with the parents to determine what is best for both the child and the family. The professional must understand that a family-centered approach to intervention and habilitation is individualized on the basis of each family's resources, priorities, and concerns (Baily, 1994). According to Roush and McWilliam (1994), the family-centered approach assumes that (1) outside social supports will affect family functioning, (2) the child's needs are best met by meeting family needs, and (3) families have the right to retain as much control as they desire over the intervention process.

The basic tenet underlying family-centered counseling is the understanding that what affects one member of the family affects all family members, and that the child's needs are best met by meeting family needs. The following basic principles provide a good summary of the family-centered approach to intervention (Dunst, Trivette, Starnes, Hamby, & Gordon, 1993):

- Recognize that the family, not the individual, is the unit of intervention.
- Foster the family's sense of competency and independence.
- Respect the parents' right and responsibility to decide what is best for their child.
- Help mobilize resources for coordinated, normalized service delivery.
- Develop a collaborative relationship with the family.

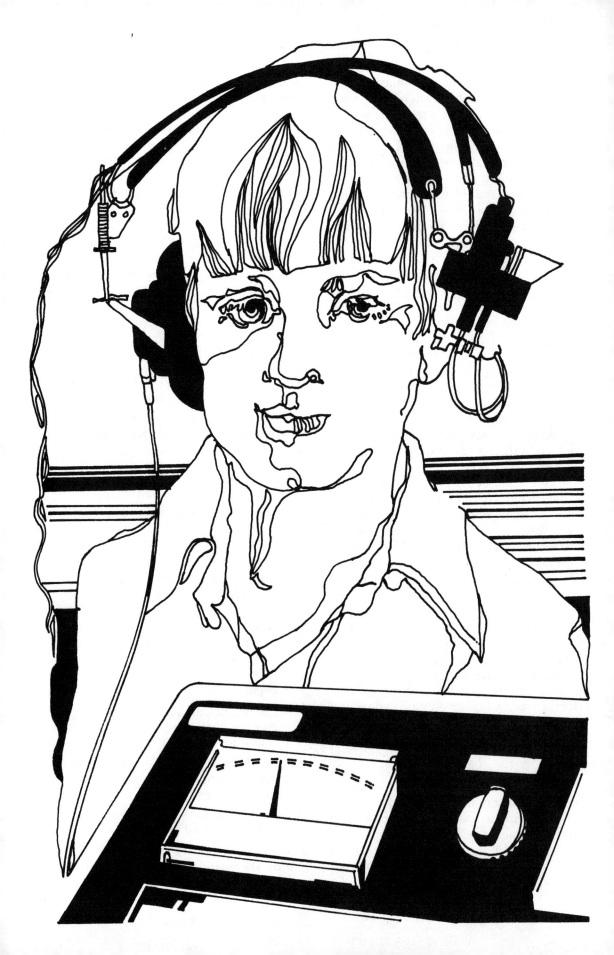

CHAPTER 6

Behavioral Hearing Testing

Modern technology has greatly increased the number of options available to test the hearing of infants and young children. However, regardless of how sophisticated testing techniques become, there will always be need for the behavioral hearing evaluation. Many of the newer testing procedures require expensive equipment or lengthy time commitments. Audiologists must be cautioned regarding the false sense of confidence provided by hearing test results obtained with physiologic "objective" techniques. Every clinician must be well versed in the understanding and the application of basic behavioral pediatric audiometry. With experience in pediatric audiology, a battery of special testing procedures becomes available for use in the daily clinical setting, and decisions need to be made for cost- and time-effective protocols to be used with each infant and child. Electrophysiologic tests can be used to estimate auditory sensitivity but are not true tests of hearing; thus, they should never be a substitute for behavioral audiometry in children.

Auditory evaluation of hearing in children should not be considered complete until specific thresholds are obtained for octave interval frequencies from 250 to 4000 Hz in each ear. A variety of testing procedures might be needed to obtain this final result, and more than one test session may be necessary to achieve the complete hearing examination. Parents need to be advised that the pediatric hearing examination, especially when hearing impairment is suspected, is an ongoing, age-specific activity, so that as the child grows older, more accurate hearing results can be obtained.

Jerger and Hayes (1976) advocate use of the cross-check principle in pediatric audiometry. They caution that simple behavioral observation of auditory behavior in children can be misleading and result in misdiagnosis of auditory problems and, ultimately, mismanagement of the hearing-impaired child. The cross-check principle uses physiologic test procedures, especially auditory brainstem response (ABR) audiometry, acoustic immittance, and otoacoustic emissions procedures as cross-checks of behavioral test results. They reason that behavioral test results need to be confirmed by independent test measures to reduce the potential errors of using behavioral results alone. In most cases, acoustic immittance audiometry and otoacoustic emissions will serve as cross-checks for behavioral audiometry. However, when these measures are in disagreement, ABR should be used to resolve the controversy (see Chapter 7).

The authors strongly recommend the use of insert earphones that are placed into the ear canal of the patient to perform air-conduction testing. In some children, the anatomy of the concha-meatus opening creates collapse of the ear canal from pressure of traditional earphones against the pinna, producing a pseudoconductive-type hearing loss. Audiometric testing will show an erroneous air-bone gap from the supposed conductive hearing loss. The pseudoconductive hearing loss will not be confirmed by the cross-check of test results with acoustic immit-tance measures, otoacoustic emissions testing, or otologic examination. The use of insert earphones, or even sound field testing, will eliminate any potential for the collapsed ear canal problem.

The experience of the audiologist is the main key to successful evaluation of the pediatric patient. A broad test battery ap-proach with children is the recommended clinic protocol. Audiologists who work with pediatric patients must have the skills and flexibility to incorporate any and all of the testing procedures at a mo-ment's notice as well as the knowledge and experience to know when to change approaches during the testing period.

TESTING PROCEDURES

Considerable progress has been made in recent years in the development of bet-ter, more accurate procedures to evaluate hearing in infants and young children. Wilson and Thompson (1984) classified the behavioral audiologic testing of chil-dren into two major divisions: techniques used without reinforcement, and proce-dures based on reinforcement of the in-fant's or child's responses. During the early 1970s, considerable research was devoted to defining the most effective stimulus-response characteristics to be used in the assessment of a child's hear-ing abilities. Test procedures that do not incorporate reinforcement principles are known as *behavioral observation audiom-etry* (BOA). Procedures that use reinforce-ment to develop repeatable responses are known as conditioned audiometry and may be further described by the type of reinforcement used, such as visual rein-forcement audiometry (VRA).

BOA is a common nonreinforcement subjective procedure used in the hearing screening of infants and young children between 6 and 12 months of age. This technique can also be used to screen the hearing of older children through 24 months of age. In general terms, the audi-ologist presents some type of calibrated auditory stimulus and observes the in-fant's or toddler's response to the pres-ence of the sound, which the audiologist then interprets as the child "hearing" the stimulus. BOA requires a reflexive or ac-tive response from an infant or toddler passively standing by or quietly involved in a simple task. An example of this tech-nique is the presentation of an auditory stimulus to a lightly sleeping infant while observing behavioral changes that are time-locked to the stimulus presentation. BOA has numerous limitations, including rapid habituation of responses. The rein-forcement used and the response magni-tude are dependent on many variables, including the state of the infant or child during the procedure, the parameters of the acoustic stimulus, the definition of an acceptable response, and the subjective decision by the audiologist as to whether a response occurred.

The *conditioning approach* to assess-ing hearing levels in infants and children uses a stimulus-response-reinforcement paradigm to elicit repeatable responses. In these procedures, the response is clearly defined and cued by the presenta-tion of auditory stimulus. The response is actually strengthened through the use of various reinforcements. In this approach, the infant or child is an active participant in the testing situation. Although studies have shown that infants as young as 6 months can be evaluated with condition-ing techniques, typically these techniques are used with children between 12 and 48 months of age. As an example of a condi-tioning technique, VRA is used to rein-force the head-turning, localization re-sponse of an infant or child with an at-tractive, illuminated stimulus.

The use of behavioral and conditioning procedures with infants and young chil-dren may lack sufficient precision to es-tablish valid auditory sensitivity thresh-olds. Accordingly, Matkin (1977) sug-gested the use of minimum response level (MRL) to describe the lowest intensity of auditory stimulus that produces the desired response. Use of the term "minimal response level" rather than "auditory threshold" for pediatric hearing evaluations serves as a reminder that improvement in response behavior might be anticipated as the child matures and test results become more accurate.

PARENT INTERVIEW

In addition to the actual hearing test, audiologists can contribute insight into the auditory and oral behavior of the child. No one understands better than the experienced clinician the effect of a certain degree of loss on the child's behavior and how the history of auditory development relates to the onset and degree of loss. The audiologist's time will most valuably be spent in analyzing these aspects of the child's history. Very often, simple questions presented to the parent will help the audiologist anticipate and understand problems presented by the pediatric patient. Therefore, the sequence of the audiologic parental interview might be as follows:

1. Question the parents as to the chief concern that precipitated the visit: "Who referred the child?" "Do you believe your child has problems in hearing?"
2. If a hearing loss appears evident, query the parent as to the child's auditory and oral development:
   - At 0–4 Months. When the infant was sleeping quietly, did sudden noises awaken the baby momentarily? Did the infant jump to sudden loud noises?
   - At 4–7 Months. Did the baby begin at 4 months to turn toward sounds that were out of sight? Did the infant repetitively babble a large variety of sounds at 5 and 6 months? By 7 months did the baby turn directly to sounds or voices that were out of sight? What kinds of babbling

sounds were made at 6 and 7 months? Could the infant sit alone at 6 months?
   - At 7–9 Months. Did the baby turn to find the source of sounds out of direct sight? Did the baby gurgle or coo to voices or sounds that the baby could not see? Did the baby make sounds with rising and falling inflections?
   - At 9–13 Months. Did the baby turn and find a sound coming from behind? Did the infant begin to imitate some sounds and have a large variety of different sounds? Were some of them consonant sounds (buh, guh, duh)? Did the baby say "ma-ma-ma-ma" or just "mama?" What specific sounds did the baby say?
   - At 13–24 Months. Did the toddler hear you when you called from another room? Did the toddler make a noise in response or come to you? What words or sounds other than "mama" were made? Did the voice sound normal?

   AFrom this line of questioning and from listening to the child's voice quality and speech, the audiologist can derive clues as to the onset of the hearing loss and its degree. If the voice quality is strident and only vowel sounds are made, an early severe hearing loss would be suspected. If the voice quality is good, in the presence of an evidently severe loss, a later onset would be suspected. Particularly if the child has some words or even sounds in normal intonation, a later onset is suggested. Such clues are helpful in determining the etiology and onset of the hearing loss.
3. Administer a pediatric audiology test battery to determine if the child has hearing within normal limits or if a hearing loss is present.

To help in understanding the etiology of the hearing loss, an informal, brief case history may reveal what aspects should be pursued in detail. Table 6-1 contains a list of questions that comprise a basic history that includes the primary items that place a child at risk for hearing loss. Table 6-2 presents a more detailed medical assessment questionnaire for children with sensorineural hearing impairment.

Table 6-3 shows the rapid development checklist approved by the American Academy of Pediatrics. Care should be taken in

Table 6.1.
Audiologic Case History Questionnaire for Parents of Children With Hearing Loss

I. *Chief complaint* _____

  When was problem first noted? _____

  Extent of problem _____

  Previous examinations and evaluations _____

  _____

II. *Prenatal history* _____

  Exposure to viral diseases during pregnancy? _____

  Which viral disorder? _____

  During which pregnancy month? _____

  Drugs during pregnancy? _____

  Trauma during pregnancy? _____

III. *Birth history* _____

  Gestation age at birth _____

  Birth weight _____ Bilirubin level high? _____

  Asphyxia? _____ Meningitis? _____

IV. *Family history* _____

  Childhood deafness in family? _____

    Relationship to patient _____

  Birth defect or abnormalities _____

    In any other relatives? _____

V. *Developmental history* _____

  Age of first smile response? _____

  Age when sat up alone? _____

  Age when first crawled? _____

  Age of "stranger anxiety?"_____

  Age of walking? _____

VI. *Physical history* _____

  Cleft lip or palate _____ Submucous cleft

  Low-set ears _____ Poorly formed ears

  High fevers with illness _____ Seizures

  Ear infections _____ How many?

  Previous treatment for ear conditions? _____

VII. *What do you (parents) really think caused this hearing problem?*_____

  _____

  Name of child's pediatrician _____

  Names of other physicians who have seen this child_____

  _____

Table 6.2.
Sensorineural Hearing-Impaired Child Assessment

Name _____

Age _____

Date of Birth _____

Hospital # _____

Age child identified by M.D. (months) _____

Age suspected of loss by mother (months) _____

Family History

Were parents relatives before marriage	Yes	No
Family history of kidney disease	Yes	No
Family history of thyroid problems	Yes	No
Family history of progressive blindness	Yes	No
Family history of previous stillbirths or miscarriages	Yes	No
Family history of hearing loss	Yes	No
Another affected child in family	Yes	No
Mother worked outside home	Yes	No
Specify		
Father worked during pregnancy	Yes	No
Specify_____		

Maternal Factors

Drugs (inc. antibiotics)	Yes	No
Specify_____		
Exposure to chemicals	Yes	No
Specify_____		
Exposure to radiation	Yes	No
Specify_____		
Amniocentesis	Yes	No
Rh immunoglobulin given Rh or ABO incompatible	Yes	No
Maternal illness during pregnancy	Yes	No
Specify_____		
Bleeding	Yes	No
Anemia	Yes	No
Diabetes	Yes	No
Toxemia	Yes	No
Paternal illness during pregnancy	Yes	No
Specify_____		

During pregnancy, mother exposed to:

Measles	Yes	No
Mumps	Yes	No
Chickenpox	Yes	No
German measles	Yes	No

During pregnancy, mother diagnosed with:

Syphilis	Yes	No
Herpes virus	Yes	No
Influenza	Yes	No
Cytomegalovirus (CMV)	Yes	No
Toxoplasmosis	Yes	No
Other	Yes	No
Specify_____		

Delivery/Labor

Full-term pregnancy	Yes	No
Labor induced	Yes	No
Labor less than 3 hr	Yes	No
Labor longer than 24 hr	Yes	No
Premature membrane rupture	Yes	No

Bleeding	Yes	No
Forceps/assisted delivery	Yes	No
Cesarean section	Yes	No
Other	Yes	No
Specify_____		

Infant/Newborn Factors

Small birthweight (<2 kg/5 lb)	Yes	No
Birthweight (lb/oz) _____		
Apgar low at birth	Yes	No
In an intensive care unit	Yes	No
How long (wk) _____		
Breathing problems	Yes	No
O_2 given	Yes	No
How long (wk)		
Bilirubin >15 mg/100 ml	Yes	No
Congenital rubella	Yes	No
Defect of ear, nose, throat	Yes	No
Specify_____		
Congenital heart disease	Yes	No
Drugs (inc. antibiotics)	Yes	No
Specify_____		
Exposure to chemicals	Yes	No
Specify_____		
Exposure to radiation	Yes	No
Specify_____		
Paralysis	Yes	No
Seizures	Yes	No
Septicemia	Yes	No

Infant/Childhood History

Eye problems	Yes	No
Specify_____		
Balance/gait/incoordination		
Dizziness problems	Yes	No
Cerebral palsy	Yes	No
Seizures	Yes	No
Head trauma/skull	Yes	No
Ever hospitalized for:		
Meningitis	Yes	No
Encephalitis	Yes	No
Measles	Yes	No
Influenza	Yes	No
Rubella	Yes	No
CMV	Yes	No
Chickenpox	Yes	No
Septicemia	Yes	No
Diabetes	Yes	No
Sickle cell disease	Yes	No
Other (including conductive loss)	Yes	No
Specify_____		

Table 6.3.
Rapid Developmental Screening Checklist

NAME: . . . . D.O.B. . . . . 1st Visit . . . .

AGE			DATE	
1 mo:	Can he raise his head from the surface in the prone position?		Yes	No
	Does he regard your face while you are in his direct line of vision?		Yes	No
2 mo:	Does he smile and coo?		Yes	No
3 mo:	Does he follow a moving object?		Yes	No
	Does he hold his head erect?		Yes	No
4 mo:	Will he hold a rattle?		Yes	No
	Does he laugh aloud?		Yes	No
5 mo:	Can he reach for and hold objects?		Yes	No
6 mo:	Can he turn over?		Yes	No
	Does he turn toward sounds?		Yes	No
	Will he sit with a little support (with one hand)?		Yes	No
7 mo:	Can he transfer an object from one hand to another?		Yes	No
	Can he sit momentarily without support?		Yes	No
8 mo:	Can he sit steadily for about 5 minutes?		Yes	No
9 mo:	Can he say "ma-ma" or "da-da"?		Yes	No
10 mo:	Can he pull himself up at the side of his crib or playpen?		Yes	No
11 mo:	Can he cruise around his playpen or crib, or walk holding onto furniture?		Yes	No
12 mo:	Can he wave bye-bye?		Yes	No
	Can he walk with one hand held?		Yes	No
	Does he have a two-word vocabulary?		Yes	No
15 mo:	Can he walk by himself?		Yes	No
	Can he indicate his wants by pointing and grunting?		Yes	No
18 mo:	Can he build a tower of three blocks?		Yes	No
	Does he say six words?		Yes	No
24 mo:	Can he run?		Yes	No
	Can he walk up and down stairs holding rail?		Yes	No
	Can he express himself (occasionally) in a two-word sentence?		Yes	No
2½ yr:	Can he jump lifting both feet off the ground?		Yes	No
	Can he build a tower of six blocks?		Yes	No
	Can he point to parts of his body on command?		Yes	No
3 yr:	Can he follow two commands involving "on," "under," or "behind" (without gestures?)		Yes	No
	Can he build a tower of nine blocks?		Yes	No
	Does he know his first name?		Yes	No
	Can he copy a circle?		Yes	No
4 yr:	Can he stand on one foot?		Yes	No
	Can he copy a cross?		Yes	No
	Does he use the past tense properly?		Yes	No
5 yr:	Can he follow three commands?		Yes	No
	Can he copy a square?		Yes	No
	Can he skip?		Yes	No

Developed by the Committee on Children with Handicaps, American Academy of Pediatrics, New York Chapter 3, District II. This checklist is a compilation of developmental landmarks matched against the age of the child. These are in easily scored question form and may be checked "Yes" or "No." "No" responses at the appropriate age may constitute a signal indicating a possible developmental lag. If there is a substantial deviation from these values, then the child should be evaluated more carefully, taking into consideration the wide variability of developmental landmarks. (Adjust for prematurity, prior to 2 years, by subtracting the time of prematurity from the age of the child, i.e., a 2-month-old infant who was 1 month premature should be evaluated as a 1-month-old infant.)

interpreting some of the landmarks as indicative of normal hearing (see Chapter 5 for a discussion of babbling development in normal-hearing and hearing-impaired babies). A deaf infant coos and chuckles quite normally at 2–3 months, laughs aloud at 4 months, babbles in two sounds before 6 months, says something like "ma-ma" at 9 months, and may have a vocalization that sounds like "da-da" by 12 months. This sequence of events can be misleading. The parents of one deaf child in our clinic insisted that their boy had normal hearing at 1 year of age because, they reported, he said "mama" and "dada." Yet radiographic studies of the child's mastoids showed congenital gross bony abnormalities of the both inner ears that precluded the possibility of any hearing at birth. It is well to view such reports of early speaking with healthy skepticism.

THE AUDIOLOGIST AND THE CHILD

Too often audiologists say, "I don't like to work with young children—I can't depend on their responses, and they are too inconsistent to be relied upon." Nothing could be less true. Babies do just what they are supposed to do; the clinician often does not. The audiologist has to give the right stimulus in the right structured situation to get the right response. There are no poorly responding babies—only inadequately prepared clinicians.

What are the general rules about working with children of all ages? The audiologist should quickly establish an easy relationship with the parents by speaking pleasantly and in a relaxed manner with them. During this "hallway conversation" (as named by Renshaw & Diefendorf, 1998), the child will look back and forth between the audiologist and the parent(s). As the child watches the interaction develop, he or she will finally recognize that all is well and will likely relax. In other words, the child absorbs the cathexis between the audiologist and the parents and becomes at ease. Many clinicians prefer to work with a child alone without the parents present in the testing sound suite. This is fine if there is enough time to establish a relationship with the child. It may be quicker and easier to include the parents in the testing situation so that the child is less apprehensive and stays relaxed during the session. Parents are usually (although not always) quite cooperative, genuinely concerned, and entirely rational.

The most important piece of advice for every pediatric audiologist is to tell the child what the audiologist wants him or her to do—not to ask. In this respect, the very young and the very old are alike, and one handles them both not by asking whether they would like to do something (they never do) but by telling them firmly and pleasantly that this is what they are going to do. Children do just what is expected of them, and if the audiologist firmly expects them to do what he or she wants them to, they usually oblige. Occasionally, of course, a child balks and yells like a banshee anyway—you can't win them all, but give it a try! Children are a great deal easier to handle than most people think.

The audiologist should develop a staunch and fervid belief that when children hear a sound, they will react in a stereotyped way that is consistent with their level of mental functioning. This holds true for the hearing-impaired child and for the normal-hearing child. The child with a threshold of 80 dB for a given sound will respond at 85 dB like the normal-hearing child who hears the same sound at 5 dB above the normal-hearing threshold. A 2-year-old cognitively impaired child with a mental age of 1 year will respond near his or her threshold in the way a normal-hearing child of 1 year responds near his or her threshold. There is no mystique about observing the hearing-impaired child's responses; the answer, if there is any, is to become confidently familiar with the auditory behavior of normal-hearing children so that the lack of normal responses will be immediately evident and suggest the need for additional testing.

At the risk of becoming maudlin, another principle should be added—love every child as a human being. The clinician is often hard-put to develop any charitable feelings toward the wall-climber, the temper tantrum expert, and the withdrawn child, or in some cases the syndrome-ridden child with misshapen, contorted face and limbs. The same humanity underlies all these children, the kicker, the screamer, the silent one—all of them humanly acting out their protests at a world that has given them less than it has to others. They too can be loved.

BEHAVIORAL OBSERVATION AUDIOMETRY: BIRTH TO 2 YEARS OF AGE

Behavioral testing of children and infants is the cornerstone and foundation of pediatric audiology (Madell, 1998). During BOA, the testing of infants and young children is accomplished without reinforcement of responses and depends on the audiologist's subjective observation of responses under structured conditions. The major advantages to BOA are efficiency in time required and the lack of need for specialized equipment. The disadvantages of BOA include the fact that it is difficult to eliminate tester bias, the responses of infants and young children are quick to reach extinction without reinforcement, and a wide variance of responses are noted in such youngsters. BOA is useful for initial hearing screening but some form of operant reinforcement audiometry should be used in the establishment of specific hearing threshold data.

The use of noise-makers and sound field signals as acoustic stimuli in evaluating hearing responses in infants and young children can be extremely useful during BOA. Situations and circumstances will exist that require that the audiologist be able to administer and interpret simple behavioral responses to auditory noise-makers. Hearing tests of infants and young children with noise-makers and sound field signals without conditioning and reinforcement is often a first-level indicator of the presence of normal hearing or the suggestion of hearing impairment. Pediatric BOA is certainly the most cost- and time-effective way of evaluating hearing in newborns and children through 2 years of age. The intensity

levels and the expected behavioral responses of the normal-hearing newborn to 2-year-old child are shown in the Auditory Behavior Index shown in Table 6-4 and in Figures 6-1 and 6-2.

Kevin Murphy of Reading, England, (1962, 1979) developed the original concept for an auditory behavior index. This remarkable observer of infants and children diagrammed the quality of the behavioral responses of children to noise-makers. The value of such an index lies in its description of the normal maturation process that all normal-hearing infants go through during specific periods in their development. Some variability is to be expected around the age periods described for each auditory behavior, but one must be impressed with the consistency and predictability of the age limits at which certain auditory responses are noted. The information below on testing infants at various age levels is based on a firmly established auditory maturation sequence that all normal-hearing infants go through as they develop from birth to 12 months of age. The audiologist who works with infants, babies, and very young children must become familiar with the normal auditory maturation and know well the average age in months at which higher levels of responses occur.

The auditory responses of infants and young children can also be described in terms of *reflexive* or *attentive* behaviors. Reflexive behaviors include the startle (body) response, arm or leg jerks, slow limb movements, the auropalpebral reflex, change in sucking behavior, eyeblinks, and facial twitches. Attentive behaviors are described as quieting responses (decrease in ongoing activity), increase in ongoing activity, breath-holding or a change in breathing rate, onset of vocalization, sudden stopping of vocalization, starting or stopping crying, eyewidening, searching or localization, head-turning as in searching or localizing the sound source, smiling or other change in facial expression, brow-furrowing, or shriek of surprise. A commonly seen at-

Table 6.4.
Auditory Behavior Index for Infants: Stimulus and Level of Response[a]

Age	Noise-makers (Approximate dB SPL)	Warbled Pure Tones (dB HL)	Speech (dB HL)	Expected Response	Startle to Speech (dB HL)
0–6 weeks	50–70	75	40–60	Eye-widening, eye-blink, stirring or arousal from sleep, startle	65
6 weeks– 4 months	50–60	70	45	Eye-widening, eye-shift, eye-blink, quieting; beginning rudimentary head-turn by 4 months	65
4–7 months	40–50	50	20	Head-turn on lateral plane toward sound; listening attitude	65
7–9 months	30–40	45	15	Direct localization of sounds to side, indirectly below ear level	65
9–13 months	25–35	38	10	Direct localization of sounds to side, directly below ear level, indirectly above ear level	65
13–16 months	25–30	30	5	Direct localization of sound on side, above and below	65
16–21 months	25	25	5	Direct localization of sound on side, above and below	65
21–24 months	25	25	5	Direct localization of sound on side, above and below	65

Modified with permission from McConnell, F., & Ward, P.H. (1967). *Deafness in childhood*. Nashville, TN: Vanderbilt University Press.

[a]Testing done in a sound room.

tentive behavior in response to the presentation of a sound is when the child looks directly at the parent's face as though in expectation of finding the source of the sound.

As normal-hearing infants grow older, they respond to auditory stimuli at lower (softer) levels. The authors have developed guidelines shown in Table 6-4 that we call the Auditory Behavior Index, estimating the approximate sound level necessary to elicit responses from infants through toddlers for various stimuli. Audiologists are urged not to accept the Auditory Behavior Index as the final word for every child. Nor should the auditory behavior levels presented be depended on as absolute thresholds. Audiologists must gain experience testing normal-hearing infants and young children to recognize the expected responses with various noise-makers and sound field auditory stimuli. The value of the Index is enhanced for each clinician by determining individual style of eliciting auditory re-

sponses with acoustic stimuli at hand and performing the test on literally hundreds of normal-hearing infants and young children. Only then can the audiologist feel confident with this simple but effective means of separating normal-hearing children from those with possible hearing problems.

For the kinds of responses described above, audiologists generally rely on carefully selected toy noise-makers or sound field speech and narrowband noise stimuli with sudden, rapid signal onset. Obviously, the frequency spectrum of such toys is difficult, if not impossible, to control, but the appeal of the sounds to youngsters probably has to do with the rich complexity of the frequency spectrum. Clearly, some toys, such as a tiny Hindu metal bell, have a higher frequency representation than a baby rattle. Audiologists must be aware that the lack of frequency specificity with toy noise-makers must be recognized as a limitation of this technique. On the other hand, frequency spec-

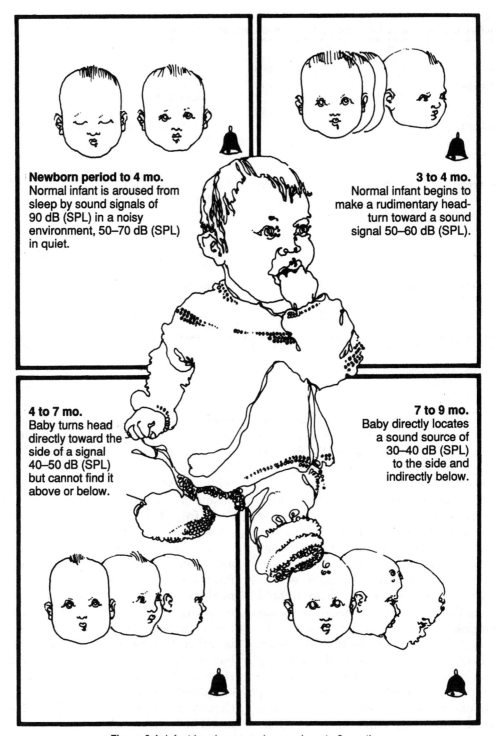

Newborn period to 4 mo.
Normal infant is aroused from sleep by sound signals of 90 dB (SPL) in a noisy environment, 50–70 dB (SPL) in quiet.

3 to 4 mo.
Normal infant begins to make a rudimentary head-turn toward a sound signal 50–60 dB (SPL).

4 to 7 mo.
Baby turns head directly toward the side of a signal 40–50 dB (SPL) but cannot find it above or below.

7 to 9 mo.
Baby directly locates a sound source of 30–40 dB (SPL) to the side and indirectly below.

Figure 6-1. Infant hearing screening: newborn to 9 months.

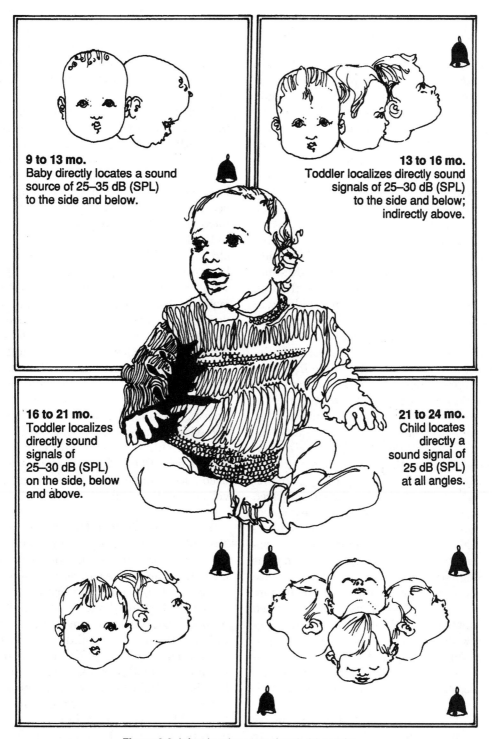

9 to 13 mo.
Baby directly locates a sound source of 25–35 dB (SPL) to the side and below.

13 to 16 mo.
Toddler localizes directly sound signals of 25–30 dB (SPL) to the side and below; indirectly above.

16 to 21 mo.
Toddler localizes directly sound signals of 25–30 dB (SPL) on the side, below and above.

21 to 24 mo.
Child locates directly a sound signal of 25 dB (SPL) at all angles.

Figure 6-2. Infant hearing screening: 9–24 months.

trum measurements should be made from each toy noise-maker to define the frequency content of the signal.

Premeasurement of the intensity as a function of distance from the infant's ear is requisite for this procedure. It should be noted that "calibration" of the noise-makers is not used; these toys can obviously not be "calibrated" like an electronic device. However, they must be measured for signal intensity output, at some specific distance typical of the hearing test situation, so that an estimate can be made about the level of the signal necessary to elicit expected behaviors from the infant or child. Typical toys used for auditory localization evaluation include small bells, plastic blocks or rattles with sand inside that can be shaken suddenly, a rubber squeeze toy, and a louder impulse toy, such as a bicycle horn.

A spin-off of the use of the Auditory Behavior Index has been its value in identifying developmental delay in children. Zigler (1969) described two theories of childhood maturation in handicapped children that are known as the *developmental theory* and the *difference theory*. The difference theory predicts that the auditory responsiveness displayed by developmentally delayed children compared with normal children will be unexpected, deviant from the normal, and nonpredictable. The developmental theory assumes that the retarded child passes through the same maturation sequence as the normal child, although much more slowly. Flexer and Gans (1985) verified the developmental theory for the auditory behavioral testing of multihandicapped children, showing that the expected auditory responses follow the normal sequence of auditory maturation in normal-hearing children but are significantly delayed. Thus, if an 8-month-old baby shows only arousal and basic eye-widening to acoustic stimuli but does not show even rudimentary head-turning for localization, his or her auditory behavior is less than expected for the age level. If an 18-month-old toddler shows only lateral head-turning localization behavior and does not seek out sound sources presented below or above eye level, the child is performing on a 6- to 9-month auditory maturation stage.

Further logic suggests that if one can correlate auditory behavior with mental age, with a reasonable level of confidence, then the audiologist who is testing a mentally retarded youngster with a chronologic age of 6 years but a mental age of 2 years or less should expect the child to have the auditory responses appropriate to the limited mental age. Thus, a 6-year-old with an IQ of 60 will not respond with hand-raising behavior but will respond with the auditory localization responses expected from a child of approximately 2 years of age. The auditory responses of retarded and developmentally delayed children are much closer to their mental age than to their chronologic age. Wilson and Thompson (1984) state that even though BOA lacks precision as an indicator of hearing thresholds, it is the only available behavioral procedure for some profoundly retarded children. Gans (1987) reported results from BOA minimal response levels used successfully to test 82 profoundly involved handicapped children.

BOA in the 0- to 6-Month-Old Infant. Typically, infants are presented either in a hospital bassinet or in the arms of a parent. Although reactions to sounds in an awake baby can be observed, as Ling et al. (1970) pointed out, the chance is too high for observing random responses and judging them to be valid responses to sound. The authors prefer to use noise stimuli to elicit responses while the infant is in a light sleep. In the observation of responses it is useful for the audiologist to be able to see the baby's face clearly, with both ears visible and with all blankets, wraps, coats, etc. peeled off the infant so that responses of the body, limbs, hands, and facial expressions can be noted.

For sleeping infants between 0 and 4 months of age, an intense sound is usually required to elicit behavioral responses. The only legitimate, acceptable responses to the auditory stimuli need to be obvious and easily observable. In clinical practice, the best behavioral response is arousal from the sleep state. By arousal we mean even a brief, transitory movement from the infant that indicates a marked change from the quiet, motionless sleep condition. Acceptable responses include a definite eye-blink immediately following the presentation of the noise-maker stimulus, a slight shudder of the whole body, an opening of the eyes (even briefly), or a marked movement of the body, arms, or legs. The response should be seen within 2 seconds of the noise-maker stimulus presentation to be considered valid.

Before the presentation of the noise-maker sound, maintaining complete quiet for at least 1 minute helps to "set the stage" for the sudden onset of the stimulus to evoke a response of large magnitude. Although these noise-maker procedures can be conducted in any situation, performing the evaluation in a quiet background, especially within a sound-treated booth, heightens the chance for successful observation of clear responses. If the infant is in deep sleep, there is less chance for good behavioral responses than when the baby is in a lighter stage of sleep.

The authors recommend that following 1 minute of complete silence, the toy noise-maker be held motionless within 3 inches of the infant's ear. Naturally, the toy and the motion necessary to create the sound stimulus should carefully be kept out of the baby's visual field. Effort should be made to initiate the sound as quickly as possible, and it may be necessary to maintain the sound stimulus at the same intensity for 2–5 seconds before a response is noted. The authors follow a specific presentation sequence beginning with the softest (lowest intensity) noise-maker followed sequentially by different and louder noise-makers, ending the test session with the loudest signal to elicit a startle response. The startle response noise-maker is best saved for the final presentation, as this signal may actually frighten the infant into crying. Behavioral responses should be noted with each of the noise-makers, and time should be permitted to elapse between noise-makers to ensure a new, brisk response. If there is doubt about the presence of a response, the noise-maker can be repeated after a brief period of quiet or rotated to be used again later in the sequence. However, these sound stimuli lose their novel effect very quickly, the infants habituate, and their responses soon extinguish. In fact, sometimes a single behavioral response is all that will be made to each noise-maker presentation, so the audiologist must be prepared and alert for accurate observations. If the evaluation with noise-makers takes too long, the baby's sleeping state may change into a deep sleep from which the audiologist must shake the crib, or the infant, to raise the awareness level into the light-sleeping condition again.

It has been our experience that nearly all normal-hearing infants—even those at risk for hearing loss—can be quickly identified as having hearing within normal limits during a single test session with careful noise-maker evaluation. Babies will often "fail" the noise-maker test if conducted in a noise background such as that found in the nursery. However, when proper quiet background conditions are established, the same baby will respond briskly and clearly as expected for maturation level. In completing the hearing screening of an infant, the audiologist must of course confirm the presence of normal hearing with otoacoustic emission tests (OAEs) as described in Chapter 7.

Thompson and Thompson (1972) noted that for infants of 7–12 months of age, speech and high-pass filtered speech produced the most behavioral responses over other types of auditory stimuli. They recommended the use of the high-pass filtered speech signals as a useful stimulus for assessing high-frequency hearing in infants. They found that with 22- to 36-month-old infants there is no longer an advantage in one auditory stimulus over another. Samples and Franklin (1978) observed the responses of 7- to 9-month-old infants to speech signals, warble tones, and noise bands. They found that the intensity level required for a response was lower, and the number of responses were significantly higher, to speech signals than to either the warble tones or broadband noise stimuli.

BOA in the 4- to 7-Month-Old Infant.

As the infant passes 4 months of age, he or she takes a giant step toward auditory maturation. The infant now begins to turn the head and eyes toward the sound source—a response that occurs now to a lower level of sound than during the first 4 months of life. From an average minimal response level of 45 dB hearing level (HL) to a sound field speech signal, the baby now becomes aware of speech at about 20 dB HL. During this period of growth, muscle strength and eye-motor coordination also show great improvement. By 6 months of age, the baby now laughs out loud, holds a rattle tightly, reaches for objects and grasps them, can turn over without help, and sits with only minimal support. By 7 months of age, the baby can transfer an object from hand to hand and sit up without support momentarily.

The audiologist should be aware of the visual acuity of the child as testing begins. Does the baby track a bright object visually from side to side? Does the baby have good eye contact with the audiologist for even brief periods? If the audiologist smiles at the baby and nods his or her head, is there integrity in the way the infant returns this attentive behavior? The improved muscular coordination at this age allows the child soon after 4 months of age to begin to turn toward sound with

the entire head, but only on a lateral plane. The head turn at 4 months is a wobbly one that is probably not a full 90°. By 6 months of age, the head turn should be stronger and under better control, but the baby will still not find the sound source if it comes from above or below eye level.

Auditory localization testing can be accomplished by having the baby sit in the parent's lap, facing the audiologist. The audiologist working alone kneels in front of the baby, with the noise-maker toy array previously set up out of sight, perhaps under the parent's chair. The audiologist may prefer to stand or kneel unobtrusively behind the parent's chair, totally out of sight of the baby, as shown in Figure 6-3. A small, not-too-attractive, passive toy (such as a book or a soft animal doll) can be given to the baby as an entertaining device. The parent should be instructed not to talk to the baby, not to provide any cues to the baby during the test, and not to make any undue noise. In fact, the authors sometimes put hearing conservation earmuffs on the parent to ensure that the parents not participate in any way when the sound stimuli are presented.

Babies at this age will also localize to sound field speech and narrowband noise stimuli presented from loudspeakers. Behavioral observation can be made of the child's responses, or conditioning techniques as described later in this chapter can be included to reinforce the head-turning response. Typically, sound stimuli (speech or narrow bands of pulsed noise) are presented from one loudspeaker at a 45° angle to the child until a head turn response is elicited. Then a similar or different stimulus is quickly presented from a loudspeaker located 45° on the other side of the child until a head-turn is noted. At this age, an effective speech stimulus is to use the child's name: "Hi, Johnny! Hi, Johnny! Look this way, Johnny." Of course, always find out exactly what name the parents use with the child, as it does little good to say, "Hi,

Johnny!" to John Edwin who is called "Eddie" by his family. As the baby approaches 7 months of age, the infant may now become responsive to a speech stimulus of "bye-bye," and in fact, a voluntary (but somewhat reflexive) wave is often elicited from the baby. Normal minimal response levels to speech stimuli at this age are approximately 20 dB HL.

The startle response at 65 dB HL may also be included at the end of the test period, as shown in Figure 6-3. A sudden onset speech stimulus presented through the sound field loudspeaker system, with the baby seated quietly on the parent's knees as far forward as possible with minimal support, should provide the clinician with a brisk, whole-body startle response as the baby hears the loud speech signal. The lack of a strong startle response following doubtful auditory localization behaviors is suggestive of severe

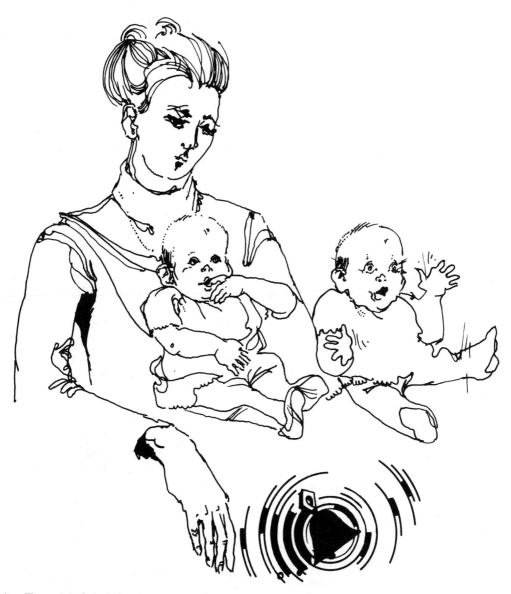

Figure 6-3. Quiet baby shows startle response to sound presentation heard at 65 dB sensation level.

to profound hearing loss, and additional hearing evaluation tests including acoustic immittance, otoacoustic emissions, and ABR must be performed to determine a repeatable minimal response level to auditory stimulation.

BOA in the 7- to 9-Month-Old Infant.

During the 7- to 9-month period, the improvement in strength and motor coordination allows the infant to sit steadily and to change position without falling. The child can now manipulate two objects simultaneously and transfers objects from hand to hand to mouth. This is the explore-everything-in-the-mouth stage, and the well-advised clinician only gives the infant clean items. This stage is not uncommonly seen in older developmentally delayed children who function at this mental age. The child of 7–9 months is able to play peek-a-boo and perhaps pat-a-cake. At this age, a child begins to be initially shy with strangers and may take a few moments to warm up to the audiologist. The baby probably can respond to "bye-bye" with a wave of the hand and arm but may need some encouragement to perform this act for a new person. "Dada" and "mama" may be heard in vocalizations but without specific referents. Imitation of gross sounds should be in place by the age of 9 months.

In terms of auditory maturation, the 7- to 9-month-old is able to find a sound source located below eye level and off to the side but only by looking first to the lateral side and then down to the sound source. This behavior is known as *indirect fixation* of a sound source. The transitional stage of the auditory maturation sequence is clearly evident in this age range. Be warned, however, as this young child is normally visually very alert, and it is difficult to introduce the noise-maker signals without attracting visual attention from the baby before the sound is actually produced. The use of two noise-maker toys, with one held in front of the child's face and the other held off to the side, permits one to elicit a head-turn to the side with the presentation of the auditory signal, without worrying about the child "sighting in" on the stimulus toy (Fig. 6-4).

With sound field localization stimuli presented from loudspeakers, the minimal response for speech awareness is now approximately 15 dB HL. A child of this age will usually sit quietly in the parent's lap and be mildly amused with a passive toy, book, or a few blocks. As in all of the tests with young children, the audiologist needs to develop a calm presence and steady pace and to be fully aware of an opportune moment to present the auditory stimuli. If the child is still exploring the environment, the audiologist should allow a few moments until the child is comfortable and relaxed before starting the testing sequence. If the child becomes too engrossed in the toy to be aware of the auditory environment, it may be necessary to change toys (if possible) or to wait until the enthusiasm for the item diminishes.

The use of calibrated sound field speech stimuli, alternating from the loudspeakers on either side of the sound suite, may actually turn the child's head from side to side like that of a person watching a tennis match. Not for long, however, without reinforcement of some type, as this is not an interesting enough activity to sustain the child's interest. The audiol-

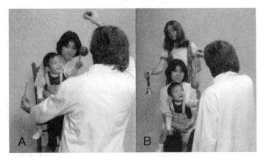

Figure 6-4. Demonstration of BOA with screening noise-makers. **(A)** The testing technique with one tester. **(B)** The utilization of a two-tester team.

ogist may elicit some vocalization response to the speech stimuli, and the child may actually imitate the speech sounds, such as "oh-oh," if presented with singsong inflection. At this age, the child is normally happy and outgoing and very curious about everything going on in the environment. Once again, the cross-check techniques of acoustic immittance, otoacoustic emissions, and ABR when necessary should be used to confirm behavioral observations.

BOA in the 9- to 13-Month-Old Infant. It is normal for the baby of this age to be somewhat afraid of strangers if they come too close or offer to hold the child. "Strangeness" is one of the psychic organizers described by Spitz (1959). In fact, the child who comes easily to the arms of a complete stranger at this age may suffer a lack of psychic development. The parent should be permitted to handle the child exclusively for the auditory evaluation period. The audiologist may need to do his or her work from outside the sound-treated booth in a darkened room, because as long as the child can see this "stranger," suspicion reigns. Without this visual presence, the child will relax and feel secure in the lap of the parent. Normal babies do not object to the quiet of the sound-treated booth, and only occasionally have the authors seen a youngster object violently to going into the sound-treated booth.

By 11 months of age, the baby is standing firmly and perhaps walking by holding on to furniture or the parents. The child may begin making single-word utterances, perhaps with an appropriate referent. The baby knows his or her own name easily by now, and a speech awareness response level can be determined by using the name in an ascending intensity approach until the child localizes briskly to the correct loudspeaker. The auditory localization behavior noted during this maturation stage progresses from the indirect to the direct fixation of the sound source on the lower level. By the upper age limit of the stage, at 13 months, the child should also be able to localize with indirect fixation (initial lateral head-turn with subsequent looking up) to auditory stimuli presented above eye level and to the side. Typically, the child in this age range is extremely interested in the environment and will localize rather briskly and quickly to your auditory signals. The average minimal response level at this age is 10 dB HL.

BOA in the 12- to 24-Month-Old Child. Once the child has reached 12 months, the auditory orientation response should be fully mature. The child of 12 months or older can be conditioned with VRA; accordingly, it is possible to obtain frequency-specific minimal response levels for each ear in the sound field situation. Some audiologists may choose to perform an initial hearing screening with toy noise-makers just to establish some idea of the child's response patterns and behaviors, as well as a means to develop rapport with the child and the parent. Remember, however, the ultimate goal of the hearing test is to obtain as much audiometric frequency-specific information as possible in each year, verified by speech awareness minimal response levels in each ear, before the child grows tired and becomes irritable about the testing situation. Time should be taken at the end of each test session to cross-check the behavioral test results with immittance audiometry.

By 18 months of age, the toddler should know a few simple objects well enough to look for them. This skill and ability can be used in the speech stimulus by asking the child, at lower and lower intensity levels, to identify by looking at a few simple toys, such as, "Where is the kitty cat?" or "Where is the doll baby?" or at the appropriate parent, such as "Where is mama (or daddy)?" By 24 months of age, it may be possible to have the child pick up certain simple toy objects and hand them to the parent at the audiologist's instruction through the loudspeakers. Some children at this age are clever enough to identify simple body parts on suggestion, such as "Where is your nose?" or "Show me your teeth," or "Show mama (or daddy) your shoes." A final behavioral response may be obtained by asking, "Do you want to go bye-bye?" To establish minimal speech response levels it is necessary to present the carrier phrase in the sound field ("Give mama [or daddy] the . . .") at 20 dB speech level and then quickly to shift down to the level you want to test for the keyword (". . . doggy."). The minimal response level for speech audiometry in a child of this age is 5 dB HL for normal hearing.

After 24 months, the child may actually inhibit response behaviors, especially without reinforcement of some type. It is good to question the parents at this time about the vocalization skills of the child so they can be related to normal speech development milestones. It may also be important to ask the parents about possible previous history of ear infections with medical or surgical treatment and to consider referral for language assessment in children with significant history of recurrent otitis media.

It is not surprising for a child to suddenly stop responding because he or she has lost interest in the activity. Part of the challenge of pediatric audiology is to learn when the child has had enough and the limits of attention have been exceeded. The audiologist must be prepared to change the game or activity to reinterest the child so that additional information about the hearing response levels can be obtained. The use of a darkened instrument room is still indicated for children up to 24 months of age. The purity of the child's responsiveness is an unquestioning reaction to the voice signal. Between 13 and 24 months, the child may be confused by the presence of a voice originating in loudspeakers without visualizing a person doing the speaking. However,

it is likely that the unquestioning obedience of a child of this age will serve the practitioner of pediatric speech audiometry well.

The need to apply the cross-check of immittance audiometry with tympanometry and acoustic reflex measurements, otoacoustic emissions, and ABR when necessary to confirm behavioral observations cannot be emphasized enough. Children who appear to have hearing loss by their behavioral audiometry evaluations should be scheduled for ABR testing.

REINFORCEMENT AUDIOMETRY PROCEDURES

Liden and Kankkonen (1961) first coined the term *visual reinforcement audiometry* (VRA), based on a technique described by Suzuki and Ogiba (1961) and termed by them "conditioned orientation reflex" (COR) audiometry. These procedures use lighted transparent toys hidden in smoked Plexiglas boxes that are flashed on simultaneously with the presentation of the auditory signal during a conditioning period. During the testing phase, the lighted toy is flashed immediately following the response of the child looking toward the light (Fig. 6-5). Thompson and Folsom (1984) found no difference between 30 and 60 dB HL conditioning trials before exploring minimal response levels in 1- and 2-year-old normal-hearing children.

The technique of VRA is to establish conditioning through the use of a few training trials during which the child's attention should be directed toward the stimulus (auditory sound) at the onset of the trial and held there until the reinforcer (flashing lighted toy) is presented. The visual reinforcers should be at least 90° from the midline and require a full head-turn to observe the lighted toy. Babies will respond as minimally as possible to see the reinforcer, so if a slight head-turn is reinforced, that may be the extent of future responses. On the other hand,

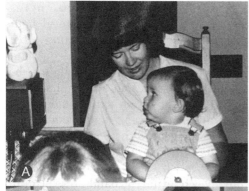

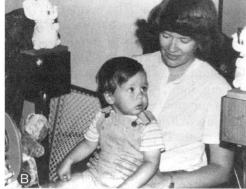

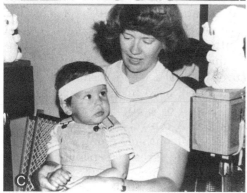

Figure 6-5. VRA. Note the head localization to either side when the auditory stimulus is heard. The flashing, lighted toy reinforces the head-turn. Bone-conduction testing can also be performed with this technique following the Weber localization concept.

limited head-turns can be shaped into bigger head-turns by the experienced audiologist controlling the reinforcement to require more overt responses with each stimulus presentation.

Diverting the child's attention toward the stimulus and away from the reinforcer may require prompting or physical assistance, which, it is hoped, can be diminished with each successive training trial. The stimulus and response must always precede delivery of reinforcement. Although the "on" time between trials for stimulus presentation should be varied, the reinforcement should immediately follow the desired response, and the stimulus should not be terminated until the response occurs. Culpepper and Thompson (1994) recommend short stimulus duration of 0.5 seconds rather than longer presentations of 4 seconds to decrease habituation time and increase the overall number of responses from the child. Primus (1992) reported that the most valid responses from a child during VRA occur within 4 seconds after the stimulus onset.

The *observer-based procedure* uses reinforcement (such as a video display or moving, lighted mechanical toy) following any change in the infant's behavior related to the onset of an auditory stimulus. This testing procedure depends on the observer's skills to reliably detect spontaneous responses in an infant or young child's behaviors following presentation of a sound. To keep the infant responding to the sound, whatever response that the infant makes is reinforced by some visual token. In practice, the observer-based technique with reinforcement must keep the observer blinded to control trials in which no sound is presented. Observer-based procedures make it possible to estimate reasonable thresholds in infants who are too young to make nice crisp, short-latency head-turns toward a sound source, but who nonetheless can learn the association between a sound, their response, and the reinforcer (Rovee-Collier, 1987; Werner et al., 1994).

The training trials will only be successful when the audiologist is absolutely sure that the child hears the stimulus. Therefore, stimulus presentations for a hearing-impaired youngster may, of necessity, be quite loud. Parents or other observers in the test room with the child may wish to wear ear defenders during these loud training trials. The VRA technique can also be used to test the child's responses with hearing aids.

Matkin (1977) found that VRA is successful with 90% of both normal-hearing and hearing-impaired children between the ages of 12 and 30 months. Furthermore, he found that speech stimuli are more effective than the warble tones. In sound field, VRA will only test the child's better ear, even when loudspeakers on each side of the child produce the signals. Hodgson (1985) stated that the child with a severe hearing loss would not have learned to localize sound. He suggested that where there is confusion in localization, it is best to use only one loudspeaker in testing. To distract the child from looking constantly at the loudspeaker, an animated toy can be activated in another direction.

Children with unilateral hearing loss and one normal-hearing ear typically have difficulties in localizing the source of a sound, and this is certainly a consideration in children who seem to have diffi-

culty with VRA for no other apparent reason. Children who have unilateral hearing loss can actually localize sound, albeit more slowly than normal-hearing children, by moving their head slightly between the presentation of stimuli. We believe that localization skills among children vary considerably and seem to be a function of age and the parameters of the stimulus. For example, warble-tone signals are much more difficult to localize than speech or narrowband noise stimuli. Moore, Wilson, and Thompson (1977) determined rank order of signals according to their effectiveness in producing VRA localization responses in 12- to 18-month-old infants: (1) an animated toy, (2) a flashing light, (3) social reinforcement, and (4) no reinforcement (Fig. 6-6).

Moore, Wilson, Lillis, et al. (1976) and Moore et al. (1977) affirmed the success of VRA in eliciting responses in infants as young as 5 months. They used a complex noise centered between 1000 and 4000 Hz and maintained at 70 dB as a stimulus. Each of 60 infants between 4 and 11 months of age were given this stimulus 40 times, reinforced by a toy animal that moved in place. Their technique used a conditioned head-turning response that was shaped by a stimulus-reinforcement paradigm. A control trial was also given. The 2- to 5-month-old group and the 7- to 11-month-old group responded significantly more frequently to the signals that were reinforced visually than to the nonreinforced signals.

Wilson and Thompson (1984) established auditory thresholds in 90 infants between 5 and 18 months of age who were divided into groups of 15 according to age. Threshold level was first obtained by using behavioral observations of responses to a complex noise signal. The VRA protocol was begun at that level, with a protocol of attenuating the signal 20 dB after each positive response and increasing it 10 dB after each failure to respond. The results showed the VRA responses to be significantly better than the

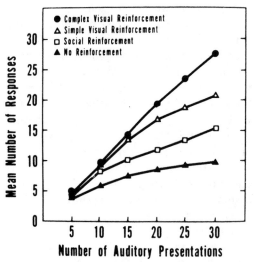

Figure 6-6. Response curves for operant conditioning audiometry. (Reprinted with permission from Moore, J.M., Wilson, W.R., & Thompson, G. [1977]. Visual reinforcement of head-turn responses in infants under twelve months of age. *Journal of Speech and Hearing Disorders 42,* 328.)

behavioral observation even for the 5-month-olds. Gravel and Traquina (1992) utilized VRA to evaluate hearing in a cohort of 211 babies and toddlers ranging in age from 6 to 24 months, obtaining ear and frequency-specific thresholds from more than 80% of these children.

Eilers, Wilson, and Moore (1977) used VRA techniques in a speech discrimination paradigm designed to show developmental changes of discrimination ability and termed Visually Reinforced Infant Speech Discrimination (VRISD). They demonstrated that 1- to 3-month-old infants and older infants could discriminate certain easier phonemic contrasts such as sa-sa and sa-va, but that other contrasts are more difficult for very young children than for older infants as they approach 14 months (e.g., fi-i, sa-za). Thus, the use of VRA techniques can be useful in the study of the development of auditory prelinguistic skills.

VRA and COR techniques are powerful tools for assessing minimal response levels in young children when used correctly with acknowledged conditioning protocols. These techniques are the evaluation procedures of choice in children between 6 and 24 months of age, although it should be obvious that the older children in this range will condition more easily and quicker than the younger children. As described by Primus (1987), the COR response requires detection of the sound, localization of the auditory image, coordination of auditory and visual space, and subsequent orientation to the appropriate reinforcer with a motor response (i.e., a head-turn). The VRA response requires only a detection of the auditory signal as prerequisite to an appropriate head-turn. The difference between the response modes is that VRA defines one criterion response (i.e., a head-turn toward a single loudspeaker/reinforcer location). The COR response requires that the child localize the test signal to determine which of two reinforcers (left or right) is the appropriate response. Close proximity of loudspeakers and reinforcers is advantageous in both VRA and COR procedures, according to Primus, because most unconditioned children turn spontaneously toward initial presentation of the sound stimulus.

Commercially available VRA systems have a pair of illuminated and/or animated reinforcement boxes. These systems may be especially useful for the audiologist working without an assistant as the equipment includes a third (orientation) toy, in front of the child, which can be illuminated between stimulus presentation trials to bring the child's head back to the center position in readiness for the next VRA stimulus and head-turn response. VRA is especially viable for the older, developmentally delayed patient who may be functioning at a level too low for the hand-raising response task (Fig. 6-7).

Computerized and automated VRA systems are available that use interactive video images as the reinforcement for correct responses in an application of Visual Reinforcement Operant Conditioning Audiometry (VROCA). Keith and Smith (1987) described a system designed to facilitate hearing assessment in 3- to 7-year-old children (Fig. 6-8). This computer-controlled audiometer provides

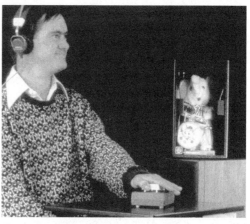

Figure 6-7. VRA system as used with a developmentally delayed youngster.

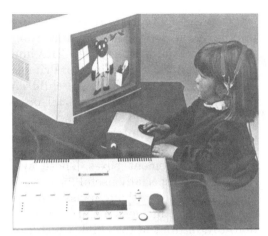

Figure 6-8. Computer-based audiometer designed to use interactive video images as the reinforcement for correct responses. (From Life-Tech Instruments, Houston, Texas.)

practice trials, hearing screening, and auditory threshold tracking. The child is conditioned during practice trials to quickly depress a bright red button on the response box immediately following presentation of an auditory stimulus. A brief, animated color video presentation occurs after each correct response made within a short time window. False responses produce no visual reinforcement of any kind. This pediatric audiometer adapts the test signal presentation speed to the response speed of the child and in the automatic mode includes several validity checks. Such systems can also include silent control trials interspersed at random intervals.

Other computer-mediated VRA procedures have been reported to obtain complete audiometric data more efficiently than is possible using standard behavioral techniques. Tharpe and Ashmead (1993) evaluated several parameters in computerized simulations leading to various test outcomes using adaptive testing procedures. Berstein and Gravel (1990) described a three-frequency Interweaving Staircase Procedure, and Eilers, Widen, Urbano, Hudson, and Gonzales (1991) developed a four-frequency Optimized Hearing Test Algorithm. These computer-as-

sisted assessment techniques require a minimum of 50 test trials lasting approximately 15 minutes. Use of these innovative VROCA systems suggests great promise for pediatric hearing assessment.

OPERANT REINFORCEMENT AUDIOMETRY

Operant reinforcement audiometry for children between 6 and 24 months of age is particularly valuable as a clinical tool for the pediatric audiologist. Stimulus, response, and reinforcement parameters and techniques have been developed to be consistent with each child's developmental level and response capability. The use of reinforcement for responses made to audiometric stimuli strengthens the test paradigm, maintains the child's responses longer, reduces habituation to the stimulus, and thus allows for a more precise estimate of hearing thresholds in young children.

Wilson and Thompson (1984) recommended the operant discrimination paradigm in hearing testing. They described two modes of operant conditioning termed *operant discrimination* and the *conjugate procedure*. In operant discrimination, the stimulus precedes the responses and acts as a discriminative signal that reinforcement is available. In the conjugate procedure, the stimulus follows the response as a consequence. The intensity of a continuously available reinforcing stimulus varies as a function of the rate of the response. Since the stimulus is a consequence of the response, in the conjugate procedure the stimulus itself must have reinforcing value to the child.

An example of a conjugate reinforcement technique is the innate sucking response in infants, which was originally developed by Siqueland and DeLucia (1969) and enthusiastically endorsed by Madell (1998). This procedure relies on a natural newborn response and capitalizes on the reinforcing properties of the stimulus. The spontaneous behavior (sucking) is brought under stimulus control through the use of response-contingent stimulation. The auditory stimulus is then made contingent on a criterion-level sucking response, and the auditory stimulus takes on reinforcing properties for the infant. Disadvantages to the sucking response is the physical demand placed on the infant, a baseline criterion level of 20–40 sucks per minute so that criterion level changes may be noted, and the fact that the general length of time required to complete studies is substantial. Eisele, Berry, and Shriner (1975) generated threshold hearing data from 100 infants by observing the rate of sucking as a function of stimulus intensity.

Aslin, Pisoni, and Jusczyk (1983) summarized four versions of the BOA head-turning technique that have been used to evaluate auditory abilities in infants. The first version is a simple auditory threshold procedure in which the infant's task is to respond to any just detectable sound emitted from a single loudspeaker. In a second version, the same task is involved for the infant, except that two sound field speakers are used. The infant is centered between the speakers, and the silence is interrupted by a signal presented from one of the two speakers. The first directional head-turn response is scored and correlated with the location of the sound source. A third technique is somewhat more complex, as it involves the addition of a background stimulus that is interrupted by the presentation of a different (or target) stimulus. This is then a discrimination procedure to evaluate an infant's ability to differentiate between two suprathreshold auditory stimuli. A "catch trial" is essential in this technique, which consists of informing the observer that a scoring interval is occurring but not letting him or her know if the target stimulus was included in this tone interval. This is done as an attempt to eliminate experimenter bias. A fourth version of the head-turning technique involves the addition of a trial-to-criterion measure to the basic discrimination response procedure. Kuhl (1979) and Kuhl and Miller (1982) used these discrimination techniques to evaluate speech perception in infants.

Primus (1987) investigated response and reinforcement features of two operant discrimination paradigms with normal-hearing 17-month-old children. He found more success in a paradigm that based the response task on complex central processing skills (i.e., localization and coordination of auditory/visual space) over a simple detection task. His use of animated toy reinforcement resulted in more than a two-fold increase in responses. In a 1985 research project, Primus and Thompson tested the response strength of young children in operant audiometry. One- and 2-year-old children reinforced on a variable-ratio schedule of intermittent reinforcement and a 100% schedule demonstrated equivalent response habituation and consistency. Primus reported that the use of novel reinforcement had a strong influence in eliciting conditioned responses from normal-hearing 2-year-old children and that an audiologist can delay the habituation of responses by the use of novel (different) reinforcements.

Procedures using computer technology have influenced operant conditioning paradigms (Eilers, Miskiel, Ozdamar, Urbano, & Widen, 1991). Computerized stimulus presentations include preprogrammed catch trials or control presentations when no auditory signal is actually presented. Computerized scoring response criteria can be established to limit the time window of the child's response in other ways and can be used to define the "correctness of response," with the observer(s) blinded as to the presentation of control (no signal) trials.

Tangible Reinforcement Operant Conditioning Audiometry (TROCA). During this operant conditioning paradigm, the auditory stimulus cues the child that a behavior-specific response will immediately produce a positive reinforcement. The positive reinforcement is a tangible item such as candy, cereal, or a trinket of some sort that is automatically dispensed from specifically designed audiometric equipment. Visual stimulation, in the form of a blinking light array, moving cartoon video, or animated puppets may also be used as positive reinforcement. Negative reinforcement (mild punishment), such as "time out" for false-positive responses from the child, might be incorporated in demanding situations. Lloyd, Spradlin, and Reid (1968) described success with TROCA, using edible positive reinforcement, with a group of developmentally delayed children.

Typically, the child's behavior is conditioned to push a response button whenever a sound is perceived, initially in sound field and subsequently under earphones. The tangible reinforcement item is usually accompanied by an outburst of secondary social approval reinforcement by the audiologist and parents or caretaker. Fulton, Gorzycki, and Hull (1975) reported success using the TROCA technique to assess hearing levels in young children. TROCA is useful with children between 2 and 4 years of age and generally requires more total testing time than traditional conditioning techniques.

TESTER-OBSERVER BIAS

Response bias by testers and observers is one of the most difficult errors to avoid in the clinical hearing evaluation of children. Several studies have confirmed that there is a tendency for judges to score responses when no auditory signals were presented (Moncur, 1968; Ling et al., 1970; Langford, Bench, & Wilson, 1975). Weber (1969) suggested using two persons to test the child, with one observer in the room with the child while the tester operates a tape recorder in the control room. The operator selects a randomized stimulus schedule with 20 stimulus presentations—10 of which are heard only by the child. The observer wears earphones and hears all 20 stimulus presentations but cannot tell which sounds are presented to the child under evaluation. The operator and observer each make judgments about the responses of the child, which are compared with the stimulus presentation schedule following the test session.

In our clinic, we use only one audiologist to work with each child during the hearing evaluation process, incorporating the parents' help, when necessary, to shape the child's conditioning behavior. Although we prefer having the audiologist outside the test room, many audiologists prefer sitting in the test room with the child (and parent). Understanding the potential observer bias that can exist with a single tester presenting stimuli and judging the child's responses, our experience has been that this technique is cost- and time-effective and does not significantly alter the results of the hearing test. The audiologist engages the infant's (or child's) forward attention with a simple toy, selects and presents a test signal, varies its presentation intensity as appropriate, judges the child's behavioral response, and activates directly the reinforcement for correct head-turning. A careful and thoughtful clinician guarding against the potential hazards of single-examiner assessment may obtain reliable and accurate audiograms (Gravel, 1989).

Gans and Flexer (1982) investigated observer bias in BOA with profoundly involved multiple-handicapped children. Their findings implicated clear observer bias in 85% of children. At low test intensities, observers aware of the stimulus events tended to score fewer responses than those judges unaware of stimulus intensity. In cases of high sound intensities, judges tend to "see" more behavioral changes to sound than actually occur. Gans and Flexer were disappointed that even when observers were told that they exhibited biased scoring responses, this information did not influence the observer's subsequent scoring tactics.

CLINICAL TESTING OF THE CHILD AGED 2–4 YEARS

Between 2 and 4 years of age the child grows into the independence of early maturity. The child begins to separate from mother without much fuss and to dress alone, first with supervision and then without. The youngster now becomes a wanderer and can quickly delve into the audiologist's toys and equipment. The child begins to understand some abstract words, such as cold or hungry, and can give a full name when asked. Actually, the child becomes an eager beaver, happy to please the audiologist. As a result, the child may give the clinician a hard time in testing. Once children know that cooperation in play conditioning pleases the audiologist, they may forget what they are supposed to listen for, in eagerness to be praised. Strangely enough, this attitude is often found in older deaf children—even teenagers—who will give false responses to please or to give a "good" test.

The learning of play-conditioning techniques starts at 2 years of age. However, one should not be deceived by the bright, talkative 2-year-old who appears certain to be able to learn the procedure. The clinician should still obtain all the information possible from the observation of behavior as the child waits in the waiting room, walks into the sound booth, and watches the interaction with the parents. Until the child is 4 or 5 years old, the audiologist's ingenuity is challenged to complete the hearing test. Remember that the goal is to achieve pure tone thresholds at all test frequencies in each ear. However, the child should not be traumatized so much that he or she will be frightened the next time. There is always another day.

The darkened instrument room should not be forgotten even for these older children. A shy, immature child of 2.5 years may learn play-conditioning techniques easily, but the odd situation of a stranger's face in the window may create too much distracting stress. The bodiless voice over the speaker can be coped with; it takes the stranger out of the situation. All the necessary instructions to the child can be given through the speech circuit (earphones or loudspeakers) without being seen.

Speech Reception Threshold. The authors generally begin the hearing evaluation of the 2- to 4-year-old with behavioral speech testing, establishing a speech reception threshold (SRT) for each ear to obtain an initial impression of the hearing levels of the child. This is done because it incorporates the child immediately into the test activity, thereby reducing any apprehension the child has about the test environment. Although the SRT task can be accomplished easily with most 3- and 4-year-olds through insert earphones, the authors typically start the 2-year-old by speaking through the sound field loudspeaker system to determine a binaural SRT. Once it has been shown that the 2- to 3-year-old can perform the required tasks, an attempt is made to replicate the activity with insert earphones so that an SRT can be established for each ear.

In the sound-treated room, the armamentarium of the audiologist should include a carefully selected array of toys, the names of which approach spondaic principles as closely as possible. However, to present children with easily recognizable toys, some compromise may be necessary (Fig. 6-9). It is more important for the child to know and recognize the toy than for the clinician to worry if the toy name conforms to the equal-stress-on-each-syllable principle. Typical "spondaic" toys might include an airplane, baseball, toothbrush, hot dog, cowboy, and fire truck. Suggestions for nonspondaic toys include a baby (small doll), kitty, doggie, horsie,

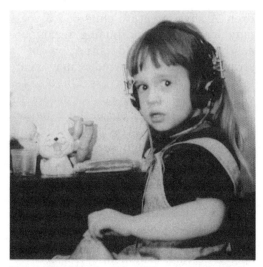

Figure 6-9. Speech audiometry measurement using earphones and toys.

car, and truck. The authors have found that toys from pet departments are more substantial than variety store items.

No more than four or five of these toys need be used to determine the SRT for the 2- or 3-year-old; the 4- or 5-year-old can select from among 6–8 items. The toys can be presented via picture boards, but it is much more interesting to the child if actual toys are involved. The authors wire the toys to a perforated board and have the parent hold the board while the child responds with a pointing response. Sometimes, very confident and mature 4- and 5-year-olds will repeat the SRT words verbally.

With the speech circuit of the audiometer set at 50 dB HL (or as high as necessary to be sure the child can hear), the audiologist should say, "Hello there. Can you hear me? Show me the airplane." When the child makes the correct response, social reinforcement with exaggerated praise should be given. The audiologist should then descend in 10 dB steps, asking at each level for the child to identify a different toy. When the child no longer responds, the clinician should ascend 5 dB but set the carrier phrase "Show me . . ." at a 10 or 15 dB higher level and switch quickly to the lower level

for the test word. Too long a silent period will lose the child, so when searching for threshold the louder carrier phrase should be given. Two valid responses on the ascending presentation should be accepted, and testing should then quickly switch to the other ear. Listening at low levels is not easy for a child, and one must work quickly for the sake of holding the child's attention. If discrepancies appear later, a recheck can always be done. It need hardly be said that the tester's mouth should not be visible to the child while saying the words.

Thompson, Thompson, and Vethivelu (1989) noted a paucity of information about the relative effectiveness of audiometric procedures for testing hearing in 2-year-old children. They evaluated 2-year-old subjects with VRA, VROCA, and play audiometry. Their results indicated that a higher percentage of children could be conditioned to VRA than to either VROCA or play audiometry. However, in terms of response habituation, play conditioning had a longer response activity period. In their conclusions, these researchers noted that under general clinical conditions, the question regarding hearing levels in 2-year-olds is whether hearing loss might be a factor in speech/language development. Under this circumstance, VRA is recommended because the vast majority of 2-year-olds will readily condition to this task for purposes of hearing screening.

CONDITIONED PLAY AUDIOMETRY

Conditioned play audiometry is the most consistent behavioral technique to determine ear-specific and frequency-specific hearing thresholds in young children from 3 years of age. Because this technique is such an important part of the pediatric audiologist's skills, a detailed step-by-step description of the authors' recommended protocol, along with numerous clinical tips, is presented. The child should sit on the parent's lap. The more confident 3- or 4-year-old may prefer to sit alone at a small, child-size table with a parent nearby in another chair. The parent's closeness may be important even at an older age.

The audiologist should sit down and talk to the parents first, developing an easy rapport. "What seems to be Johnny's (or Debbie's) problem?" The parents should be given time to tell briefly why the child is being tested, but the child's history should not be belabored. The child is the chief interest and target. The audiologist should turn casually to the child and ask some simple questions such as, "How old are you?" Comments can be made about the child's clothing, hair, or a toy that the child brought along. The child should then be informed that there are some special games to play today.

During this period many observations can be made. Attention should be paid to the child's voice quality and articulation of words. Does the child substitute for the high-frequency consonants? If he or she omits or substitutes for the unvoiced consonants, either mild sensorineural or a conductive loss can be suspected. If the child misses the voiced consonants and some of the vowel sounds in addition, a more severe sensorineural loss may be predicted. Is the child able to repeat words readily but not to identify the corresponding toy?

The audiologist should maintain control of the session and gently tell the child what is going to happen in simple, clear terms that are easily understandable for the language-age of the child (the child should not be asked if he or she wants to play the game). "Now we're going to play a telephone game. We'll let you listen through this special telephone (earphones), and you can talk to me. Hello!" The clinician should then put the earphones gently but firmly on the child's head or insert the earphones into the ear canals, saying "Hello, how are you? Now wait, and I'm going to talk to you from the other room." The audiologist should move

quickly before the child balks at the earphones. If he or she balks, however, the parent can hold the earphones to the child's ear ("Like a real telephone."). With the very young and the shy child, it may be preferable not to start with earphones at all. A trial run can be done in sound field first, allowing the child to become familiar with the situation, then the placement of earphones may be attempted. Another way to start the test session is for audiologists to put the earphones on themselves.

There should be a number of sets of motivational toys geared to different ages: plain blocks for building a tower, a graduated ring tower, beads to throw into a container, and a peg board with colored pegs (put a horse or a car in the center and build a fence or a garage). A popular game is to drop pennies into a bank. The ingenious audiologist can devise other motivational games. Usually, a single game is sufficient to accomplish the task, but one must be ready to switch to another game at the first sign of boredom. It is largely the enthusiasm of the clinician that keeps the child attending, but occasionally novelty must be used.

The audiologist needs to show the child what the game is about, and instructions can be communicated without talking much. Facial expression, body language, and clear demonstrations can transmit even to the nonverbal child what is to be expected. The child can also be told in words, "We're going to hold this peg (or block, etc.) up to our ear and listen for a little bell. Oh! I hear it, so I can put the peg in the board. Now I'm going to listen for a little one. Oh! I hear it, so I put the peg in. Now you can do it, and build a fence for the horse." In the case of the 2- and 3-year-old, the parent should be instructed to hold the child's hand with the peg at the test earphone (or ear if using sound field) and to guide the hand to the pegboard when the sound is heard. This should be practiced through sound field even to the extent of establishing a quick threshold for a 2000 Hz tone or narrow-band noise stimulus so the clinician is sure that the task is understood. Three or four trials should be sufficient for the child to learn. The novelty of the task should not be worn out with too many practice trials.

The child should then be instructed to perform the task alone, preferably with earphones testing one ear at a time. The tone should be presented at 40–50 dB above the expected threshold. The audiologist should quickly switch to the speech circuit and praise the child for a correct action. The parent should be instructed to have another peg ready to give to the child the moment the child has responded accurately. Testing should descend in intensity as rapidly as possible from 40 to 50 dB HL in 10- or 15-dB steps, indicating that the child is to listen for a "tiny little bell (or beep)." Again, work should be done quickly to obtain threshold, accepting two responses on the ascending presentation. The clinician must guard against presenting the test stimuli in any sort of pattern. He or she should occasionally wait a few seconds after the urge to present the tone. Babies and children are very good at anticipating a pattern or picking up subtle cues as to when they are "supposed" to respond.

It is most important to establish hearing thresholds at 500 Hz and 2000 Hz in each ear as quickly as possible. The initial practice tones should be loud enough for the child to hear easily based on their SRT levels. Sometimes a child will seem to be cooperative at first but soon forget what to do. In this case, the child should be reconditioned, with the parent's help, at levels at which it is certain that he or she can hear. Several reconditioning periods may have to be run during a test. The audiologist should not give up until it is apparent that the child is not about to stay with the task. If the child stays with the task nicely, the clinician should fill in the 1000 Hz and 250 Hz thresholds and then 4000 Hz threshold for each ear. It is important for the clinician to know when

to stop, because there is likely additional testing to be done, and there must be some reserve of attention to carry the child through it.

When the child persistently refuses to wear the earphone headset or even one insert earphone, the audiologist should move quickly to sound field audiometry. Warbled pure tones or narrow bands of noise, precalibrated to the location where the child is sitting, should be presented by using the play-conditioning techniques. The thresholds will represent the hearing in the better ear only but will give essential information about how the child is hearing, at least in the better ear.

Play conditioning audiometry can also be used to determine bone-conduction thresholds. The bone conduction oscillator is placed on the child's mastoid ("We're going to use another kind of telephone—one that goes behind the ear. But you can hear the sounds just like the other telephone. That's like airplane pilots (or astronauts) use!") The clinician should repeat the procedure as described above for air-conduction testing, doing the more important frequencies first and filling in with the others where possible. It is possible to estimate bone-conduction thresholds by presenting speech spondees used in the SRT through the bone-conduction oscillator. It is critical that the bone-conduction SRT has been precalibrated on normal-hearing people. Bone-conducted speech can be masked effectively in the opposite ear without affecting the validity of the child's responses. The bone-conducted speech test is one of the most useful of the audiologist's tools. At the end of each test procedure, the child should be praised with some token such as a sticker. This is insurance for future cooperation. The audiologist may have to see this child many times, so groundwork should be laid for a happy return visit.

Audiologists must remember that adequate confirmation of an infant's or child's hearing status cannot be obtained with a single test. Rather, a test battery is required to cross-check the results of both behavioral and physiologic measures as described by Jerger and Hayes (1976). The cross-check procedures include tympanometry, acoustic reflex measurement, and otoacoustic emissions. When test results are still questionable about the child's actual hearing levels, an ABR evaluation may be in order. However, ABR evaluation is not incorporated into every pediatric patient's workup. Because of the time and expense associated with ABR evaluation, this technique is reserved for those children whose hearing levels cannot be determined precisely through any other method.

SPEECH DISCRIMINATION TESTING IN YOUNG CHILDREN

Speech discrimination testing (Table 6-5) in children is an area that has yet to be fully developed, although research is currently underway to rectify this situation. As Olsen and Matkin (1979) point out, the selection of receptive vocabulary competency, the designation of an appropriate response task, and the utilization of reinforcement are primary factors that may affect the reliability and validity of pediatric measurements. The results ob-

tained during speech discrimination measures may actually be more a reflection of the child's interest and motivation for the task at hand than a real indication of higher auditory speech discrimination abilities.

There is no standard technique or test of auditory discrimination in children. Although numerous tests have been developed for this purpose, apparently none of them "fits the bill" well enough for all clinicians to agree generally on which is most suitable for clinical work. One major problem with most current speech discrimination procedures is that the data base underlying the development of the test has not been standardized well enough on a broad spectrum of children of varying ages and backgrounds, and few implications can be generalized between normal-hearing and hearing-impaired children.

Many children are too shy to speak in the test room environment, and, of course, articulation problems are common in children, so it may be difficult for the audiologist to score speech discrimination tests as done with adults. The most practical method of testing auditory discrimination in children has been to use some form of picture identification task. The child

Table 6.5.
Selected Pediatric Speech Audiometric Procedures

Test	Materials	Message Set; Response Mode	Task Domain	Minimum Age (yr)
SERT	30 environmental sounds (train, telephone)	Closed; picture identification	Unrestricted: 4 alternatives	3
ANT	Numbers 1 through 5	Closed; picture identification	Restricted: 5 alternatives	3
NU-CHIPS	50 monosyllabic words (food, school)	Closed; picture identification	Unrestricted: 4 alternatives	3
PSI	20 monosyllabic words (dog, spoon)	Closed; picture identification	Restricted: 5 alternatives	3
PSI	10 sentences, 2 syntactic constructions (Show me a bear brushing his teeth. A bear is brushing his teeth.)	Closed; picture identification	Restricted: 5 alternatives	3

From Jerger, S. (1984). Speech audiometry. In: J. Jerger (Ed.): *Pediatric audiology*. San Diego: College Hill Press.

SERT, Sound Effects Recognition Test (Finitzo-Hieber et al., 1980); *ANT*, Audio Numbers Test (Erber, 1980); *NU-CHIPS*, Northwestern University Children's Perception of Speech (Elliott & Katz, 1980); *PSI*, Pediatric Speech Intelligibility (Jerger et al., 1980, 1981).

hears the test word and attempts to identify an appropriate picture.

Jerger (1983) published an excellent discussion and review of current speech audiometry materials for children. She points out that two basic principles have been important in the history of speech testing in children: vocabulary restriction in the selection of test material and limited response set definition. To these basic tenets she adds two more important considerations necessary in pediatric speech test development and administration: the need to control the influence of receptive language ability on test performance, and the need to consider the effect of extraauditory (cognitive) factors on children's performance.

For nearly 50 years the most widely used speech discrimination test for children has been an open-ended set of stimulus words known as the Phonetically Balanced Kindergarten (PBK-50) word lists (Haskins, 1949). The PBK is usually administered via live-voice and is composed of three lists of phonetically balanced words selected from the spoken vocabulary of kindergartners. Children younger than 4.5 years may not do well with them. Smith and Hodgson (1970) did show that tangible reinforcement (i.e., candies, toys, pennies) was an effective method of maintaining the interest of young children in the PBK-50 test. In fact, token reinforcement created significant improvement in speech discrimination scores from children aged 4–8 years. Olsen and Matkin (1979) recommend that clinicians use caution with this test unless there is relatively good assurance that the receptive vocabulary age of the youngster under evaluation approaches at least that of a normal-hearing kindergartner. Meyer and Pisoni (1999) concluded that children with limited vocabulary skills, such as very young or profoundly deaf children, may score poorly on the PBK Test because the specific words used on the test are simply too difficult and not within the vocabulary of these children.

One of the earliest attempts was the Discrimination by Identification of Pictures (DIP) test developed by Siegenthaler and Haspiel in 1966. Their test consists of 48 cards with 2 pictures on each card. One can quickly surmise that chance selection would produce fairly high scores, because only two choices are involved in each presentation. The investigators selected test words on the basis of contrasting acoustic dimensions rather than the traditional phonemic balance approach. The test was standardized on 295 normal-hearing children between the ages of 3 and 8 years and was administered at sensation levels of 0, 5, and 10 dB.

Ross and Lerman (1970) developed a picture identification test for hearing-impaired children known as the Word Intelligibility by Picture Identification (WIPI) test. They evaluated the test on 61 hearing-impaired children of ages 5 and 6 and caution about the use of the test with children younger than 5 years of age. The test consists of 25 picture plates with 6 pictures per plate used as test stimuli. The test is thus a closed-response set. The lists are reported to have high reliability coefficients, and the tests are simple and rapid to administer.

In 1976, Sanderson-Leepa and Rintelmann compared the speech discrimination performance of 60 normal-hearing children on the WIPI test, the PBK-50 test, and the Northwestern University Auditory Test No. 6 (NU-6). They found that the WIPI test yielded the highest discrimination sources; the PBK-50 test, intermediate scores; and the NU-6, the lowest scores.

Erber (1980) noted that the traditional speech discrimination tests developed for children are often inadequate for real diagnostic purposes or too difficult for children with severe hearing impairment. He developed a simple auditory test to determine whether a young hearing-impaired child can perceive spectral aspects of speech or only gross temporal acoustic patterns. Known as the Auditory Numbers Test (ANT), this live-voice test requires the child to identify counted sequences and individual numbers. The ANT requires only that the child be able to count to five and be able to apply these number labels to sets of from one to five items. Picture cards are used that are color-coded and depict groups of one to five ants with the corresponding numerals. Erber recommends this test for rapid evaluation of speech perception in young severely and profoundly hearing-impaired children to aid in the planning of auditory training and habilitation activities.

The Northwestern University Children's Perception of Speech (NU-CHIPS) test developed by Elliott and Katz (1980) uses 50 monosyllabic words that were documented to be in the recognition vocabulary of normal children older than 2.5 years of age. The test includes 65 word pictures and interchanges 50 words as test items and foil items. Simple words, such as "food" and "school," are represented in a four-alternative picture set, and the child responds by "picture painting." In a review article regarding the effects of noise on perception of speech by children, Elliott (1982) pointed out that young children have poorer levels of performance than do adults when listening at low levels in quiet to words within their receptive vocabularies. For normal-hearing 3-year-olds to perform with nearly 100% accuracy on the NU-CHIPS test, the words had to be presented at levels more than 10 dB greater than the level at which 5-year-olds scored 100%, approximately 15 dB greater than the level at which 10-year-olds score 100%, and nearly 25 dB greater than the level at which adults score 100%. Chermak, Pederson, and Bendel (1984) questioned the reliability of the NU-CHIPS when it is administered in a noise background.

Finitzo-Hieber, Gerlin, Matkin, et al. (1980) described the development and evaluation of a Sound Effects Recognition Test (SERT) for use in the pediatric audiologic evaluation. They point out that such a test may be the only available standardized measure of auditory discrimination in children with limited verbal abilities. The test is composed of three equivalent sets, with each containing 10 familiar environmental sounds (such as a dog barking, a toilet flushing, a mother singing, someone hammering, a cat meowing, and a baby crying). The authors indicated that the SERT is not intended to be a substitute for traditional speech discrimination tests but is expected to supplement them, especially when the child has very limited verbal abilities.

Jerger, Lewis, Hawkins, et al. (1980) and Jerger, Jerger, and Lewis (1981) described their use of realistic speech materials to control the receptive language factor in children by incorporating the actual responses of normal youngsters between the ages of 3 and 6 years in the new Pediatric Speech Intelligibility (PSI) test. The children composed both monosyllabic word and sentence test items elicited by picture stimulus cards selected from lists of words and actions comprising children's early vocabularies. The PSI test is composed of 20 monosyllabic words and a 10-sentence procedure. The word lists include simple nouns such as "dog" and "spoon" and two types of sentence construction identified as Format I and Format II. An example of a Format II sentence is, "A bear is brushing his teeth." The different sentence formats represent the different speech patterns of normal children between 3 and 6 years of age. The test materials are applicable for children as young as 2.5 or 3 years old.

The Jerger group's approach to PSI test development documented information regarding the utilization of the test items in the presence of a competing message and the definition of performance-intensity functions for children of varying chronologic and receptive language age groups. Their results confirmed the ability of children to perform these tasks that were previously applied only to adults.

They have focused attention on the importance of variables such as predetermination of receptive language ability and cognition skills, rather than considering only chronologic age (Figs. 6-10 and 6-11).

With the advent of cochlear implants and their success with young deaf children, a need was identified for speech perception tests that could be used to evaluate the preimplant and postimplant status of speech recognition skills. Accordingly, a number of word recognition tests were developed for children with severe and profound hearing loss who would, by definition, have extremely poor discrimination abilities. Decisions regarding the selection of candidates for cochlear implantation in young children must include evaluation of speech perception that might lead to estimates of outcome predictions. In fact, there is an overwhelming amount of information on the large number of speech tests developed to assess speech perception in children with profound deafness as reviewed by Busby, Dettman, Altidis, Blamey, and Roberts (1990), Tyler (1993) and Plant and Spens (1995). Miyamoto et al. (1996, 1997) published results from studies of the speech perception and speech production skills of children with cochlear implants. A brief overview of these special word recognition tests for children is presented below.

The Monosyllabic, Trochee, Spondee (MTS) Test developed by Erber and Alencewicz (1972) consists of 2 presentations of 12 pictured words: 4 monosyllables, 4 trochees (2-syllable words with stress on the first syllable), and 4 spondees (2-syllable words with equal stress on each syllable). The pictures are placed in front of the child, who is asked to point to the correct picture requested by the examiner. Two scores are obtained that reflect the number of times the correct stress pattern was recognized and the number of words correctly identified.

The Glendonald Auditory Screening Procedure (GASP) developed by Erber (1982) is a closed-set of 12 words and is similar to the MTS. The GASP uses 3 monosyllables, 3 trochees, 3 spondees, and 3 polysyllables as well as 10 common, everyday sentences and a phoneme detection task.

The Early Speech Perception (ESP) Test was developed by Geers and Moog (1990) at the Central Institute for the Deaf to meet the needs of the very young, profoundly hearing-impaired child with limited vocabulary and language skills. The test is composed of three sections. Part I is a pattern perception subtest and 2-word identification subtests. Part II is a 12-item spondee identification test with each word featuring a different vowel sound. Part III is a 12-item monosyllabic word identification test containing similar words. A low-verbal version of the test is the Four Choice Spondee subtest that includes four words represented by pictures or objects. Each word is presented three times in random order. The words commonly used are "baseball," "hot dog," "airplane," and "popcorn." Geers and Moog used the ESP to separate skills into categories: (1) no pattern perception, (2) consistent pattern perception, (3) inconsistent word identification, (4) consistent word identification, and (5) open-set word recognition.

The Test of Auditory Comprehension (Los Angeles County, 1980) is a closed-set, recorded test that evaluates perception of environmental sounds and speech. It has 10 subtests beginning with elementary differences between linguistic and nonlinguistic sounds, and proceeding to speech recognition in competing messages. The response mode requires the child to point to pictures.

The Minimal Auditory Capabilities Battery, widely known as the MAC (Owens, Kessler, Raggio, & Schubert, 1985), has 13 auditory tests and 1 speech-reading test to evaluate phonemic discrimination, sentence identification, suprasegmental features, environmental sounds, and visual enhancement with

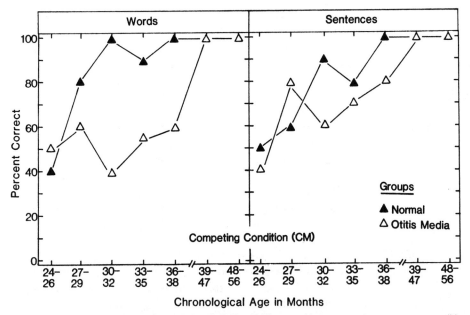

Figure 6-10. Data from the Pediatric Speech Intelligibility (PSI) test with a competing message condition for a group of normal-hearing children and a group of children with otitis media. Note the disparity between the two groups, shown with the word materials. Although the sentence materials also bring out perceptual differences between the two groups, the poorer performance by the otitis media group is especially evident with the word test. (Courtesy of Susan Jerger, Baylor School of Medicine, Houston, Texas.)

and without amplification. The test is demanding and cannot be used with young children.

The Vowel Perception Test (Fryauf-Bertschy, Tyler, Kelsay, Gantz, & Wood-

worth, 1997) consists of five plates of four pictured consonant-vowel-consonant words. On each plate the words are contrasted by medial vowel only (e.g., "bite," "boot," "boat," and "bat"). Each word is

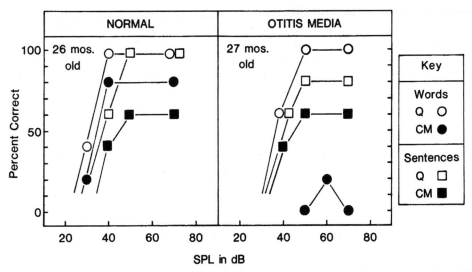

Figure 6-11. PSI data from two children of equivalent chronologic age and receptive language ability. PSI performance-intensity functions in quiet (Q) look quite similar between the two patients, but note the performance-intensity function for the otitis media child when words are presented with a competing message (CM) background. (Courtesy of Susan Jerger, Baylor School of Medicine, Houston, Texas.)

presented in the sound-only condition twice for a total of 40 test items.

TESTING THE OLDER CHILD

By 5 years and older, the child of normal intelligence can cooperate in the standard adult pure tone techniques and can repeat simple words. These youngsters will attend for fairly long periods of time to traditional hand-raising responses when they hear the test stimuli, given sufficient praise and encouragement. Beware of too much encouragement, however, as the child may begin to give false responses in order to please. The pure tone audiometric technique that is chosen is a matter of preference, so long as it fulfills the requirements of the descending-ascending bracketing technique. Carhart and Jerger (1959) described the most commonly accepted techniques for obtaining thresholds.

A method proposed by Berlin and Catlin (1965) has some advantages over traditional procedures. The initial tone presentation is given at 0 dB HL and ascends in 10 dB steps until the level is reached at which the subject responds. Another signal is given at 5 dB above that level to confirm its validity, and then another presentation is given at 10 dB below the previous one. A second ascent is then made. If a response is given, the next tone is presented at 10 dB below that level, and the next tone ascends 5 dB. Two or three responses must be seen at "threshold." Advantages to this method are as follows: (1) it structures the bracketing of threshold; (2) it confirms the first response at a higher level; (3) it eliminates the taking of false responses as the threshold, by confirming the lowest response level through a 5 dB higher level; (4) it accustoms the child immediately to listen for softer tones rather than louder tones; and (5) in the case of a functional hearing loss, it minimizes the "measuring stick" of the child by the presentation of lower hearing levels at the start.

Regardless of the pure-tone testing technique used, the experienced clinician will routinely use the confirmatory procedure of presenting a 5 dB higher level than the presumed threshold. False responses can be spotted rapidly with this maneuver.

The younger child in the 5- to 10-year age group requires motivation to keep his or her attention on the test. This can usually be done by social approval (e.g., smiling, nodding the head, clapping the hands). The time spent in gaining rapport with the child is worth the effort. The audiologist should talk to the child briefly about clothes, interests, toys, or activities, displaying a real interest in each youngster. During this time, useful observations are made about voice quality, articulation, extent of vocabulary, and degree of cooperation. The audiologist can then explain to the child exactly what is going to happen, telling the child what he or she is going to do—not "Will you do this for me?" It must also be explained to children that they need to raise their hand (or finger) even when the tone sounds very faint and far away. It should also be stressed that the child must "listen hard for these little tiny sounds because they are a long way off."

The child and teenager between 10 and 16 years of age can be treated very much like an adult patient. Very few modifications of standard audiometric procedures are ever required for the 10- to 16-year age group. The development of rapport, the complete explanation of the test procedure, and the use of mild motivational techniques are usually sufficient for a valid test. If the clinician has been presented with an audiogram from elsewhere showing a 30- to 60-dB loss, yet the youngster responds perfectly well to soft speech levels, he or she should be prepared to conduct the hearing tests very carefully. In this case, testing should start with a slow, ascending presentation of both pure tones and speech. Time will be saved in arriving at an accurate understanding of the hearing problem.

The hearing-impaired child may over-respond when no sound is actually heard in an attempt to appear to have more favorable hearing than really exists. It is best not to let such children see the audiologist during the test presentation. The child should face completely away from the clinician. Such children are so visually alert that they can catch even a raised eyebrow out of the corners of their eyes. During the test, there should occasionally be long periods of silence. If the child responds falsely, they should be reproved for the false response. Gentle reprimands are sometimes helpful to counteract this enthusiastic response behavior.

At this and younger ages, the child has a right to understand what it means to have a hearing loss, providing the child has any receptive language at all. Too often, professionals tend to "talk over" the child to the parents, in words that the child does not understand. In the meantime, the child is sitting there, wondering what is wrong. The clinician should take time to explain in words that the child can understand about the hearing loss, how severe it is, and what is going to be done about it. Often the clinician's explanation of the problem will ease the way toward accepting the amplification and habilitation that will follow. Parents may be unable to explain these things to the child or may try to gloss over the facts, leaving the child bewildered and sometimes antagonistic. The child may be worried about what the other children will think and say in school. It should be explained that the hearing loss does create special problems but that the audiologist is going to be sure that the child can do everything "other kids" can do and that the child will now be able to hear his or her friends and the teacher better.

USING A TESTER ASSISTANT

Although many audiology clinical settings require that the audiologist work alone, the hearing testing of children is often enhanced by the use of an extra observer or an assistant to the tester. This tester assistant remains in the test room with the child to help control the test paradigm, to monitor and direct the behavior of the child under evaluation, and to communicate with the tester as necessary. Guidelines are in order so that the tester assistant can be of maximum use in the audiologic evaluation.

To be a successful team, the tester and the assistant must have clearly defined roles and areas of responsibility understood before testing begins. One person is identified as the "tester" and typically is the person responsible for the task at hand. The other person is the "assistant" and follows the directives of the tester. Both are in continuous contact by earphones and the talkback circuit of the audiometer, through the sound field system, or even by closed circuit video. The designated person has the task of all major communication with the parents. It is very disruptive to have both the tester and the assistant talking to the parents at different times during the test session.

The assistant is in charge of the test room as much as possible and maintains the behavior of the child and the parents. It may be appropriate for the assistant to talk briefly to the parents during the session to warn them of what is about to happen in the test sequence, to guide their communication with the child, or to caution them about influencing the responses of the child unless specifically asked to do so. The team must often make an educated estimate about whether to include the parents in the sound room during the test session, based on a number of observations including the behavior of the parents, the relationship between the parents and the child, and the number of accompanying relatives, friends, neighbors, and siblings.

Before the start of the test session, the sound room environment needs to be well organized. Toys must be kept out of sight until they are ready to be introduced to the child, one at a time, under control of the assistant. The test room should be as visually bland as possible to keep distractions to a minimum. Careful consideration must be given to the arrangement of chairs, tables, sound field speakers, and visual reinforcers as well as the positions of the parent(s), assistant, and child, all so that the tester will have an unobstructed view of the child.

The test session should be started when the infant or child is showing a moderate amount of interest in a quiet toy used as a distractor. The timing of the test signal presentations and the time interval between signal presentations are very important to the success of the test session. Generally, the initial test presentations are slow, and as the child's performance improves, trials can be generated with much shorter intertrial intervals. "Time out" may be used following false responses from the child, allowing the youngster to "settle down" again. One of the most common errors made by inexperienced testers is to run through the test session too quickly too soon. Well-trained infants and children can perform quite well with rapid trial presentations, but the tester must be sure that the desired response relative to the stimulus presentations has been adequately shaped.

The assistant's task is to keep the child in a moderate state of alertness—not so absorbed in the toys that he or she will not be responsive to the auditory stimulus, yet not so uninterested that he or she will continuously visually search the room or fixate on the reinforcer. It is to be expected that there is tremendous variability among children's behavior in the test room environment. There is also wide variation in the child's attention level during the test session. The real challenge is for the assistant to judge precisely and anticipate the state of the child and to have the ability to manipulate and maintain the child's state at the desired level.

The choice of toys is important. Toys vary in how much attention they demand from children. Sometimes a child will have no preconceived idea of what a specific toy is supposed to do, so the imagination of the assistant has much to do with how successful a toy can be during the test session. Toys that generate noise and action toys that become too intriguing should be avoided. Toys should be introduced only one at a time, with all other toys being kept out of sight. When a child is done with a toy, it should also be put out of sight and out of reach. Toys in use should be kept directly in front of the child to eliminate false head-turns. The manipulation of the toys by the assistant is very important to the timing and the eventual success of the hearing evaluation.

TESTING THE DIFFICULT-TO-TEST CHILD

The difficult-to-test child is a child with special needs. The child's behavior or level of functioning may be so erratic that standard techniques of audiometry cannot be used. To apply appropriate tests for hearing, the clinician must be able to recognize the dysfunction present and to adjust the tests to it. The classic disorders to be differentiated are mental retardation, cerebral dysfunction, and autism (Myklebust, 1954). More than one of these may be present in one child. The clinician trained in evaluating any of these disorders may also test the child's functioning in that specific area as well as in the hearing area. At the very least, the audiologist has the responsibility of recognizing the disorder that exists, being able to apply the proper tests for hearing, and making a referral for diagnosis and treatment of the other disorder.

In discussing the entities that must be recognized, it is necessary to reiterate an important fact, that is, neither cerebral dysfunction, nor central auditory disorders, nor mental retardation, nor autism itself results in a decrease of auditory acuity as represented by the audiogram.

The responses that can be elicited certainly require more ingenuity to obtain. The clinical audiologist's task is to choose the appropriate test procedures that will reveal the presence or absence of peripheral hearing loss and/or central auditory disorder. It is not always a simple task to make this distinction.

Children With Multiple Handicaps. Children with multiple handicaps present difficult testing problems for audiologists. By definition, profoundly multihandicapped children cannot function independently at the most basic skill levels including self-presentation, self-care, mobility, and communication (Baker, 1979). When viewed within the context of developmental theory, the profoundly multihandicapped child responds to the same stimulation parameters as the normal child of the same developmental age (Kamhi, 1982). The developmental theory implies that the retarded child passes

through the same auditory developmental states as the normal child, except that the retarded child develops more slowly and with less potential.

The evaluation of hearing in profoundly multihandicapped children requires the utmost in audiologic skills and application of the cross-check test battery. Although the ABR procedure is usually required for definitive hearing assessment, these patients cannot always be successfully tested with ABR because central nervous system drainage and severe neurologic abnormalities often confound their problems. Accordingly, behavioral measurement of hearing must be included as a basic component of the auditory evaluation. On occasion, the uncontrollable behavior of the multihandicapped child makes it extremely difficult to structure the testing situation properly (Table 6-6).

In the most severe cases of multiple involvement (including blindness and retar-

Table 6.6.
Suggestions for Audiologic Testing of the Multihandicapped Child

Concern	Adaptation
These children vary in their capabilities for selective attention	May need to reduce extraneous visual or auditory distraction to avoid "overload" (e.g., reduce demands for motoric or visual activity when eliciting auditory response)
State of arousal may vary during interaction	If child becomes lethargic, change in positioning may heighten arousal (e.g., rock from supine to sitting position); parent or teacher may suggest strategy
Child often requires more than the usual amount of response time	Careful pacing of stimulation to allow for latent responses
Interfering self-stimulatory behaviors	Provide alternative action; ask parent and teacher for input regarding methods for reducing these behaviors
Tactile defensiveness may affect interaction with examiner	Inquire and observe for incidence of this behavior; approach the child carefully if touch is nonreinforcing
VRA response requires many prerequisites that may not be in the child's repertoire	Note if the child has self-regulated looking, sufficient head-neck control, cognitive prerequisites; explore adaptive positioning (can the child lie on the floor and roll to a sound source? While in standing board, can the child shift eye gaze to light stimulus?) Are the visual and auditory stimuli reinforcing enough?
Child may exhibit subdued or noncharacteristic behavior in new environment	Observe the child in a natural setting (school or home) if possible; allow "visits" to the suite before testing; provide warm-up/exploration time and sufficient practice trials

Adapted from Moeller, M.P. (1988). *Sensory organizational issues: Multi-handicapped child.* Omaha, NE: Boys Town National Institute, Coordinator for Aural Rehabilitation.

dation), the authors have found it useful to rely on the simplest of behavioral commands, presented through the sound field speaker system, of "sit down," "stand up," various orienting stimuli, and observation of quieting responses to specific stimuli presentations. At the most rudimentary level, these response behaviors may suggest the presence of near-normal hearing, although the absence of consistent responses can, in no way, be interpreted as the presence of hearing loss.

Flexer and Gans (1982, 1985, 1986) studied the auditory responsiveness of profoundly multihandicapped children and support the practice of determining auditory function of these children in relation to their development age. These researchers noted that narrow bandwidth auditory signals are simply not as effective in eliciting responses from multihandicapped children as are broader bandwidth stimuli, including speech stimuli.

Accurate assessment of hearing level in developmentally delayed persons is crucial to optimal efforts at rehabilitation, intervention, and follow-up. A comparative study of audiometric testing techniques with 61 moderately and 103 profoundly mentally retarded children from a large institution was conducted by Benham-Dunster and Dunster (1985). These clinicians compared BOA responses with VRA, Sensitivity Prediction with the Acoustic Reflex (SPAR) test technique, and ABR (sedation was required for 66% of moderately delayed and 91% of profoundly delayed children). The BOA was more reflective of developmental capabilities than of hearing loss, especially among the profoundly delayed. The acoustic reflex SPAR procedure overpredicted hearing loss and was problematic because of uncooperative behavior.

ABR, acoustic immittance measures, and the otoacoustic emissions test are the best bets for the measurement of hearing loss among the profoundly delayed. For a thorough investigation of the auditory mechanism and hearing in the developmentally handicapped, a full battery of tests offers the most complete assessment. A wide range of data help overcome gaps in information that result from difficulties inherent in testing developmentally delayed individuals.

Mental Retardation. One principle should be kept in mind when dealing with the mentally retarded child: if generalized developmental retardation is the only disorder, the child will behave in all areas at the level of his or her age. This principle will hold up in all cases except those in which autistic behavior or cerebral dysfunction is superimposed on the general retardation. Then the testing problem is further compounded, although not insoluble. Of course, this group of difficult-to-test children must absolutely be cross-checked with acoustic immittance measures, otoacoustic emissions tests, auditory brainstem response (ABR), and acoustic immittance measurements described in Chapter 7. Dahle and McCollister (1983) have reviewed all of the procedures for evaluating mentally retarded children, including an appropriate review of the physiologic tests of hearing. They point out that normal ABR tracings in this group of children give valuable information about their auditory peripheral sensitivity. However, when the ABR is abnormal and a central nervous system abnormality is obvious, the ABR results are ambiguous (Worthington & Peters, 1980).

If previous developmental scales or IQ test results are available, the clinician will have no difficulty in correcting the auditory test results for mental age. It is when the intellectual status is unknown that the clinician must anticipate auditory responses based on observations of developmental landmarks. After 4 months of age, the infant with mental retardation can be identified through auditory behavior responses as well as through the developmental landmarks present. If by 5 months of age the child is not making even a partial head-turn toward the sound, developmental milestones such as reaching and holding objects and laughing aloud need to be determined. The mentally delayed child may not hold the head erect or be able to follow a moving object—behavior that would place the child below the 3-month level of functioning. In this case, one can expect only the auditory responses listed for a child less than 4 months old. If all behaviors are consistent for a certain age level and the auditory indices are within the normal limits listed for that age level, the hearing level is judged to be normal.

Wilson, Folsom, and Widen (1982) evaluated VRA in testing infants who had Down syndrome and reported poor success until the developmentally delayed infants reached at least 10 months equivalent age. Werner et al. (1996) reported success in testing the hearing of infants with Down syndrome using an observer-based procedure for babies as young as 2 months of age.

A period of pretest observation will reveal what can be expected of the youngster. The child should be presented with toys and observed to see how familiar he or she is with them. Can the child hand them to the clinician on command? If the child recognizes most of the toys and can give them to someone on command, the audiologist can probably expect to obtain both an SRT and play-conditioned thresholds. Many older developmentally delayed children will have a level of functioning that permits behavioral conditioning techniques or speech audiometry tests to be used. Depending on the degree of accuracy required during the hearing test, the audiologist must be prepared to cross-check the subjective auditory thresholds with additional independent tests. When precise thresholds are desired in a borderline functioning child, the techniques of VRA and ABR should be used.

The Centrally Disordered Child. The suggested techniques for testing the brain-damaged child rest on two basic assumptions:

- Any reduction in auditory sensitivity for pure tones, or decreased acuity for speech intelligibility is caused by lesions in the peripheral auditory system, not in the midbrain or higher pathways (see Chapter 5).

- Only in the extremely severe centrally damaged child with gross motoric involvement will one see the complete absence of all of the four basic auditory reflexes: head-turn, eye-blink, startle response, and arousal from sleep.

The first rule in testing such a child is to determine the level of behavior through some means of pretesting. The audiologist should sit and talk quietly and play with the youngster in the sound room. Can the child attend for any length of time to anything that is said or done? Can the child give his or her name, age, or other appropriate information? Can the child hand the audiologist toys or repeat words on request? In the case of a very young child, as well as an older one, is eye contact steady and does it have integrity? Can the child sit still for any length of time? Is the child hyperactive? Does the child throw things around?

The child who has auditory perceptual dysfunction may be able to sit quietly and attend to visual stimuli but not be able to repeat words or to pick up objects on command. Such a child may, however, be perfectly able to participate in play-conditioned audiometry with pure tones and speech signals. If it is evident that formal testing techniques will not be successful, it is best to start at the lowest level of testing procedure, as has been described for infants. The entire battery of observations should be made, from localization procedures to startle reactions. It should be remembered that this child may be inconsistent in responses to various stimuli and at various times.

It is rare for the entire array of behavioral auditory reflexive responses to be absent in a child. These auditory behavioral reflexive responses are mediated at the level of the brainstem and are usually intact in the presence of higher cortical dysfunction. Auditory reflexes only tell us about the integrity of the peripheral auditory system and the central auditory system through the brainstem. They tell us nothing about the higher orders of perception and integration.

Only in the presence of degeneration of the brainstem at the olivary complex can the absence of the head-turn and eye-blink be expected. Even then the startle reflex, mediated at a low brainstem level, should be active, unless there is widespread motoric damage that prevents the muscular system from coordinating. Although the startle or eye-blink reflexes to a 65 dB (speech level) signal do not eliminate the presence of a sensorineural loss, it is likely that the hearing loss is not of a degree that would produce the severe degree of symptoms found in a child with profound or total deafness.

Stein et al. (1987) evaluated 122 profoundly retarded children from a single residential institution over a 4.5-year period. Most of the children were nonambulatory and had multiple handicapping conditions. The children ranged in age from infants to 18 years, with a mean age of 7.8 years. By definition, this group represented the most profoundly retarded subpopulation of the retarded described as untestable or difficult to test by behavioral audiometry. This study noted that 32% of the population showed hearing loss (by ABR testing) of 20 dB or greater in one or both ears, with 12% conductive loss and 20% sensorineural hearing loss. Some 8% of the study sample showed bilateral severe to profound hearing loss. Although the authors caution that the data reported are limited in generalization to the institutionalized profoundly retarded, this study confirms the presence of a high incidence of hearing loss in such populations. Six of nine children in this group fitted with hearing aids accepted and appeared to benefit from the use of personal amplification.

Autistic-Like Child. It is seldom that one sees the purely autistic-like child, but when one does, the bizarre behavior displayed can be recognized almost immediately: refusal to meet any person's eye gaze, disregard of all human speech stimuli, long-term fixation on some object, and refusal of physical contact with humans. This child will consistently fail to attend to any speech stimulus, yet will attend to some other acoustic signals. One such child will look for pure tone signals at low intensities, another will search for a novel sound field speech signal at soft levels, and another will localize to a white or a complex noise signal. All will startle or eye-blink to a 65 dB HL voice in a structured sound room situation if hearing is normal. All the stimuli described for testing from birth on should be tried. Some stimulus will likely produce a response if the hearing is normal, even if it is only a startle response.

The real testing problem arises when autistic behavior is superimposed on central dysfunction. Indeed, one wonders whether all brain damage is not accompanied by some degree of autistic behavior. The symptoms are often so similar that they defy separation. In addition to the behavior described above, there may be the heightened activity and lashing out at humans. If such a child is difficult for the neurologist and psychiatrist to understand, so too is the child for the audiologist.

The testing procedures described for mental retardation for central nervous system disorders are applicable here. It should be kept in mind that autistic symptoms are sometimes found in the deaf child, so the clinician should not let anything mislead him or her in the search for peripheral hearing loss. The cross-check principle is especially important in the evaluation of hearing in these children. The physiologic tests, such as ABR and immittance measurements, with special attention to acoustic reflex thresholds, are extremely valuable.

The Deaf-Blind Child. It is the authors' opinion that the evaluation of hearing in deaf-blind children is the most difficult task faced by the audiologist. These cases are most often confounded by central nervous system damage that makes it difficult to structure the testing situation properly.

In severe cases of multiple involvement, the authors have found it most expedient to rely again on the auditory reflexes, on orientation responses, and on quieting responses. In the absence of speech and language, one must apply the tests as for the infant, proceeding to the upper limits of the auditory abilities present. Application of the cross-check principle using the independent measures of acoustic immittance, otoacoustic emissions, and ABR will most likely be required with these children.

Stein, Ozdamar, and Schnabel (1981) published an excellent report on the neurologic handicaps, degree of hearing and visual disability, and the level of language and developmental characteristics of a young deaf-blind population. These authors reviewed data from 141 deaf-blind children evaluated at their clinic. Of these children seen for diagnostic hearing evaluation, 38 were found to have normal or near-normal hearing and, therefore, were technically not "deaf." The diagnosis of normal hearing in most of these difficult-to-test children was accomplished only through the use of the ABR technique (Stein et al., 1981). The previous diagnosis of deafness given these children was based largely on behavioral testing, and these children simply failed to respond behaviorally to sound.

Stein et al. summarized the findings in their study as follows:

- A high incidence of neurologic handicapping conditions, including neuromuscular disorders, is associated with congenitally deaf-blind children.

- Severe hearing disability was more common than severe vision disability in this sample of deaf-blind children. Sixty-eight percent of children had so little usable hearing that the potential benefit of wearable amplification was minimal at best.

- Many of the "deaf-blind" children referred for evaluation proved to have normal peripheral hearing without normal behavioral responses to sound. The use of the ABR as part of the audiologic evaluation is thus an absolute necessity with these children.

- The combination of hearing and visual problems together with neurologic handicapping conditions has a profound effect on the language level, cognitive skills, and general development of these children.

- The severe hearing loss and neurologic problems will require that most, if not all, of these children will need supervised care for the rest of their lives.

Summary for Difficult-to-Test and Special Needs Children. It is the audiologist's responsibility to make the decision about the multihandicapped child's hearing abilities. It must, perforce, be a bold decision, for any equivocation is not useful to the child. The conservative hearing aid trial with careful observations by all concerned during a diagnostic therapy period may be helpful. Hesitation may deprive the child of critical time for learning auditory skills and thus do him or her a disservice. Little textbook information or standardized developmental scales are available regarding techniques for evaluating the hearing response in these children. It is often useful to the audiologist to discuss the hearing potential of the difficult-to-test child with the parents and teachers who are with the child for long periods.

CENTRAL AUDITORY PROCESSING DISORDERS

Children with either organic lesions of the central auditory pathways or auditory perceptual and language disorders are diagnosed with tests of central auditory function. An understanding of the current research and its implications, diagnostic testing, and management of central auditory processing in children is necessary for pediatric audiologists. A complete discussion of this topic is beyond the scope of this section, and the reader is referred to a number of reference sources including Bellis (1996), Chermak and Musiek (1997), and Masters, Stecker, and Katz (1998).

Central auditory processes, as described by ASHA (1996), are the *auditory system* mechanisms and processes responsible for the behavioral phenomena listed below. A central auditory processing disorder (CAPD) is an observed deficiency in one or more of the listed behaviors and is assumed to apply to nonverbal and verbal signals affecting many areas of speech and language. For some persons, CAPD is presumed to result from dysfunction of processes and mechanisms dedicated to audition; for others, CAPD may stem from some more general dysfunction, such as an attention deficit or neural timing deficit.

- Sound localization and lateralization
- Auditory discrimination
- Auditory pattern recognition
- Temporal aspects of audition, including:
  - temporal resolution
  - temporal masking
  - temporal integration
  - temporal ordering

- Auditory performance decrements with competing acoustic signals
- Auditory performance decrements with degraded acoustic signals

After more than 20 years of dealing with issues related to central auditory processing, CAPD still lacks uniform consensus on definition, identification procedures, and intervention practices. A number of issues remain unresolved which continue to make the topic of central auditory testing somewhat "fuzzy." A major problem is the lack of data on the cause-and-effect relationship of auditory-perceptual deficits and language, reading, and learning disorders. The lack of standardized terminology and diagnostic techniques raises doubt about the validity of remediation for such problems. The development of adequate remediation programs for children with auditory processing disorders continues to be a problem for those who work with this population. Although CAPD touches multidisciplinary areas of expertise, recent years have seen the profession of audiology step forward and claim the diagnosis of CAPD as their own scope of practice, working with speech-language pathologists to develop remediation and management plans. Teachers look to audiologists and speech-language pathologists for guidance in helping children with these problems.

Keith (1986) defined an auditory processing disorder as an "impaired" ability to attend to, discriminate, recognize, remember, or comprehend information presented auditorily even though the person has normal intelligence and hearing sensitivity. These difficulties are more pronounced when listening to low redundancy (distorted) speech, when there are competing sounds, or when there is a poor acoustic environment. Keith (1988) hypothesizes that some basic auditory-perceptual skills (e.g., appreciation of frequency, intensity, and duration of sounds) exist in every child and serve as building blocks of audition, leading to language development through imitation. As language skills are acquired, children also acquire other linguistically dependent auditory-perceptual skills, such as memory, discrimination, closure, and blending. In addition, as the child's neuroanatomic pathways mature, the ability to cope with higher-level auditory tasks such as dichotic listening, binaural release from masking, and other nonlinguistically based listening skills begins to improve.

Controversy exists about the difficult (if not impossible) differential diagnosis between attention deficit hyperactivity disorder (ADHD) and CAPD. Professionals debate whether both disorders represent the same or separate developmental disorder(s). Children with CAPD are known to exhibit a wide range of behaviors as they experience a number of language and learning problems, expressing some of the following characteristics as described by Keith (2000a):

- Normal pure-tone hearing thresholds with a possible history of recurrent otitis media
- Inconsistent responses to auditory stimuli
- Inability to follow auditory instructions
- Difficulty with auditory localization of sound and inability to differentiate soft and loud sounds
- Unexplainable fear of loud noises, with children often holding their hands over their ears to stop the sounds
- Difficulties in remembering phonemes and manipulating them in tasks such as reading, spelling, and phonics
- Difficulty understanding speech in noisy backgrounds
- Difficulty with auditory memory, either span or sequence, and poor auditory memory
- Poor listening skills with decreased attention, increased distractibility, and restlessness
- Frequent requests to repeat information
- Significant reading problems, poor spelling, and poor handwriting
- Withdrawal tendencies and shyness with poor self-concept resulting from multiple failures

A number of available tests are designed to measure these auditory abilities. It is necessary to select carefully the appropriate test for the ability to be measured and to evaluate the results against appropriate normative standards. Recent developments in electrophysiologic techniques indicate promising approaches to assessing central auditory processing abilities in children. These techniques, including middle latency responses and various other cortical evoked potentials, will require substantial investigation before they can be applied for clinical purposes.

It is helpful to review the definitions of the most common central auditory abilities that test developers attempt to measure in order to identify central auditory processing problems in children. To be complete, every central auditory test battery should include (1) patient history; (2) observation of auditory behaviors; (3) an extended audiologic evaluation to include auditory pure tone thresholds and speech recognition tests as well as tests for temporal processing skills, localization and lateralization, low redundancy monaural speech, dichotic stimuli, binaural interaction procedures, and electrophysiologic tests as appropriate; and (4) speech language evaluation. The definitions of terms used in CAPD evaluation are provided below:

- **Auditory Localization.** The ability to locate the source of a sound through hearing only. This ability requires binaural stimulation.
- **Binaural Synthesis.** The ability to integrate centrally incomplete stimulus

patterns presented simultaneously or alternately to opposite ears.

- **Figure Ground.** The ability to identify a primary signal or message in the presence of competing sounds. Auditory figure ground can be a monaural or a binaural task.

- **Binaural Separation.** The ability to listen with one ear while ignoring stimulation of the opposite ear. Dichotic listening, as a binaural separation task, requires the listener to attend to and report back different signals presented simultaneously to two ears.

- **Memory.** The ability to store and to recall auditory stimuli, including length or number of auditory stimuli, and sequential memory or the ability to recall the exact order of auditory stimuli presented.

- **Blending.** The ability to form words out of separately articulated phonemes.

- **Discrimination.** The ability to determine whether two acoustic stimuli are the same or different. In speech, auditory discrimination is the ability to recognize fine differences that exist among phonemes.

- **Closure.** The ability to perceive the whole (word or message) when parts are omitted.

- **Attention.** The ability to persist in listening over a reasonable period.

- **Association.** The ability to establish a correspondence between a nonlinguistic sound and its source.

- **Cognition.** The ability to establish a correspondence between a linguistic sound and its meaning. Cognition is the highest level of auditory perception and results from a summation of all auditory (and all sensory) tasks.

An enormous number of tests have been developed over the years to test central auditory processing. The available tests vary considerably in the scientific rigor under which they were developed. Many have limited comparative norm data and many are out of date, being supplanted by more current testing procedures. Certainly, before any attempt is made to administer tests for CAPD, the audiologist must be certain that no conductive or sensorineural hearing loss is present in either ear of the child. Generally, patients with CAPD show no hearing loss for traditional audiometric tests, although that is not to say that CAPD does not coexist in children who do have substantiated hearing disorders.

Most tests of CAPD are based on some form of challenging auditory signal for the auditory nervous system to identify as in speech-in-noise or distorted speech tests. These tests, known as "sensitized speech tests," use various means of distortion of speech to reduce the intelligibility of the message. Distortion can be accomplished in many ways including high- or low-pass filtering that reduces the range of frequencies (filtered speech testing). Another technique is to reduce the intensity level of speech above a simultaneously presented background noise (auditory figure ground testing). Speech can be distorted in the time domain by interrupting the speech at different rates, and by increasing the rate of presentation (time-compressed speech). Persons with normal hearing and normal auditory pathways can understand distorted speech messages; however, when a central auditory processing disorder is present, speech intelligibility under difficult circumstances is poor. The construct of sensitized speech testing is extremely powerful and forms the basis of all behavioral speech tests of central auditory function (Keith, 1999a).

Included in the list of possible test battery inclusions for the CAPD child are tests of temporal processing and resolution such as assessment of thresholds for brief tones, auditory fusion tests, testing for temporal ordering and sequencing of tonal or click stimuli, and discrimination of time-compressed speech. Speech-in-noise testing is used to identify when the child's ability to communicate in the presence of noise is substantially below the performance achieved by normal children. Dichotic tests are delivered binaurally, and the child must respond to whatever was heard in either ear or report what was heard in one or both ears. Dichotic tests are available that use digits, words, spondees, syllables, and sentences. The masking level difference test (MLD) is a measure of binaural interaction. In terms of physiologic tests to evaluate CAPD, the ABR is sensitive to brainstem (and auditory pathway) abnormalities: the middle latency auditory evoked response (MLR) is used in cases in which CAPD is suspected, and the P-300 cognitive evoked potential is a measurement of general cortical activity. Results from these evoked potential procedures have been used to study auditory information processing, but interpretation of results leading to definitive conclusions about CAPD must be made with caution.

One of the most thoroughly developed, most carefully normed, and frequently used tests of CAPD is the SCAN-C: Test for Auditory Processing Disorders in Children-Revised (Keith, 2000b). The SCAN, developed in 1986 by Robert W. Keith, is designed for use with children from ages 3–11 years. The SCAN-C presents test materials on compact disc from four subtests: filtered words, auditory figure ground, competing words, and competing sentences. Admittedly, the SCAN-C is difficult for some 3- and 4-year-olds who are unable to complete the testing, and results for these younger children are inconsistent. It is important to remember that the diagnosis of a central auditory disorder is best accomplished using a team approach to assessment and a variety of test measures.

Remediation and Management of the Child With CAPD. Intervention strategies may be the easiest and yet the most diffi-cult tasks to achieve success with the CAPD child. Management strategies have focused on two approaches. The first strategy is to improve the acoustic environment to enhance the listening situation by improving the signal-to-noise ratio. This is accomplished by preferential seating and treatment of the home and classroom to reduce reverberation and increase sound absorption. The use of classroom amplification systems, or even personal FM systems, is a means of improving the signal-to-noise ratio and making speech more audible.

The second strategy, described in detail by Keith (1999b), is compensatory auditory skills development, that is, using various approaches to teaching auditory skills that will assist the child with CAPD. Cognitive therapy includes language and auditory training, vocabulary development, and the teaching of organizational skills. Butler (1983) suggested the teaching of mnemonic strategies, rehearsal, paragraphing, imagery, networking, analysis of new ideas, and the use of key words to think systematically. Cognitive therapy may include a return-to-basics approach of how to follow directions, how to use written notes, how to listen and anticipate, how to ask relevant questions, and other self-improvement techniques. Newer perceptual training techniques such as **"FastForward"** and **"Earobics"** as well as computer-assisted training have been used with reported success for children with CAPD (Merzenich et al., 1996; Tallal et al., 1996; Battin, Young, & Burns, 2000).

AUDIOLOGIST'S SELF-UNDERSTANDING

In his or her zeal to help the hearing-handicapped child and the child's parents, the audiologist often overlooks his or her own motivations and how they will affect relations with the parents. These relations may be critical to the parents' acceptance of the problem. Quite without meaning to, he or she may leave the parents with fears and pent-up emotions that can adversely affect the habilitation process. At some point the audiologist must look inward to see what his or her own feelings are in relation to the way information is given to the parents and how he or she handles them. If the audiologist has entered the audiologic profession with an emotional zeal to "do good," he or she may see himself or herself as the authoritarian figure who directs the lives of people and thus will not permit the parents to express themselves, because he or she is in charge of operations. If the audiologist has entered the field through an objective interest in the scientific manifestations of hearing, he or she may shrink from becoming emotionally involved and committed to the parents' problems.

So the audiologist, too, may have problems in feeling comfortable in his or her role as protagonist in the drama of the parent-clinician interplay. This subject deserves extensive coverage because it is vital to the ultimate emotional health of the child. Dr. Brian Hersch, a psychiatrist, and Carol Amon, an instructor of deaf children, prepared a most meaningful exposition on parent management. We are indebted to them for permission to use their analysis of the dynamics of the parent-clinician relationship presented below.

To parents who are anxious to hear that their idealized child is perfect, the statement that "Your child has a hearing impairment" may be painful words. In order to avoid this uncomfortable experience, many audiologists today choose a painless method of reporting the diagnosis—a way that, although it is painless for them, may have devastating effects on the parents and their child. After listening to many parents relate their experiences and frustrations, we realized that the act of reporting the diagnosis was not only of paramount importance, but also that it was the beginning of a process that would include the habilitation and education of the child and the crucial involvement of the parents.

An approach toward lessening the trauma of the initial contact is proposed. It is an out-

growth of an idea that an interdisciplinary approach to understanding hearing-impaired infants and their families (the disciplines being audiology, deaf education, and psychiatry) is far superior to an isolated fragmented approach of one profession (Schlesinger & Meadow, 1972).

Schlesinger and Meadow describe four ineffective professional stances which are often seen today in the reporting of the diagnosis:

1. The "hit-and-run" approach. The diagnosis is reported very quickly and matter-of-factly in passing. "Your child didn't respond too much today . . . his hearing loss is probably severe to profound. I'll see you in 6 months for another evaluation." The parents are left with their feelings of bewilderment as to what to do next. The reporting of the diagnosis appears to be a dead end with no source of help.

2. Minimizing the problem. The clinician infers that there is really nothing to worry about. "In this day and age, deaf children can be given hearing aids and go to regular school just like any other child." These words give false hope to the parents, but the audiologist says them in order to make the parents feel better.

3. The objectivity approach. Many audiologists are hidden behind objectivity, using the "big word" technique. In 1 hour's time, they report the diagnosis, explain the audiogram and the hearing mechanism, and how their child differs from normal, describe methods of habilitation, demonstrate the use and maintenance of a hearing aid, and schedule the child for the first habilitation session. The audiologist does most of the talking, often using professional jargon which leaves parents confused and feeling lost. The audiologist avoids listening.

4. The action-oriented approach. This fourth approach is also a popular one. The audiologist states the problem, and almost before he completes the reporting of the diagnosis he tells the parents what they are going to do to take care of the problem. The action part is essential, but only if there is adequate provision for exploring the feelings of the parents.

Such approaches by the audiologist greatly interfere with the process of acceptance of the handicap. A lack of acceptance prohibits the parents from helping their child grow both emotionally and educationally. The parents may deny the information and shop around for a professional who will tell them that their child is normal. Meadow (1968) pointed out that parents are more likely to listen and to integrate painful and unpleasant information from interested and "feeling" individuals.

The ineffective approaches used by the audiologist stem from a number of complex variables. First, he may lack knowledge and understanding of the habilitative process, and of the effect of his initial report. Second, he may be uncomfortable with the range of emotions that these parents may feel. Often audiologists state that they simply do not have the time to devote to reporting. This reasoning, however, may actually be a way of avoiding a more significant factor . . . that is, the audiologist has not yet worked out in his own mind what it means to him to tell someone some painful news. It is natural for people to avoid pain. The audiologist and the parents in a way become secretly and jointly involved in an agreement to avoid dealing with feelings.

There is no painless way to inform parents that they have a child with a hearing loss. However, pain does not have to be regarded negatively. It is part of a process that facilitates and encourages a family's involvement. Even though there is no way of softening the blow, there is a way to help parents accept the realities of the situation and to make use of the resources available to them. The goals of this important first discussion of the diagnosis are multifold.

1. Statement of the facts. Initially, it is important to state the facts as clearly and as emphatically as possible. These parents want up-to-date and accurate scientific information about their child's problem presented to them authoritatively, but in language they can understand. If an alliance is going to be created with these parents, it is most important that the audiologist admit any lack of information or knowledge about the problem that he has, doing so confidently and without strain. Throughout the giving of this information, the audiologist must convey a true interest in this family. The tone of voice and nonverbal behavior of an audiologist can convey callousness, or it can convey concern. It is essential to convey concern rather than the idea that you are just doing your job.
2. Support through listening. Perhaps the most important goal is to provide support through listening. By listening patiently and nonjudgmentally, you may be able to bring some of the parents' feelings out into the open—feelings of which they may not have been aware. Many parents have indicated during the initial conference that they had been anxious about their child for a long period of time, but had never shared that anxiety with anyone, not even the spouse. This may be the first opportunity they have had to express what they have been feeling for months.

In order that these feelings be expressed by both parents together, they should both be present to discuss the diagnosis unless it is physically impossible. During this discussion, we can begin to assess the parents' interactions and begin to decide whether they have the kind of relationship that will provide support to one another or whether they will require some help from outside. It is important that the audiologist note and report his initial impression of the parents, as these notes may be valuable to others involved with the family.

3. Giving the parents a role. Another important goal of this first contact is to convey to the parents that they have a great deal to offer, even thought they may have little formal knowledge about hearing loss and child development. Focusing on the parents' interaction with their child during that initial contact can give them some confidence. "You seem to sense Joey's needs very well." "That's beautiful, you called Joey's attention to that sound." "That's one of the most important ideas you will learn and you already appear comfortable with it." You can provide initial reinforcement of attributes that the parents are already equipped with, that will help their child's development.

During the initial discussion, the parents need to be made aware of the resources available to them—not only resources for habilitation and educational programming, but also resources available to help with emotional needs. Ideally, the audiologist will remain in contact with the family periodically, in order not only to give repeated evaluations, but also to act as a coordinator of professionals working with this family. It is vital that there be an interface between the person delivering emotional supportive services and those people primarily responsible for the habilitation program. This interaction will provide an opportunity to share and be aware of mutual concerns and will prevent the traditional approach of professionals working in isolation of each other.

In order for these goals to be realized, four criteria need to be present: First, the clinical audiologist must have some knowledge of the rehabilitative process; second, he must be comfortable dealing with feelings; third, adequate time must be provided for the reporting; and fourth, an atmosphere of mutual respect must be created.

For many years, the clinical audiologist has accumulated experience in diagnosing and fitting hearing aids, but has known little about the habilitation process. There is a trend today to provide audiologists with more information about habilitation, a trend that we see as positive. Perhaps as audiologists become more familiar with rehabilitative methods, they can objectively direct parents toward programs suited to their child's needs and alleviate the emotional controversy of the deaf.

Many audiologists are sensitive and concerned about their role in helping these families, but this does not necessarily mean that they feel comfortable in dealing with feelings. Sensitivity in raw form can potentially be a valuable tool and an asset for the audiologist, but just because the potential is there does not mean that it will automatically be used in a facilitative way. To learn how to use one's sensitivity effectively is a delicate process and cannot be taught. This exemplifies the necessity for an interdisciplinary approach where the audiologist who is uncomfortable in this area may take advantage of the mental health professions that deal with feelings routinely.

A seemingly minute detail in the criteria for effective reporting of the diagnosis is the allotment of time; however, this is probably an essential factor in reporting. One of the most consistent complaints of parents in their dealings with audiologists initially is that the situation was regarded lightly and not enough time was devoted to this important problem. It is our feeling that the audiologist must allocate a minimum of 45 minutes to this initial reporting. Should this not be possible, or should both parents not be available during this initial session, it is critical that an appointment be scheduled within the next 24 hours to discuss the problem thoroughly. As was indicated earlier, parents may experience a number of feelings at the outset, the most frequent being shock. Then may come anger, guilt, or depression. It is very important not to tell parents what they may feel because people experience different emotions. It is important to provide an open-ended approach, however, such as, "Today I have told you about your son's hearing loss. Over the weeks and months to follow, you may or may not experience some uncomfortable feelings as many parents naturally do. We will be available to you to discuss whatever feelings you may be having. Let's plan to talk again in a month or anytime before that, should you desire."

The approach to effective reporting of the diagnosis is not only dependent upon the audiologist's knowledge, his comfortable feelings and the allotment of adequate time but also upon the atmosphere created. It is the universal observation of those who have constructed programs for special groups of young disabled children that unless the parents' emotional needs are adequately dealt with, the programs themselves have limited benefit for the children (Mindel & Vernon, 1971). Thus, it is critically important that an atmosphere of mutual respect and honesty be created—an atmosphere that allows the expression of feelings in nonjudgmental and accepting ways.

Often the atmosphere of mutual respect is interrupted when the parents' depression explodes into external anger that sometimes is directed at the audiologist. If the audiologist does not understand that this expression of anger is only an indication of the parent's internal struggles, he may become defensive. The parents will be aware of his defensiveness even if it is only conveyed nonverbally, and thus the climate of mutual respect is destroyed.

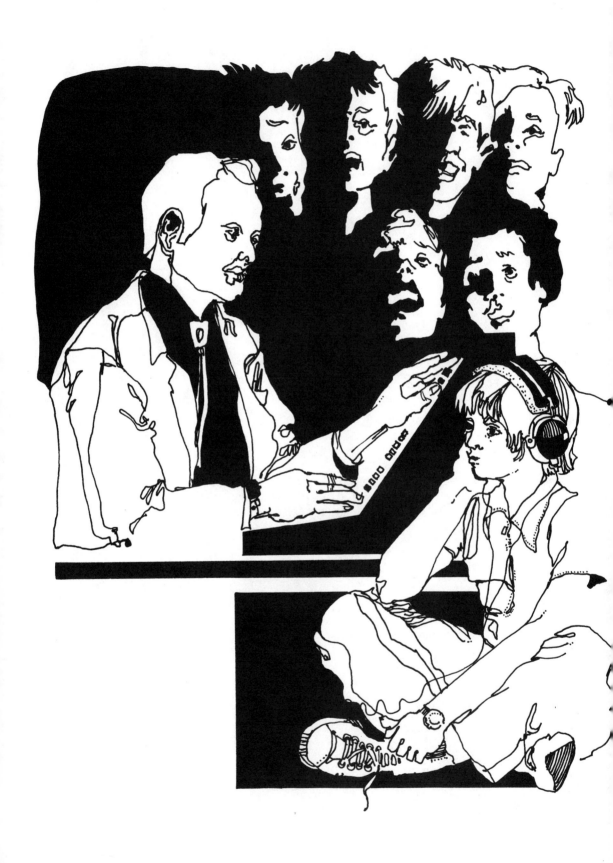

CHAPTER 7

Physiologic Hearing Tests

Nothing can be more frustrating to an audiologist than to work with a 2-year-old child who needs to have his or her hearing evaluated but who refuses to cooperate with any of the testing procedures. It seems impossible that the youngster who sat quietly and politely in the patient waiting area can suddenly turn into a crying, yelling, totally uncooperative subject in the sound-treated booth. What causes a child, who has been happily playing while waiting for his or her hearing test, to suddenly become an overly self-conscious, introverted, and unworkably shy patient? How does a clinician establish rapport with a youngster who is hidden in mother's skirt or wrapped around father's leg? Every clinician ultimately faces the child who cannot be tested. There are, indeed, means of handling such children, but the skills necessary to evaluate the hearing in uncooperative children are gained through experience and insight.

One may expect the behavior of "normal" children occasionally to be obstinate. What about testing the hearing of a hyperactive, developmentally delayed child? How does one elicit cooperation and establish play-conditioning techniques with an autistic or emotionally disturbed youngster? How can one fit earphones on a child with hydrocephaly? Play-conditioning techniques are obviously not possible with a child who will not even sit down! Just when the audiologist thinks that every conceivable situation has occurred, a child shows up who baffles every attempt to evaluate his or her hearing. Audiologists continue to seek a simple and accurate objective hearing test that can be used with any uncooperative child, much like the early Spanish explorers continued to hunt for the Fountain of Youth! Almost no other aspect of audiology stimulates interest in the same manner as a new report describing a promising objective hearing test to solve problems associated with testing the hearing in difficult-to-test children.

To deal with these difficult-to-test patients, the field of audiology has worked long and hard in the development of "objective" tests of hearing. An objective hearing test is one that *defines a patient's hearing ability without the patient's active participation in the test.* A physiologic hearing test relies on an autonomic response not based on the child's behavioral action. In the case of children, many factors may influence or suppress the child's ability to cooperate. The child may not have the mental or physical capabilities to cooperate fully or to attend to the hearing test task required by the clinician. The child's interest span may be too short. A clinician's skill in evaluating the hearing of these children often depends on the ability to establish rapport with the youngster and, at the same time, make an accurate evaluation of the child's capabilities in performing some task. A false start with these children may alienate them toward the testing situation, making additional test sessions necessary and possibly more difficult.

Many "objective" hearing tests, usually related to an autonomic physiologic response, have been suggested and reported.

The Ewings of England in the early 1940s used various percussion sounds and pitch pipes to elicit "aural reflex responses" in infants (Ewing & Ewing, 1944). They observed eye-blinks, squinting, involuntary jumping, and sound localization with body or head movements while testing young children. Froeschels and Beebe (1946) evaluated the auropalpebral reflex (defined as the involuntary closing of eyelids due to acoustic stimulation) in children and infants. More than a decade later, Froding (1960) of Sweden used a small gong and mallet that produced a sound of 126–133 dB SPL to evaluate the auropalpebral reflex in sleeping infants. Froding pointed out that the infants showed "a lack of consistency" in their responses to his gong and mallet stimulus despite the loudness of his signal.

New objective hearing tests are formulated with older children or cooperating adults, and these results are then generalized to young children. Somehow, the generalization that procedures that work well with adults should therefore also apply to children lacks credibility when the clinician comes face to face with a noncooperative 3-year-old. This chapter orients the student to a variety of physiologic, or as they are known by audiologists "objective," testing procedures commonly used in the pediatric audiology clinic. There are now complete textbooks devoted to each of the tests described in this chapter, so of course, it is not possible to describe every technical aspect of each physiologic test.

The presence of some physiologic response, seemingly related to the presence of an auditory signal, does not ensure that the child does indeed "hear." Hearing, in this sense, implies meaningful interpretation of the sound so as to produce thought and language with verbal or nonverbal encoding and decoding. The toughest test for a new clinical procedure is to withstand clinician criticism by proving itself to be reliable, quick, easy to administer, inexpensive, and worthwhile over a long period.

ACOUSTIC IMMITTANCE MEASURES

Acoustic immittance measurement is an objective means of assessing the integrity and function of the peripheral auditory mechanism. Acoustic immittance provides a number of important measures used to determine middle ear pressure, tympanic membrane mobility, eustachian tube function, continuity and mobility of the middle ear ossicles, acoustic reflex thresholds, and nonorganic hearing loss (Northern, 1996). The clinical application of acoustic immittance measurements has come to be known as *immittance audiometry*.

The testing techniques are especially well suited for children, because they are objective, accurate, quick, and easy to administer and create little discomfort to the patient. Children who will not cooperate with conventional audiometric techniques may not object to the immittance test battery. Immittance audiometry results are of special benefit to the physician who is unable to perform adequate otoscopic examination on a youngster, as well as to the audiologist who has difficulty in establishing valid hearing thresholds on an uncooperative child. Vast numbers of children have been tested with the immittance technique, and a wide variety of normative immittance test values are available.

The acoustic immittance technique in the evaluation of the auditory mechanism was originally proposed by Metz in 1946 and has been used routinely in Scandinavia since that time. North Americans, however, were slow to accept the clinical utility of this testing procedure until Alberti and Kristensen (1970) and Jerger (1970) independently published articles exalting impedance audiometry as a valuable routine procedure for assessing the nature of hearing loss. Jerger succinctly stated the significance of impedance audiometry by commenting, "We frankly wonder how we ever got along without it." Immittance measurements are now essential testing techniques in the evaluation of children's hearing and middle ear status.

Early publications by Brooks (1968, 1971) and Jerger (1970) validated the important benefits of acoustic immittance measures in children. Northern (1978c, 1980c, 1986, 1992) published numerous reviews on the use of immittance measurements in populations of special needs children, including those with hearing disabilities, the developmentally delayed, emotionally disturbed, the deaf-blind, those with cleft lip and palate, those with Down syndrome, and those with craniofacial disorders. Wiley and Fowler (1997) published a useful primer of acoustic im-

mittance measurements for clinical audiology testing.

The literature in this area uses the terms "impedance" and "immittance" somewhat interchangeably. Impedance is a measurement of resistance to movement, while immittance is a measurement of compliance or ease of motion. The acoustic immittance technique is based on the principle that sound pressure level (SPL) is a function of closed cavity volume. Regardless of whether acoustic immittance measures are expressed in terms of acoustic admittance (ease of sound flow) or acoustic impedance (resistance to sound flow), the method of clinical measurement is the same.

The hand-held immittance probe system is shown in Figure 7-1. An airtight seal is obtained with a soft rubber cuff

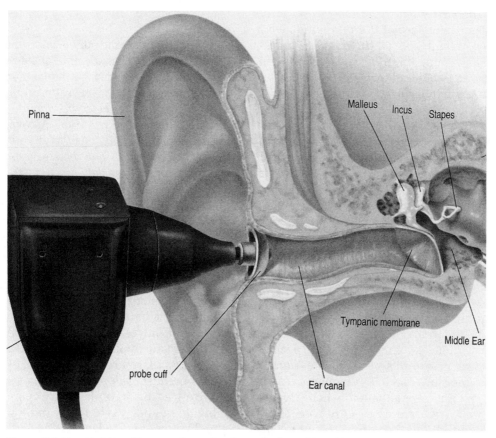

Figure 7-1. Hand-held immittance probe system hermetically positioned into the external auditory canal.

placed around a small probe that is inserted into the external auditory canal. A stimulus tone is emitted from the probe. The probe also controls an air pressure pump capable of creating positive, negative, or atmospheric air pressure in the ear canal cavity between the probe tip and the tympanic membrane. The probe system also includes a microphone that measures the SPL of the probe tone in the canal cavity. Specifically, the SPL of the ambient probe signal is an indirect measure of the acoustic immittance of the middle ear system. The middle ear is a stiffness-dominated mechanical system that is sensitive to low-frequency tones. Thus, most electroacoustic immittance instruments use a low-frequency probe tone of approximately 220 Hz. Some instruments have the capability to emit higher-frequency probe tones, or to produce multifrequency measurements, in addition to the 220 Hz signal.

The compliance of the tympanic membrane and integrity of the middle ear system determine the SPL of the probe tone in the external auditory canal cavity. The pickup microphone quantifies the SPL of acoustic energy that is reflected back into the external auditory canal. A high amount of reflected energy is measured when the middle ear system is stiff, as in such pathologic conditions as ossicular fixation, otitis media, or cholesteatoma. In contrast, discontinuity of the middle ear system creates a flaccid tympanic membrane that absorbs most of the probe tone sound energy and reflects very little sound back into the external auditory meatus.

The basic immittance test battery includes tympanometry, the ear canal physical volume test (PVT), and acoustic reflex threshold measurement. Although each of the test procedures can provide significant information, their diagnostic capabilities are strengthened when results from all three procedures are considered together (Table 7-1). For example, although tympanometry by itself is useful,

Table 7.1.
Summary of Immittance Audiometry Applications in Children

Tympanometry

    Objectively measures tympanic membrane mobility

    Measures middle ear pressure

    Confirms patency of ventilation tubes in tympanic membrane

    Estimates static compliance

Static compliance

    Differentiates middle ear fixation from disarticulation

Acoustic reflex threshold

    Objectively measures cochlear pathology

    Validates nonorganic hearing loss

    Validates conductive hearing loss

    Aids in the differential diagnosis of conductive hearing loss

    Provides objective inference of hearing sensitivity

Ear canal physical volume test

    Identifies nonintact tympanic membrane, perforation, and patency of ventilating tubes

interpretation of the physical volume measurement is crucial, and absence of the acoustic reflex may be due to any of several reasons. Yet, interpretation of results from all of the tests will provide important and valid information. An experienced audiologist can easily administer the entire battery of four tests in approximately 1 minute per ear.

Audiologists using immittance measurements must follow three general rules: (1) recognize overall patterns in the tests of the impedance audiometry battery, (2) pay little attention to the absolute value of any of the immittance test battery results, and (3) beware of the implicit diagnostic conclusions based only on the immittance test battery (Northern, 1980b). Jerger and Hayes (1980) stated that in the "diagnostic application of immittance audiometry there are no absolutes... [use caution because] the results of any single immittance measurement are usually ambiguous and have little individual value." Wiley and Fowler (1997) point out that audiograms and acoustic immittance measures can be used together to determine the cause of middle ear pathology, particularly when either measure alone does not provide adequate differential information. Similar conductive losses noted on audiograms may be differentiated by appropriate interpretations of acoustic immittance test results.

Tympanometry. Tympanometry is a dynamic and objective technique for measuring the compliance or mobility of the tympanic membrane as a function of changing air pressures in the external auditory canal. The general term "tympanometry" refers to methods and techniques for measuring, recording, and evaluating changes in acoustic impedance (or resistance of the auditory mechanism) with systematic changes in air pressure. The compliance of the tympanic membrane at specific air pressures is plotted on a graph known as a tympanogram, which represents the compliance-air pressure function. Tympanometry uses minute air pressure changes ranging from +200 Pascals (daPa) to −400 daPa. Tympanic membrane mobility is of particular interest, because almost any pathology located on or medial to the eardrum will influence its movement.

Physicians typically identify children with middle ear effusions through otoscopic examination. Physicians vary in their ability to examine visually the tympanic membrane. Although otologists teach that pneumatic otoscopy is absolutely necessary to identify the presence of middle ear effusion, not all physicians use the pneumatic otoscope. Tympanometry, however, may be considered more "objective" than the otolaryngologist's eye through an otoscope. The air pressures used in the tympanometry technique are very small compared with the air pressures created with a pneumatic otoscope. Eardrums noted to have normal mobility by pneumatic otoscopy examination can be shown to have abnormal mobility with tympanometry.

The compliance of the tympanic membrane is at its maximum when air pressures on both sides of the eardrum are equal. That is, the eardrum is most mobile when the air pressure in the external auditory canal is exactly the same as the air pressure in the middle ear (Fig. 7-2). Tympanometry can thereby provide an indirect measure of middle ear pressure through the determination of the air pressure in the external auditory canal at which the eardrum shows maximum mo-

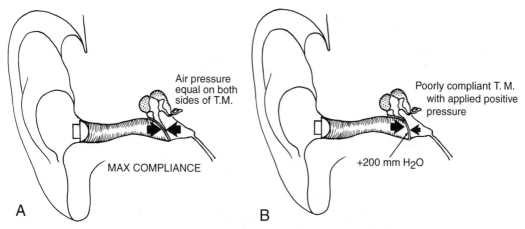

Figure 7-2. The compliance, or mobility, of the tympanic membrane is at its maximum when air pressure is equal on both sides of the tympanic membrane as shown on the left. When air pressure on either side of the eardrum is unequal, as shown on the right, the tympanic membrane does not move well (poorly compliant) and is often associated with conductive-type hearing loss.

bility (admittance). Thus, when the examiner finds the air pressure value at which the eardrum reaches its maximum compliance, it can then be inferred that the middle ear pressure is the same as the ear canal air pressure. Research has shown the accuracy of tympanometric measurements of the middle ear pressure to be within 15 daPa of the actual middle ear pressure.

Middle ear pressure is important clinical information. When the process of aeration in the middle ear is halted, as in closure of the eustachian tube, the now static air in the middle ear space is absorbed by the blood vessels in the mucosal lining. This situation produces negative air pressure in the middle ear space, causing transudation of fluid and retraction of the tympanic membrane. If the aeration process of the middle ear cavity is blocked for an extended period, fluid may totally fill the middle ear space. Thus, the early identification of negative middle ear pressure may permit the physician to practice preventive medicine and avoid the condition of otitis media.

The presence of unequal pressures on either side of the tympanic membrane typically occurs when negative pressure develops in the middle ear space. This may be sufficient to cause a retraction of the eardrum accompanied by mild conductive hearing loss although no fluid may be observed in the patient's middle ear. The most explicit example of this occurs when air pressures are changed in the passenger cabins of commercial aircraft. A passenger will first experience mild ear discomfort as the air pressure in the cabin is changed, thus creating a positive ear canal pressure relative to the passenger's middle ear air pressure. When the passenger forces open his or her eustachian tube to alleviate this discomfort (i.e., to equalize the pressure on both sides of the eardrum), the environmental sounds in the aircraft become suddenly louder along with relief of the mild ear discomfort. This is a practical explanation of the numbers of children who have negative middle ear pressure as noted by tympanometry, accompanied by mild conductive hearing loss, and by the time they are evaluated by a physician, found to have no evidence of an otologic problem.

Jerger (1970) described basic tympanogram patterns and related them to conditions of the middle ear. Jerger's classification system of tympanometry curves, which he also calls "pressure-compliance functions," is summarized in Figure 7-3. For simplicity, Jerger ascribed alphabetical letters to each type of curve. This classification is convenient, but it may be more explicit to describe each tympanogram in terms of its dynamic compliance and the air pressure at which maximal compliance is noted.

Types of Tympanograms. *Type A.* Type A curves are found in patients with normal middle ear function. The curve shows adequate relative compliance and normal middle ear pressure at the point of maximal compliance. Some controversy exists concerning the limits of normal middle ear pressure values. Alberti and Kristensen (1970) recommended the use of ± 50 mm H_2O as normative values, but the authors have noted many instances of negative middle ear pressure as great as -150 mm H_2O in patients who demonstrated normal audiograms and normal otoscopic examination. Brooks (1969) evaluated 1053 children in England and determined "normal" middle ear pressure from a statistical distribution to be from 170 to 0 mm H_2O. Decisions regarding "limits of normal" in terms of middle ear pressure will undoubtedly vary depending on the clinical situation and circumstances.

Type A_S. This pressure-compliance function is characterized by normal middle ear pressure and less than normal amplitude of the tracing relative to the mobility of the normal tympanic mem-

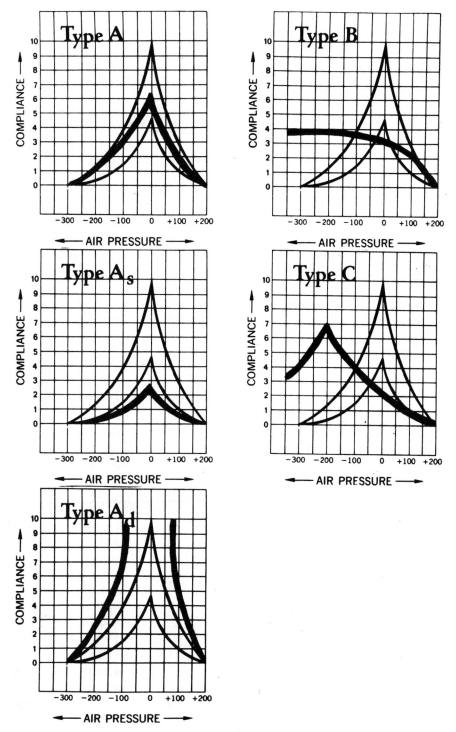

Figure 7-3. Classification of tympanograms according to Jerger (1970). See text for clinical significance of each type of tympanogram.

brane. This type of curve may be seen in cases of otosclerosis, thickened or heavily scarred tympanic membranes, and some cases of tympanosclerosis. The subscript "S" nomenclature is indicative of "stiffness" or "shallowness" of the tympanogram.

Type A_D. This curve is represented by large changes in relative compliance with small changes of air pressure. The A_D curve is noted in middle ears in which discontinuity of the ossicular chain has occurred or the eardrum demonstrates a large monomeric membrane. The significance of this curve is its representation of an extremely flaccid eardrum, with the subscript "D" indicating "disarticulation," "discontinuity," or a "deep" tympanogram curve.

Type B. The type B tympanogram is characterized by a function representing little or no change in compliance of the middle ear as air pressure in the external ear canal is varied. Often no point of maximal compliance is observable with air pressure as low as -400 mm H_2O. This curve is seen in patients with serous and adhesive otitis media and some cases of congenital middle ear malformations (Northern & Bergstrom, 1973). Although a type B, or "flat" tympanogram may be noted in patients who have perforations of the tympanic membrane, ear canals totally occluded with cerumen, or with a patent ventilating tube in the eardrum, this represents a false reading. Because air pressure is not changing the compliance of the nonintact tympanic membrane, a true tympanogram is not recorded.

Type C. This tympanogram is represented by near-normal compliance and middle ear pressure of -200 mm H_2O or worse. This curve may or may not be related to the presence of fluid in the middle ear, but one can conclude that the eardrum still has some mobility. Blue-

stone, Beery, and Paradise (1973) reported a very low incidence of middle ear effusion in children with type C tympanograms upon whom they performed myringotomies. Paradise, Smith, and Bluestone (1976) published an impressive set of data dealing with the use of tympanometry and detection of middle ear effusion in infants and young children. They reported that a poorly compliant negative pressure tympanogram is approximately three times more likely to be associated with middle ear effusion than a negative pressure tympanogram that is highly compliant.

Persistence of the type C tympanogram infers poor eustachian tube function in the presence of an intact tympanic membrane. Sometimes, patients can be instructed to "pop their ears" or perform the Valsalva procedure (patient holds nose and forces positive air pressure into the middle ear cavities). If the patient can open his or her eustachian tube, a repeat tympanogram may show that the type C curve has changed to a type A curve. Youngsters with upper respiratory infections, however, seldom can alleviate the type C tympanogram with the Valsalva maneuver.

A drawback to the use of such categories to classify tympanograms is that the clinician inevitably comes across a tympanogram that does not clearly fit into one of the expected categories. Such tympanograms may be few, but they do exist. In addition, audiologists do not always agree on the same precise definitions of the tympanogram patterns. It has been suggested that we describe the mobility of the eardrum in absolute terms of compliance (or admittance) and the middle ear pressure or perhaps draw the tympanogram or place the recorded result into the patient's medical records, if possible. Margolis (1979) suggested that we express acoustic immittance clinical results in quantitative physical measurements rather than in arbitrary units.

Tympanogram Procedure. The technique for obtaining a tympanogram is quite simple; in fact, modern equipment may automatically perform the test. Initially, the test begins when the eardrum is put into a position of known poor mobility with positive air pressure from the instrument of +200 mm H_2O. Then the positive air pressure is slowly removed, and relative changes in the compliance of the eardrum are noted and measured. The compliance change is actually monitored by the instrumentation as a decrease in the SPL of the enclosed cavity. As the positive air pressure against the tympanic membrane is decreased, the compliance of the eardrum is increased. With the release of air pressure, more of the sound energy is transmitted through to the middle ear, creating a decrease in the SPL of the enclosed ear canal cavity.

As the positive air pressure decrease approaches the point at which it matches the existent air pressure of the middle ear, the mobility of the tympanic membrane increases. Maximal compliance is, of course, achieved when the air pressure in the external auditory canal equals the existing air pressure in the middle ear space. As the air pressure continues to be withdrawn from the external ear canal, a point is reached that unbalances the previously equalized air pressure on either side of the tympanic membrane, thereby creating a decrease in eardrum compliance again.

Tympanometry evaluation is a useful technique to monitor the progression and resolution of serous otitis media in children. Typical tympanograms obtained under such circumstances are shown in Figure 7-4. Figure 7-4 shows results from a child who demonstrates a type A tympanogram under normal healthy conditions. As the otologic disease process begins with a closed eustachian tube, negative pressure is created in the middle ear space which retracts the eardrum and produces a type C tympanogram. As fluid develops in the middle ear, the compliance of the eardrum is decreased, and the child demonstrates a type B tympanogram. If prescribed medications are effective and the fluid condition of the middle ear begins to resolve, one would expect to see the type C tympanogram once again. Finally, the type A tympanogram is recorded when the middle ear is back in its normal healthy condition (Northern, 1978).

Paradise (1982) published an editorial retrospective review of tympanometry in which he states that tympanometry has instructional, practical, and intellectual value for the physician. Tympanometry (1) separates infants and children into two subgroups, those with suspected or nearly certain disease who require careful examination and those virtually certain to be free of disease; (2) refines and clarifies questionable otoscopic diagnoses; and (3) objectifies the follow-up evaluations of patients with diagnosed middle ear disease.

Studies have been conducted to show the influence of negative middle ear pressure (identified with tympanometry) to elevate hearing thresholds. Cooper, Langley, Meyerhoff, et al. (1977) examined 1133 children with middle ear pressures between −150 and −400 mm H_2O and found their hearing thresholds to be elevated as much as 25 dB. An orderly relationship exists between the degree of negative middle ear pressure and hearing threshold shift. An approximately 8 dB shift in hearing thresholds will be noted in the speech frequency range with a middle ear pressure of −100 mm H_2O. This shift in hearing thresholds increases to at least a 20 dB shift when middle ear pressure is −400 mm H_2O.

Static Immittance. The concept of acoustical impedance, or static immittance, is a direct outgrowth of applications made by electrical engineers and physicists to describe the willingness of

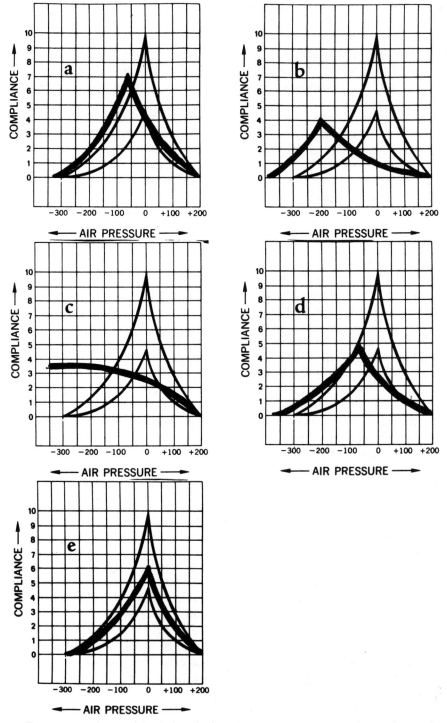

Figure 7-4. Tympanometry is a useful technique for following the pathophysiology of a middle ear effusion. (**a**) A near-normal tympanogram. (**b**) Negative middle ear pressure and reduced compliance often accompany an upper respiratory problem. (**c**) Middle ear effusion. (**d**) Improved compliance due to reduced negative middle ear pressure. (e) Return of the middle ear to its proper normal control condition.

an electrical system to permit electron flow and the ease with which a mechanical system moves.

The impedance of any mechanical system involves a complex relationship between three factors—the mass, friction, and stiffness of the system. In the middle ear mechanical system, mass is represented primarily by the weight of the three ossicles. The weight of the three ossicles, however, as is immediately obvious to one who has ever held the ossicles in his or her hand, constitutes very little mass. Friction in the middle ear is due primarily to the suspensory seven ligaments and two muscles that support the ossicular chain. This intricate suspension of the ossicles, however, lends to ease of mobility; thus, friction as a factor in mechanical impedance constitutes meager influence in the impedance of the middle ear. The third element of impedance, stiffness, has a much more prominent role in the middle ear. The stiffness element has been identified as occurring at the footplate of the stapes, where a large resistant component must be overcome to move the fluids of the cochlear ducts. Thus, the impedance of the middle ear mechanical system is stiffness-dominated (Zwislocki, 1963).

Compliance is technically the inverse of impedance. A system with a great deal of mobility, or high compliance, has very little resistance to motion, or low impedance. Likewise, a poorly mobile system has low compliance and high resistance. This small equivalent volume in cubic centimeters of compliance is equal to large impedance in acoustic ohms, and vice versa. In the middle ear, pathologies (e.g., serous otitis media) create a middle ear system of very low compliance or very high impedance. On the other hand, a disarticulated ossicular chain in the middle ear creates a condition of high compliance or low impedance.

The major weakness of static immittance is its wide variance in values related to specific pathologies of the auditory mechanism. In clinical patient populations, the variation in static immittance values creates considerable overlap among normal middle ears, otosclerotics, and ears with discontinuity. Stach and Jerger (1990) find the usefulness of static immittance to be limited to differentiate only between normal and extreme pathologic conditions. As a guideline, the middle ear is abnormally stiff when the static compliance is less than 0.28 cc of equivalent volume and abnormally flaccid when the static compliance is greater than 2.5 cc of equivalent volume. Serous otitis media often creates poor compliance of 0.1 cc of equivalent volume or less. Jerger, Jerger, Mauldin, et al. (1974) found static compliance to be the least informative test of the immittance battery in children younger than 6 years of age. The static immittance measure is too variable for accurate diagnosis, although it can be used to support the other measurements in the immittance test battery.

Ear Canal Estimated Volume Test. Because the immittance meter is able to measure volume in cubic centimeters, information about the absolute cavity size medial to the probe tip can be quite significant. This measurement is known as the *physical volume test (PVT)*. The acoustic immittance instrumentation relies on the physical principle that the intensity of a sound in a closed cavity is a direct function of the cavity size. Thus, a signal of fixed intensity introduced into a large cavity and into a small cavity will produce different SPL values in each cavity. The larger cavity will have a lower SPL, the smaller cavity will have a higher SPL.

In the presence of an intact eardrum, the typical enclosed ear canal cavity between the probe tip and the tympanic membrane should be 0.65–1.75 cc in an adult or 0.5–1.0 cc in a child. In infants the PVT value may be as low as 0.5 cc. This value may vary depending on how far the probe tip cuff is inserted into the ear canal or how large or small the diameter of the external canal might be (Fig. 7-5). Ear canal volume estimation is a routine component of most current commercially available immittance instruments.

When the physical volume size is considerably greater than these norms in light of a hermetically sealed probe tip and cuff, the audiologist can reasonably assume that the "cavity" includes the external ear canal, middle ear space, and possibly even the mastoid air cells and entrance to the eustachian tube orifice. In circumstances of a nonintact (perforation or with tympanostomy tube in place) tympanic membrane, the PVT value may be 3 or 4 times greater than normal volume values, often exceeding 5.0 cc. The authors use the PVT as a means to rule out the presence of a perforation. The PVT measurement has been useful in forecasting the presence of a hidden perforation behind an exaggerated anterior external ear canal wall overhang or beneath an adherent crust on the eardrum. The PVT can be used to identify obstruction of ventilation tubes and blind attic retraction pocket perforations.

Knowledge of the physical volume in cubic centimeters will help clarify the etiology responsible for type B tympanograms: (1) nonmobile tympanic membranes with volumes larger than 2.0 cc in children are usually indicative of a perforation or patent ventilation tube; (2) type B tympanograms with a normal volume measurement are indicative of a nonmobile intact tympanic membrane; and (3) abnormally small physical volumes may be related to cerumen occluding the external canal or probe tip, or they may suggest that the probe tip is closed off against the external ear canal wall (Table 7-2).

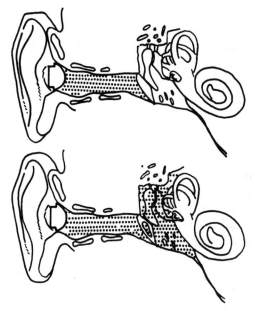

Figure 7-5. Utilization of the immittance meter to estimate volume. (**Top**) Volume between probe tip and intact eardrum. (**Bottom**) Greater volume measurement when eardrum is perforated or has a patent ventilating tube in place. (Reprinted with permission from Northern, J.L. (1980b). Clinical measurement procedures in impedance audiometry. In J. Jerger & J. L. Northern (Eds.), *Clinical impedance audiometry*, (2nd ed.). Acton, MA: American Electromedics Corp.)

Acoustic Reflex Thresholds. The acoustic reflex test is based on the signal threshold level at which the stapedial muscle contracts. The classic research of Otto Metz, reported in 1952, determined that in normal-hearing persons a bilateral acoustic muscle reflex can be elicited with pure tone signals between 70 and 100 dB hearing threshold level (HTL) and 65 dB HTL for a broadband noise stimulus. The lowest signal intensity capable of eliciting the acoustic reflex is the acoustic reflex *threshold* for the *stimulated* ear.

Because the stapedial muscles contract bilaterally in response to an appropriate acoustic stimulus represented in either ear, both an *ipsilateral* (uncrossed) and a *contralateral* (crossed) acoustic reflex may be measured (Fig. 7-6). Most current immittance meters will measure the acoustic reflex in ipsilateral or contralateral mode. In ipsilateral reflex measurement, the eliciting acoustic stimulus is presented through the probe tip itself and the acoustic reflex is monitored in the same ear. Under conditions of contralat-

Table 7.2.
Tympanometry and the Physical Volume Test in Children

Tympanogram	Physical Volume	Etiology
Type A	0.8–1.0	Normal middle ear
Type B	<0.3	Cerumen or canal wall
	0.8–1.0	Serous otitis; middle ear congenital anomaly
	>2.5	Tympanic membrane perforation or patent ventilation tube
Type C	0.8–1.0	Negative middle ear pressure; inadequate eustachian tube function

eral acoustic reflex measurement, the acoustic stimulus is presented through an earphone to one ear while the probe tip in the opposite ear verifies the resultant change in immittance. Regardless of whether measuring ipsilateral or contralateral (crossed or uncrossed) acoustic reflexes, it is standard practice to *record* the acoustic reflex for the stimulated ear—noting in writing, of course, as to which lateral mode (contralateral or ipsilateral) was used for the measurement.

The major advantage of ipsilateral reflex measurement is that confusion is eliminated regarding which ear is being tested. Utilization of hand-held ipsilateral reflex techniques virtually eliminates the need for the cumbersome head-band-earphone arrangement used in contralateral reflex measurement. The use of ipsilateral reflex measurement and the hand-held probe tips are especially useful with pediatric patients and in mass screening programs. Research reports that compare acoustic reflex threshold sensitivity between contralateral and ipsilateral stimuli have been published, indicating that ipsilateral thresholds are 3–6 dB more sensitive than contralateral thresholds (Moller, 1962; Fria, LeBlanc, Kristensen, et al., 1975).

The function of the stapedial muscle is still open to question, but the classic interpretation offered by Wever and Lawrence (1954) is that the stapedial muscle reflex is responsible for protection

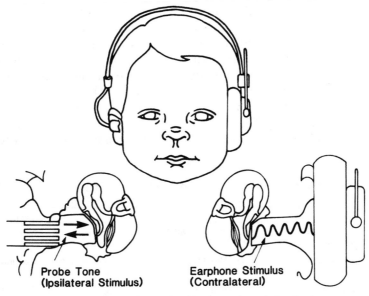

Probe Tone
(Ipsilateral Stimulus)

Earphone Stimulus
(Contralateral)

Figure 7-6. Acoustic reflex measurements may be made with a contralateral stimulus from an earphone or with an ipsilateral stimulus presented through the probe tip.

of the inner ear from loud sounds. Anatomically, the stapedial muscle is attached from the neck of the stapes to the posterior wall of the middle ear cavity. When the stapedial muscle contracts, it pulls posteriorly on the ossicular chain, thereby decreasing the compliance of the middle ear system and attenuating the intensity of the sound that actually reaches the cochlea. Thus, contraction of the stapedial muscle creates an increase in the reflected SPL of the probe tone.

Acoustic reflex threshold testing should be carried out at frequencies of 500, 1000, 2000, and 4000 Hz. However, acoustic reflex responses at 4000 Hz are often absent for no apparent reason even in normal-hearing patients, so pathologic conclusions may not be valid if only the 4000 Hz reflex is not present. Acoustic reflex thresholds are difficult to interpret in isolation, because absence or elevated acoustic reflex thresholds may occur in a wide variety of conditions. Comparison of contralateral (crossed) and ipsilateral (uncrossed) acoustic reflexes increases confidence in interpreting the audiogram and immittance audiometry results (Table 7-3).

Much emphasis has been placed on the clinical value of the acoustic reflex measurement. Because the acoustic reflex is mediated by loudness, it is a sensitive indicator of cochlear pathology. The acoustic reflex threshold level in patients with cochlear pathology usually occurs at sensation levels less than 60 dB above the auditory pure tone threshold. The patient with cochlear pathology hears the test signal as though it were much louder, as a result of abnormal appreciation of loudness. Thus, the acoustic reflex threshold provides an objective, simple technique to identify the site of pathology to the cochlea.

The ability to establish the presence of the loudness recruitment phenomenon permits the clinician to localize the site of auditory lesion to the cochlea. Anyone who has ever attempted the traditional psychophysical loudness balance procedures on a child younger than 6 years of age to identify a cochlear site of lesion will immediately appreciate the simplicity and objectivity of this technique.

The informed audiologist can achieve considerable diagnostic information through the subtleties of acoustic reflex interpretation. For example, the acoustic reflex sensation level shows an inverse relation to the degree of sensorineural hearing loss. The acoustic reflex sensation level decreases from approximately 70 dB for patients with a 20 dB sensorineural hearing loss to approximately 25 dB for patients with an 85 dB sensorineural hearing loss. Jerger, Jerger, Mauldin, et al. (1972) concluded that as long as the cochlear hearing loss is less than 60 dB, there is a 90% likelihood for the presence of the acoustic reflex being observed. As the sensorineural loss increases above 60 dB, chances of observing the acoustic reflex grow less. With an 85 dB hearing loss, the chances are only 50% of observing the acoustic reflex; if the loss is 100 dB hearing level (HL), only a 5–10% chance exists of the reflex being

Table 7.3.
Interpreting Crossed and Uncrossed Acoustic Reflexes With the Audiogram to Identify Site of Lesion of Hearing Impairment

Reflex Pattern	Audiogram	Predicted Site
Neither crossed nor uncrossed can be elicited from either ear	Bilateral air-bone gap	Middle ear
Neither crossed nor uncrossed can be elicited from either ear	Bilateral severe sensory loss	Cochlea
Neither crossed nor uncrossed can be elicited from either ear	Normal	Brainstem

Reproduced with permission from Stach, B., & Jerger, J. (1990). Immittance measures in auditory disorders. In J. Jacobson & J. Northern (Eds.), *Diagnostic audiology* (p. 118). Boston: College-Hill Press.

present. Thus, the presence of acoustic reflex thresholds, in light of hearing loss, provides a powerful indication for sensorineural diagnosis. In patients with unilateral cochlear hearing loss less than 85 dB, the acoustic reflex should be easily observable bilaterally.

In children with conductive hearing problems, the contralateral acoustic reflex can be observed only in mild *unilateral* conductive hearing loss. When the unilateral conductive hearing loss exceeds 30 dB HL, the acoustic reflex is typically obscured bilaterally. Thus, when the stimulating sound is presented to the conductive hearing loss ear, the 30 dB+ hearing loss is sufficient to prevent the signal from being perceived loudly enough to elicit the acoustic reflex. Then when the earphone is on the normal ear and the probe is in the unilateral conductive loss ear, the pathology causing the conductive loss prevents the eardrum from showing a change in compliance. Naturally, in a bilateral conductive loss, the acoustic reflexes will be absent bilaterally because the pathology in *each* ear prohibits the probe from noting a compliance change when the opposite ear is stimulated with sound. The ipsilateral acoustic reflex will also be absent bilaterally.

Because conductive-type pathology precludes tympanic membrane compliance change, the acoustic reflex can be expected to be absent when the probe tip is in a conductive loss ear, regardless of how small an air-bone gap exists. The presence of a small air-bone gap of only 10 dB is sufficient to obscure the reflex to the probe ear 80% of the time (Jerger, Burney, Mauldin, et al., 1974b). Conversely, if acoustic reflexes can be noted in the probe ear, it is virtually impossible for a conductive hearing loss to exist in that ear. Thus, even a very mild conductive hearing loss will obscure the acoustic reflex. Interpretation of acoustic reflexes in hearing loss can be diagnostically important and of particular value when the patient is a youngster in whom audiometric masking is impractical or impossible.

Clinical Application of the Immittance Battery With Children. Whereas tympanometry, static immittance, the ear canal physical volume measurement, and the acoustic reflex threshold each provide some information about the function of the auditory system, their results become more meaningful when relationships between the tests are considered. Diagnostic judgments and patient referrals are made with greater authority and assurance when the overall pattern is considered. Tympanometry alone is useful to only a limited degree, static compliance norms are too variable for accurate diagnosis, and the absence of the acoustic reflex may occur from several factors. When considered together, however, the limitations of each test are reduced while their combined implications are enhanced (Table 7-4).

Table 7.4.
Use of Immittance to Help Confirm Audiometric Impression in Evaluation of Young Children

Tympanometry	Static Compliance	Acoustic Reflex	Confirm Behavioral Audiometric Impression
Type A bilaterally	Within normal range bilaterally	Normal bilaterally	Bilateral normal hearing or bilateral mild to moderate sensorineural hearing loss or unilateral mild to moderate sensorineural hearing loss
Type A in one ear; type B or C in other ear	Normal in A ear; low in B or C ear	Absent bilaterally	Unilateral conductive loss
Type B or C bilaterally	Low bilaterally	Absent bilaterally	Bilateral conductive loss

From Jerger, J. (1970). Clinical experience with impedance audiometry. *Archives of Otolaryngology, 92*, 311–324.

Examples of the immittance test battery and its relation to clinical diagnosis are shown in Figures 7-7 and 7-8. Immittance test results from a case of negative middle ear pressure in a youngster's right ear are demonstrated in Figure 7-7. The audiogram shows a mild hearing loss with a 20 dB air-bone gap in the patient's right ear and normal hearing in the left ear. The audiogram gives no clue as to the etiology of the unilateral conductive hearing loss. The tympanogram for the left ear is superimposed on the normal tympanogram pattern, while the tympanogram for the right ear shows slightly reduced compliance and middle ear pressure of -200 mm H_2O. Static compliance is reduced in the right ear, suggesting stiffness, thereby corroborating the re-

duced compliance noted in the tympanogram. Static compliance in the left ear is within the normal range. The contralateral acoustic reflexes are present but show elevated thresholds when the stimulating earphone is on the involved ear. The 20 dB air-conduction hearing loss in the right ear is not severe enough to prohibit loudness from eliciting the acoustic reflex when the earphone is on this ear. When the earphone is placed over the normal-hearing left ear, the acoustic reflexes are absent. The probe tip is now in the involved conductive loss ear, and the conductive loss element prohibits compliance change in the right tympanic membrane. Knowledge of only the immittance test battery results, accompanied by experience in test interpretation,

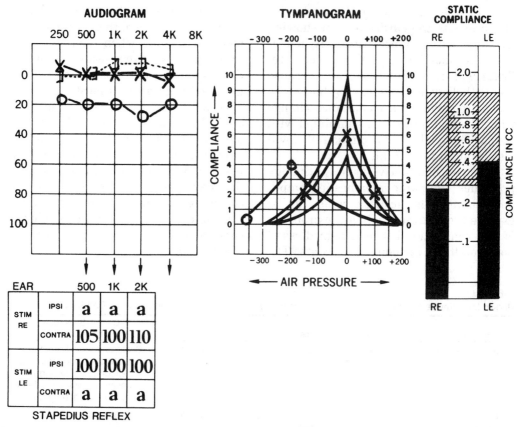

Figure 7-7. Audiometrics and acoustic immittance results accompanying a right-sided conductive hearing loss caused by significant negative middle ear pressure. Note contralateral and ipsilateral acoustic reflex findings. See text for full explanation.

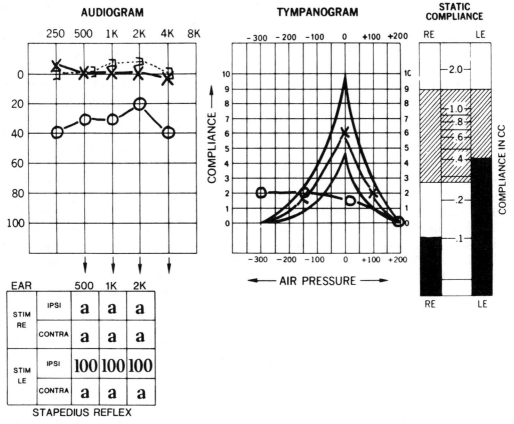

Figure 7-8. Audiometrics and acoustic immittance results in a unilateral conductive hearing loss of otitis media etiology. Note contralateral and ipsilateral acoustic reflex findings. See text for full explanation.

would permit a close estimation of this patient's audiogram if audiometry could not be accomplished successfully.

Figure 7-8 demonstrates findings in a patient with unilateral otitis media. The audiometric results show a stiffness-type air-conduction curve with an approximate 30 dB air-bone gap in the right ear. Hearing in the left ear is normal. The tympanogram of the involved right ear shows a type B pattern, substantiated by a rather low static compliance measure. These results ensure the presence of a stiffness component to the etiology of the right conductive hearing loss. That the contralateral stapedius reflex is absent bilaterally, in view of a unilateral hearing loss, confirms that the loss must be conductive in nature. This overall pattern could also represent cerumen packed in

the right ear canal, a perforation of the right tympanic membrane, or otitis media. Diagnosis is in the realm of the physician, but these immittance test findings, even without the audiogram, would suggest referral of this child to a physician.

Bluestone et al. (1973) compared air-conduction audiometry and tympanometry in 84 youngsters with concurrent or recent middle ear disease to determine which procedure could better predict the presence of middle ear effusion. They concluded that tympanometry is far more sensitive than air-conduction audiometry for detecting common conduction defects in children. They caution, however, that tympanometry cannot detect sensorineural hearing loss and thus cannot be substituted for pure tone audiometry as a screening technique. They suggest that tympanometry in combination with air-conduction audiometry appears to constitute the best method for detecting middle ear disease and hearing impairment in large groups of children.

Immittance and Infants. There is contradictory evidence in the literature regarding the merits of performing acoustic immittance measurements in infants, as shown by Northern's reviews of studies of immittance in infants (1988). Margolis (1978) described the situation with a statement that acoustic immittance measurements in infants have provided results that are "both promising and perplexing." In an effort to determine whether immittance could be used effectively with newborns, Keith (1973, 1975) tested healthy infants from the newborn nursery. Keith reported normal tympanograms in 33 of the infants and a "W-shaped" tympanogram in 7 infants. Keith also examined stapedial reflex measurements in these 40 infants, using a 220 Hz probe tone with stimulus presentations of 100 dB HTL at 500 and 2000 Hz. He reported that behavioral movement of the infants often contaminated stapedial reflex responses. In fact, from 160 stimulus presentations, only 33% resulted in clear stapedial reflex responses. No acoustic reflex responses were noted in 26% of the stimulus presentations, and 4 of the 40 infants showed no acoustic reflex in either ear initially, although all 4 babies were later confirmed to have normal hearing responses. The author warned that immittance findings cannot stand alone and that immittance should only be interpreted in combination with some independent assessment of hearing sensitivity level. Unfortunately, this warning has been largely unheeded to the detriment of the technique.

Acoustic immittance measurements in infants seemed to be a reasonably well-accepted clinical tool until the publication of an article by Paradise et al. (1976).

Their evaluation of 280 children ranging in age from 10 days to 5 years showed a high positive correlation (86%) between tympanometry and otoscopy for subjects older than 7 months of age. Poor correlation, however, was found between the two measures in infants younger than 7 months of age. In fact, in 43 infants younger than 7 months of age, 40 of 81 ears had confirmed middle ear effusion (determined by myringotomy), yet 24 of the 40 abnormal ears displayed *normal tympanograms*. The authors concluded that although the use of tympanometry had much to offer in the diagnosis of middle ear effusion, its use (tympanometry) was not recommended in infants younger than 7 months of age.

In contrast to the studies that question the efficacy of tympanometry in infants, successful tympanometric results with 91 infants between 4 weeks and 17 months were reported by Groothuis, Altemeier, Wright, et al. (1978) and Groothuis, Sell, Wright, et al. (1979). These clinicians used otoscopy and tympanometry in 549 evaluations to study the pathogenesis of acute and chronic otitis media. Normal tympanograms and normal otoscopy findings correlated highly in 92% of the evaluations; flat tympanograms and abnormal otoscopy findings were correlated 93% of the time. However, the intermediate negative pressure tympanograms and otoscopy correlated only 59% of the time. The authors reported that no flat tympanograms were found in otitis-free infants.

The Groothuis studies provide some especially interesting findings. First, because of the report of Paradise et al. (1976) regarding the shortcomings of tympanometry in infants younger than 7 months of age, Groothuis et al. (1978, 1979) examined their data separately for infants older and younger than 7 months. They found that the high correlation of tympanometry and otoscopy findings were similar in infants older and younger than 7 months of age. Second, when a nonmobile tympanogram appeared in an asymptomatic infant who had not previously had otitis media, acute otitis media developed within 1 additional month. Third, the resolution of otitis media was often prolonged as long as 6 months in 60% of infants. The authors concluded that tympanometry is a most useful tool and may be used for the earlier identification and more accurate follow-up of acute otitis media in infants.

Reichert, Cantekin, Riding, et al. (1978) examined 878 3-month-old infants with otoscopy and tympanometry. All infants were examined tympanometrically while being held in their mothers' arms and being comforted with a pacifier or bottle. The authors concluded that tympanometry produced a low diagnostic specificity (accuracy in identifying nondiseased individuals) with a high number of false-positive results—16 flat tympanograms were found in ears that were otoscopically normal. In their discussion, Reichert et al. recognized that inclusion of the measurement of the acoustic reflex may have provided different results than were obtained only with the use of tympanometry.

Studies published by Orchik, Dunn, and McNutt (1978a) and Orchik, Moroff, and Dunn (1978b) clearly show that prediction of middle ear effusion on the basis of tympanometric data alone is difficult at best, unless the tympanogram is a flat, nonmobile pattern where a 90% occurrence of effusion is present. Wright et al. (1985) followed 210 infants during the initial 2 years of life with routine pneumatic otoscopy and immittance at each physician encounter. Tympanometry proved to have high predictive value (86%) for confirming normal ears but relatively poor predictive value (58%) for detecting abnormal ears. In general, the tympanometrically abnormal ear often appears normal during otoscopic examination. The problem is the determination of which procedure is really the criterion against which the other procedures

should be compared. Otoscopy is most often accepted as the criterion test against which to compare other screening techniques, although it is well known that the accuracy of otoscopy depends on the person using the otoscope. Because otoscopy is so subjective, it can be argued that acoustic immittance should be the criterion procedure because of its objectivity and test-retest reliability. Generally speaking, otoscopy used as the criterion (as reported by Wright et al., 1985) produces higher sensitivity agreement because fewer subjects "fail" otoscopy, while many subjects "fail" tympanometric screening.

Schwartz and Schwartz (1978, 1980) published data that supported the combined use of tympanometry and acoustic reflex measurement to identify middle ear effusion in infants. They concluded that while a normal tympanogram cannot be considered evidence of a mobile tympanic membrane or effusion-free middle ear, the presence of an acoustic reflex with a normal tympanogram supports normal middle ear function.

Keith (1978) summarized the situation by stating that it is imperative that tympanometry and stapedial reflex testing always be performed together. According to Keith, to do less results in erroneous statements that "tympanometry is neither accurate nor reliable for use in screening infants." Keith expressed concern that such statements will be interpreted by some as indicating that the immittance *battery* is not valid or reliable for infants younger than 7 months of age. Based on the information provided above, the general consensus among audiologists is to use caution when performing acoustic immittance measurement with infants younger than 6 months of age.

Acoustic Reflexes in Infants. An intriguing finding concerning infant acoustic reflexes was reported by McCandless and Allred (1978), who showed that with a 220 Hz probe tone only 4% of 53 infants younger than 48 hours of age demonstrated an acoustic reflex. When the probe tone was increased to a frequency of 660 Hz, an astounding 89% of the same infants had an acoustic reflex. McCandless and Allred opened the door for subsequent research on immittance measurements in infants by suggesting that although a 220 Hz probe tone was superior for infant tympanometry tracings, the 660 Hz probe tone was clearly better for acoustic reflex evaluation.

In a series of studies of acoustic reflexes in infants, Bennett and Weatherby (1979, 1982; Weatherby & Bennett, 1980) used a two-component variable probe tone immittance meter to record contralateral acoustic reflexes in newborns. Their studies showed that as the probe tone frequency is raised, the prevalence of the reflex increases while the threshold of the acoustic reflex decreases. With a maximum intensity of 96 dB SPL, no reflexes were detected with a 220 Hz probe, whereas with probe tones above 8000 Hz all newborns exhibited acoustic reflexes. Bennett (1984) pointed out that calibration of the contralateral earphone stimulus in infants is important because of the smaller volume of newborn ear canals and that differences in SPLs between adults and infants under earphones can easily exceed 6 dB. Bennett found the optimal probe tone frequency for detecting acoustic reflexes in neonates to be 1400 Hz.

In a thorough study of tympanometry and acoustic reflexes in neonates, Sprague, Wiley, and Goldstein (1985) reported 80% observable reflexes with the 660 Hz probe tone and 50% observable reflexes with a 220 Hz probe tone with ipsilateral and contralateral activating stimuli. Instead of a standard earphone cushion for the contralateral stimulus, these researchers used insert receivers and found lower acoustic reflex thresholds than previously reported in other studies. McMillan, Bennet, Marchant, and Shurin

(1985) investigated ipsilateral and contralateral acoustic reflexes in neonates with probe tones of 220 and 660 Hz. Their results indicated that ipsilateral and contralateral reflexes to pure tone activators occurred three times more frequently with a 660 Hz probe tone (76%) than with the 220 Hz probe tone (24%). In their review of research articles dealing with acoustic reflex measurements in infants, Hodges and Ruth (1987) concluded that "the acoustic reflex mechanism is functional for infants as young as 9 hours after birth, and both crossed and uncrossed acoustic reflex thresholds can be measured."

Practical Pediatric Considerations. Nearly anyone can be trained to turn the dials and read the meters of an acoustic immittance meter, and most clinicians have little difficulty testing cooperative adults. The real challenge occurs when the clinician is face-to-face with an uncooperative youngster. A prime requisite for clinicians faced with a difficult youngster is confidence. Persistence has its reward when working with children, so the clinician should not give up easily if difficulty is encountered—a second, third, or fourth effort may yield important results. The clinician who manages each child with a matter-of-fact attitude of self-assurance will often triumph.

On occasion, the clinician must be willing to compromise the entire acoustic immittance test battery for less than optimal information. Although it is desirable to complete the immittance test battery whenever possible, with some difficult-to-manage children the clinician may have to settle for a quick tympanogram and a single acoustic reflex measurement in each ear. Clinicians must be prepared to work rapidly and efficiently; a smooth, effective initial effort is often surprisingly successful.

The main limitation of immittance measurements in young children is that

the test battery cannot be completed while the youngster is vocalizing—speaking, crying, yelling, or any combination of these noises. Acoustic reflex contraction and eustachian tube changes during vocalization cause the compliance of the tympanic membrane to alter wildly, thereby making immittance measurements impossible. The clinician's most challenging task is to make the youngster stop vocalizing for just the few necessary moments to obtain impedance data. Each clinician must devise his or her own techniques to momentarily distract the screaming child (Fig. 7-9).

For children younger than 3 years of age, it is helpful and essential that a second or even third person be recruited for obtaining impedance measures. Practice and coordination of these personnel are helpful, and they must be in constant communication during all aspects of the test to ensure rapid and reliable results. It is difficult for one person to manipulate the ear insert while operating the pressure pump and other dials on the immittance devices. It is preferable to have one person operate the impedance instrument

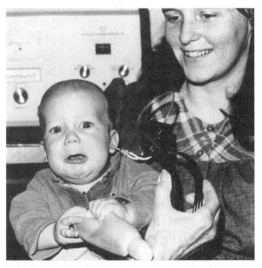

Figure 7-9. Acoustic immittance testing is an essential part of every pediatric hearing evaluation.

while a second stabilizes the child's head and inserts the probe tip. This latter person must be appraised at all times as to whether a seal has been obtained or the pressure manometer must be in a position to be observed directly by him or her. Sometimes it works well for an assistant to hold the probe tip in place by hand during the entirety of the test to prevent a loss of pressure seal due to head movement.

The age range between 2 and 12 months presents one of the most difficult periods in which to obtain acoustic immittance tests. The children are not old enough to understand the test or to respond to verbal enticements, yet they are old enough to react (sometimes decisively) both to the test situation and to the insertion of the probe tip in particular. The authors have found that it is most effective to employ a distractive technique to redirect the youngster's attention from the test. The form of distraction is relatively unimportant so long as it is sufficiently novel to compel the infant to disregard the insertion of the probe tip. The external stimuli can be visual, tactile, auditory, or a combination of these. Before assuming a distractive procedure to be necessary in immittance testing, one should try first to place the probe tip quickly, but gently, in the ear. Frequently, this takes the child by surprise, and further games are not necessary. Often, the entire immittance battery can be completed before the child really has time to react or respond; however, at the first hint of reaction from the child, the clinician should be prepared to present a visual distraction. If habituation to one mode of distraction occurs, other diversionary tactics should be introduced instantly. If the diversions fail, it may be possible to apply passive restraint of the child's body, head, or hands to complete the test.

The following are examples of the many possible distractive techniques that can be used with children younger than 3 years of age. The number and type of devices are limited only by the ingenuity of the examiner.

- **Animated Toys**. Animated toys should be introduced only as required at critical times necessary to complete the test. Movement artifacts can be avoided by keeping the toy well out of the reach of the child.

- **Cotton Swab.** The back of the child's hand, arm, or leg can be brushed gently in a slow, even motion. The distraction can be made visual and tactile by making oscillatory or exaggerated movements of the swab.

- **Pendulum.** Using a bright and unusually shaped object, the examiner can make a pendulum with an 18-inch string. This technique is highly effective if the examiner swings the pendulum around in various motions within various areas of the infant's vision.

- **Mirror.** To an infant younger than 1 year who is capable of reacting and attending to faces, a large mirror is sometimes irresistible.

- **Toys That Produce Sounds.** Toys or other devices that elicit intense sounds should be avoided if at all possible, because they may evoke an acoustic or other reflexive response from the child. Toys that produce softer sounds in no way interfere with the test and can be used effectively.

- **Watch.** In front of the child, simply remove one's wrist watch, manipulate or wind it well out of reach of the child, or point to it.

- **Shoe.** A simple yet effective technique is to begin lacing and unlacing a child's shoe either on or off his or her foot. The clinician should move slowly and methodically and not appear to have any objective in mind except to lace and unlace the shoe.

- **Action Toys.** A variety of toys are available that perform repetitive actions.

- **Wad of Cotton or Tissue.** A cotton ball or pledget can facilitate effective passive attention by balancing the cotton on the hand, arm, or knee of the subject or on the hand of the assistant. It can be squeezed or otherwise manipulated; it can be blown or allowed to fall repeatedly from the hand. A tissue can also be used as a parachute, torn slowly into strips, rolled into small balls and be placed in the child's hand, waved, and punctured.

- **Tape.** A roll of adhesive or paper surgical tape is one of the most effective distractive devices available in the clinic. Bits of tape can be torn off or stuck on various parts of the child's or examiner's anatomy. The child can be allowed to pull the tape off, objects can be picked up with the adhesive side of the tape, fingers can be bound together, links can be made with small strips, rings can be formed, fingernails covered, and innumerable other totally nonmeaningful manipulations can be performed.

- **Miscellaneous Devices.** Tongue blades, cotton swabs, colored yarn, or similar devices are all effective as distractive devices. They are best used when manipulated or "played with" by the examiner. If the child insists, he or she can be allowed to manipulate tape or string, but care must be taken to permit only passive action so as to reduce movement artifact while the test is proceeding.

The audiologist should beware of a too-elaborate array of toys or gadgets because the child may want to play with the toys and not be bothered with the test procedure. For impedance testing, extensive entertainment is usually not warranted.

There is no way to predict the behavior or reaction of children between 1 and 3 years of age. Their reaction to the test situation is influenced by past exposure to other tests, by past exposure to other health professionals, by their age, by their personalities, and by their general evaluation of what they see is about to happen to them. In many instances they are most concerned about whether the procedure will be painful. For these reasons some general rules apply when testing children in this age group. First, the audiologist should never ask a child for permission to perform impedance tests; he or she should calmly assume that the test is going to be administered and proceed to do so. Second, undue explanation regarding the test procedure should be avoided. Instructions to the child contribute nothing to the test results unless they help reduce physical movement. Besides, the child would not understand explanations even if given. It is sufficient to say something like, "Here, listen to this," or "Hold still," or "Listen to this radio," and then proceed with the test. Most often it is better to say nothing unless the child reacts to the placement of the headset or insert. Explanations usually take longer than the test itself.

For most children older than 3 years of age, no special distraction is required when applying immittance measures unless the child is particularly apprehensive in an unfamiliar clinical situation. Only a few children in this age category will demonstrate adverse reactions to immittance testing. Where necessary one can reduce anxiety by saying simply, "We are going to test your hearing, so please hold still," or other uncomplicated statements of reassurance. Most 3-year-olds can be tested by a single examiner. Allowing the child to observe other children or adults being tested helps to allay any fears that pain will occur. When working with children, remember the cardinal rule to refrain from asking permission to perform the test. Distractive techniques are viewed with suspicion by children older than 3 years. Therefore, children in this age category may be treated essentially as adults, except with occasional mild words of instruction or encouragement.

Immittance Audiometry With Developmentally Delayed Children. The evaluation of hearing in the developmentally delayed patient presents a most difficult task. Depending on the severity of the delay, many of these children do not condition well to pure tone play audiometry. They may not have sufficient maturation to perform auditory localization tasks or may even lack a consistent startle response. They may be too hyperactive to cooperate or too lethargic to be aware of changes in the environment. Studies have established that there is a higher incidence of hearing impairment among the retarded than among the nonretarded. Lamb and Norris (1969, 1970) and Borus (1972) published the earliest acoustic impedance studies with retarded children. Although it was reported that considerable variability in reflex thresholds was noted among the mentally delayed, the authors endorsed the acoustic immittance test battery as a critical component of the hearing evaluation (Fig. 7-10).

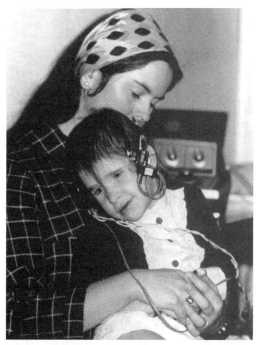

Figure 7-10. Acoustic immittance testing can be accomplished with difficult-to-test patients such as this multiply disabled youngster.

Central nervous system damage in children often makes physiologic auditory responses unreliable. Yet, accurate assessment of hearing function or middle ear status of developmentally delayed children may be critical for educational placement or medical/surgical treatment. Sometimes even a tympanogram or acoustic reflex measure can be valuable, since the clinician can then make reasonably accurate assumptions regarding the presence or absence of middle ear problems and the need for medical referral. Acoustic immittance measures are also valuable in the evaluation of nonmobile children with severe developmental delay, who are virtually impossible to test with any other testing procedure. These youngsters are certainly at high risk for developing chronic middle ear disease.

Jordan (1972) pointed out that even a mild degree of hearing loss might have a disproportional impact on a child with developmental delay because he or she is less capable of compensating cerebrally with the aid of other senses. As early as 1971, the Accreditation Council for Facilities for the Mentally Retarded, required that all residents of institutions be given audiometric screening at regular intervals. Audiologists in such facilities find themselves faced with great numbers of disabled patients of all ages and functioning levels. Certainly, acoustic immittance audiometry should be a part of every hearing evaluation.

Immittance With the Congenitally Deaf Child. The workup of patients with substantial sensorineural deafness will usually not identify superimposed middle ear anomalies. Immittance audiometry provides a useful means of evaluating the conductive hearing mechanism in patients with sensorineural hearing loss (Northern, 1980c). Children attending schools for the deaf are not routinely evaluated by otolaryngologists. These deaf children seldom complain about their ears or of changes in their hearing sensitivity due to otologic pathology. Bone-con-

duction measurements are of limited usefulness in this special population with severe to profound sensorineural hearing impairment.

Rossi and Sims (1977) reported the use of acoustic reflex measurements in the severely and profoundly deaf in an effort to evaluate the validity of audiometrically determined air-bone gaps. They conducted immittance studies on 85 deaf students, showing that approximately 80% of the "air-bone gaps" produced by audiometry were, in fact, invalid. They recommended the use of the acoustic reflex to resolve the ambiguity of responses due to probable tactile-vibratory stimulation with the audiometric bone oscillator from true conductive components.

Acoustic immittance testing provides a useful means of evaluating the conductive mechanism in patients with profound deafness. The Brooks (1975) study brought out an important additional fact about the increase in hearing loss that accompanies middle ear problems. In deaf children this additional hearing loss may have significant deleterious effects on hearing aid performance. If the child is mature enough to recognize the need to turn up the hearing aid gain, problems may be created with distortion and feedback; if the child is too young to note the change in hearing, poor performance with the hearing aid may also result. Immittance audiometry should, by all means, be a routine procedure for children attending schools for the deaf.

Hearing Loss Prediction by the Acoustic Reflex. Niemeyer and Sesterhenn (1972) developed a procedure to determine air-conduction hearing thresholds from stapedial reflex measurements. They noted that the acoustic reflex threshold for white noise was lower than the acoustic reflex threshold for pure tones, and that the difference in decibels between the two thresholds is related to the degree of sensorineural hearing impairment. Jerger et al. (1974b) simplified the procedure into a test he called sensitivity prediction with the acoustic reflex (SPAR). SPAR is an attempt to ascertain sensorineural hearing loss within four categories of impairment (normal hearing, mild loss, severe loss, and profound loss). The Jerger technique calls for establishment of pure tone acoustic reflexes at 500, 1000, and 2000 Hz and broadband noise threshold difference to predict the degree of hearing loss. In a series of more than 1000 patients, Jerger et al. (1974b) reported that the predictive error of SPAR was clinically insignificant in 63% of the group, was moderate in 33%, and was serious in only 4%.

Hearing loss prediction from the acoustic reflex is apparently influenced by a number of variables including chronologic age, minor middle ear abnormalities, and audiometric configuration. Jerger, Hayes, Anthony, et al. (1978) concluded that predicting the presence of hearing loss of any degree can be accomplished by relying on the broadband noise and pure tone acoustic reflex difference, whereas the absolute acoustic reflex threshold level for broadband noise stimuli may be used to predict the degree of hearing loss. In the Jerger et al. (1978) study, 100% of children predicted to have normal hearing did, indeed, show normal audiograms. Severe hearing loss was accurately predicted in children 85% of the time. Prediction of moderate hearing loss in children was somewhat less accurate (54%). Clearly, the prediction of hearing loss with the acoustic reflex can be a useful tool in hearing evaluations with difficult-to-test children. Objective prediction of hearing loss in children has numerous applications in daily clinical testing, and all audiologists should be familiar with and able to implement the technique when appropriate.

OTOACOUSTIC EMISSIONS

Otoacoustic emissions (OAEs) are a relatively recent adjunct to nonbehavioral physiologic-based auditory response measurements. OAEs are low-level "leakage" of acoustic energy associated with the normal hearing process that can be detected with specialized equipment from the external ear canal. A probe microphone system, similar to that used in acoustic immittance measurements, is placed into the external ear canal of the patient to measure low-level, inaudible sounds reflected back by vibratory motion in the cochlea. Otoacoustic emissions are actually a by-product of sensory outer hair cell transduction and are reflected as "echoes" into the external auditory canal. OAEs are preneural in origin and are directly dependent on outer hair cell integrity (Jacobson, 1996). These audio frequencies are transmitted from the outer hair cells in the cochlea as a release of sound energy that in some cases is spontaneous, but most likely is evoked in response to external acoustic stimulation. Although Thomas Gold, an English physicist, theorized the concept of extraneous acoustic energy reflected externally from the cochlea as early as 1948, it was 30 years later when David Kemp (1978) was able to verify the presence of OAEs in the human external ear canal.

Kemp (1980) developed a computerized system that used a sound source and a miniaturized microphone mounted in a probe tip and sealed in the external ear canal to measure otoacoustic emissions. Kemp used acoustic transients (clicks) as the stimulus and then recorded an acoustic response beginning 5 msec following the onset of the presentation of the rapidly repeating clicks. This discovery was especially important to hearing theories because of the long-held belief that the cochlear vibrations transmitted energy only upward through the auditory system. It was Brownell's research (1983, 1985) demonstrating the outer hair cell's active electromotile response that helped explain the mechanics of how OAEs are generated within the cochlea and reflected back into the ear canal. Thus, OAEs actually follow a reversal pathway of what has previously been considered normal acoustic transduction.

Common middle ear disorders in young children that cause conductive hearing loss will eliminate the presence of otoacoustic emissions. It is therefore prudent to perform acoustic immittance tests (tympanometry and acoustic reflexes) before OAE tests. In addition, otoacoustic emissions cannot be elicited from patients with severe to profound sensorineural hearing loss. Robinette and Glattke (1997) and Hall (2000) have published textbooks with complete discussions and extensive literature reviews of otoacoustic emissions. These textbooks document the extremely important and valuable application of OAEs in the hearing evaluation of pediatric patients.

From the flurry of research activity that followed the discovery of otoacoustic emissions, two broad classes of OAEs emerged. First, there are spontaneous emissions, which are naturally present in approximately 60% of persons with normal hearing (Martin et al., 1990). Spontaneous OAEs (SOAEs) are low-intensity sound reflections measured in the ear canal when there is no external sound stimulation present. Bright (1997) reviewed the literature about spontaneous otoacoustic emissions to note that it has been suggested that SOAEs might be the result of some minor structural irregularities within the cochlea which are sufficiently significant to affect audiometric thresholds. Because of the inability to predict which patients might have SOAEs, there has been limited suggestion as to their clinical utility.

The second category of OAEs includes low-intensity sound emissions elicited by low to moderate levels of acoustic stimulation presented through an ear canal microphone. This category includes two types of measurements known as transient evoked otoacoustic emissions (TEOAEs) and distortion product evoked otoacoustic emissions (DPEOAEs). Each type of evoked otoacoustic emission measurement is different, and each has differ-

ent advantages and disadvantages. The primary differences between the TEOAEs and DPEOAEs techniques lie in what the cochlea is doing during the measurement and which parts of the whole OAE response are captured and which parts are rejected (Kemp, 1997). Both of these evoked otoacoustic emissions, the TEOAEs and the DPEOAEs, are clinically useful measurement tools.

TEOAEs. TEOAEs are stable, frequency-dispersive responses to brief acoustic stimulation presented repeatedly (clicks or tone pips) that begin 4–15 msec after presentation of the stimuli (Kemp & Ryan, 1993). TEOAEs are easy to record and interpret with only a single stimulation channel that requires inexpensive synchronous averaging technology, which has been readily available since the 1970s. The technique samples the noise in the ear canal synchronously with stimulus presentations, and events that are time-locked to the stimuli are preserved in the resulting averaged response (Glattke & Fujikawa, 1991). An example of a typical TEOAE is shown in Figure 7-11. TEOAEs are especially useful in clinical hearing evaluations because they can be recorded in all non-pathologic ears that have hearing better than approximately 30 dB HL regardless of age or gender. TEOAEs can be measured in 60 seconds or less per ear and are present in nearly all normal hearing ears. In the most important clinical application, TEOAEs are used to quickly and accurately identify normal-hearing ears from ears with hearing loss. The most common reason for absence of the TEOAE, in light of normal middle ear function, is sensorineural hearing loss greater than 30–40 dB HL.

TEOAEs show increases in amplitude in infants from 1–9 months of age, whereas decreases in amplitude have been observed in older children aged 4–13 years (Norton & Widen, 1990; Widen,

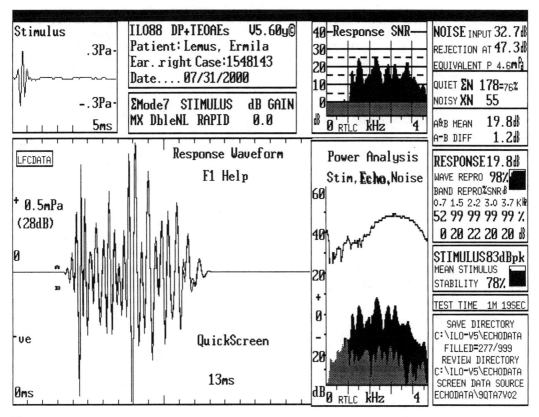

Figure 7-11. Example of a normal (**top**) and abnormal (**bottom**) hearing transient evoked otoacoustic emission (TEOAE) recording.

1997). Although it is impossible to estimate the threshold of hearing from characteristics of the TEOAE response, measurement of TEOAEs provide a highly sensitive technique for separating a normal-hearing ear from an abnormal-hearing hear (Fig. 7-12). In the absence of any middle ear pathology, one should be able to elicit otoacoustic emissions from any patient with hearing better than 30–40 dB (Hood, 1998).

Although infants tend to show OAE response patterns that are inherently physiologically "noisier" than noted with adults, this technique has tremendous application in hearing screening programs as described in Chapter 6, and in the identification of children with auditory neuropathy disorder as described later in this chapter.

DPEOAEs. DPEOAEs may be detected in the external ear canal when two different pure tone stimuli at frequencies f_1 and f_2 are presented simultaneously. DPEOAEs are tonal responses located at precise frequencies determined by the f_1 and f_2; the resulting DPEOAEs occur at specific distortion product frequencies such as $2f_1-f_2$, and $2f_2-f_1$, as well as at $3f_1-2f_2$ (Lonsbury-Martin & Martin, 1990). The measurement of DPEOAEs requires specialized equipment with two separate high-quality stimulus channels and two transducers with elaborate signal and processing technology. DPEOAEs are always present in ears with normal hearing sensitivity. Their primary advantage is that they offer the audiologist the capability of objectively evaluating frequency-specific regions of the cochlea. Therefore,

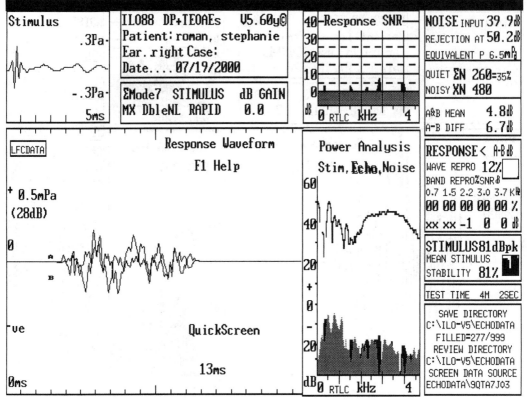

Figure 7-12. Example of an abnormal transient evoked otoacoustic emission (TEOAE) recording.

DPEOAEs represent a method of frequency sampling along with a level of auditory sensitivity pattern related to the threshold audiogram. According to Jacobson (1996), the primary disadvantage is that the DPEOAE is not recordable at frequency regions that show hearing loss greater than 50 dB HL. DPEOAEs can be used to identify frequency-specific regions that have hearing thresholds within normal limits. DPEOAEs may take slightly longer to establish than TEOAEs and may be measured in either or both of two techniques. During one procedure, the results of the DPEOAE measurement are plotted on a DPgram as shown in Figure 7-13. The DPgram is obtained by maintaining a constant stimulus intensity level and varying the frequency response. The frequency range of the DPgram is approximately 500–8000 Hz, and the relatively extensive dynamic range of response amplitude ($\cong$50 dB) allows cochlear evaluation at or near threshold and suprathreshold levels of stimulation (Lonsbury-Martin and Martin, 1990).

The second DPEOAE technique may be used to establish an input/output function where frequency is held constant and intensity is varied. The noise levels below 1000 Hz significantly affect the recording of the DPgram. The degree of separation of the noise floor levels and the actual DP emissions is an indicator of normal outer hair cell motility. Although no standard of measurement criteria exist, it is generally agreed that the amplitude of the DPEOAE must be 3 dB or greater than the noise floor to be accepted as a true response with either of the two measurements. Collet et al. (1989) confirmed, with a study of 76 subjects with sensorineural hearing loss, that OAEs are never found when hearing loss at 1000 Hz exceeds 40

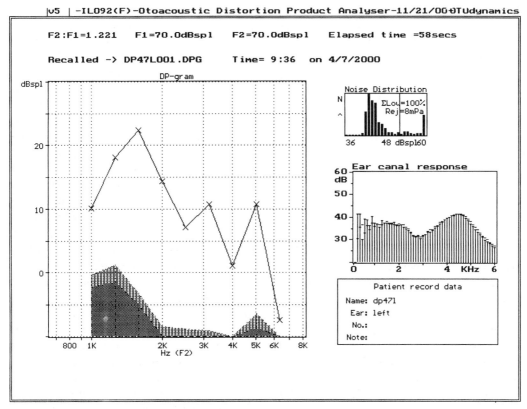

Figure 7-13. Example of a normal and abnormal distortion product evoked otoacoustic emission (DPEOAE) recording.

dB HL or when the mean audiometric hearing loss at 500, 1000, 2000, and 4000 Hz exceeds 45 dB HL. According to Norton (1993), when outer hair cells are structurally damaged or nonfunctional, OAEs cannot be evoked by acoustic stimulation. These findings opened the door for OAE measurement to become an important asset in the hearing screening of newborns (see Chapter 8).

Although for the most part otoacoustic emissions are relatively easy to establish in infants and young children in a matter of a few minutes, the procedures are not without problems. Obtaining a proper fit of the ear cuff for the probe tip into the ear canal can be difficult. Both external and physiologic noise is often a contaminant in the testing procedures, suggesting that testing for OAEs should be conducted in a quiet setting. Although the various sizes of the ear canal permit external noise to interfere with the OAE test, the well-fitted probe tip will seal the ear canal, helping to eliminate the noise contamination. A poorly fitted probe tip also permits loss of the low frequencies of the stimulus. Widen (1997) suggests that the test be considered valid if the response spectrum contains 3 dB or more power than the noise spectrum in each of 3 1000-Hz frequency bands centered at 1500, 2500, and 3500 Hz.

Successful OAE measurement does require some passive cooperation from the patient. Older children are likely to hold still, while distraction techniques may be necessary for the toddler. Some suggestions for testing infants with OAEs might be providing a comfortable chair in which the parent can relax and hold the infant, darkening the room to induce the child to sleep, or reserving the test to follow the infant's feeding. Careful thought should be given when scheduling infants early in the morning or following nap times to increase success with audiometric testing. OAEs are not influenced by sedation, but seldom is such an extreme step necessary for this quick procedure. On the other hand, if the child was sedated for other physiologic testing, it would be wise to perform the OAEs at the same time.

EVOKED AUDITORY RESPONSE AUDIOMETRY

More than 60 years ago, Davis (1939) noted that the electrical activity of the brain, as indicated by electroencephalographic recordings, showed a change when the subject heard a loud sound. This led numerous clinicians to attempt to use the standard electroencephalographic technique as a test for hearing sensitivity. Results, however, were universally disappointing. The electrical response in the cortex to auditory stimuli is so small that it is nearly impossible to see with any consistency the normal ongoing electrical activity of the brain, particularly when the stimuli are low-intensity pure tones.

In the early 1960s a number of special purpose computers appeared on the commercial market. These computers, known generally as signal-average computers, utilized a summation technique to cancel out random ongoing background physiologic "noise." This created an improved signal-to-noise condition to enhance specific, time-locked potentials of small magnitude. These computers store and average potentials related in time to the onset of a stimulus. The "random" noise consists theoretically of an equal number of positive and negative electrical potentials and is averaged out. Thus, only the wanted potential activity summates in the computer (Fig. 7-14).

The averaged evoked response is not a unitary response, but rather is a composite response reflecting various activities from the auditory pathway. An idealized

auditory evoked potential is presented in Figure 7-15, which shows the component potentials as they are commonly described in terms of latency. Davis (1976) identified these potentials in terms of their latency "epoch" as *first components* (0–2 msec, including the cochlear microphonic and summating potential); *fast components* (2–10 msec, the acoustic nerve and auditory brainstem responses [ABRs]); middle latency components (8–50 msec, thalamus and auditory cortex activity); *slow components* (50–300 msec, primary and secondary areas of the cerebral cortex); and *late components* (300 msec and longer from the primary and association areas of the cerebral cortex).

The amplitude of these auditory evoked responses is generally related to the intensity of the stimulus; the more intense the stimulus, the larger the average evoked response to a certain point. The growth in amplitude of the wave is accompanied by a decrease in latency of the peak components. As the stimulus signal is decreased toward threshold levels, the presence or absence of the averaged evoked response becomes difficult to separate from the biologic baseline activity. The clinical applications of evoked potential measurements are quite varied and include auditory, visual, and somatosensory evaluations. Evoked potentials may also be used for surgical monitoring by otolaryngologists, ophthalmologists, and orthopedic surgeons.

The evoked potential literature grew by leaps and bounds during the 1970s and 1980s. These studies were the beginning of a tremendous change in the field of physiologic evoked potential measurements. Improvements in equipment and computer technology have helped clarify the various evoked potentials in humans and, in turn, greatly influenced the field of audiology.

The objective nature of this physiologic evaluation of auditory evoked response has been especially helpful in estimating hearing levels in pediatric patients and special needs populations. Stein and Kraus (1988)

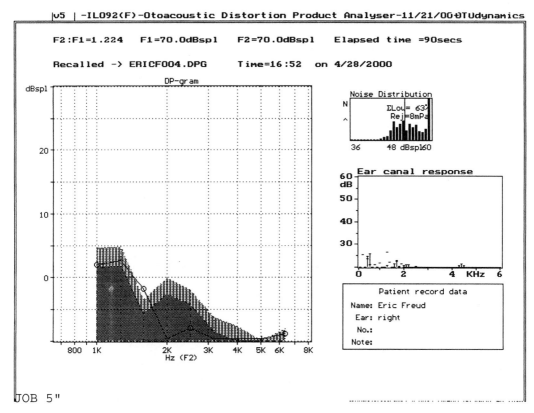

Figure 7-14. Signal-average computers utilize a summation technique to cancel out random ongoing background physiologic "noise," which creates an improved signal-to-noise condition to enhance specific, time-locked potentials of small magnitude. (Courtesy of Laszlo Stein, PhD, Northwestern University.)

described the use of auditory evoked potentials (AEPs) as tests of both hearing and neurologic dysfunction common to many pediatric disorders including mental retardation, deafness-blindness, hydrocephalus,

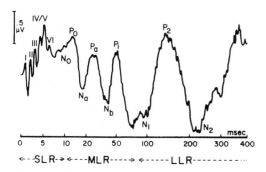

Figure 7-15. An idealized full auditory evoked potential representing the short-latency response (SLR), the middle-latency response (MLR), and the long-latency response (LLR). (From American Speech-Language-Hearing Association. (1987). *The short latency auditory evoked potentials* (p. 29). Rockville, Maryland: American Speech-Language-Hearing Association.)

meningitis, and infantile autism. The authors comment that although the audiologist is primarily interested in AEPs as tests of hearing, abnormal neuropathologic conditions may hinder the diagnosis of hearing loss. Thoughtful interpretation of AEP results must take into account the effect of potential peripheral hearing loss and neurologic conditions.

Most audiology and otolaryngology textbooks now include complete materials devoted to descriptions of AEPs. The task in this chapter is to present a current overview of the early evoked potentials and their application in the clinical evaluation of hearing in children. The discussion has drawn heavily from the materials of Jerger, Jerger, and Lewis (1981), Jacobson (1996), and Hood (1998).

Auditory Brainstem Evoked Responses. In 1967, an important discovery was reported by two Israeli physicians, Sohmer and Feinmesser, who used click stimuli to evoke a polyphasic response recorded with electrodes on the vertex of a human subject. This evoked potential was of very short latency, within the initial 12.5 msec poststimulus, and consisted of a specific pattern with five positive-direction waves. In 1971, Jewett and Williston noted seven positive peak waveforms that occur within the initial 10 msec poststimulus showing remarkable stability and consistent waveform latencies (Fig. 7-16).

Jewett and Williston (1971) systematically recorded the early ABR human responses to varying stimulus and recording parameters. They labeled their seven positive peaks from I to VII, as shown in Figure 7-16. Waves VI and VII are not always readily apparent, so general clinical interpretation has focused on waves I through V. Wave V has proven to be the most prominent component of the response pattern and is often seen combined with wave IV to form the *IV-V complex*. The normal latency of each wave is about 1 msec longer than its designated number, so wave I has a latency of about 2 msec, while wave V has a latency of about 6 msec, as shown in Figure 7-17. Although the amplitude of the waves is easily influenced by numerous variables, the latency of the peaks is very stable.

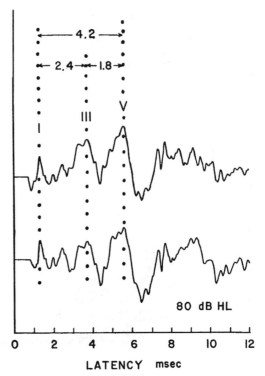

Figure 7-17. Typical latency measurements and interwave latency measurements for a high-intensity ABR. (Courtesy of Laszlo Stein, PhD, Northwestern University.)

The neural generators for the ABR were postulated to be the peripheral acoustic nerve and the various nuclei of the ascending auditory brainstem pathway. Experimental studies in animals and studies of ABR in humans with confirmed lesions have led to the general conclusion that wave I represents the auditory nerve site and that waves II and III are associated with the medulla and pons, specifically the cochlear nucleus and superior olivary complex. Changes in the wave forms of IV and V are associated with lesions affecting midbrain auditory structures, the lateral lemniscus and the inferior colliculus (Fig. 7-18). Although controversy exists over the exact specification of origin sites for each wave of the ABR, Picton, Hillyard, Krausz, et al. (1974) suggested that waves I through IV represent activity from the auditory nerve and brainstem auditory nuclei, but

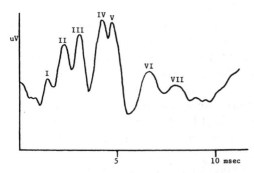

Figure 7-16. An idealized example of the peaks in the early component evoked response according to Jewett and Williston (1971).

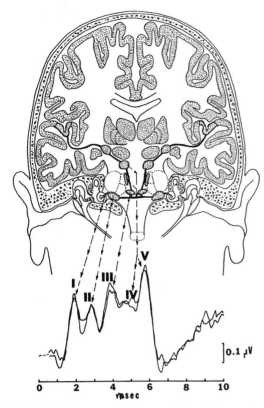

Figure 7-18. Diagrammatic representation of the auditory brainstem response waves and their generator sites. Wave I is associated with the auditory nerve, wave II comes from the cochlear nucleus, wave III comes from the superior olivary complex, wave IV is thought to come from the area of the lateral lemniscus, and wave V is from the inferior colliculus. (Courtesy of Laszlo Stein, PhD, Northwestern University.)

avoid confusion with the cochlear microphonic, yet fast enough to avoid being masked by muscle reflexes. The ABR is widely known for its freedom from the effects of central nervous system state and the replicability of the waveform pattern. In fact, the validity of an ABR tracing is usually verified by repeating the test and comparing both runs. Because ABR is relatively unaffected by the physiologic state of the patient, the measurement is accomplished with excellent results in both awake and sleep stages, thereby making the technique especially valuable with children.

ABR measurements provide information regarding the identification of the site of a lesion in the auditory brainstem pathways (including acoustic nerve tumors), assessment of auditory function in patients with stroke or trauma, assessment of infant hearing, prediction of hearing sensitivity in difficult-to-test children, evaluation of aided versus unaided auditory performance, evaluation of neurologic disease and/or dysfunction, and provision of central auditory processing information. ABR measurements are used by numerous medical specialists such as otolaryngologists, neurologists, ophthalmologists, neurosurgeons, anesthesiologists, and audiologists.

ABR Parameters. The ABR is optimally recorded differentially from the vertex scalp to the ipsilateral mastoid or earlobe with an electrode on the contralateral mastoid serving as ground. The ABR is usually evoked with click stimuli, repetitively presented (n = 2000) at 30 clicks per second and summated by computer analysis. Click stimuli provide a sufficiently short rise time to ensure a synchronous neural burst from the auditory system (Hecox, Squires, & Galambos, 1976). Therein, however, is the main shortcoming of the ABR technique—the lack of frequency-specific information about the hearing of the patient. The spectral energy of the transient click

that the total wave pattern is influenced by the composite contribution of multiple generators. Jerger et al. (1981) pointed out that with such a "farfield" recording technique with electrodes on the scalp, it is too simple to assume site specification of each wave to a unique generator. It is more reasonable to assume the ABR represents a "complex interplay and interaction of evoked potential activity from multiple overlapping dipoles involving all the structures of the auditory system."

The clinical attributes of the ABR were summarized by Davis (1976) to include waveform consistency, easy recordability with proper equipment and technique, and optimal latency—slow enough to stimulus is shaped by the earphone resonant characteristics and the duration of the click. Because clicks fail to allow frequency specificity in the auditory system, the ABR reflects predominantly the basal turn of the cochlea or hearing information between 1000 and 4000 Hz.

Several techniques have been developed with stimuli other than clicks to enable ABR results to be more frequency-specific. Tone pips, filtered clicks, or the subtractive masking procedure can be used as frequency-specific stimuli, although there is some question about the spread of energy around each of these transient sudden onset signals. The use of these frequency-specific stimulus techniques is typically more demanding and time-consuming than the use of unmasked tone bursts or filtered clicks.

Stimulus factors have an interactive influence on the ABR waveform which can be demonstrated by varying individual parameters of the stimulus and observing modifications of the wave pattern (Stockard & Stockard, 1979). Increasing stimulus intensity influences the ABR waveform by increasing the amplitude and decreasing wave latencies. The relationship between stimulus intensity and wave peak latencies is used to plot *latency-intensity functions* for each of the waves. Figure 7-19 demonstrates typical latency-intensity functions as used in differential diagnosis of hearing losses compared with the normal range of latency-intensity responses.

The latency-intensity function is usually plotted for waves I, III, and V, and the patterns of all three functions are approximately parallel. This indicates that the interpeak intervals (sometimes called interwave latency intervals) are relatively constant over the entire intensity range. Thus, the interpeak intervals (i.e., I–III, III–V, or I–V as shown in Fig. 7-18) can be measured at any intensity level without concern that the measurement will be affected. In older children and adults, the I–III interpeak interval is about 2 msec, the III–IV interpeak interval is approximately 2 msec, and thus the I–V interval is about 4 msec.

At high stimulus intensity (80 dB HL or greater), all five waves are usually seen with clarity in normal persons. As stimulus intensity is decreased, below 60 dB HL for example, waves I, II, and IV tend to become difficult to identify with certainty. When stimulus intensity nears auditory threshold, wave V is often the only remaining landmark in the response tracing. In this fashion, as shown in Figure 7-20, ABR is used to estimate auditory threshold. The tester must keep in mind the lack of information provided from traditional audiometric test frequencies below 1000 Hz. Likewise, the ABR is very sensitive to peripheral high-frequency hearing loss and central auditory pathway disorders. These conditions, either singularly or together, can make the ABR waveform difficult to interpret.

Gorga, Worthington, Reiland, Beauchaine, and Goldgar (1985) compared ABR responses with pure tone audiograms obtained from patients with cochlear hearing loss. The click-evoked ABR thresholds were most closely related to behavioral audiometric thresholds at 2000 and 4000 Hz, with poor agreement at 1000 and 8000 Hz. The ABR latency-intensity function slope was related to the configuration of the hearing loss so that patients with high-frequency sensorineural hearing losses had steeper slopes than patients with flat hearing losses or normal hearing.

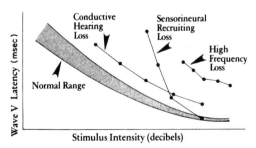

Figure 7-19. Characteristic latency-intensity functions obtained from normal-hearing patients and patients with various types of hearing loss. (Courtesy of Nicolet Biomedical, Madison, Wisconsin.)

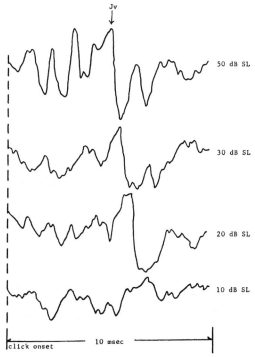

Figure 7-20. Summed brainstem evoked responses at decreasing intensities. Each response represents 2048 click presentations. (Courtesy of Steven Staller, PhD, Cochlear Corporation.)

An increase in the stimulus click rate increases the latency and reduces the amplitude of the ABR waves. The amplitude of wave V is constant up to 30 clicks per second, although the peak latency of wave V may change about 1.0 msec as the stimulus click rate is increased from 10 to 100 clicks per second. These technical considerations make it mandatory that all clinical facilities that wish to perform ABR establish their own norms for their particular test parameters and procedures before testing patients.

Maturation of the ABR. Starr, Amlie, Martin, et al. (1977) reported the results of ABR studies on infants as young as 28 weeks of gestational age and believed that the brainstem response wave complexes could be identified if the stimuli were sufficiently loud. However, an important variable in the interpretation of

ABR tracings, especially in premature infants, is the effect of maturation on the waveforms. The effect of maturation in infant populations is significant, and without proper normative standards, misinterpretation of peak wave latencies can easily occur. Several leading laboratories have evaluated both neonatal normal and high-risk populations with ABR techniques in an attempt to determine the reliability, sensitivity, and accuracy of the procedures. Gorga, Kaminski, and Beauchaine (1988) recommended the use of insert earphones for use with infants to prevent erroneous conductive hearing loss due to collapse of the external ear canals, a common occurrence when circumaural earphones are used.

Stockhard and Westmoreland (1981) identified several limitations of ABR evaluations in a neonatal population. A heightened vulnerability of the neonatal wave potentials to certain technical and subject factors should be of concern. Stimulus intensity calibration can be a major source of variability in peak and interpeak latencies. Uncertainty about the conceptual age versus gestational age of the infant may confuse the interpretation, because of the rapid change of maturational levels in auditory transmission time. Between the ages of 18 months and 25 years of age, ABR shows little change in latency or amplitude.

Many waveform criteria of AEPs—including the absolute latency of waves I and V, the latency-intensity function, the wave I–V interwave interval, and the amplitude ratio of wave V to wave I—are used to identify hearing-impaired infants and to distinguish peripheral hearing loss from intracranial pathology (Finitzo-Hieber, 1982). Accurate infant assessment requires age-specific norms for each of the measurements. These waveforms are first visible in a premature infant at 28–30 weeks *after conception* (or 28–30 weeks gestational age), not after birth. However, latencies are prolonged and thresholds are elevated when compared with those of a full-term newborn. The maturation of the ABR is not complete until 12–18 months postterm (with term being 38–40 weeks gestational age). Figure 7-21 illustrates the maturation of wave V and wave I over time. Note that the critical time is expressed in time after conception rather than in time after birth.

Finitzo-Hieber (1982) made the following recommendations for conducting ABR in premature infants. First, if a premature infant is tested far in advance of hospital discharge, the baby can present with a significant, but transient, impairment that may show partial or complete recovery at the time of discharge. If ABR is to be effective, assessment should take place near discharge time, when the infant is in an open crib and is not less than 37 weeks of gestational age. Second, a single ABR assessment is not sufficient in premature infants. Both improvement and deterioration in auditory function have been documented on follow-up testing. Therefore, at-risk infants should be monitored with ABR every 3 months in the first year of life.

Figure 7-22 shows the general maturation of the ABR from newborn to adulthood (Hecox & Jacobson, 1984). Gorga, Reiland, Beauchaine, Worthington, and Jesteadt (1987) contributed substantially

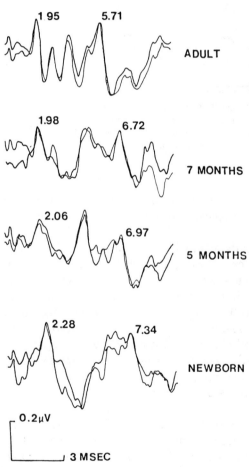

Figure 7-22. Maturation of the auditory brainstem response from postnatal newborn period to adulthood. (Reprinted with permission from Hecox, K. & Jacobson, J. [1984]. Auditory evoked potentials. In J. L. Northern (Ed.), *Hearing disorders*. Boston: Little, Brown & Co.)

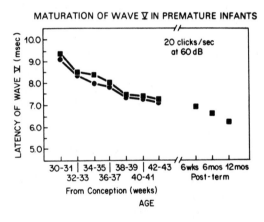

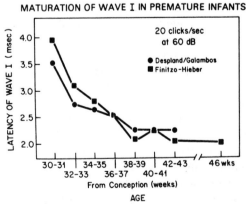

Figure 7-21. Maturation of wave V and wave I over time. (Reproduced with permission from Finitzo-Hieber, T. [1982]. Auditory brainstem response: Its place in infant audiological evaluations. *Seminars in Speech, Language and Hearing, 3,* 76–87.)

to the establishment of ABR normative standards in infants and young children. Their comprehensive study of 585 graduates of an intensive care nursery showed small, systematic decreases in response component latencies occurring with increasing age. The normal distribution of results, therefore, makes it possible to identify an individual infant's wave V latency or interpeak latency difference that might fall below the 5th or 10th percentile of the respective cumulative distribution. Their results also confirmed the importance of taking chronologic age of the infant into account when evaluating ABR latencies.

As an extension of the above-described study of ABR with intensive care nursery infants, Gorga, Kaminski, Beauchaine, Jesteadt, and Neely (1989) reported normative data on 535 normal-hearing children from 3 months to 3 years of age. Wave V latency decreased as age increased at least to 18 months, while little or no change was noted in wave I latencies over the same age range. Interpeak wave latency differences followed the same developmental time course as wave V. More information on the maturation effect in premature infants may be found in Chapter 8 (ABR Infant Hearing Screening).

Binaural stimulation is often useful when testing children (Fig. 7-23). Binaural stimulation with clicks produces waveforms that are approximately 1.5 times greater in amplitude than noted with monaural stimulation of either ear. The latencies of the waves are essentially the same for monaural and binaural stimulation. The binaural stimulation technique is good for approximating auditory threshold, because the response to binaurally presented clicks is the same as the response to monaurally presented clicks in the better hearing ear.

A major disadvantage in ABR with children is that most children between the ages of about 6 months and 4 years must be sedated for the duration of the testing session. This requires the use of a professional medical staff to be on hand during the session. The authors allow a minimum of 1 hour for each test session, although they are always prepared to carry on longer if necessary to obtain adequate information about the hearing of the patient. Most children older than 4.5 years can be entertained during the session or will sit fairly quietly until the test is completed.

Jerger and Hayes (1976) have brought out the value of the cross-check principle in young children who may yield a behavioral audiogram, the validity of which is under question because of conflicting speech audiometry results or impedance audiometry findings. No ABR study should be undertaken without first attempting behavioral audiometrics and impedance audiometry. Shimizu (1981) warns that ABR is only a part of the whole diagnostic process for clinicians, whose responsibility must cover history taking, traditional audiometrics, evaluation of the patient's overall communicative abilities, parent counseling, and overall case disposition. It must be emphasized that the ABR does not test "hearing" in the perceptual sense, nor can it identify a specific neurologic lesion at a given location (Table 7-5). Consequently, the ABR results cannot stand alone and must be interpreted in the context of other clinical information. Jerger, Hayes, and Jordan (1980) cite overinterpretation of ABR results and failure to consider other test findings in the whole clinical picture as the most common error made by clinicians.

Auditory Middle-Latency Evoked Responses. The auditory middle-latency evoked responses (MLRs) are so called because their latency lies between that of the early or brainstem evoked responses and the late cortical evoked responses. The latencies of the MLR peaks are found between 12 and 60 msec poststimulus. The discovery and the major investigation

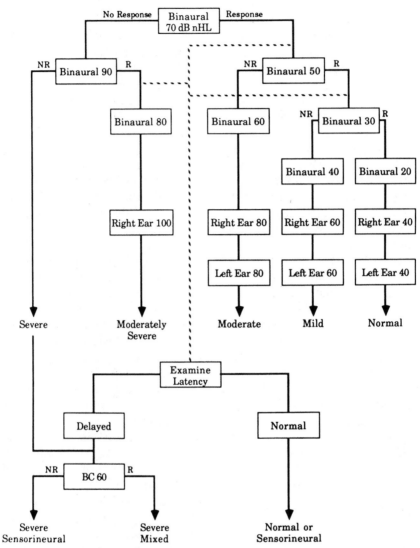

Figure 7-23. Flow diagram of Jerger's "binaural strategy" technique to obtain time-efficient ABR hearing threshold estimates in children. (From Jerger, J., Oliver, T., & Stach, B. (1985). Auditory brainstem response testing strategies. In J. Jacobson (Ed.), *The auditory brainstem response* (pp. 371–388). San Diego: College-Hill Press.)

of auditory middle-latency evoked potential are associated with Goldstein and Rodman (1967), Mendel and Goldstein (1969), and Mendel (1980). The site of generation has not been identified precisely, although Beagley and Fisch (1981) believe it to be situated in the auditory radiations in the thalamic region and in the primary auditory cortex in the temporal lobe.

Hood (1975) described the nature of the MLR to be two major positive peaks (P_o with a latency of 12 msec, and P_a with a latency of 32 msec) and three negative troughs (N_o, N_a, and N_b) occurring at 8, 18, and 52 msec, respectively. Hood suggests, based on the works of Goldstein and associates, that with the finding of close agreement between MLR thresholds and behavioral thresholds for the same stimuli, the MLR may serve to be an indicator of auditory sensitivity (Fig. 7-24).

Table 7.5.
Candidate Pediatric Populations for ABR Tests

Age Group	Definite Candidates	Possible Candidates
Newborns (0–2 months)	Conditions leading to intensive care nursery admission	
	Conditions leading to high-risk register enrollment	
	Failure of behavioral hearing screening in normal nursery	
	Meningitis	
Infants (3–23 months)	Meningitis	Recurrent apnea
	Congenital atresia	Failure to thrive
	Persistent otitis media with effusion	Infantile autism
	Sepsis and ototoxic drug therapy	Developmental delay
	Delayed speech	
	Parental suspicion of hearing loss	
Children (24 mo+)	Mental retardation	Autism
	Emotional disturbance	Developmental delay
	Learning disability	Sudden and progressive sensorineural hearing loss
	Suspicion of retrocochlear lesion	
	Meningitis	

From Fria, T. (1980). The auditory brainstem response: background and clinical applications. *Monographs in Contemporary Audiology, 2* (2), 37.

Mendel and Goldstein (1971) showed that the amplitude of the MLR is influenced dramatically through various sleep stages and wakefulness. Subsequent studies have verified the sleep effect on the MLR. Work by Kraus, McGee, and Comperatore (1989) shows that wave P_a detectability is especially poor during certain stages of sleep. Jerger, Chmiel, Frost, and Coker (1986) point out that since young children must typically be sedated to carry out evoked response testing, the effects of natural and/or induced sleep are a crucial factor in limiting the MLR in pediatric applications.

Kraus et al. (1989) stated that the occurrence of MLR in children ages 4–9 years is not haphazard and that the MLR in children can be reliably obtained during certain states of arousal. These authors routinely measure simultaneously the ABR and the MLR in children to obtain a measure of low-frequency hearing. When MLRs are present, they provide a useful test of auditory threshold estima-

tion at 500 and 1000 Hz. However, because of the inconsistency of the detectability of the MLR in children, absence of the MLR cannot be interpreted as an indication of hearing loss in the low frequencies.

Kavanagh, Gould, McCormick, and Franks (1989) compared low-intensity ABR and MLR in a group of 48 developmentally delayed persons. Although the ABR measurement generally showed less test-retest variability than the MLR, several of the subjects with hearing loss were noted to have recordable MLRs when no ABR could be detected. These authors suggested that this is evidence that the ABR and MLR have different neurologic centers and that perhaps a loss of neuronal synchronization may result in the absence of the ABR but still allow recording of the low-frequency MLR.

Although early investigations reported MLRs in babies, attempts to use the MLR for infant hearing screening have been unsuccessful. Jerger, Oliver, and Chmiel

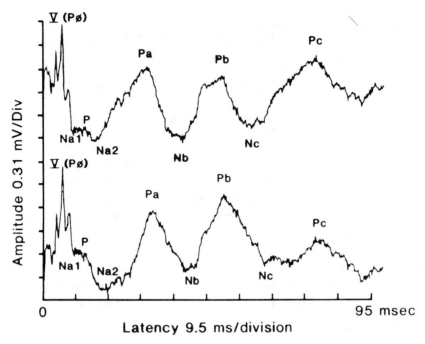

Figure 7-24. Normal MLR curves. The upper waveform was recorded with standard-phase shift settings, whereas the lower waveform was recorded with zero-phase shift (filter setting = 15 Hz, 24 dB/octave). (From Kavanagh, K.T., & Domico, W.D. (1987). High pass digital and analog filtering of the middle latency response. *Ear and Hearing, 8* (2), 102.)

(1988) point out that the MLR is observed in babies only under very slow stimulus rates and is a "very fragile" response at best. The Jerger group concludes that the MLR parameters (large number of average responses, slow rate of data acquisition, and the dependence of stimulus rate) limit the clinical value of this evoked potential.

Ozdamar and Kraus (1983) published a study of auditory MLRs and ABRs in the same persons. They found that mild sedatives did not appear to affect either MLR or ABR and that MLR differed from ABR in their stimulus-related properties, implying that the neuronal mechanisms underlying their generation are not the same. In contrast to previous studies (Mendel, Hosick, Windman, et al., 1975), they found that MLR wave components were not as readily identifiable at low stimulus levels as the ABR wave V, and they concluded that the ABR appears to be the test of choice when hearing sensi-

tivity is in question. Finally, they suggest that MLRs are likely to be most clinically useful in patients with neurologic or central auditory processing disorders.

Late AEPs. The late AEPs have had a long and colorful history beginning in the 1960s. In fact, during the mid-1960s, the late evoked potentials were being hailed as "the answer" to audiometric testing problems and the difficult-to-test patient. The success of the technique was related to the fact that under the best of conditions, auditory thresholds obtained with this "objective" procedure agreed within 20 dB of adult auditory behavioral thresholds! Unfortunately, the late potentials are extremely sensitive to even minor alterations in subject state of awareness, level of consciousness, and changes in stimulus parameters. Technical problems, equipment expense, and lack of clinical precision made routine use of auditory late potentials impractical for most clinical facilities. Thus, efforts to use late cortical potentials in clinical measurements were largely abandoned in the early 1970s.

The cortical evoked response results from generalized electrical activity on the cortex because of the presentation of various sensory stimuli including light, vibrotactile stimuli, and sound. The presentation of any sensory stimulus of sufficient intensity or the abrupt change of any stimulus produces a widespread evoked potential from the human brain during the 300 msec following the stimulus presentation (Fig. 7-25).

The late cortical potentials are receiving renewed interest because of their presumed relationship to the perceptual attributes of sound and interhemispheric differences and because of their various neurologic and psychiatric applications. One particular wave, the P300 component, has been studied in various cognitive tasks and is thought by some to hold

promise for investigating how the brain processes information (Mendel, 1985). At present, however, the late cortical potentials are not used in routine clinical audiometric evaluations (Figs. 7-26 and 7-27).

AUDITORY NEUROPATHY

The recently described disorder known as *auditory neuropathy* came to light shortly after the clinical utilization of otoacoustic emissions. The diagnosis refers to patients who demonstrate normal OAEs and absent or grossly abnormal ABRs. The normal otoacoustic emissions suggest normal outer hair cell function, and the abnormal ABRs are consistent with neural disorder. According to Hood (1998), infants and children with auditory neuropathy may appear to have repeatable ABR responses, but their ABR latency does not increase with decreasing intensity as expected with nor-

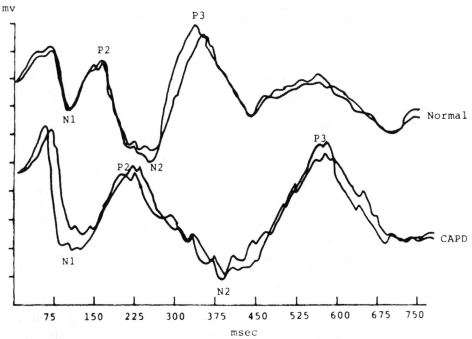

Figure 7-25. Normal long-latency auditory potentials from a normal control group (**top**) and a group of children with central auditory processing disorders (CAPD) (**bottom**). Note the shift in P_3 component latency. (From Jirsa, J., & Clontz, K. [1991]. Long latency auditory event-related potentials from children with auditory processing disorders. *Ear and Hearing, 11* (3), 225.)

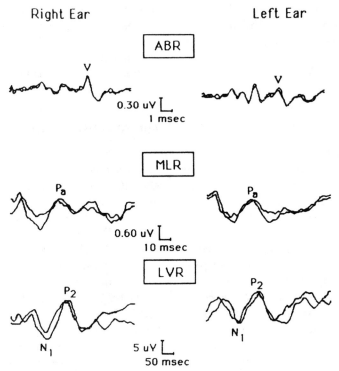

Figure 7-26. Auditory evoked potential series from a child with delayed speech and language development. Auditory evoked potential testing included the auditory brainstem response (ABR) to a click presented at 70 dB nHL, the middle-latency response (MLR) to a click presented at 70 dB nHL, and the late vertex response (LVR) to a 500 Hz tone burst presented at 50 dB nHL. All auditory evoked potential components were of normal latency, amplitude, and morphology. (Courtesy of B. Stach, PhD, Baylor School of Medicine, Houston, Texas.)

mal ABR testing. When the polarity of the stimulus is reversed (i.e., changed from condensation to rarefaction clicks), the recorded responses also reverse, which is characteristic of the cochlear microphonic rather than an ABR.

Sininger, Hood, Starr, Berlin, and Picton (1995) suggested a set of salient clinical features that distinguish the patient with auditory neuropathy, including mild to moderate sensorineural hearing loss, absent to severely abnormal ABR to high-level stimuli, normal otoacoustic emissions that do not suppress with contralateral noise, absent acoustic reflexes to both ipsilateral and contralateral tones at 110 dB HL, and inconsistency of middle and late evoked auditory potentials. These patients may also show a loss of speech comprehension in quiet that is out of proportion to their pure tone auditory threshold

configuration. Although neither organic evidence of auditory neuropathy nor the exact anatomic loci of the disorder have been identified, the symptoms are not unlike disruption of neural synchrony. Presence of normal otoacoustic emissions and cochlear microphonics leads to the conclusions that the outer hair cells and general cochlear mechanics are normal, while the absence of the auditory nerve action potential (no wave I of the ABR) suggests a more central lesion (Stein et al., 1996).

Rance, Beer, Cone-Wesson, Shepherd, et al. (1999) published a thorough examination of the clinical findings for a large group of infants and young children with auditory neuropathy in an effort to determine the prevalence of this newly described disorder. Their results suggest that auditory neuropathy is more common in the infant population than previ-

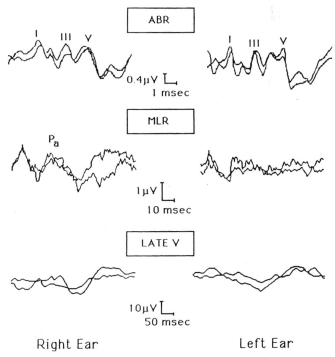

Figure 7-27. Auditory evoked potential series from a child with central auditory processing disorder. Auditory brainstem response (ABR) to a click presented at 70 dB nHL, the middle-latency response (MLR) to a click presented at 70 dB nHL, and the late vertex response (Late V) to a 500 Hz tone burst presented at 60 dB nHL. Wave V is identifiable at normal latencies on the ABRs, and peak P_a is identifiable on the right-ear MLR. The P_a on the left ear was degraded. No waveform peaks were identifiable on the LVRs. (From Stach, B.A., Loiselle, L.H., Jerger, J.F., Mintz, S.L., & Taylor, C.D. (1987). Clinical experience with personal FM assistive listening devices. *The Hearing Journal, 40* (5), 24–30.)

ously suspected. In the future, the incidence of pediatric auditory neuropathy is likely to increase even further as strategies for the care of premature and low-birthweight babies improve. Because the subjects evaluated in this study varied significantly in both their audiometric findings and general response to sound, it was recommended that the management of children with auditory neuropathy must be flexible and take into account individual differences.

Harrison (1998) described a research study of auditory neuropathy in which chinchillas with extensive, but not total (i.e., scattered), inner hair cell degeneration showed normal OAEs (and normal cochlear microphonics) while their ABR thresholds were severely elevated. However, in the same animal subjects, central auditory neurons (in the inferior collicu-

lus) showed response thresholds that were considerably lower (by up to 50 dB) than ABR thresholds. Harrison concluded that these findings parallel the characteristics of auditory neuropathy in humans, in which absent or abnormal ABRs are recorded in patients with only mild to moderate audiometric thresholds and preserved OAEs. The conclusion is that one possible etiology of scattered inner hair cell damage is a likely candidate for the etiology of auditory neuropathy in humans. The author further suggests that one of the causes of such pathology is related to long-term cochlear hypoxia, such as might be present in some infants with high-risk factors present during birth.

Treatment and management of children with auditory neuropathy is unclear and presents a confusing picture. This disorder is often confused with sensorineural hearing loss treated in the usual manner with hearing aids but marked by unsuccessful use and progress with personal amplification. Some children with auditory neuropathy have used hearing aids with fair success, and a few children have undergone cochlear implant. Success in learning language using a purely auditory mode seems questionable in light of the suggested neural dysfunction. Proper identification of this disorder calls for careful and routine use of a cross-check plan based on acoustic immittance, otoacoustic emissions, and ABR evaluation.

ELECTROCOCHLEOGRAPHY

Investigators have long been intrigued by the electrical potentials generated within the auditory system. Clinicians have made many efforts though to utilize these auditory potentials in some form of clinical procedure. These measurements were termed "electrocochleography" (ECochG) by Lempert, Wever, and Lawrence (1947). The electrocochleogram (ECochGm) consists of more than one auditory electrical potential including the whole nerve action potential (AP), the cochlear microphonic (CM), and the summating potential (SP). The AP is the most obvious and easily recorded component of the ECochGm (Fig. 7-28).

The electrical potential from the auditory nerve is the AP, noted initially by Derbyshire and Davis as early as 1935. The AP consists of nerve impulses in the eighth nerve triggered by the CM. The AP response consists of a well-synchronized volley of impulses called N_1, which may be followed by smaller waves known as N_2 and N_3. Although initial clinical attempts to use auditory electrical potentials centered around the CM, the compound AP response is currently proving most valuable in clinical use. The compound AP has a latency of about 2 msec when the cochlea is stimulated by an abrupt sound stimulus. Although the in-

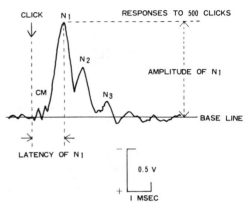

Figure 7-28. Electrocochleographic (ECochG) averaged response as recorded by Yoshie and Ohashi (1969) from an electrode in the wall of the external auditory canal. This figure illustrates the definition of N, latency, and amplitude of the ECochG response.

dividual AP in each auditory nerve fiber is a diphasic spike potential, the response of the whole auditory nerve is a compound potential that gives information from the basal turn of the cochlea and, to a lesser extent, from the middle turn (Beagley and Fisch, 1981).

The CM originates from the hair cells in the organ of Corti as originally described by Wever and Bray (1930). The CM reproduces faithfully the waveform of the stimulating auditory signal and is usually measured by an electrode from the round window niche. The CM has no threshold other than the lower limits of the recording apparatus (i.e., the CM is produced to any auditory signal, no matter how slight).

The ECochG is a powerful electrophysiologic index of cochlear integrity—when a response is present, one can be assured that there is at least some residual hearing, and when there is no response, one can be reasonably certain that no residual hearing exists. With transtympanic recording (through the tympanic membrane with the needle electrode positioned on the otic capsule), the large promontory responses require relatively few samples to obtain useful data; an entire input-output function for click stimuli can be generated very quickly. In fact, most early work with ECochG involved inserting a needle electrode through the tympanic membrane, touching the promontory of the otic capsule. This "surgical" invasive procedure obviously greatly limited the clinical utilization of the technique in the United States.

It has been shown that electrodes placed in the ear canal, touching or very near to the tympanic membrane, may yield acceptable ECochG results. Placement of the electrode is crucial as there is a direct relationship, of course, between the voltage amplitude of the ECochG and the recording site; that is, the closer the electrode to the source of generation, the larger the recorded amplitude (Jacobson, 1996). A variety of extratympanic electrodes are available as shown in Figure 7-29. The extratympanic electrodes can be used in children with appropriate sedation, and current auditory evoked potential recording systems allow for either in-dependent or simultaneous recording of ECochG and ABR potentials.

Ear canal ECochG is not used often in the testing of children because it is not possible to estimate auditory thresholds from the technique. In fact, ECochG has largely been replaced in the United States with widespread use of ABR. The ABR requires less technical expertise, is less expensive, is less traumatic to the patient, and offers more extensive information about the auditory system and hearing threshold estimation. With ABR, however, it is sometimes difficult to identify wave I, and under such circumstances it may prove useful to utilize ECochG measurements to demonstrate the presence of wave I. Ferraro (1986) and the American Speech-Hearing-Language Association (1987) have published excellent descriptions of ECochG techniques and clinical applications.

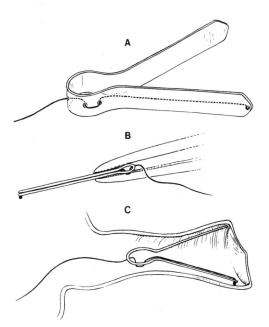

Figure 7-29. Examples of (**A**) special electrode developed for recording from the external ear canal silver ball electrode, (**B**) electrode assembly held by forceps for placement into the ear canal, and (**C**) placement in the ear canal. (From Coats, A.C. [1974]. On electrocochleographic electrode design. *Journal of the Acoustical Society of America, 56,* 79.)

SEDATION

It may occasionally be necessary to sedate a noncooperative child to conduct the necessary physiologic auditory tests to determine the presence or absence of hearing or to further define a suspected hearing loss. Medications used for sedation and anesthesia may have undesirable side effects that place patients at risk for adverse medical complications and reactions. The American Speech-Language-Hearing Association published safe practice procedures for the use of sedation and topical anesthetics in audiology and speech-language pathology. The guidelines urge practitioners who participate in such procedures to be fully aware of the complex factors that may expose their patients to risk or harm. Of course, administration of medications to achieve a desired patient state is a medical procedure requiring physician or dentist prescription, monitoring, and supervision. Audiologists should define in writing specific protocols developed in collaboration with a physician. The protocols should specify responsibility for each aspect of care and limit procedures to professional settings with immediate access to emergency medical care. In all instances, both in development of written protocols and in actual professional practice, the comfort and safety of the patient must be paramount ASHA, 1992).

Audiologists need be aware of the terminology and definition of the various levels of sedation and anesthesia in common practice in outpatient surgery and during operative procedures:

- *Conscious sedation* describes a minimally depressed level of consciousness that retains the patient's ability to maintain a patent airway independently and continuously as well as to respond appropriately to physical stimulation and/or verbal commands.

- *Deep sedation* is a controlled state of depressed consciousness or unconsciousness from which the patient is not easily aroused, which may be accompanied by a partial or complete loss of protective reflexes. The patient maintains the ability to maintain a patent airway independently and responds purposefully to physical stimulation and verbal command.

- *General anesthesia* is a controlled state of unconsciousness accompanied by a loss of protective reflexes, loss of the ability to maintain a patent airway, and loss of the ability to respond to physical stimulation or verbal command.

Sedation may be administered in the pediatric office or the otolaryngology clinic to help achieve complete audiometric test results, especially for the physiologic procedures that require passive cooperation such as immittance audiometry, otoacoustic emissions tests, ABR, and ECochG. Chloral hydrate or secobarbital are commonly used because of their ease of administration and general effectiveness. The action of chloral hydrate and secobarbital is such that drowsiness, quieting, and sometimes deep sleep is achieved within 1 hour. Following the auditory evaluation the youngster can be aroused, observed during the recovery period, and taken home. The disadvantage to chloral hydrate and secobarbital is that both drugs are long-acting sedatives. Acoustic reflexes can be observed in patients sedated with chloral hydrate or secobarbital, but researchers have suggested that the acoustic reflex thresholds may be elevated (Robinette, Rhodes, & Marion, 1974; Mitchell & Richards, 1976).

Clinicians must be aware that a child's reaction to such medication is not always as expected. Children vary considerably in their response sensitivity to sedatives, and the recommended dosages may not be sufficient to induce the desired effect. The same dosage in other children may actually increase activity and excitement levels so that the desired physiologic study is still not possible. Developmentally delayed children may be maintained with medications for management of behavioral or convulsive disorders. Thus, the absence of acoustic reflexes in this population may be drug-related. Acoustic immittance and otoacoustic emissions can be obtained under conditions of sedation, but may not be successful under general anesthesia. Middle ear pressure is increased under inhalation of some gases such as nitrous oxide, thereby decreasing the compliance of the tympanic membrane and obscuring the acoustic reflex (Thomsen, Terkildsen, & Arnfred, 1965).

EVALUATION OF CHILDHOOD DIZZINESS

There is a scant array of literature regarding vestibular evaluation of children with complaints of dizziness or vertigo. Considerable time and effort are exerted on the problem and prevention of hearing loss in children, yet we often ignore concurrent or subsequent vestibular disorders. This neglect could be due to several factors, perhaps the most common being the fact that vertiginous crises in childhood are often attributed to clumsiness or behavior problems. When a child describes vertigo, the very real possibilities for etiology include brain tumors, brainstem lesions, or epileptic seizures. In addition, because of the relatively rare incidence of childhood dizziness, one should also consider the possible presence of a functional disorder. The child with verifiable vertiginous complaints may be subjected to a series of lengthy and expensive medical tests.

More attention should be directed to the likelihood of peripheral disturbances, rather than central etiologies, in children suffering from vertigo or disequilibrium. Basser (1964) described a syndrome called benign paroxysmal vertigo of childhood. He reported that it was common in children but differed significantly from the benign paroxysmal vertigo found in adults. The distinction rests on the childhood prevalence and on the pure paroxysmal nature of the attacks, their brevity, recurrence, absence of any prolonged disequilibrium, and the absence of the febrile illness or upper respiratory infection at the onset. Utilizing electronystagmography (ENG) (Fig. 7-30), Basser successfully documented vertiginous com-

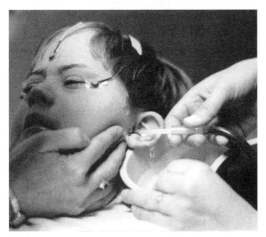

Figure 7-30. Water caloric irrigation with ENG electrodes in place on a cooperative youngster.

plaints from children. Koenigsberger, Chutorian, Gold, et al. (1970) also reported successful application of ENG testing in children with benign paroxysmal vertigo. Cyr (1983) published an excellent overview and discussion of pediatric vestibular evaluation.

Within the population of vertiginous children that the authors evaluate, there are postmeningitis patients and those with combined renal dysfunction and decreased visual acuity, as in Alport's syndrome. Children displaying visual and vestibular disturbances are of particular concern because of the risk of permanent damage to two of the three systems necessary for maintenance of balance. The authors also test children who have received long-term and/or high doses of ototoxic drugs that are particularly toxic to the vestibular portion of the inner ear (e.g., gentamicin and streptomycin).

The development of a clinically feasible battery for evaluating vestibular function in infants and preschool children has been described by Cyr, Brookhouser, Valente, and Grossman (1985). Their procedures involve modifications of standard ENG testing and the use of the low-frequency rotary chair. They report that the vestibular test battery is easy to administer, takes a minimal amount of time, and is the preferred evaluation method for most children. The test battery includes pediatric ocular motor testing, positional testing, caloric testing with simultaneous binaural bithermal stimulation through a closed-loop irrigation system, and computerized rotational chair testing (harmonic acceleration). Infrared video technology can also be used to provide ongoing monitoring of the child's head and eye position in a darkened test enclosure during the examination.

An ENG should be performed on any child for whom there is strong suspicion of vestibular dysfunction. The child who develops bilateral vestibular weakness in infancy or childhood will often be asymptomatic and may adapt to the loss in a few days. However, when this child is left in the dark, begins to swim underwater, or grows up to be a deep-sea diver or a construction worker on high buildings, the loss of vestibular function will very quickly and suddenly become apparent. Audiologists should be able to recognize and understand the implications of vestibular dysfunction in childhood and be prepared to undertake appropriate evaluation or referral.

PHYSIOLOGIC AUDITORY TESTING

The availability of auditory physiologic tests adds an extra dimension to pediatric audiology. The physiologic tests serve a two-fold purpose: first, to provide an estimate of audiometric hearing thresholds when necessary, and second, as a differential diagnostic technique for otologic disorders (Fig. 7-31). Although these physiologic procedures are commonly categorized as "objective," many believe that because the interpretation of the test results depends on the skills and experience level of the audiologist, the procedures are more "subjective" than first thought. Seldom is it appropriate that the physiologic tests are the audiologist's mainstay to evaluate and verify the hearing of infants and young children in place of traditional behavioral testing. Although acoustic immittance measurements and otoacoustic emissions are readily included in the routine pediatric test bat-

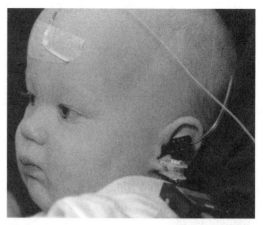

Figure 7-31. Brainstem evoked potential screening being performed on a neonate with the use of insert receiver earphones.

tery, the evoked response and electrocochleography techniques are usually reserved for especially difficult-to-test patients.

Skinner and Glattke (1977) presented an excellent overview article on electrophysiologic response audiometry (Table 7-6). They categorized evoked responses that occur within a latency range of 1–5 msec as originating from the cochlea and auditory nerve. Responses in the 4–8 msec latency ranges have the brainstem as their origin. Responses with latencies from about 8–50 msec presumably arise from the upper brainstem and primary projection areas. Slow wave responses from 50 to 300 msec originate as a secondary discharge from the primary corti-

Table 7.6.
Electrophysiologic Response Classifications

Response Latency Classification	Site of Origin	Response Waveform	Response Latency (msec)	Amplitude (μV)
Electrocochleography	Auditory nerve	Fast	1–5	0.1–10
Early	Brainstem	Fast	4–8	0.001–1
Middle	Brainstem/primary cortical projection	Fast	8–50	1.0–3
Late	Primary cortical projection and secondary association areas	Slow	50–300	8.0–20
Very late	Prefrontal cortex and secondary association areas	Very slow	300 and greater	20–30

From Skinner, P., & Glattke, T.J. (1977). Electrophysiologic response audiometry: state-of-the-art. *Journal of Speech and Hearing Disorders, 42,* 180.

cal projection areas and surrounding secondary and association areas. The longest latency potentials, about 300 msec, are slow shifts that appear to arise from the prefrontal and secondary or association areas of the cortex. Audiologists have found that the early, or brainstem, potentials have the widest application, since they can be easily and reliably detected in young individuals and are not affected by sedation. The MLRs may be of secondary importance, and late potentials are not reliable for use with young children and are significantly affected by sedation. ECochG is one of the most reliable of all physiologic measures, but because of the intricate requirements for administering the procedure, should only be considered after behavioral and other physiologic tests have proven inconclusive.

The use of the array of physiologic auditory tests helps make the term "sensorineural" archaic. With today's procedures and tests, hearing loss can be confirmed as either "sensory" or "neural" in terms of the origins of the pathology. Knowledge of the precise anatomic location of a child's etiology of deafness is very important to overall management and prognosis. Future research into the prevention and treatment of deafness depends on the ability to identify accurately the anatomic location of the disorder.

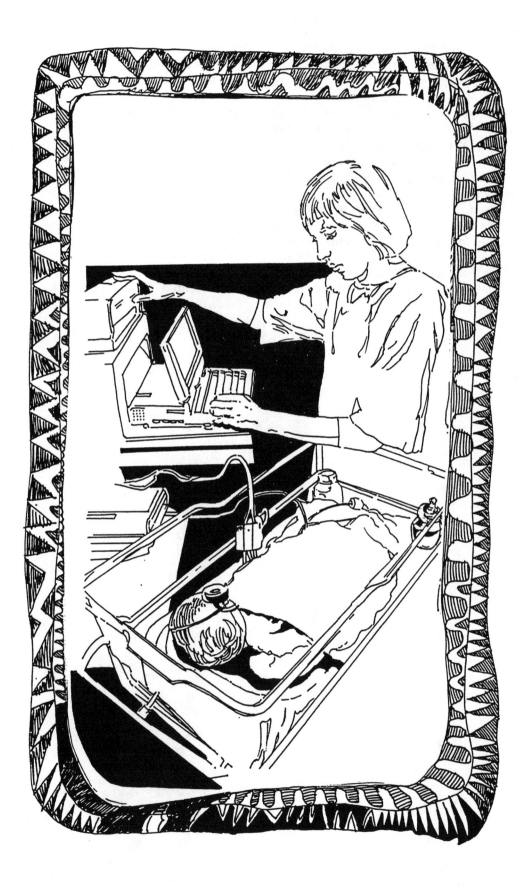

CHAPTER 8

Hearing Screening in Children

Screening is the process of applying certain rapid and simple tests, examinations, or other procedures to generally large numbers of persons which will identify those persons with a high probability of a disorder from those who probably do not have the disorder. A criterion measurement cutoff point is always involved, below or above which the disorder is suspect. Screening is not intended as a diagnostic procedure; screening merely surveys large populations of undiagnosed and typically asymptomatic persons to identify those who are suspected of having the disorder and who require more elaborate diagnostic procedures. Persons identified with positive or suspicious findings are referred to their physician for diagnosis and, if necessary, appropriate treatment.

Because hearing impairment is relatively invisible, hearing screening tests have been in use for at least 60 years to identify children for further auditory evaluation. Screening for hearing loss in U.S. public schools has been in practice since the 1930s, and nearly every state has some sort of mandated hearing screening program to identify children with educationally handicapping hearing impairments. The literature of audiology abounds with descriptions of various group and individual hearing tests designed for use in schools, dating from the introduction in 1927 of the Western Electric 4-C group speech test (McFarlan, 1927). Currently, either by order of legislative mandate or through some type of coordinated statewide program, hearing screening of school-aged children is conducted in nearly all U.S. states (Penn, 1999).

Screening for disease as early as possible in a child's life is now an accepted public health mandate. In a separate focus of hearing screening, the past 35 years has seen hearing screening programs for newborns developed to identify those newborns with hearing loss so that habilitative measures can be instituted. The historical development of hearing tests for infants has evolved from early behavioral observation techniques to today's sophisticated physiologic hearing screening technologies. Out of approximately 4,000,000 live births in the United States each year, it is estimated that 10% are at risk for congenital hearing loss. Of these infants, 30–50 of every 1000 are hearing impaired (Northern & Hayes, 1994).

A more difficult problem has been the development of simple, efficient, and valid hearing screening techniques for young children between 2 and 4 years of age. The effect of mild to moderate hearing impairment in this age group has been shown to be detrimental in speech/language development, but no hearing screening technique has gained universal acceptance for use in Head Start Programs, primary care physician offices, or public or private preschool grades.

Inasmuch as a wide variety of material relative to all aspects of hearing screening in children is presented, it is useful to look at the philosophy of screening from the vantage point of all the health sciences. A great deal of effort has been expended by public health agencies and epidemiologists to analyze the performance characteristics of all types of screening procedures. This chapter also examines the construct and evaluation procedures for individual screening procedures, as these are important concepts for audiologists to understand. Such discussions will help professionals to evaluate the present status of their approaches to children's hearing screening programs and specifically to provide the tools to critique individual hearing screening tests.

PRINCIPLES OF HEARING SCREENING

The following two aspects of screening philosophy are relevant to the current discussion of screening theories and how they relate to hearing conservation programs: (1) the selection of the disorder or disease, and (2) the evaluation of the screening procedures. The first question that must be asked is whether there should be a screen for a certain disease. If the answer is yes, then specific criteria described below should be applied to the selection of disorders (Frankenburg and Camp, 1975; ASHA, 1995).

Occurrence Frequent Enough or Consequence Serious Enough to Warrant Mass Screening. How prevalent is the disease in the population to be screened? Some balancing of cost with the number of children who have the disease must be made. Cunningham (1970) stated, "From the point of view of a public health program, in order to justify a mass screening program, the condition must be reasonably frequent or if rare it must have seri-

ous consequences if not detected." In the case of hearing, screening neonates for congenital deafness can be justified on the basis of its severity and resultant disastrous consequences; the screening of the young child can be justified on the basis of numbers alone and on consequences. Table 8-1 illustrates the relative status of hearing screening compared with other commonly screened newborn diseases. Hearing screening not only yields the highest returns among these diseases, but also is more productive of results once the problem is identified.

Amenability to Treatment or Prevention That Will Forestall or Change the Expected Outcome. What would be the prognosis for the person if treatment is instituted or if it is not instituted? It perhaps matters little if such a disorder as color blindness is detected early, as no treatment will change it. But the tragic consequences of untreated hearing losses are all too commonly seen: the complete lack of speech or language development at ages when these functions should be well-implanted; the deterioration of the parent-child relationship into subtle rejection or bewildered overprotection; and personality deviations of a wide variety, ranging from autistic-like withdrawal to hyperactivity and acting out. So long as a disease state can be accurately identified, its severity should at the very least be lessened by treatment if mandatory screening is going to be regarded as a profitable endeavor. There is no question that the sequelae of a true hearing loss can be ameliorated if the disorder is given proper treatment.

Table 8.1.
Matrix Analysis for Test Performance Characteristics

Test Results	Impaired	Normal	Total
Positive	TP	FP	TP + FP
Negative	FN	TN	FN + TN
Totals	TP + FN	FP + TN	TP + FP + FN + TN

From Jacobson, J., & Jacobson, C. (1987). Application of test performance characteristics in newborn auditory screening. *Seminars in Hearing, 8* (2), 133.
TP, true positive; *TN,* true negative; *FN,* false negative; *FP,* false positive.

Availability of Facilities for Diagnosis and Treatment. If there is a suspicion that a child has a certain disorder, can the child be properly assessed and treated without unreasonable expenditure in money and effort? This question largely concerns the state of the art and the number of trained professionals who can be depended on to produce accurate evaluations and remediation for the child. If 1-year-old Johnny is found in a rural area to have profound deafness, there may not be a facility for his diagnosis and training for hundreds of miles. Even in a big city, critical fellow professionals may view the facilities available with a jaundiced eye. When these situations occur—and they certainly do—can screening for the disorder in that location be justified? The concerned professional must answer, "Yes" to that question.

Cost of Screening Reasonably Commensurate With Benefits to the Individual. Is the screening equipment costly to purchase and to maintain? Do the personnel administering the screening tests require expensive training or high-level salaries? It is very difficult to designate any costs as excessive when the health and welfare of many individuals are at stake, but there are limitations to the funds available in any area. Some equipment can continue to be used for long periods and for many thousands of tests before any repair or calibration is required. In addition, as the trend toward the use of nonprofessional aides continues, the cost of screening continues to decrease. The cost-analysis of screening the infant and preschool population also varies, but in no case would it be considered exorbitant when compared with the benefits accrued.

Cooper, Gates, Owen, et al. (1975) published data regarding efficiency and cost of school screening programs. They reported that the ongoing rate for audiometric screening was about 5 minutes per student, or 12 students per hour. They also reported data for immittance screening to be approximately 1.1 minute per child, or

21 children per hour. Cooper and associates determined the cost of their screening program by establishing an index of cost per accurate referral of failures. To compute the cost per accurate referral, the following formula was developed:

$$\text{Cost per Child} = \frac{S}{R} + \frac{C + (M \times L)}{(N \times L)}$$

S = salary of person screening, in dollars per hour
R = screening rate in children per hour
C = cost of equipment in dollars
M = annual maintenance cost of equipment in dollars
L = lifetime of the equipment in years
N = number of children screened per year

Mehl and Thomson (1998) calculated the cost for universal newborn hearing screening in Colorado. Their analysis can be summarized with their description that "...the true cost for each infant screened is estimated to be $25 per infant, including labor costs, disposable supplies, and amortized capital equipment costs [page 4]." They further explained that the costs of screening actually ranged from $18.30 per infant when performed by supervised volunteers, to $25.60 per infant when performed by a paid technician, and to $33.30 per infant when performed by an audiologist. Considering the entire program and the number of infants identified to have significant hearing loss, Mehl and Thomson present their entire cost-analysis documentation and state that the screening costs to identify correctly one new case of congenital hearing loss are calculated to be $9600.

Screening Test Performance Characteristics. The success of a screening program depends on the effectiveness of the measures used to identify those who are likely to have the target disorder and to pass over those who do not have the target disorder. It is no longer sufficient to evaluate a test procedure critically by simply reporting the percentage of positive results in patients with the "disease" and the percentage of negative results in patients without the disease (Jerger, 1983). More rigid and critical performance characteristics must be applied to each screening test to evaluate fully its effectiveness in the overall attempt to identify infants and children with hearing problems. Jacobson and Jacobson (1987) provided an excellent discussion of screening test performance characteristics, and the current authors are grateful for their permission to use their material as the basis of the following discussion.

It must be kept in mind that the principle objective of any hearing screening program is to correctly identify hearing loss in those persons who truly have a problem, while ruling out hearing loss in normal-hearing persons. Screening tests should identify high-risk persons who are predisposed to develop disease or who are asymptomatic (undiagnosed), so that they can be effectively treated. Thus, the validity of a screening test is based on the proportion of test results that are confirmed diagnostically. If a hearing screening test too often passes infants or children who, indeed, have hearing impairment or it too often mistakenly identifies normal-hearing infants or children as hearing-impaired, the screening test will not stand up to critical performance evaluation and should be considered invalid and economically unfeasible.

Decision Matrix Analysis. A decision matrix is typically a 2 × 2 table that describes the results of a test procedure to the actual presence or absence of the disease (i.e., hearing impairment [Table 8-1]). The four components of the matrix table are *true positive* (TP), the number of hearing-impaired persons correctly identified by the test; *true negative* (TN), the number of persons with normal hearing who are correctly identified; *false positive* (FP), the number of persons with normal hearing incorrectly labeled as hearing-impaired; and *false negative* (FN), the number of persons truly impaired but in-

correctly identified as normal. A screening test of choice would result in a high proportion of true-positive rates and in a low proportion of false-positive rates, because those with the disease would be identified, whereas healthy participants would pass the screen. It is the formulation of actual screening pass-fail results to this decision matrix that allows the calculation of test performance validity.

The validity of a screening test that is dependent on diagnostic confirmation for every person under consideration is determined by the relationship of three components: (1) sensitivity, the ability of a test to correctly identify patients with the disease (hearing loss); (2) specificity, the ability of a test to correctly identify those without the disease (normal hearing); and (3) disease prevalence, the total number of patients with the disease in a given population. Thus, it is the actual test results that define these terms.

Sensitivity. When a test operates at a 70% sensitivity rate, only 7 of every 10 patients who are hearing-impaired are correctly identified. The remaining three impaired patients are improperly classified. This concept is illustrated in Table 8-2, which uses a hypothetical group of 1000 screened newborn infants. In this example, a total of 100 babies are truly hearing-impaired; however, only 70 (70%) were correctly identified as such. Thus, for this example 70% (70/100) represents the true-positive rate, whereas 30%, the misclassi-

Table 8.2.
Matrix Analysis for Hypothetical Test Results

Test Results[a]	Impaired	Normal	Total
Positive	70	180	250
Negative	30	720	750
Totals	100	900	1000

From Jacobson, J., & Jacobson, C. (1987). Application of test performance characteristics in newborn auditory screening. *Seminars in Hearing, 8* (2), 133–141.
[a]Sensitivity, 70/100 (70.0%); specificity, 720/900 (80.0%); predictive value of positive test, 70/250 (28.0%); predictive value of negative test, 720/750 (96.0%); overall, 790/1000 (79.0%); incidence, 100/1000 (10.0%).

fied (those who passed the screen), represents the false-negative rate.

In hearing screening it is most desirable to use a test that gives the highest possible rate of sensitivity. For example, if a child passes a hearing screen but presents with significant impairment, the abnormality may hold serious behavioral, developmental, and educational consequences if it goes undetected even for a short period early in the child's life.

Specificity. If all children with normal hearing passed a screening, the test would perform at a 100% specificity rate. However, as the test begins to fail normal-hearing children, the rate of specificity decreases. For example, if 8 of 10 infants were correctly identified as having normal hearing, the test would operate at 80% specificity. The remaining two incorrectly classified normal-hearing infants would be subjected to subsequent diagnostic follow-up. In Table 8-2, 720 of 900 normal-hearing babies passed the screen, resulting in 80% (720/900) test specificity. Those 180 normal-hearing newborns who were incorrectly classified rendered a 20% false-positive rate. This situation may result in parental stress and anxiety; however, misdiagnosis is usually ameliorated by further diagnostic assessment. Table 8-2 demonstrates that the terms sensitivity and specificity represent the true-positive and true-negative rates, respectively. It is evident that a reciprocal relationship exists between sensitivity and the false-negative rate and, similarly, between specificity and the false-positive rate.

Prevalence Versus Incidence. Both of these characteristics describe disease frequency rate. Prevalence rate is a census measure that expresses the presence of diseased patients per 100,000 population at the time of investigation. The rate of prevalence is calculated by dividing the number of diseased patients in the population at a specified time by the number of individuals in the population at that spec-

ified time. In contrast, incidence rate is the frequency of new outbreak of a disease condition in a population for a given period. To calculate incidence rate, two variables must be defined: (1) the beginning and end of the time period under study, and (2) the population at risk for developing the disorder under study. Incidence rate is calculated by dividing the number of new diseased patients in a population during a specified period by the number of persons exposed to the risk of developing the disease during that same period.

The relationship between prevalence and incidence is clarified by the following example. The incidence of an acute disease such as middle ear effusion in high-risk infants may be high, because large numbers of neonates contract the disease during convalescence. The prevalence is usually low, however, because the disease has a relatively short duration. Conversely, the incidence of a chronic disease such as sensory hearing loss may be low in newborns, but the prevalence in the population may be high. Although only a small percentage of babies are identified as sensory-impaired each year, sensory hearing loss is irreversible and therefore cumulative. Thus, the incidence of sensory hearing loss in children increases cumulatively, as the average age of the sample cohort grows older.

Predictive Value. Performance characteristics (i.e., sensitivity and specificity) define the ability of a test to estimate disease or nondisease in a given population accurately and, therefore, are of primary importance in the selection of a screening test. In contrast, predictive values, which are related to disease prevalence, examine the percentage of patients correctly labeled diseased or healthy by the test and provide information about test result interpretation. The predictive value of a positive test (PVP) is defined as the percent of all positive results that are true positive when the test is applied to a population containing both healthy and diseased subjects (TP/(TP + FP) × 100). The predictive value of a negative test (PVN) represents the percent of all negative results that are true negatives (TN/(TN + FN) × 100).

It is important to recognize that predictive values are dependent on test performance characteristics and disease prevalence in the population under study. Once measures of sensitivity and specificity are tabulated, it is then possible to establish probability statements regarding the presence or absence of disease, because predictive values relate directly to test outcome. Predictive value measures can be derived from Table 8-2. Of the total 250 patients who failed the screen, 70 were true positive. The remaining 180 patients were false positive, leaving a PVP of 28% (70 of 250). The PVP results mean that approximately three-fourths (180 of 250) of all patients who failed the test were false positive. The PVN result was 96% (720 of 750), meaning that this test correctly identified 720 members of the normal-hearing population. Thus, for persons who were determined to have passed the screen, only 4 of every 100 negative results were false negative. Finally, the overall efficiency (i.e., a measure of the percent of all true-positive and true-negative results) was 79%.

Disease prevalence within a target population will influence predictive values. Table 8-3 presents a hypothetical example of such an effect. By decreasing the prevalence of the disease from 5% (50/1000) to 1% (10/1000) to 0.1% (1/1000) while maintaining relatively high performance characteristics (sensitivity 90%, specificity 90%), predictive values change correspondingly. The PVP result decreased from 32.1% to 8.3% to less than 1.0%, whereas the PVN result in this case remained stable. When disease prevalence is 0.1% (1/1000), it is similar to that reported in mass auditory screening. The false-positive rate is 99.1%. This example clearly points to the importance of applying screening tests to high-prevalence populations. If not, the false-positive rate will be so great that it may be indefensible.

Pass-Fail Criteria. Given the inherent differences in biomedical investigation, it is unlikely that any test, screening or diagnostic, will be designed that can separate all patients with disease from

Table 8.3.
Effects of Disease Prevalence on Predictive Values When Sensitivity (90%) and Specificity (90%) Remain Constant

Test Results	Impaired	Normal	Total
Disease prevalence 5%			
Positive	225	475	700
Negative	25	4275	4300
Totals	250	4750	5000
PVP = 32.1%			
PVN = 99.4%			
Disease prevalence 1%			
Positive	45	495	540
Negative	5	4455	4460
Totals	50	4950	5000
PVP = 8.3%			
PVN = 99.9%			
Disease prevalence 0.1%			
Positive	4.5	499.5	504
Negative	0.5	4495.5	4496
Totals	5	4995	5000
PVP = 1.0%			
PVN = 100%			

From Jacobson, J., & Jacobson, C. (1987). Application of test performance characteristics in newborn auditory screening. *Seminars in Hearing, 8* (2), 133141.

those without disease. The result is that there will always be those screened who are inaccurately labeled. Thorner and Remein (1967) have addressed this integration of normal and pathologic patients in the theory of overlapping distributions. The selection of a cutoff point within the overlapping distribution will directly influence the anticipated yield (incidence) of identified patients with disease as well as affect test performance characteristics. The determination of pass-fail criteria is a critical factor in the establishment of eventual test outcome.

Figure 8-1 illustrates the concept of overlapping distribution. In this hypothetical hearing screening population, a cutoff score was initially established. Using this stated pass-fail criteria (i.e., a predetermined intensity level) a certain proportion of patients passed the screen, whereas others did not. Depending on individual test outcome, measures of sensitivity and specificity, false-positive rates, and false-negative rates were established. However, if the cutoff score for hearing screening was adjusted either up (higher intensity level) or down (lower intensity level), performance values would change correspondingly. If the cutoff score was increased so that more hearing-impaired persons pass the test, sensitivity would decrease because the false-negative rate (hearing-impaired persons who pass the test) would increase. Conversely, as sensitivity decreased, specificity rate would increase as a result of the reduced number of false-positive (normal-hearing persons who fail the test) results. If, on the other hand, the cutoff point was lowered, fewer hearing-impaired persons would pass the test, and the false-negative rate would decrease. By doing so, specificity would decrease as the false-positive rate would increase. The result is a reciprocal relationship between sensitivity and specificity—as sensitivity increases, specificity decreases; and as specificity increases, sensitivity decreases.

A cutoff score is an arbitrary point that can be set to favor a specific test outcome. The PVP and PVN results also change as the pass-fail cutoff point is manipulated. Because both test performance characteristics and disease prevalence influence the predictive value, an increase in the cutoff point (e.g., using a more stringent or rigorous definition of hearing loss) will reduce the "overall incidence" of hearing impairment. Finally, the overall test efficiency will be influenced, since the cutoff point may also determine the correct identification of hearing-impaired and normal-hearing persons.

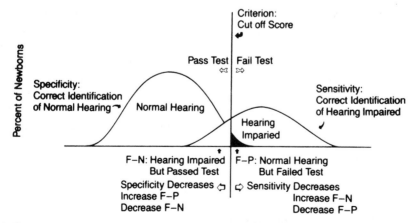

Figure 8-1. Graphic representation of a hypothetical newborn screened population. Illustration displays an overlapping subject distribution and its effect on specific operating characteristics. (From Jacobson, J., & Jacobson, C. (1987). Newborn auditory screening. *Seminars in Hearing, 8* (2), 139.)

The ideal hearing screening test would correctly differentiate 100% of the time between normal-hearing and hearing-impaired persons. Unfortunately, the development of such a hearing screening test that would meet the requirements of objectivity, ease of administration, rapid and simple technique, and economic feasibility is unlikely. Therefore, as each specific population targeted for hearing screening is determined, the selection and implementation of a hearing screening tool must depend heavily on the various measures of test validity and desired performance characteristics. The use of sensitivity, specificity, and their reciprocal counterparts can provide information about the number of persons correctly identified as hearing-impaired or normal-hearing as measures against predetermined pass-fail criteria. Predictive values that are dependent on the prevalence or incidence of hearing disorders describe the test's ability to separate correctly true-positive and true-negative results in those with and without hearing loss. Of course, the final validation of any screening test measure must account for the diagnostic confirmation of all individuals screened, regardless of initial test outcome.

NEONATAL AND INFANT HEARING SCREENING

Prevalence of Newborn Hearing Loss.
Stein (1999) asked the critical question concerning how many newborns might be expected to be found with significant hearing loss in the annual U.S. population of 4 million births. The prevalence of newborns with hearing loss is currently under reexamination, with new data being generated from universal infant hearing screening programs underway in more than 20 states. For many years, it was widely held that the prevalence of hearing loss in the newborn population is approximately 1 in 1000 live births, or 4000 infants per year. It was argued by many that this estimate was understated

as it was based only on congenital, profound bilateral hearing loss. Further, early surveys failed to include newborns at risk for developmental disabilities in whom the prevalence of hearing loss is now known to be significantly greater than the well-birth infant population. Hearing loss of mild, moderate, or severe degree or unilateral hearing losses were not taken into account simply because of the difficulty in accurately assessing hearing in infants before the advent of otoacoustic emission (OAE) and auditory brainstem response (ABR) screening.

It has been long known that the number of babies with hearing loss identified in the newborn intensive care unit (NICU) is considerably higher than in the general well-baby population. Several studies estimated the incidence of hearing loss in this NICU targeted population at 20–50 times greater than in the newborn nursery, or at least 1 in 150 babies (Schulman-Galambos & Galambos, 1979; Simmons, 1982; Davis & Wood, 1992). Although more and more research studies are underway to establish the true prevalence of hearing impairment in newborns and children, as this information is crucial for long-term planning and funding of intervention and special education programs, it is clear that the answer to the question is complex. In each study, consideration must be given to the specific description of the target population; the definition of hearing loss in terms of degree, type (sensorineural and/or conductive), and unilateral or bilateral presence; technique of identification and protocol followed; criteria for what degree of hearing loss constitutes pass or failure; and the success of follow-up and diagnostic confirmation of each hearing loss (Stein, 1999).

The incidence of congenital hearing loss in the general newborn population is high and is a relatively common occurrence. Mehl and Thomson (1998) compared the incidence of bilateral hearing loss in newborns in Colorado against

Table 8.4.
Yield in Infant Health-Care Screening Tests

Disease Screened	Yield
Phenylketonuria	7 in 100,000 births
Combined immunodeficiency disease	25 in 3 million births
Maple syrup urine disease	1 in 300,000 births
Neonatal hyperthyroidism	25 in 100,000 births
Cystic fibrosis	50 in 100,000 births
Hemoglobinopathy	13 in 100,000 births
Bilateral sensorineural hearing loss	260 in 100,000 births

Adapted from Mehl, A., & Thomson, V. (1998). Newborn hearing screening: The great omission. *Pediatrics, 101* (1), e4.

other existing disease screening programs as shown in Table 8-4. They reported that congenital bilateral hearing loss is present in 200 of 100,000 newborns. For comparison, the incidence in galactosemia is 2 per 100,000 births; phenylketonuria, 10 per 100,000 births; and hypothyroidism, 25 per 100,000 births. The prevalence of newborn and infant hearing loss has been estimated in other studies from 1.5 to 6.0 per 1000 live births (Watkin, 1996; Parving, 1993; White & Behrens, 1993; Northern & Hayes, 1994). Risk factor screening identifies only 50% of infants with significant hearing loss (Pappas, 1983; Elssman, Matkin, & Sabo, 1987; Mauk, White, Mortensen, & Behrens, 1991), and failure to identify the remaining 50% of children with hearing loss results in diagnosis and intervention at an unacceptably late age.

Review of the literature of the past 35 years confirms that substantial data exist to support irrefutable facts delineated by Northern and Hayes (1994) about hearing impairment in early childhood:

- Sensorineural hearing impairment in infants and young children is a serious condition that results in life-long disability.
- Continued dependence on the high-risk registry approach to screening infants

will identify less than 50% of infants with significant hearing loss.

- Valid techniques, with proven acceptable sensitivity and specificity, are currently available to detect moderate, severe, and profound hearing loss in infants.
- Early intervention is essential for facilitating speech, language, and cognitive skills; social-emotional development; and academic achievement.

Early identification and habilitation of all infants with hearing impairment must continue to be a major goal for health-care systems.

Joint Committee on Infant Hearing Screening. In 1969, at the suggestion of Marion Downs, a national committee formed of representatives from the Academy of Pediatrics, the Academy of Ophthalmology and Otolaryngology, and the American Speech and Hearing Association met to make recommendations for newborn infant hearing screening. The Joint Committee at that time addressed itself to the use of behavioral observation hearing screening tests for use with infants which had been developed and described by Downs and Sterritt (1964) and Downs and Hemenway (1969). The Joint Committee developed a *high-risk register for deafness* that identified five major criteria that would put newborn infants at risk for having severe to profound hearing impairment. The five criteria were family history; intrauterine fetal infection; defects of the ear, nose, or throat; low birthweight; and high bilirubin level. These risk factors could be identified by interviewing the birth mother or by examining the medical records of each infant to see whether there was any history or physical finding that would give a high probability of hearing loss. The Downs and Sterritt project mass-screened 17,000 newborns in Denver, resulting in the identification of 17 infants with profound hearing loss. The high-risk register approach was an attempt to focus attention on those infants most likely to have significant hearing loss rather than screening every baby. The high-risk concept assumes that one can identify a small group of children whose history or physical condition results in a high chance of having the target handicap.

The Joint Committee on Infant Hearing met again in 1982, 1990, 1994, and 2000 to review and update new position statements, based on new knowledge and reviews of current literature relevant to practices of identifying the hearing-impaired neonate and infant. The evolution of recommended infant hearing screening practices presents an interesting look at the growth and application of new technologies and knowledge in continued efforts to improve the efficiency and accuracy of early identification of infants with hearing impairments. Interested readers are referred to Hayes and Northern (1996), in which a complete history of the Joint Committee meetings, as well as the complete position statements, is published.

The decade of the 1990s will no doubt be remembered for the return to the concept of implementing hearing screening for all newborns, now known as *universal newborn hearing screening*. As described by Hayes (1999), during the first half of the 1990s, three important activities stimulated interest in early detection of infants with hearing loss. First, in 1990, with support of federal funding, the Rhode Island Hearing Assessment Project was developed to evaluate systematically the feasibility of using the new technique of transient evoked otoacoustic emissions to screen infants for hearing loss. The success of the Rhode Island Project stimulated the occurrence of the second activity, the NIH-sponsored Consensus Conference, which met and issued a statement recommending that "universal screening be implemented for all infants within the first 3 months of life." The third important activity was the development and release of a new position statement of the Joint Committee on Infant Hearing (JCIH) in 1994, which endorsed "the goal of universal de-

tection of infants with hearing loss as early as possible. All infants with hearing loss should be identified by three months of age, and receive intervention by six months of age." Finally, even the American Academy of Pediatrics (1999) published an independent endorsement of universal newborn hearing screening calling for pediatricians to take a more active role in pediatric hearing screening programs.

The Rhode Island Project was the first statewide effort to attempt the goal of universal newborn hearing screening (Vohr, Carty, Moore, & Letourneau, 1998). A universal infant hearing screening program was established in eight maternity hospitals in Rhode Island based on a two-tiered approach of TEOAEs for all infants, with those failing the initial screening referred for ABR. Review of the first 4 years of the project, 1993–1996, showed a steady improvement in the percentage of infants completing the two-stage screen process with compliance in the rescreening and diagnostic testing stages as well as significant improvements in the age of identification and age of intervention for infants with confirmed hearing loss. Results were reported for the identification and habilitation of 111 infants with permanent hearing loss identified from more than 53,000 total babies screened and an amazing 99% of all babies born in Rhode Island. The study showed an impairment rate of 2 per 1000, with the mean age of hearing loss confirmation decreased from 8.7 months to 3.5 months, and the age of initial amplification declined from 13.3 months to 5.7 months during the 4 years of the study.

Recognizing that the high-risk register screening approach to the identification of infants with congenital hearing loss that was used in the late 1980s and early 1990s was missing some 50% of young children later identified who had none of the risk factors at birth, the federal government convened a special meeting of experts to evaluate existing evidence and to recommend improved screening protocols. Although the 1993 NIH Consensus

Conference provoked considerable debate regarding the feasibility of, and justification for, universal newborn hearing screening, recommendations were issued to clearly define the approaches and timetables for universal detection of infants with hearing loss. Based largely on the success of the Rhode Island Project, the NIH Consensus Conference recommended universal newborn hearing screening using a two-stage physiologic test approach of an initial TEOAE screen for all newborns and ABR screening for those infants not passing the initial screening procedure.

The Joint Committee in Infant Hearing 1994 Position Statement supported the NIH Consensus Conference by endorsing the goal of universal detection of infants with hearing loss. The 1994 Joint Committee, however, specifying that infants should be screened with established physiologic testing techniques, encouraged continuing research to evaluate existing screening techniques and to develop new protocols. The 1994 JCIH statement expanded the role of high-risk factors (termed "indicators") associated with sensorineural and/or conductive hearing loss in newborns and infants.

The current guidelines and recommendations for early identification of hearing loss were developed by the Joint Committee on Infant Hearing. The 2000 document is a masterful statement concerning the status and the future directions of infant hearing screening. Although the entire document is too lengthy to reproduce in these pages, the background information, general principles, and salient information are presented below.

JOINT COMMITTEE ON INFANT HEARING YEAR 2000 POSITION STATEMENT

PRINCIPLES AND GUIDELINES FOR EARLY HEARING DETECTION AND INTERVENTION PROGRAMS

The Joint Committee on Infant Hearing (JCIH) endorses early detection of and intervention for infants with hearing loss (early hearing detection and intervention, EHDI) through integrated, interdisciplinary state and national systems of universal newborn hearing screening, evaluation, and family-centered intervention. The goal of EHDI is to maximize communicative competence and literacy development for children who are hard of hearing or deaf. Without appropriate opportunities to learn language, children who are hard of hearing or deaf will fall behind their hearing peers in language, cognition, and social-emotional development. Such delays may result in lower educational and employment levels in adulthood (Gallaudet University Center for Assessment and Demographic Study, 1998). Thus, all infants with congenital or neonatal hearing loss should be identified using objective, physiological tests before 3 months of age and should begin an intervention program before 6 months of age. Regardless of prior hearing screening outcomes, all infants who demonstrate risk indicators for delayed onset or progressive hearing loss should receive ongoing audiologic and medical monitoring for 3 years and at appropriate intervals thereafter to ensure prompt identification and intervention (ASHA, 1997). EHDI systems should guarantee seamless transitions for infants and their families through the process of screening, confirmation of hearing loss, medical diagnosis of hearing loss and related disorders, and intervention. To achieve informed decision making, families should have access to professionals and educational and consumer organizations, and they should have opportunities to interact with adults and children who are hard of hearing and deaf. Families should have access to general information on child development and specific information on hearing loss and language development. To achieve program accountability, individual hospital, agency, and state programs should assume the responsibility for coordinated, ongoing measurement and improvement of EHDI process outcomes.

BACKGROUND

Hearing loss in newborns and infants is not readily detectable by routine clinical procedures (behavioral observation), although parents often report the suspicion of hearing loss, inattention or erratic response to sound before hearing loss is confirmed (Arehart, Yoshinago-Itaono, Thomson, Gabbard, & Stredler Brown, 1998; Harrison & Roush, 1996; Kile, 1993). The average age of identification in the United States is being reduced with EHDI programs; until very recently, it had been 30 months of age (Harrison & Roush, 1996). While children who have severe to profound hearing loss or multiple disabilities may be identified before 30 months, children with mild to moderate losses often are not identified until school age because of the nature of hearing loss and the resultant inconsistent response to sound (Elssmann, Matkin, & Sabo, 1987). For this reason, the National Institute on Deafness and Other Communication Disorders (of the National Institutes of Health) released a *Consensus Statement on Early Identification of Hearing Impairment in Infants and Young Children* in 1993. The statement concluded that all infants admitted to the neonatal intensive care unit should be screened for hearing loss before hospital discharge and that universal screening should be implemented for all infants within the first 3 months of life (NIDCD, 1993). In its 1994 Position Statement, the JCIH endorsed the goal of universal detection of infants with hearing loss and encouraged continuing research and development to improve methodologies for identification of and intervention for hearing loss (Joint Committee on Infant Hearing, 1995). In the ensuing years, considerable data have been reported which support not only the feasibility of universal newborn hearing screening (UNHS) but also the benefits of early intervention for infants with hearing loss. Specifically, infants who are hard of hearing and deaf who receive intervention before 6 months of age maintain language development commensurate with their cognitive abilities through the age of 5 years (Yoshinaga-Itano, 1995; Yoshinaga-Itano, Sedey, Coulter, & Mehl, 1998). Numerous investigators have documented the validity, reliability, and effectiveness of early detection of infants who are hard of hearing and deaf through universal newborn hearing screening (Finitzo, Albright, & O'Neal, 1998; Spivak, 1998; Vohr et al., 1998; Vohr & Maxon, 1996). Cost-effective screening is being undertaken in individual hospitals and in numerous statewide programs in the United States (Arehart et al., 1998; Finitzo et al., 1998; Mason & Hermann, 1998; Mehl & Thomson, 1998; Vohr et al., 1998). As of fall 1999, approximately half of the states have enacted legislation supporting universal newborn hearing screening. Working groups convened by the National Institute on Deafness and Other Communication Disorders (NIDCD) in 1997 and 1998 offered recommendations on Acceptable Protocols for Use in State-Wide Universal Newborn Hearing Screening Programs and Characterization of

Auditory Performance and Intervention Strategies Following Neonatal Screening (NIDCD, 1997). Given these findings and empirical evidence to date, the JCIH considers that accepted public health criteria have been met to justify implementation of universal newborn hearing screening (American Academy of Pediatrics, 1999; ASHA, 1989 a, b; Spivak, 1998). The JCIH issues the year 2000 Position Statement, describes principles underlying effective EHDI programs, and includes an accompanying guideline on implementing and maintaining a successful EHDI program.

PRINCIPLES

The Joint Committee on Infant Hearing (JCIH) endorses the development of family-centered, community-based early hearing detection and intervention (EHDI) systems. EHDI systems are comprehensive, coordinated, timely, and available to all infants. The following eight principles provide the foundation for effective EHDI systems. Each of the principles is discussed in the Guideline, which follows the delineation of the principles.

1. All infants have access to hearing screening using a physiologic measure. Newborns who receive routine care have access to hearing screening during their hospital birth admission. Newborns in alternative birthing facilities, including home births, have access to and are referred for screening before one month of age. All newborns or infants who require neonatal intensive care receive hearing screening before discharge from the hospital. These components constitute universal newborn hearing screening (UNHS).

2. All infants who do not pass the birth admission screen and any subsequent rescreening begin appropriate audiologic and medical evaluations to confirm the presence of hearing loss before 3 months of age.

3. All infants with confirmed permanent hearing loss receive services before 6 months of age in interdisciplinary intervention programs that recognize and build on strengths, informed choice, traditions, and cultural beliefs of the family.

4. All infants who pass newborn hearing screening but who have risk indicators for other auditory disorders and/or speech and language delay receive ongoing audiologic and medical surveillance and monitoring for communication development. Infants with indicators associated with late-onset, progressive, or fluctuating hearing loss as well as auditory neural conduction disor-

ders and/or brainstem auditory pathway dysfunction should be monitored.

5. Infant and family rights are guaranteed through informed choice, decision-making, and consent.

6. Infant hearing screening and evaluation results are afforded the same protection as all other health care and educational information. As new standards for privacy and confidentiality are proposed, they must balance the needs of society and the rights of the infant and family, without compromising the ability of health and education to provide care (AAP, 1999).

7. Information systems are used to measure and report the effectiveness of EHDI services. While state registries measure and track screening, evaluation and intervention outcomes for infants and their families, efforts should be made to honor a family's privacy by removing identifying information wherever possible. Aggregate state and national data may also be used to measure and track the impact of EHDI programs on public health and education while maintaining the confidentiality of individual infant and family information.

8. EHDI programs provide data to monitor quality, demonstrate compliance with legislation and regulations, determine fiscal accountability and cost effectiveness, support reimbursement for services, and mobilize and maintain community support.

RISK INDICATORS

Since 1972, the JCIH has identified specific risk indicators that often are associated with infant and childhood hearing loss. These risk indicators have been applied both in the United States and in other countries and serve two purposes. First, risk indicators help identify infants who should receive audiologic evaluation and who live in geographic locations (e.g., developing nations, remote areas) where universal hearing screening is not yet available. The JCIH no longer recommends programs calling for screening at-risk infants because such programs will identify only 40% to 50% of infants with hearing loss; however, these programs may be useful where resources limit the development of universal newborn hearing screening. Second, because normal hearing at birth does not preclude delayed onset or acquired hearing loss, risk indicators help identify infants who should receive on-going audiologic and medical monitoring and surveillance.

Risk indicators can be divided into two categories: those present during the neonatal period and those that may develop as a result of certain medical conditions or essential medical interventions in the treatment of an ill child. Risk indicators published in the 1994 Position Statement are revised in 2000 to take account of current information. Specifically, data have been considered from an epidemiological study of permanent childhood hearing impairment in the Trent Region of Great Britain from 1985 through 1993 (Fortnum & Davis, 1997) and the recent NIH multicenter study "Identification of Neonatal Hearing Impairment" (Norton et al., 2000). Cone-Wesson et al. (2000) analyzed the prevalence of risk indicators for infants identified with hearing loss in that study. Three thousand one hundred thirty four infants evaluated during their initial birth hospitalization were reevaluated for the presence of hearing loss between 8 and 12 months of age. The majority of these infants were NICU graduates (2,847) and the remaining 287 infants had risk indicators for hearing loss that did not require intensive care, such as family history or craniofacial anomalies. Infants with history or evidence of transient middle ear dysfunction were excluded from the final analysis, revealing 56 with permanent hearing loss.

Cone-Wesson et al. (2000) determined the prevalence of hearing loss for each risk factor by dividing the number of infants with the risk factor and hearing loss by the total number of infants in the sample with a given risk factor. Hearing loss was present in 11.7% of infants with syndromes associated with hearing loss—which included Trisomy 21; Pierre Robin syndrome; CHARGE syndrome; choanal atresia; Rubinstein-Taybi syndrome; Stickler syndrome; and oculo-auriculo-vertebral (OAV) spectrum (also known as Goldenhar syndrome). Family history of hearing loss had a prevalence of 6.6%, meningitis 5.5%, and craniofacial anomalies 4.7%. In contrast, aminoglycoside antibiotics had a prevalence of hearing loss of only 1.5%, consistent with data of Finitzo-Hieber, McCracken, and Brown (1985). Analyzing risk indicators, such as ototoxicity, by prevalence points out that while a large number of NICU infants with hearing loss have a history of aminoglycoside treatment, only a small percentage of those receiving ototoxic antibiotics actually incurred hearing loss. In fact, 45% of infants treated in the NICU received such treatment (Vohr et al., 2000).

1. Given these current data, the JCIH risk indicators have been modified for use in neonates (birth through age 28 days) where universal hearing screening is not yet available. These indicators are:

a. an illness or condition requiring admission of 48 hours or greater to a NICU (Fortnum & Davis, 1997)
b. stigmata or other findings associated with a syndrome known to include a sensorineural and or conductive hearing loss
c. family history of permanent childhood sensorineural hearing loss (Fortnum & Davis, 1997)
d. craniofacial anomalies, including those with morphological abnormalities of the pinna and ear canal (Fortnum & Davis, 1997).
e. in-utero infection such as cytomegalovirus, herpes, toxoplasmosis, or rubella (Demmler, 1991; Littman, Demmoer, Williams, Istas, & Griesser, 1995; Williamson, Demmler, Percy, & Catlin, 1992).

Interpretation of the Cone-Wesson et al. (2000) data reveals that 1 of 56 infants identified with permanent hearing loss revealed clear evidence of late-onset hearing loss by one year of age. The definition of late-onset hearing loss for this analysis was a present ABR at 30 dB in the newborn period and hearing thresholds by visual reinforcement audiometry at age 8-12 months greater than 40 dB for all stimuli. The infant with late-onset loss passed screening ABR, TOAE, and DPOAE during the newborn period but had reliable behavioral thresholds revealing a severe hearing loss at one year of age. Risk indicators for this infant included low birthweight, respiratory distress syndrome, bronchio-pulmonary dysplasia, and 36 days of mechanical ventilation. While these data are valuable, additional study of large samples of infants is needed before risk indicators for progressive or delayed onset hearing loss can be clearly defined.

2. The JCIH recommends the following indicators for use with neonates or infants (29 days through 2 years). These indicators place an infant at risk for progressive or delayed-onset sensorineural hearing loss and/or conductive hearing loss. Any infant with these risk indicators for progressive or delayed-onset hearing loss who has passed the birth screen should, nonetheless, receive audiologic monitoring every 6 months until age 3 years. These indicators are:
a. parental or caregiver concern regarding hearing, speech, language, and or developmental delay
b. family history of permanent childhood hearing loss
c. stigmata or other findings associated with a syndrome known to include a sensorineural or conductive hearing loss or eustachian tube dysfunction

d. postnatal infections associated with sensorineural hearing loss including bacterial meningitis (Ozdamar, Kraus, & Stein, 1982)
e. in-utero infections such as cytomegalovirus, herpes, rubella, syphilis, and toxoplasmosis
f. neonatal indicators—specifically hyperbilirubinemia at a serum level requiring exchange transfusion, persistent pulmonary hypertension of the newborn associated with mechanical ventilation, and conditions requiring the use of extracorporeal membrane oxygenation (ECMO) (Roizen, 1999)
g. syndromes associated with progressive hearing loss such as neurofibromatosis, osteopetrosis, and Usher's syndrome
h. neurodegenerative disorders, such as Hunter syndrome, or sensory motor neuropathies, such as Friedreich's ataxia and Charcot-Marie-Tooth syndrome
i. head trauma
j. recurrent or persistent otitis media with effusion for at least 3 months (Stool, Berg, Carney, et al., 1994)

Because some important indicators, such as family history of hearing loss, may not be determined during the course of UNHS programs, the presence of all late-onset risk indicators should be determined in the medical home during early well-baby visits. Those infants with significant late-onset risk factors should be carefully monitored for normal communication developmental milestones during routine medical care.

The JCIH recommends ongoing audiologic and medical monitoring of infants with unilateral, mild, or chronic conductive hearing loss. Infants and children with mild or unilateral hearing loss may also experience adverse speech, language, and communication skill development, as well as difficulties with social, emotional, and educational development (Bess, Dodd-Murphy, & Parker, 1998; Tharpe & Bess, 1999; Blair, Petterson, & Viehweg, 1985; Davis et al., 1986; Roush & Matkin, 1994). Infants with unilateral hearing loss are at risk for progressive and/or bilateral hearing loss (Brookhouser, Worthington, & Kelly, 1994). Infants with frequent episodes of otitis media with effusion (OME) also require additional vigilance to address the potential adverse effects of fluctuating conductive hearing loss associated with persistent or recurrent OME (Friel-Patti & Finitzo, 1990; Friel-Patti, Finitzo, Meyerhoff, & Hieber, 1986; Friel-Patti, Finitzo-Hieber, Conti, & Brown, 1982; Gravel & Wallace,

1992; Jerger, Jerger, Alford, & Abrams, 1983; Roberts et al., 1995; Stool et al., 1994; Wallace et al., 1988).

The Multidisciplinary Team. The evaluation and assessment of an infant identified with hearing loss should be performed by a team of professionals working in conjunction with the parent/caregiver as described by the earlier JCIH 1994 Statement. The team should consist of the following:

1. A *physician* with expertise in the management of early childhood otologic disorders.
2. An *audiologist* with expertise in the assessment of infants and young children to determine type, degree, symmetry, stability, and configuration of hearing loss and to recommend amplification devices appropriate to the child's needs (e.g., hearing aids, personal FM systems, vibrotactile aids, or cochlear implants).
3. A *speech-language pathologist, audiologist, sign language specialist, and/or teacher* of children who are deaf or hard-of-hearing with expertise in the assessment and intervention of communication skills.
4. Other professionals as appropriate for the individual needs of the child and family. This team should work together to develop a program of early intervention services Individualized Family Service Plan (IFSP) that is based on the infant's unique strengths and needs and is consistent with the family's resources, priorities, and concerns related to enhancing the child's development. This multidisciplinary team must include the parent/caregiver. Team planning should be cognizant of and sensitive to the range of available communication and educational choices, and parents should be given sufficient information regarding all options to enable them to exercise informed consent when selecting their child's program.

Trained Volunteers. Individual volunteers, or volunteers from various community service groups, can be trained by the audiologist to perform many of the functions required in an infant hearing screening program. Not all volunteers actually want to test the hearing of babies, but the personnel support from such groups can be effectively directed to interviewing mothers, reviewing hospital medical records, conducting record-keeping and other administrative tasks, and telephoning to ensure follow-up care. When volunteers are used in hospital situations, it is suggested that appropriate steps be taken to ensure legal protection and legal clearance for these nonprofessional people to examine medical charts, move babies from the nurseries to the audiologic test area, interview new mothers, and perform other tasks. The advantage to the use of volunteers is the low cost for supportive personnel; the major disadvantage of using volunteers is often a progressive lack of interest in this particular project, or a change-over in the volunteer club's officers or a change in direction of the service organization's activities. The audiologist dependent on a volunteer staff to perform the infant hearing screening program must be a master of working with people to obtain high-quality support and ingenious at maintaining the volunteer enthusiasm for the project at hand.

UNIVERSAL NEWBORN SCREENING

Following the recommendation for universal screening of newborns developed during the NIH Consensus Conference on Early Identification of Hearing Impairment in Infants and Young Children held in 1993, considerable controversy was generated over the panel's conclusions supporting mass hearing screening. Bess and Paradise (1994) characterized universal screening for infant hearing impairment as "not simple, not risk-free, not necessarily beneficial and not presently justifiable." Their commentary impugned infant hearing screening and questioned the effectiveness and need for early intervention for infants with hearing loss. Northern and Hayes (1994) took exception to their presentation and published a response in favor of universal infant hearing screening. The debate stimulated a rash of Letters to the Editor (*Pediatrics*, 94:6, 948–963, 1994), with most respondents indicating that ample data exist to support infant hearing screening and the need for early intervention. Despite Bess' and Paradise's editorials, the momentum for universal hearing screening of infants grew to involve more than 22 states by the year 2000, according to the Marion Downs National Center for Newborn Hearing Screening (Denver, CO) as shown in Figure 8-2.

The Rhode Island Hearing Assessment Project was the first major attempt at universal hearing screening of newborns and has been written about extensively (White & Behrens, 1993; White, 1996; Vohr et al.,

1998). Based on a two-stage protocol using otoacoustic emissions as the birth admission screening, followed by ABR procedure, results were reported for more than 53,000 newborns. Referral rates following the first-stage screen were 8%, decreasing to less than 3% following the second screening procedure. Other state programs followed with their own versions and protocols in efforts to establish statewide newborn hearing screening programs. Mehl and Thomson (1998) described the Colorado experience over a 4-year period involving the screening of more than 41,000 infants. They concluded that the cost (estimated at $9600 per case identified) and the positive predictive value (estimated at approximately 19% for two-staged automated ABR screening) of universal newborn hearing screening compared favorably with cost and predictive value of screening for other congenital conditions. Mason and Hermann (1998) reported results of a single

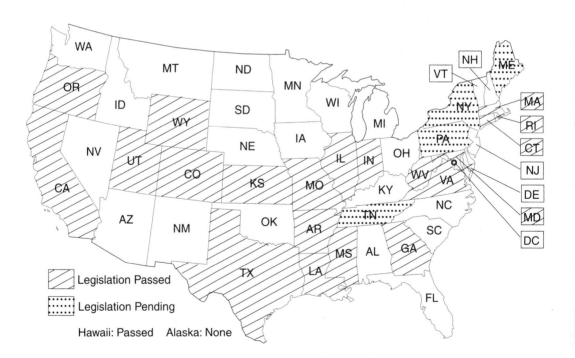

Figure 8-2. Statewide neonatal hearing screening programs. (Black) states with mandates for neonatal hearing screening. (Lined) states with no legal mandate but with neonatal screening programs widely in place. (White) no statewide screening program in place.

hospital-based program in Hawaii in which 96% of infants were successfully screened, including more than 10,000 infants over a 5-year period. In the Hawaii experience, the cost of screening was reported to be $17 per infant, resulting in an estimated cost to identify each case of true bilateral hearing loss to be $17,750 per infant. Finitzo and Albright (1998) and Finitzo and Crumley (1999) described the Sounds of Texas infant screening program. They reported that during a 3-year period in 11 Texas hospitals, 98% of all newborns were screened for hearing before discharge. Texas hospitals using a two-technology screening protocol (EOAE followed by ABR screening) averaged a 3% failure rate, while hospitals using a two-stage one-technology (either EOAE or ABR) protocol showed a 5% failure rate (Fig. 8-3).

A massive project was undertaken as the New York State Universal Newborn Hearing Screening effort to determine the feasibility of universal newborn screening in seven regional perinatal centers comprised of eight hospitals. Their results over a 3-year period have been described in a series of articles (Prieve & Stevens, 2000; Spivak et al., 2000; Prieve et al., 2000; Dalzell et al., 2000; Gravel et al., 2000). Over the 3-

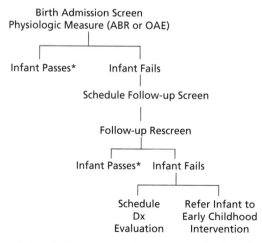

Figure 8-3. Flow diagram of the components of a universal newborn hearing screening program. (Used with permission from the Sounds of Texas Project, Terese Finitzo, Dallas, TX.)

year period in New York, nearly 70,000 newborns were screened at the 8 hospitals, representing 96.9% of all live births. The overall failure rate of 4%, combined with the miss rate of 2.6%, resulted in 6.6% of infants referred for outpatient follow-up. According to Hayes (2000), the New York State Project confirmed the necessity and demonstrated the feasibility of developing a compete audiologic system of care of newborn infants, and further established a standard of care benchmark of accountability for all universal screening statewide programs.

RISK INDICATORS FOR DEAFNESS

Despite substantial research efforts and a number of years of clinical application, limiting infant hearing screening to only those newborns with known high-risk factors proved to identify only 50% of the pediatric population with congenital hearing loss. Accordingly, use of the high-risk register is no longer recommended. However, knowledge of current risk indicators associated with childhood hearing impairment is extremely helpful in interpreting developmental history about children under evaluation. The audiologist is well advised to have an in-depth understanding of the risk indicators for deafness, because an infant with any of these factors in the neonatal history has an increased chance of having hearing impairment. The form that was used to collect information about prenatal and postnatal conditions for each infant confirmed with hearing loss in the Colorado Newborn Hearing Screening Project is shown in Figure 8-4 and is especially useful for noting the presence of risk indicators. A breakdown of the most common causes of congenital deafness is presented in Table 8-5.

Parental Concern and Family History. According to the NIH Consensus Conference on Early Identification of Hearing Impairment (1993), as many as 70% of infants and children with hearing impair-

COLORADO NEWBORN HEARING SCREENING PROJECT

Report Date ___/___/___

CONFIRMED HEARING LOSS REPORT

for Colorado resident children under 3 years of age

Audiologist _____ Hospital/Clinic _____ Phone # _____

Child's name _____ Sex: M F Birth Date ___/___/___

Mother's name _____ Father's name _____ Physician _____

Home address _____

Birth hospital _____ Previous newborn hearing screening? Y N If yes, where? _____

PRE- and POSTNATAL CONDITIONS	YES	NO
A. Severe asphyxia which may include infants with Apgar scores of 0-3 or who fail to institute spontaneous respirations by ten (10) minutes and those with hypotonia persisting to two (2) hours Apgar Score 5 min. ____		
B. Bacterial meningitis, especially H. influenza		
C. Congenital or perinatal infections present: ☐ Toxoplasmosis ☐ Cytomegalovirus ☐ Syphilis ☐ Herpes Simplex virus ☐ Rubella		
D. Anatomical defects of the head and neck (e.g. Down Syndrome, ear tags, atresia)		
E. Hyperbilirubinemia (when level in excess of specified amount below) Birth Weight (grams) Bili level ≤ 1000 10.0 1001-1250 10.0 1251-1500 13.0 1501-2000 15.0 2001-2500 17.0 2500+ 18.0		
F. Family history of childhood hearing impairment		
G. Birth weight less than 1500 grams (3.3 pounds)		
H. Persistent Fetal Circulation / Persistent Pulmonary Hypertension; Prolonged mechanical ventilation for a duration equal to or greater than 10 days		
I. Stigmata or other findings associated with a syndrome known to include SNHL (e.g., Waardenburg, Ushers)		
J. Ototoxic medications including aminoglycosides used more than 5 days (e.g., gentamicin, tobramycin, kanamycin, streptomycin) and loop diuretics used in combination with aminoglycosides		
K. Other		
Admitted to Neonatal Intensive Care Unit		

HEARING TEST RESULTS
Test Date ___/___/___
Hearing Loss: Type: Ear: Use audiogram on back of form to report degree and slope of hearing loss:
☐ Unilateral   ☐ S/N   ☐ Right   Degree (letter) ____   Slope (number) ____   (right ear)
☐ Bilateral   ☐ Cond   ☐ Left   Degree (letter) ____   Slope (number) ____   (left ear)
☐ Mixed

Figure 8-4. Sample form used by the Colorado Newborn Hearing Screening Project for each confirmed infant with hearing loss. (Used with permission, Colorado Newborn Hearing Screening Project. (1999). Colorado Department of Public Health and Environment.).

ment are identified because of parental concern about their child's hearing. Therefore, it is important to educate parents about signs of hearing impairment and familiarize them with normal develop-ment are identified because of parental opmental milestones of speech and language. This education includes calling attention to the risk indicators known to be associated with congenital hearing loss as cited by the JCIH Year 2000 Position

Table 8.5.
Causes of Deafness

Prenatal (5–10%)

    Congenital infections (TORCH)
    Teratogen exposure (alcohol, cocaine,
      methylmercury, thalidomide)

Perinatal (5–15%)
    Prematurity and/or low birth weight
    Anoxia
    Hyperbilirubinemia
    Sepsis

Postnatal (10–20%)
    Infection (meningitis, mumps)
    Otitis media complication
    Ototoxic medication

Genetic: familial or sporadic (30–50%)
    Syndromic
    Nonsyndromic

Questionable and other (5%)
    High fever, infection, trauma, seizures

Unknown (20–30%)

Adapted from Marazita, M. L., Ploughman, L.M., Rawlings, B., et al. (1993). Genetic epidemiological studies of early-onset deafness in the US school-age population. *American Journal of Medical Genetics, 46,* 486.

Statement. A very informative first question that can be asked of the parents of any child presented for hearing evaluation is, "Do you have any concerns about your child's hearing, speech, or language?"

It is well known that congenital deafness may be inherited from other family members who were deaf or hearing-impaired in childhood. The various patterns of inheritance are described in Chapter 4. Obviously, an infant with a family history of permanent childhood sensorineural hearing loss in blood relatives is at risk for inheriting that same trait.

Not so simple, however, is the task of eliciting family history from the baby's parents. Unfortunately, family history information is typically sparse for generations earlier than the infant's grandparents. Often, only one parent is available for interview, so little information is available from the other side of the family. Information about relatives with dis-

abilities is often glossed over by relatives, so that considerable uncertainty exists about the true nature, degree, onset, or diagnosis of the condition. A parent once told the authors that no deafness existed in his family, although a cousin did attend the state deaf school. The parent was quick to add that the cousin was not "deaf"—he "wore a hearing aid and could hear normally." Another parent implicated his uncle, who "was not hearing-impaired—but totally deaf since birth."

Therefore, questions must be phrased carefully to avoid misunderstandings or erroneous responses. The authors ask, "Do you know any of the baby's relatives who now have a hearing loss, which started before the age of 5 years? Please think hard about all of your family and the baby's father's (or mother's) family." If the answer is "Yes," the parent is asked who the relative was (is) in relationship to the baby. The parent is then asked, "Do you know what caused the hearing loss? What makes you think the onset of the loss was before the age of 5? Did he or she still wear a hearing aid before age 5? Does the relative still wear a hearing aid? Did he or she attend a special school for the deaf or public school?" When the family history information is positive, the infant should be identified as at risk for hearing impairment. It is important to remember the potential progressive nature or possible late onset of hereditary hearing loss. Careful follow-up and thorough parental counseling is advised for those babies who have risk indicators but who pass the initial hearing screening test.

Asphyxia. Asphyxia is a common condition in infants who might require longer stays in the hospital or admissions of 48 hours or greater in the NICU. Asphyxia (hypoxia or anoxia) is a condition in which there is a lack of oxygen and an increase in carbon dioxide in the blood and tissues. Short spells without breathing (known as apneic attacks), however, are not uncommon during the neonatal period. With the introduction of intensive care treatment for very sick babies has come increased skill and technology in resuscitation and mechanical breathing Asphyxia may be the single most important factor causing general developmental sequelae.

The clinical definition of asphyxia varies somewhat among authors. Scheiner (1980) suggests the use of multiple measures in determining clinically significant asphyxia, including the length, degree, frequency, and severity of the episodes. The occurrence of asphyxia is commonly related to a number of other medical conditions, so it is difficult to establish asphyxia absolutely as the single cause of a specific case of deafness.

The Apgar method of evaluation has proven most practical as a guide to prognosis and the need for particularly close observation or care in the delivery room and nursery (Apgar, 1953; Apgar & James, 1962). One minute, 5 minutes, and 10 minutes after the complete birth of the infant, five standardized observations (heart rate, respiratory effort, reflex irritability, muscle tone, and color) are noted. A rating of 0–2 is assigned to each observation based on the scale shown in Table 8-6. A total score of 10 indicates an infant in the best possible condition. Low Apgar scores taken at 1 minute and 5 minutes are an index of asphyxia and an indicator of the need for assisted ventilation (American Academy of Pediatrics, 1986). The 5- and 10-minute scores are more accurate indices of the likelihood of neurologic involvement such as cerebral palsy (Vaughan, McKay, & Behrman, 1979). A preterm infant is more likely to experience anoxic episodes than a full-term infant. Infants with anoxia and low Apgar scores at 1 minute and 5 minutes after birth may have low arterial pH levels, coma, seizures, or the need for resuscitation with oxygen by mask or intubation (Hegyi et al., 1998).

Craniofacial Anomalies. There is a well-recognized association between craniofacial anomalies (CFAs) and hearing loss in children. Of 71 syndromes and birth anomalies associated with deafness described in "Smith's Recognizable Patterns of Human Malformation" (Jones, 1988), 58 or 82% identify CFA as a related feature. Anomalies associated with craniofacial and skeletal abnormality range from the very obvious to slight, subtle defects of the head, ears, mouth, and neck. Typical indications of a neonate with head and neck defects include babies with syndromal stigmata including abnormalities, malformed, low-set, or aberrant pinna configurations (microtia and/or atresia); preauricular or postauricular tags and pits; cleft lip and/or palate (including submucous cleft palate); first-arch and/or second-arch anomalies including mandibular and maxillary variants; and branchial cysts. Nevertheless, not all infants with such defects will have hearing impairment. The presence of such abnormalities, however, increases the risk of hearing problems in that particular child.

An informative study by Hayes (1994) of 145 infants with CFAs included evaluation by ABR to determine the presence of hearing loss. Although the presence,

Table 8.6.
Apgar Evaluation of the Newborn Infant

Sign	0	1	2
Heart rate	Absent	Less than 100 bpm	Greater than 100 bpm
Respiratory effort	Absent	Slow, irregular	Good, crying
Muscle tone	Limp	Some flexion of extremities	Active motion
Response to catheter in nostril	No response	Grimace	Cough or sneeze
Color	Blue, pale	Body pink, extremities blue	Completely pink

From Vaughan, V., McRay, R.J., Behrman, R. (1979). *Nelson textbook of pediatrics* (11th ed., p. 393). Philadelphia: WB Saunders.

type, and degree of hearing impairment varied by the type of CFA involvement, approximately 50% of infants demonstrated at least mild bilateral hearing loss. Less than 20% of infants with isolated external ear anomalies (ear tags, pits, isolated microtia) exhibited any degree of hearing loss. In 92% of infants with hearing loss, the results of ABR evaluation were consistent with conductive dysfunction.

In Utero Infections. Also known as congenital perinatal infection, this group of infections is known by the acronym TORCH. The TORCH infections are acquired by the embryo or fetus during gestation or by the newborn at delivery. In the acronym, *T* stands for toxoplasmosis, *R* for rubella virus, *C* for cytomegalovirus (CMV), *H* for herpes simplex virus (HSV), and *O* for other bacterial infections, especially syphilis, that result in hearing impairment (Nahmias, 1974). TORCH infections are often clinically inapparent, and when the infections are identified, their associated signs and symptoms are sometimes nearly indistinguishable. A subclinical infection can result in the same serious defects as one that is clinically apparent. Prognosis for the involved infant is usually grim. Nahmias estimates that up to 5% of all deliveries are infected by one of the TORCH agents, that each year in the United States a minimum of 400 infants die due to TORCH agents, and that an additional 2000 children are left with significant sequelae.

The lack of symptomatology in the pregnant woman makes the diagnosis of TORCH infections very difficult. Even when symptoms are manifest, the diagnosis cannot be confirmed without special laboratory tests. *Toxoplasma* infections and CMV rarely cause a clinically definable syndrome in the pregnant woman; the rash associated with rubella is not specific enough to differentiate it from other entities. In the case of herpes simplex infections, it is not the readily diagnosable cold sores or fever blisters that are of particular concern, but it is the less discernible genital infections that are often missed at the cervix, the primary site of involvement.

There is no clear-cut pattern in the sensorineural hearing loss attributed to TORCH complex infections. The hearing loss can be progressive and range from mild to profound, and cases of both bilateral and unilateral losses are well documented. Virus excretions may remain active for several years following birth, constituting a contributing factor in the degenerative process. In terms of infant follow-up, it is important to realize that any pattern and degree of hearing loss may occur with the TORCH complex. The screening technique of choice with these infants is auditory evoked potentials, since the chance of detecting a mild to moderate loss is possible. The potential for progressive hearing loss requires follow-up testing each 6 months for the first 2 years of life.

Toxoplasmosis. This is a parasitic infection transmitted by pregnant women to their unborn children. Most adults who are infected with the parasite have no symptoms. However, the infected child with congenital toxoplasmosis typically has chorioretinitis (inflammation of the choroid and retina of the eye), cerebral calcification, psychomotor retardation, hydrocephalus or microcephaly, and convulsions. Although reports of hearing disorders related to toxoplasmosis are in fact sparse, the congenital infection is so serious that there is no doubt that it may cause hearing loss. Active congenital infection may be fatal in days or weeks or become inactive with residuals of medical problems in varying degrees and combinations. The full impact of the infection may not become evident until some weeks or months after its apparent cessation. Apparently, the later in pregnancy the infection occurs, the less severe the clinical symptoms. *Toxoplasma* may be responsible for premature birth, cerebral palsy, blindness, and mental retardation (Vaughan et al., 1979). Some afflicted newborns appear normal but develop blindness, epilepsy, or mental retardation in later years.

Pregnant women acquire toxoplasmosis as an active disease at a rate of 2–7 per 1000, and 30–40% of these women have infected infants, making toxoplasmosis one of the most common causes of birth defects in the United States (Babson, 1980). Humans are typically contaminated in one of three ways: by eating raw or insufficiently cooked food; by having direct contact with cat feces, because the house cat is a carrier; by eating fruits and vegetables soiled by animal carriers (Robillard & Gersdorff, 1986).

Syphilis. Technically speaking, syphilis is a bacterial infection that produces similar manifestations as the viral infections of the TORCH complex, but it can be diagnosed with routine laboratory tests—so it is not usually considered part of the TORCH family. However, it is included here so that this infection is not overlooked as an indicator for deafness. Although the incidence of syphilis steadily declined through the 1970s, syphilis is apparently now on the increase (Hayes & Northern, 1996). Syphilis is a sexually transmitted disease that is passed from an infected mother to her fetus. In early, untreated syphilis, transmission to the fetus occurs in 80–90% of cases. Approximately 30% of infected fetuses die in utero, 30% die postnatally, and 40% of survivors develop late symptomatic syphilis. Congenital syphilis may demonstrate a multitude of central nervous system abnormalities including vestibular dysfunction, sensorineural hearing loss, and cardiac complications. Possible accompanying developmental delay depends on the severity of global neurologic damage.

Auditory impairment may not be present at birth. Onset of progressive sensorineural hearing loss is generally noted in early childhood. The symptoms of hearing loss may present as a sudden onset of bilaterally symmetrical severe to profound impairment. Poor hearing function and limited use of hearing aids can be expected as a result of neural atrophy. The general treatment of congenital syphilis consists of prompt and aggressive treatment with penicillin.

Rubella. Rubella, also called German measles, is a viral infection transmitted by airborne respiration that results in a mild flu-like illness, which may be accompanied by a light, red rash. Rubella may range from mild, subclinical infection to severe disease. Congenital rubella is transmitted in utero from a pregnant female with the viral infection. A widespread congenital rubella epidemic in the United States during the 1960s left an estimated 20,000 children with handicaps and disabilities. Deafness is one of the most common manifestations of congenital rubella, with an incidence of 50%. Cooper (1969) identified other problems associated with what is known as the congenital rubella syndrome (CRS) which includes heart disease (50%), cataract or glaucoma (40%), and psychomotor/developmental delay (40%). The adult survivors of the 1960s congenital rubella epidemic developed a number of late-onset medical disorders including diabetes, glaucoma, endocrine pathology, and central nervous system infections (Vernon & Hicks, 1980). With public awareness of the 1960s rubella epidemic, immunization programs developed and the number of congenital rubella cases decreased quickly to zero incidence in the United States. As cases of any endemic disease decrease, however, so does public concern, resulting in a reduced number of immunizations (Vernon & Klein, 1982). In countries without a universal immunization program, rubella remains a major cause of congenital deafness.

The gestational age of the embryo or fetus at the time of the maternal infection is the critical factor in determining outcome. Live rubella virus, however, may persist for extended periods in the newborn infant and serve as a source for spreading the infection to susceptible pregnant women (Vaughan et al., 1979). Infants of a mother with known or suspected rubella should be followed carefully throughout childhood, because asymptomatic infants may subsequently develop defects later in life. Stuckless (1980) published an excellent monograph on the status of deafness and rubella. It is often difficult to verify rubella exposure during pregnancy in the postpartum mother, who may actually have had such mild, subclinical infection that it remained unrecognized. Children with a suspected history of rubella or rubella exposure should be followed with hearing tests until 18–24 months of age, keeping in mind the potential late-onset and progressive nature of rubella hearing loss.

CMV. Congenital CMV infection is related to the herpes family of viruses and is the most common of the TORCH complex infections, as discussed in Chapter 4. If 1% of all babies born in the United States are infected, then as many as 40,000 infants with congenital CMV infection are born in this country each year. Of this number, it can be estimated that 4000–6000 children born each year with sensorineural hearing impairments actually have asymptomatic congenital CMV infections as the cause of the hearing loss (Peckham, Stark, Dudgeon, et al., 1987).

CMV is not highly contagious. In symptomatic infants, CMV is a systemic illness characterized by enlargement of the liver and spleen, jaundice, rash, chorioretinitis, cerebral calcifications, and microcephaly. However, 10% of the infected neonates are symptomatic at birth; their neurodevelopmental outcome is well documented and includes developmental delay, visual impairment, and a significant risk for progressive sensorineural hearing loss, either of congenital or later onset. According to Dahle et al. (2000), in a longitudi-

nal study of 860 children with documented CMV infection, 40% of symptomatic children and 7.5% of asymptomatic children developed delayed onset and/or progressive and fluctuant sensorineural hearing loss. Children with sensorineural hearing loss often have no identified cause of their loss; thus, according to Williamson et al. (1992), it is likely that many of these children had asymptomatic congenital CMV infection. Early identification of hearing loss in infants with CMV is hampered by the fact that for many children, the infection leads to latent damage to inner ear structures that may not appear for months or years after birth (Dahle et al., 2000). The progressive nature of the hearing loss requires periodic audiologic assessments, regardless of the severity of the initial loss, to monitor hearing status for further deterioration.

HSV. HSV is one of the most common sexually transmitted diseases. Two types of HSV infect humans. HSV-I is acquired during childhood and isolated from the mouth, nose, and oropharynx (cold sores). HSV-II is usually acquired in adolescence or adulthood as a sexually transmitted disease and is isolated from the genitalia mucosa (genital herpes).

The transmission of HSV to the fetus is possible during birth if the mother is actively infected. HSV may cause severe generalized disease in the neonate, with high mortality rates and devastating sequelae. HSV infections in the newborn are rarely subclinical or asymptomatic. The majority of cases are acquired during passage through the birth canal. A cesarean section delivery is indicated for mothers with a known genital infection at the time of delivery. When HSV infection does occur in the neonate, more than 50% are fatal. According to Nahmias and Norrild (1979), only 4% of neonatally infected HSV infants survive without sequelae. Infants with herpes infection may demonstrate symptoms ranging from localized skin lesions to severe generalized infection involving major organ systems. Neurologic and sensory system complications are common including sensorineural hearing loss.

Bacterial Meningitis. Bacterial meningitis is an acute infectious disease of the central nervous system caused by a variety of microorganisms. Unless promptly and effectively treated, bacterial meningitis can result in death or irreversible brain damage (see Chapter 4). Sensorineural hearing loss is one of the most common complications of bacterial meningitis, and by some estimates occurs in up to 30–40% of surviving infants and children (Dodge, Davis, & Feigin, et al., 1984). By far, the most frequently occurring causative microorganism is *Haemophilus influenzae* type b, or Hib disease. Bacteria may spread from infant to infant via nursery personnel or contaminated equipment. With the advent of antibiotics, treatment of meningitis is usually successful. However, as recently as the 1980s, bacterial

meningitis is believed to have occurred in approximately 20,000 U.S. children annually (Stein & Boyer, 1994). The clinical manifestations of neonatal meningitis are often subtle and deceptive, so that verification by appropriate laboratory studies provides the only means of diagnosis in newborns (Feigin & Dodge, 1976). The degree of hearing loss associated with meningitis usually ranges from severe to profound, but mild to moderate hearing loss is also seen.

A dramatic reduction in the incidence of bacterial meningitis began in 1985 through the use of *Haemophilus* type b conjugate vaccines in infants. The rate for meningitis began to decline for infants after the introduction of Hib vaccines for progressively younger age groups. Figure 8-5 shows the decrease in the incidence of Hib meningitis in infants younger than 1 year of age from 55/100,000 persons in 1988 to 30/100,000 in 1990, and to 12/100,000 in 1991. The success of a national immuniza-

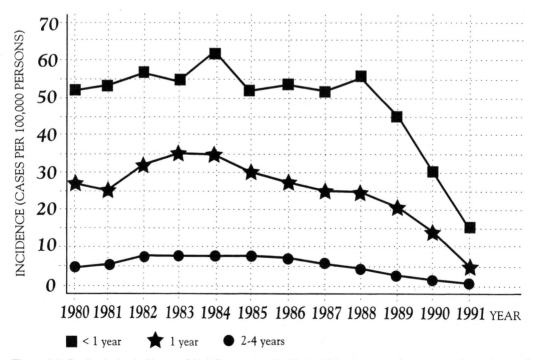

Figure 8-5. Decline in the incidence of *H. influenzae* meningitis in children younger than 1 year of age, 1 year of age, and 2–4 years of age. (From Stein, L.& Boyer, K. (1994). Progress in the prevention of hearing loss in infants. *Ear and Hearing, 15* (2), 120.)

tion program in infants may lead to complete eradication of sensorineural hearing loss in infants and toddlers attributable to *H. influenzae* type b bacterial meningitis. Further, improved antimicrobial therapy may result in reductions in hearing loss as a sequelae of bacterial meningitis attributable to pathogens other than Hib (Stein & Boyer, 1994). Of course, in developing countries, where immunization and clinical treatment programs are not readily accessible, meningitis is still a leading cause of sensorineural hearing loss in infants and young children.

Elevated Bilirubin. Hyperbilirubinemia (jaundice) occurs when there is an excess amount of bilirubin in the blood, a condition that is found in nearly 60% of normal, full-term babies born in the United States. Newborns often have some degree of jaundice following birth because their immature liver function does not adequately handle the normal breakdown of red blood cells. However, the great majority of these newborns with clinical jaundice do not require treatment because their bodies naturally expel the excess bilirubin during the first few days after birth. Because it takes more than 24 hours for bilirubin levels to rise high enough to cause severe jaundice, some newborns may be discharged from the hospital before the condition develops.

Rh or ABO blood type incompatibility between mother and child may be associated with hyperbilirubinemia, although other physiologic problems may also be responsible. Those infants with a bilirubin level that exceeds indications requiring a blood exchange transfusion are at risk for sensorineural hearing impairment. The serum bilirubin level needed for exchange transfusion is a function of the infant's birthweight.

There are two types of bilirubin, conjugated and unconjugated, which are sometimes referred to as direct and indirect bilirubin, respectively. As red blood cells break down, unconjugated bilirubin is routinely released into the plasma serum. This is observed during the healing of a bruise when the surface area under the skin becomes yellow (or jaundiced) due to the presence of unconjugated bilirubin. The unconjugated bilirubin is bound to plasma albumin and transported to the liver, where an enzyme conjugates it. That is, the potentially toxic unconjugated bilirubin is joined together with a substance in the body to form a detoxified product. The now conjugated bilirubin is normally excreted from the body through the small intestine. When bilirubin cannot be conjugated, it builds up in the serum until it crosses the plasma membrane and is deposited in the brain. *Kernicterus* is a neurologic syndrome resulting from the deposition of unconjugated bilirubin in brain cells, causing motor and sensory deficits, developmental delay, or death.

The level of bilirubin is not the only deciding factor in determining the need for an exchange transfusion. Consideration is given to several other factors including perinatal asphyxia respiratory distress, metabolic acidosis, hypothermia, low serum protein levels, low birthweight, and signs of clinical central nervous system degeneration (Levine, 1979). Although Rh incompatibility was once a major cause of deafness, increased skill in transfusion technology should reduce this factor as a cause of childhood deafness.

Low Birthweight. In the past few years, with the aid of sophisticated medical equipment, premature babies so small that they fit into an adult's hand now have a strong chance for survival. However, low-birthweight infants are more likely to have congenital defects, neurologic disorders such as cerebral palsy and seizures, gastrointestinal disorders, and respiratory problems. In the past, low-birthweight infants were often stillborn or died during delivery or soon after. Low birthweight is still the major factor associated with infant death. Compared with normal-weight infants, low-birthweight infants are almost 40 times more likely to die during their first 28 days of life, and very-low-birthweight infants are more than 200 times as likely to die during this period. Black women are more than twice as likely as white women to have a low-birthweight infant. Some babies survive at a cost of significant disabilities. The current lowest limit of viability is 24 weeks (out of full-term or 40 weeks) gestation, with a minimum weight of 500 g (just over 1 lb). Infants this small have a 5–20% chance of survival. Breathing must be accomplished with a ventilator, because the babies' lungs are not capable of breathing without mechanical aid. Improvement in technology has resulted in an increased survival rate of premature, high-risk infants. "Preemies" (technically any baby born more than 3 weeks early) have about a 70% chance of survival if they weigh less than 2 lb; 90% of preemies weighing between 2 and 3 pounds survive. A study conducted by Kenworthy, Bess, Stahlman, & Lindstrom (1987) with a sample of 266 high-risk infants with extreme immaturity revealed that approximately one-third of the population exhibited hearing impairment or speech/language problems.

Infants delivered before 37 weeks are considered to have a shortened gestation period and are *premature* or *preterm*. Historically, prematurity was defined by low birthweight. In essence, however, prematurity and low birthweight are usually concomitant, particularly among infants weighing 1500 g or less at birth (about 3 lb), and both factors are associated with increased neonatal morbidity and mortality rates. It is difficult to separate completely the factors associated with prematurity from those associated with low birthweight (Vaughan et al., 1979).

Other Risk Factors. Other neonatal hearing risk factors identified by the Year 2000 Joint Committee on Infant Hearing include syndromes associated with progressive hearing loss, neurodegenerative disorders, persistent pulmonary hypertension, conditions requiring the use of extracorporeal membrane oxygenation (ECMO), head trauma, and recurrent or persistent otitis media. Additional factors that have been suggested but lack sufficient scientific data at this time include severe neonatal sepsis, parental consanguinity, and fetal alcohol syndrome. These disorders and conditions are described in other chapters and in the appendix of this textbook.

SCREENING FOR HEARING IMPAIRMENT

Birth Through 6 Months. The JCIH Year 2000 Position Statement recommends that all infants have access to hearing screening using a physiologic measure (e.g., ABR or transient or distortion product evoked otoacoustic emission screening). The ABR is a physiologic measure of peripheral auditory function through the brainstem, and the otoacoustic emission screenings are physiologic measures of preneural auditory function. Both of these physiologic techniques are easily accomplished in neonates and correlate highly with the degree of peripheral hearing sensitivity.

A variety of hospital-based hearing screening protocols using ABR and EOAE have been successfully implemented (Arehart et al., 1998; Mason & Hermann, 1998; Vohr et al., 1998; Finitzo et al., 1998; Mehl & Thomson, 1998). For infants born in hospitals, hearing screening should be completed as close to hospital discharge as possible. Most infants pass the initial screening test or a rescreening immediately before discharge. The JCIH recommends screening technologies that incorporate automated response detection rather than those procedures that require operator interpretation and decision-making. Automated algorithms eliminate the need for individual test interpretation, reduce the effects of screener bias and errors on test outcome, and ensure test consistency across all infants. Many inpatient screening protocols provide one or more repeat screenings using the same physiologic test or a different physiologic test. Each protocol must incorporate a system for the rescreening of infants who do not pass the birth admission screening within 1 month of hospital discharge. The mechanism of rescreening is important because it minimizes the number of false-positive referrals for follow-up audiologic and medical evaluation.

Some hospital programs use automated ABR while other programs use OAE screening protocols for the admission screen. Many inpatient screening protocols use "the other" physiologic test as the rescreen procedure for all newborns who do not pass the initial screening (ASHA, 1997). The choice of screening measure depends on many factors and will certainly influence program outcomes (i.e., failure of the admission screen, referral percentages, and rescreening requirements).

The total infant hearing screening program is described as a three-part effort: (1) parent/caregiver education to ensure that they understand the relationship between hearing, speech, and language development and that they receive information to enhance their ability to observe and monitor normal development milestones; (2) the ABR or EOAE hearing screening; and (3) the follow-up evaluation and management plan to ensure that the identified hearing-impaired infant receives immediate habitation action.

ABR Infant Hearing Screening. Traditional ABR screening continues to be a practical option in many hospitals. The ABR is well established as having high sensitivity and specificity rates in the identification of hearing impairment and is generally impervious to ambient noise and sedative medications (Mason & Herrmann, 1998). Traditional ABR screening typically depends on identification of wave V at 30–40 dB nHL. The acoustic stimulus for ABR screening should include the frequency band important for speech recognition and may consist of

clicks, tone pips, or tone bursts. The pass criterion for ABR infant screening is a repeatable response from both ears at intensity levels of 35 dB nHL (normal hearing level) or lower. Alternating polarity may be appropriate in screening applications when presence or absence of wave V is the only criteria used to determine a pass/refer outcome. Wave V is enhanced in the neonate when a high-pass filter of 30 Hz is used and if an electrode montage of ground-to-the-nape-of-the-neck rather than to the traditional ipsilateral ear configuration is used. The main drawbacks to traditional ABR screening are the expense of the equipment and labor, set-up and testing time required (25–60 minutes per newborn), and necessity for a trained professional to administer the test. Failure rates generally range from 2–8% in the newborn nursery (McNellis & Klein, 1997).

Automated ABR systems have been developed and used specifically for the mass hearing screening of infants since the mid-1980s (Fig. 8-6). The automated ABR system works by comparing the online responses from the infant with a "normal" template response pattern obtained from a large sample population of newborns. If the test infant's responses falls within the normative values, the automated instrument renders a "pass" decision; if the response pattern falls outside the acceptable response template, a "refer" response is obtained suggesting the need for additional testing. Automated ABR systems do not rely on an individual to make subjective judgments regarding the presence or absence of a response. The systems are entirely objective and programmed to determine pass or refer criteria for infants younger than 6 months of age. The protocols and set-up procedures include programmable screening testing techniques for screening one or both ears simultaneously, disposable electrodes, and automatic artifact rejection systems to control for both environmental ambient noise and physiologic noise from the infant. For automated ABR, the number of repetitions is

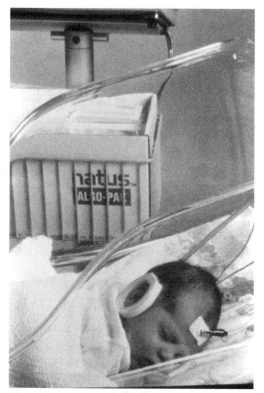

Figure 8-6. Automated ABR system used in newborn infant hearing screening.

determined automatically by manufacturer protocol. A minimum of 1000 stimulus repetitions is required under optimal recording conditions to yield reliable screening results. In less than optimum conditions (e.g., excessive noise or physiologic artifact), more stimulus presentations may be required. The infant passes the screening if reliable responses are present at the screening level of 35 dB nHL or lower. Automated ABR screening is especially efficient and practical because a trained nonprofessional can manage the simple operation. A drawback to the automated system is the expense of replacing disposable supplies. The typical screening time required to evaluate both ears in a newborn is 10–20 minutes.

It is important for parents, caregivers, and those who provide primary health care to understand that "pass" on ABR screening does not rule out development

of hearing impairment in infancy or early childhood. Infants who pass the ABR screen should receive audiologic follow-up as necessary for medical evaluation and management and/or developmental evaluation. Infants who pass the ABR screen and are at risk for progressive hearing impairment should receive audiologic monitoring on a periodic basis throughout the preschool years.

It might be questioned if continued dependence on the ABR procedure constitutes adequate follow-up for a child. According to Stein, Ozdamar, Kraus, et al. (1983a), otologic, audiologic, and neurologic examinations as well as postdischarge ABR are mandatory before any inferences can be made about hearing loss or neurodevelopmental disorders. A behavioral audiometric evaluation is ultimately necessary to obtain accurate frequency-specific information and to determine the existence or extent of a conductive hearing loss.

Evoked Otoacoustic Emissions. Evoked otoacoustic emissions (EOAEs) are extremely useful in infant hearing screening. EOAEs are low-level reflections of acoustic energy present in infants with normal hearing and absent in those with hearing loss. Two types of EOAEs are used in infant screening programs, the transient evoked otoacoustic emissions (TEOAEs) and the distortion product evoked otoacoustic emissions (DPEOAEs), as described in Chapter 7. Both types of emissions are detected in the ear canal with a hand-held probe device and are quite robust and easily measured in infants (Fig. 8-7). TEOAEs are present in the normal-hearing ear canal following presentation of brief repeated click stimuli and are easy to detect, record, and interpret. The measurement of DPEOAEs requires more sophisticated equipment with two stimulus channels. DPEOAEs are the by-product of nonlinear distortion of the basilar membrane produced by the presentation of two simultaneous pure tones. The suggested stimulus conditions

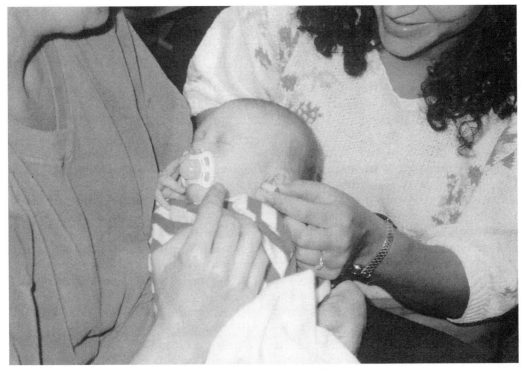

Figure 8-7. Otoacoustic emissions hearing screening with newborn infant.

for TEOAEs are broad-band clicks presented at 80 dB SPL. For DPEOAEs, the suggested stimulus conditions are $f_2/f_1 = 1.2$, with f_2 at 2000, 3000, and 4000 Hz; f_1 at 65 dB SPL; and F_2 at 55 dB SPL (ASHA, 1997).

The pass/refer criteria for evoked emissions have yet to be standardized among various infant hearing screening programs. Guidelines for the pass/refer criteria for TEOAE use a 50% or higher reproducibility score from 1000 to 4000 Hz (White et al., 1994). Salamy et al. (1996) suggest a reproducibility of 80% or higher in at least three of five frequency bands. Vohr et al. (1998) used a 75% reproducibility score between 2000 and 4000 Hz. Most researchers agree that the mid-frequency range is crucial to the pass/refer criteria, but differences exist on the waveform reproducibility measure.

DPEOAE pass/refer criteria used in infant hearing screening programs are also under investigation. Excessive ambient and physiologic noise contaminate the recording of the DPEOAE for frequencies below 2000 Hz and above 4000 Hz. This leads to concern regarding the necessary dB level the response must reach above the noise floor in order to be considered a valid measure. Salata et al. (1998) assessed a sample of newborn recordings using response levels of 5, 10, and 15 dB SPL above the noise floor and observed that screening specificity dropped from 94% to 68% to 38%, respectively. Smurzynski et al. (1993) and Smurzynski (1994) recorded DPEOAEs from preterm infants as young as 33 weeks gestation as well as term newborns and noted relatively high intersubject and intrasubject variability from preterm neonates. Most screening programs require that the response level must be at least 3 dB or greater above the noise level to be considered an acceptable DPEOAE in screening newborns. Newborns and infants who do not show a reliable OAE response from either ear following rescreening procedures should be referred for additional evaluation.

A number of researchers have administered both automated ABR and either or both types of EOAEs on large samples of well babies and infants from ICUs (Chen et al., 1996; McNellis & Klein, 1997; Doyle, Fuikawa, Rogers, & Newman, 1998; Gabbard, Northern, & Yoshinaga-Itano, 1999). The studies confirm the value of otoacoustic emissions screening in infants related to cost, time efficiency, and accuracy in identifying infants with hearing loss (Maxon, White, Behrens, & Vohr, 1995). The infants are easier to test while in deep sleep or a dozing state, and the most common problem encountered is obstruction of the tiny ear canals with vernix caseosa, which can be cleaned out before OAE testing. If the OAE response is not seen, the probe tip should be carefully inspected before it is reinserted. In addition, visual inspection with an otoscope should be standard practice before conducting OAE measurements in newborns. Gabbard et al. (1999) evaluated 110 infants (mean age, 15 hours) from the well-baby nursery with both automated ABR and TEOAE measures to determine pass/refer rates and recorded the time required for each of the measures. Significant difference was found for TEOAE measures in infants less than 10 hours of age from those infants between 11 and 24 hours of age and from those newborns older than 24 hours. Younger infants were less likely to pass the TEOAE screen, although age was not a factor with the automated ABR technique. A significantly greater pass rate of 97% was found for automated ABR birth admission screening compared with a 60% pass rate for TEOAE measures for these young infants. The average test time for both techniques was remarkably similar, at approximately 12 minutes from start to completion.

Infants and Toddlers: 7 Months Through 2 Years. This age group is particularly difficult to screen. Screening procedures to detect hearing impairment that exceeds 20–30 dB HL are available and applicable to this age group (ASHA, 1997). Developmental delays or extreme prematurity may limit applications of screening methods that rely on behavioral responses. For those children unable to participate in behavioral procedures, screening with EOAE is recommended.

Screening stimuli that lack frequency-specificity or behavioral observation techniques based on noncalibrated signals (such as rattles, music boxes, and noise-makers) are not recommended. Children who can be conditioned for visual reinforcement audiometry (VRA) can be screened by using conventional earphones or insert receivers with test frequencies at 1000, 2000, and 4000 Hz. The screening intensity level should be 30 dB HL. The ASHA Guidelines for Audiologic Screening (1997) include the use of conditioned play audiometry for those children sufficiently mature to perform the task reliably. The screening intensity level for conditioned play audiometry is 20 dB HL at 1000, 2000, and 4000 Hz. Any child who does not show reliable responses at the criterion screening level at each frequency in each ear should be referred for additional evaluation.

EOAEs are suggested as an alternative technique when behavioral methods are ineffective with this age group. The audiologist should be aware that conductive hearing loss obscures the EOAE response and requires referral for additional evaluation.

Weber (1987) described a portable VRA system that has been used extensively in a statewide program to screen infants, toddlers, and preschoolers in rural Colorado who are risk for hearing loss. The statistics from the community-wide screenings between 1977 and 1986 demonstrate the effectiveness of the VRA technique. Of the nearly 25,000 children tested during the 9-year period of the report, nearly half were younger than 2 years of age. Sixteen percent of all children screened were referred for medical consultation, and 30 children were found to have significant sensori-neural hearing loss.

Screening for Communicative Disorders. Screening for speech and language delay in children younger than 3 years of age may prove useful in identifying children who have fallen behind in normal communication development. The close relationship of auditory development in the young child with evolving speech and language skills makes it possible for screening procedures to identify those children who are significantly delayed in developmental milestones and to refer them for more complete evaluations. Because sufficient language milestones should be accessible before 36 months of age, language screening tests are useful for children at an early age. Significant delay in language development may be a sign of hearing loss.

Physicians who treat children are in a key position to identify language and hearing delay at the earliest possible age. Screening tests are customarily used when pediatricians already suspect a problem. Thus, the screening test is not being used for its intended purpose of separating from the larger population those children who are at increased risk for the disorder. Instead, the screen is being used as a post hoc confirmation of a problem. The test most frequently used for screening young children in pediatric offices is the Denver Developmental Screening Test (DDST) (Frankenburg & Dodds, 1967). A recent study compared results of performances on the language sector of the DDST with results of speech and language evaluations. With the DDST, 47% of children with delayed expressive language were not identified, thereby rendering it a questionable screen for language disorders (Borowitz & Glascoe, 1986).

The authors recommend the use of the Early Language Milestone (ELM) scale, which is a well-normed language screening instrument designed to be a rapid means of evaluating language develop-ment of children younger than 3 years of age. The test addresses both receptive and expressive language through parent report and direct testing of the child. The administration time of the ELM is 1–4 minutes. Each child's ELM profile is scored as "pass" or "fail." Walker, Downs, Gugenheim, & Northern (1989) administered the ELM in physicians' offices to more than 800 children younger than 36 months of age and found an overall failure rate of 8%. Children who failed an initial ELM screening, as well as a randomly selected sample of children who passed the ELM screening, were subsequently evaluated with a more sophisticated language test, the Sequenced Inventory of Communication Development (SICD). Based on an analysis of this evaluation procedure, it was determined that the best age range for ELM administration is between 24 and 30 months of age. Because the ELM is quickly and easily administered and because of improvement in the accuracy of parental report during a second ELM screen, it is recommended that children who fail the ELM at their appropriate age level should be rescreened with the ELM within 1–2 weeks. If the ELM rescreen is also failed, referral to a speech/language pathologist is recommended. All children with language delay should also be referred for a hearing test to rule out the possibility of hearing impairment as a cause of language problems.

Other communication screening instruments recommended for this age group by ASHA (1997) include the Communication Screen (Striffler & Willis, 1981), the Compton Speech and Language Screening Evaluation (Compton, 1978), the Physician's Developmental Quick Screen for Speech Disorders (Kulig & Bakler, 1973), the Texas Preschool Screening Inventory (Haber & Norris, 1983), the Fluharty Preschool Speech and Language Screening Test (Fluharty, 1974), the Clinical Linguistic and Auditory Milestone Scale of Infancy (CLAMS) (Capute, Shapiro, Wachtel, Gunther, &

Palmer, 1986), and the Pre-school SIFTER (Anderson & Matkin, 1996). Additional screening procedures designed for children with hearing disorders are presented by Johnson, Benson, and Seaton (1997). A thorough review of the available preschool speech and language screening tests was published by Sturner, Layton, Evans, Funk, & Machon (1994).

Preschool Children: 3–5 Years Old. Identifying hearing loss in children 3–5 years of age can be a real problem. These children are usually seen at well-baby clinics or doctors' offices. Although Head Start programs include many children who would be available for health-care screening, there are large numbers who are not seen for health visits unless special efforts are made to reach them. Nursery schools, play schools, and child care centers are prime locations for hearing screening programs.

At this age, the health care professional looks primarily for medically remediable hearing losses, on the assumption that the more severe hearing losses have been identified. The chief pathology that is being sought is otitis media; the disease can result at this age in subtle auditory disorders or middle ear disease. The tests that are adequate to identify these disorders are hearing screening, acoustic immittance testing, EOAEs, audiometry, and otoscopic examination.

Numerous efforts have been made to develop effective screening methods for the preschool child. The problems arise from the definition of screening as "rapid, simple measurements applied to large numbers of children." Any test that requires a voluntary response from 3- to 5-year-olds will be neither rapid nor simple. The preschooler can be negativistic, apprehensive, or "eager beavers"—all attitudes that hardly make for easy testing.

The task is to condition the child to the desired motor response at suprathreshold levels before initiation of the screening procedure. Conditioned play audiometry

is a form of operant conditioning in which the child is taught to wait and listen for a stimulus and then to perform a motor task in response to the presentation of the stimulus. Typically, the motor task itself serves as reinforcement. An example of a conditioned pure tone preschool screening test is described below:

1. Have available a pegboard, a ring tower, plain blocks, or other simple toys that are motivating to young children.
2. Take a block (or peg) and hold it up to one ear as if listening. Make believe you hear a sound, say "I hear it," and put the block on the table.
3. Place the earphones or insert receivers on the child's ear and hold his or her hand with the block up to the child's ear.
4. Present a 50 dB HL tone at 1000 Hz and guide the child's hand to build the block tower. Repeat once or twice and then see if he or she can do it alone. If he or she can, go on; if not, additional conditioning trials will be necessary.
5. Decrease the hearing level to 20 dB HL and repeat the test. If the child responds, repeat the procedure at 20 dB HL at 2000 and 4000 Hz. Praise the child for each correct response. After each successful tone presentation, place another block in the child's hand.
6. Switch to the opposite ear and repeat the test starting at 1000 Hz, then 2000 Hz, and then 4000 Hz.
7. The criterion for referral is when a child does not respond at 20 dB HL at least 2 of 3 times at any test frequency in either ear or if the child cannot be conditioned to the task. Those children between 3 and 5 years of age who cannot be conditioned for play audiometry should be screened by VRA.

School-Age Children: 5 Through 18 Years. The integration of hearing screening programs in schools was initiated during the 1920s but did not become a routine part of programs until the 1960s. The primary goal of the school-based hearing screening program is to keep the child functioning adequately in the class-room from kindergarten through 12th grade. In the majority of school situations, it is impossible to screen at levels less than 20 dB HL because of the presence of ambient noise. The use of otoacoustic emissions in school-aged children may be useful, although data supporting its use in this population are limited.

School hearing screening has a long and honorable history. As early as 1924, a group of dedicated otolaryngologists used a new instrument for testing the hearing of school children (McFarlan, 1927). The instrument was developed for the Western Electric Company. The Western Electric 4-A audiometer was a phonograph, connected to an assembly of 30 earphones, which would simultaneously present well-calibrated speech signals to the earphones. In the Western Electric Fading Numbers test, both a male and a female voice spoke various numbers, starting at a hearing level of 33 dB and ending at 9 dB. The reason for the change to pure tone testing was that the speech signals used in the Western Electric test did not identify children with high-frequency losses.

Although audiologists play a key role in hearing screening programs, it is generally not cost-effective for audiologists to be involved in the actual administration of the screening tests. The audiologist is responsible for the oversight of the school-based screening program and likely plans the protocol for administration of the screening tests, performs the training and supervises the technicians or volunteer screeners, and plans the implementation of follow-up procedures and protocols. Johnson, Bensen, and Seaton have presented a thorough description of hearing screening practices in their comprehensive "Educational Audiology Handbook" (1997).

Identification audiometry is only one part of a hearing conservation program. A well-planned program must go beyond initial hearing screening with consideration of rescreening, threshold audiometry, referral for audiologic and medical evaluations, education and counseling for parents and teachers, and commitment to follow-up procedures to ensure that adequate steps have been taken to alleviate or manage the hearing problem identified in each screening failure. Obviously, without concurrent follow-up programs, identification of hearing loss in children is a meaningless effort.

Recommended Hearing Screening Guidelines. The ASHA Guidelines for Audiology Screening (1997) call for hearing screening on initial entry into school, annually in kindergarten through 3rd grade, in 7th and 11th grades, and as needed, requested, or mandated by regulation. The pure tone screening procedure should be part of a program that includes an educational component designed to provide parents with information on the process of hearing screening. ASHA also recommends obtaining informed consent before the screening procedure when appropriate. Individualized, manual, pure tone screening under earphones at 20 dB HL (re: ANSI S3.6-1996) should be conducted for each ear of every child at test frequencies of 1000, 2000, and 4000 Hz. The American Academy of Audiology (1997) recommendations for school hearing screening include the addition of 500 Hz, provided the ambient noise level does not exceed acceptable levels. Frequencies of 3000 and 6000 Hz should not be included in the pure tone hearing screening protocol (Table 8-7). Penn (1999) surveyed each of the U.S. states to determine the status of their school-based hearing screening programs (Fig. 8-8).

The pass/fail criterion is the ability or failure of the child to respond to the recommended screening levels at any test frequency in either ear. All children who fail the screen should be reinstructed and rescreened during the same session in which

Table 8.7.
Recommended Guidelines for Pure Tone Hearing Screening

Test Frequencies	Intensity Level	Pass-Fail Criteria
1000–2000–4000 Hz (with acoustic immittance)	20 dB HL	Failure to respond at any test presentation in either ear
500–1000–2000–4000 Hz (without acoustic immittance)	20 dB HL and 25 dB HL at 9000 Hz	Same as above

Some parents will become overly concerned, others will show little or no concern, and still others would like to cooperate but fear the potential expense that might be involved. If parents believe that their child can "hear," despite the results of the hearing screening, special tact and persuasion will be required to convince them that a problem truly exists. The administrative and reporting aspect of the

they failed or within a 2-week period of the initial screen. Failures on rescreening should be referred for audiologic evaluation by an audiologist, with additional referrals as appropriate. Follow-up audiologic evaluation should be conducted within 1 month of the screening failure and no later than 3 months after initial screening. It is a good idea to avoid the word "fail" in reporting screening results to parents because of the negative connotation of the word. It must be remembered that many causes exist for "failing" hearing screening tests, and confirmation of the presence of hearing loss cannot be assumed until an audiometric evaluation is completed. Table 8-8 suggests a number of considerations that must be taken into account during any school hearing and middle ear screening program.

The paperwork associated with a hearing screening program can be massive, although computerized database systems certainly can help track the program in a more efficient manner. Test forms, calibration data, and student records must be carefully considered before the testing sessions. The language used in notices sent to parents and referral physicians about screening or rescreening results should avoid diagnostic conclusions and alarming predictions. Hearing impairment is not confirmed until the stage of the audiometric evaluation has been completed. It is more effective to speak directly with the parents about test results, if possible, rather than written notice.

State	With Mandates	Some Statewide Coordination	No Statewide Coordination	Authoritative Agency	Guidelines Available
AL			•	Education	
AK		•		Health	•
AR		•		Health	•
AZ	•			Health	•
CA	•			Health	•
CO	•			Education	•
CT	•			Education	•
DE			•	Program discontinued	
DC	•			Public Bur. of Benefit Coop	•
FL	•			Health	•
GA	•			Health	•
HI			•	Program discontinued	
ID			•	Local School District	
IL	•			Health	•
IN	•			Sp.-Lang.-Hearing Assn	•
IA	•			Education	•
KS	•			Education	•
KY	•			Health	•
LA	•			Health	•
ME	•			Education	•
MD	•			Health/Education	•
MA	•			Health	•
MI	•			Health	•
MN	•			Health	•
MS			•	Local School District	
MO		•		Education	•
MT	•			Local School District	•
NE	•			Health/Education	•
NV	•			Health	•
NH		•		Education	•
NJ	•			Education	•
NM		•		Education	•
NY	•			Education	•
NC	•			Education	•
ND	•			Health	•
OH	•			Health	•
OR	•			Education	•
OK		•		Education	•
PA	•			Health	•
RI	•			School for the Deaf	•
SC		•		Health	•
SD		•		Health	•
TN	•			Education	•
TX	•			Health	•
UT			•	Education	•
VT	•			Education	•
VA		•		Education	•
WA	•			Public Instruction	•
WV	•			Education	•
WI	•			Public Instruction	•
WY			•	Local School District	

Figure 8-9. Summary by state of school hearing screening programs. (From Penn, T. (1999). School-based hearing screening in the United States. *Audiology Today, 11* (6), 20.)

Table 8-8.
Pitfalls to Avoid in Hearing Screening and Acoustic Immittance Screening

Hearing screening pitfalls

Child observing dials. This should be avoided at all times, because children will respond to the visual cues. The most appropriate position at which to seat the child is at an oblique angle, so the tester and audiometer are out of the child's peripheral vision

Examiner giving visual cues (facial expression, eye or head movements)

Incorrect adjustment of the head band and earphone placement. Care must be taken to place the earphones carefully over the ears so that the protective screen mesh of the earphone diaphragm is directly over the entrance of the external auditory canal. Misplacement of the earphone by only 1 inch can cause as great as a 3035 dB threshold shift

Vague instructions

Noise in the test area

Overlong test sessions. The screening should require only 35 minutes. If a child requires significantly more time than this, the routine screening should be discontinued, and a short rest taken. If the child continues to be difficult to test, play conditioning should be used

Too long or too short a presentation of the test tone. The test stimulus should be presented for 12 sec. If the stimulus is for a shorter or longer time than this, inaccurate responses may be obtained

Acoustic immittance screening pitfalls

Clogged probe and probe tip. The probe and probe tips must be kept free from earwax

Probe tip too large or too small. Each ear canal is different and may require a different-sized probe tip. Utilization of the correct size for each child will avoid possible errors

Head movement, swallowing, or eye-blinks. The child should be kept still during testing, as a sudden abnormal movement during testing may be interpreted as a reflex

Probe tip against the ear canal wall. The probe tip must be inserted directly into the ear canal, and when the canal is not straight, the tip must be kept away from the canal wall

Debris in ear canal. The ear canal should be inspected before testing to ensure that it is clear

With permission from Roeser, R.J., & Northern, J.L. (1988). Screening for hearing loss and middle ear disorders. In R. J. Roeser and M. P. Downs (Eds.), Auditory disorders in school children (2nd ed.). New York: Thieme-Stratton.

identification audiometry program will likely require more time and thought than initially anticipated.

SCREENING FOR OTITIS MEDIA

Controversies exist regarding the need, purpose, and technique of screening for middle ear disease and hearing loss in children. Middle ear disease generally refers to otitis media, one of the most common diseases of childhood. Identification, treatment, and management of otitis media spread across the territories of numerous professional groups and thus have important economic and health-care implications in society. A special national workshop was held during 1985 during which experts in pediatrics, infectious disease, otolaryngology, epidemiology, audiology, and biostatistics gathered to as-

sess the current status of screening for otitis media in infants and children (Bluestone, Fria, Arjona, et al., 1986).

A principal problem that accompanies all cases of otitis media is hearing loss. Although usually mild, the hearing loss may be the basis of an adverse effect on the development of speech, language, and cognition of young children. (See Chapter 3 for a complete discussion of the developmental and educational aspects of otitis media.) Undoubtedly, many variables influence the outcome of otitis media and the effect it has on the development of a young child. The potential seriousness of the consequences of unidentified and therefore untreated asymptomatic otitis media is too important to overlook. The sequelae of otitis media with effusion that is of most concern to audiologists and educators are the suspected associations between frequent occurrences of otitis media during early childhood and impaired speech and language development. Some researchers have questioned whether this association is valid. Many believe that the overwhelming majority of cases of otitis media sooner or later subside spontaneously without lasting physical or developmental consequences. Nonetheless, although research continues, most speech-language specialists and audiologists believe that to wait for a definitive answer while doing nothing is an untenable position.

Because the hearing loss associated with otitis media may be episodic and mild, numerous issues concerning screening for middle ear disease exist. It is well established that traditional pure tone hearing screening testing alone may miss as many as 70% of ears with pathologic findings (Melnick, Eagles, & Levine, 1964); accordingly, tympanometry has become a critical component of mass hearing screening programs. It must be admitted that mass screening with tympanometry may indeed produce overreferrals (i.e., children referred from screening programs to physicians who have found them to have normal middle ears on examination). However, such findings are to be expected in light of the fact that otitis media with effusion is fluctuant and recurrent and that there is great seasonal variation in the presence and absence of the disorder. Acoustic immittance audiometry, especially tympanometry, is an effective screening tool, although there exists disagreement about its precise role in various screening strategies. Tympanometry is easy to use, objective, efficient, acceptable to the screening population, inexpensive, and accurate in identifying those children with significant negative middle ear pressure and effusion. Whether the child will experience serious consequences if the otitis media disorder is left untreated is not a simple and easy question, because so many other variables have influence on the final outcome.

Approximately half of U.S. states incorporate acoustic immittance as part of their recommended identification procedures (Penn, 1999). Consistent use of acoustic immittance screening is also evident in local educational agencies, day care centers, Head Start programs, well-baby clinics, and private primary care medical offices. Although there is no clear-cut resolution to the many questions that surround the immittance screening for middle ear disease and mild hearing loss controversy, the fact is that the technique has been a positive addition to hearing screening programs. To be sure, there is need for comprehensive, well-controlled research concerning the differential and cumulative effects of otitis media with effusion and mild conductive hearing loss.

Recommendations from the International Research Conference on Otitis Media (Lim, 1998) emphasized cost-effectiveness by limiting overreferrals and focusing attention on the identification of the 10% of otitis media patients in greatest need of definitive evaluation. The recommendations included the use of EOAEs, tympanometry, and pure tone audiometry for the accurate identification of otitis media in those patients who are prelingual, patients without obvious symptoms, well babies, symptomatic infants and children, and at-risk groups. The recommendation was made to conduct hearing and middle ear screening only during the initial year of school entry and 1 year later. This strategy will make screening more cost-effective and will survey children at the ages most likely to have unrecognized middle ear effusion. Middle ear screening of children 7 years of age or older will not likely identify new cases of children with significant hearing loss.

The hearing and middle ear screening should be done at least biannually, preferably early in the school year and near the end of the school year. This is recommended for two reasons: (1) children with effusion early in the fall are more likely to have chronic, persistent effusion over the winter months; and (2) screening during the winter months is likely to identify cases associated with upper respiratory tract infections. It is important to note that a *bilateral* middle ear problem is the key condition being sought by screening and is thus the basis for an immediate alerting letter to parents with a recommendation for assessment by the family's primary care physician at the earliest opportunity. A child with a *unilateral* middle ear screening failure should be rescreened at the next routine time. Two successive unilateral failures should result in an alerting letter to the parents. All children who fail unilaterally or bilaterally should be rescreened at every routine biannual screening examination.

The criteria presented for additional follow-up implicate those children with three episodes of otitis media within a 3- to 6-month period and those children who present with persistent middle ear effusion of 3 months or longer. Children identified by these criteria should be referred for audiologic evaluation (regardless of age) and screened with a formal, standardized language development assessment tool (such as the ELM scale) to ensure adequate language appropriate for age level. Children who exhibit mild language delay on the screening test may be enrolled in a home language enrichment program. Materials may be recommended for the parents which can be used in the home to enhance the child's speech and language. It is generally accepted that working with parents and instituting a home-based, moderately structured program can produce impressive short- and long-term gains for children.

ACOUSTIC OTOSCOPE

The acoustic otoscope, originally called the acoustic reflectometer, is a simple, noninvasive instrument for screening and identifying the presence of middle ear fluid in children through a technique known as *reflectometry*. The acoustic otoscope was designed as a quick and easy alternative to acoustic immittance measurement (Teele & Teele, 1984). Since the development of the original prototype the acoustic otoscope has undergone numerous modifications, and the design is now based on a digital microprocessor. The acoustic otoscope requires no hermetic seal at the ear canal and is effective even when the child is crying or when the ear canal is partially obscured with cerumen (Fig. 8-9).

The acoustic otoscope generates an input signal that consists of repeated frequency sweeps (40 frequencies per sweep) at 80 dB SPL. The pickup microphone measures the amplitude of the reflected probe tone (reflectometry) from the plane of the tympanic membrane. The instrument works on quarter-wavelength theory, so that the reflected wave completely cancels the principal wave in the external ear canal at a distance of one-quarter wavelength from the tympanic mem-

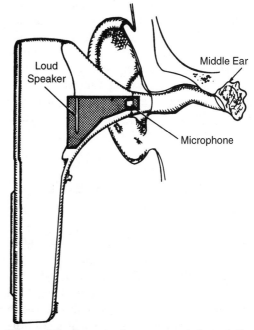

Figure 8-9. Cross-section representation of the acoustic otoscope (also known as the acoustic reflectometer).

brane. Thus, the reflected sound is inversely proportional to the total sound; a greater reflection produces reduced amplitude suggestive of middle ear effusion. To conduct the test, the examiner simply "aims" the speculum of the acoustic otoscope into the child's ear canal and presses the activator button. The instrument is positioned until the highest level of reflectometry is noted on a vertical display. The acoustic otoscope derives reflectivity from an arbitrary 0- to 9-unit scale, with 9 representing the largest degree of signal cancellation. The reflectivity reading is a function of the inelasticity of the tympanic membrane and will be low from a normal eardrum. There will be almost complete cancellation with a high reflectivity reading on the display when the eardrum is retracted or rigid with middle ear effusion. Pellette, Cox, & MacDonald (1997), in a comparative study, reported that acoustic immittance data compared more favorably with otoscopy than did results obtained from the acoustic otoscope.

Acoustic reflectometry is an interesting technique as a middle ear screening device for otitis media and is now available for home use by parents. The device requires little training or skill in its use, but considerable caution must be used in interpretation. Results are questionable in infants. Acoustic reflectometry has not proven to have sufficient performance sensitivity, specificity, and predictive ability to be recommended for use in screening programs.

ACOUSTIC IMMITTANCE SCREENING

Acoustic immittance technique is well suited for use with children, because it requires little cooperation, provides objective results, and is quick and easy to administer (Fig. 8-10). However, before being accepted as an integral part of hearing screening programs, advocates in favor of incorporating acoustic immittance measurements as part of the screening process faced outspoken critics

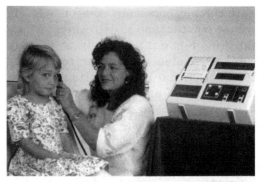

Figure 8-10. Acoustic immittance screening is an important element in the school hearing testing program.

who opposed including immittance tests as a matter of routine. The debate about the role of immittance screening was summarized in two points of view by Bess (1980) and Northern (1980b). Brooks, an early advocate of acoustic immittance screening as a supplement to the standard pure tone hearing screening test, published a comprehensive review of the pertinent literature in 1980.

It must be remembered that the goal of a hearing screening program is to identify those individuals who probably have some hearing problem from those individuals who probably do not have a hearing problem. Children who "fail" the screening tests may or may not have ear problems and are thus "tagged" for additional testing to determine the cause of screening failure. Traditional pure tone techniques for screening hearing fail to identify persons who have mild hearing loss due to the presence of middle ear disease. The immittance technique is capable of yielding more accurate screening results in the identification of middle ear disease than is possible with otoscopy or pure tone audiometry—a firm fact substantiated in numerous studies (Northern, 1992).

Opponents to the use of immittance in mass screening raise legitimate concern that the technique will identify asymptomatic children who have transient episodes of otitis media for which specific treatment may be inadvisable. Although otitis media with middle ear effusion may resolve spontaneously in many individuals, undetected and untreated middle ear effusions may indeed create serious otologic complications as well as speech, language, and educational problems.

To determine validity of a screening technique, one screening procedure is used as a criterion measure against which to compare other screening tests. Otoscopy is most often accepted as the criterion test against which to compare acoustic immittance screening, although the accuracy of otoscopy varies as a function of the person behind the otoscope (Paradise, Smith, & Bluestone, 1976; Roeser, Glorig, Gerken, et al., 1977). Otoscopy is so subjective that it can be argued that acoustic immittance measurement should be the criterion procedure because of its objectivity and test-retest reliability. Generally, the use of otoscopy as the criterion produces higher sensitivity agreement, since fewer subjects "fail" otoscopy, while many subjects may "fail" screening. Acoustic immittance measurement sensitivity with otoscopy as the criterion measure is very high, at approximately 95%, with a low specificity of about 50%. The amount of pathology in the sample population affects the sensitivity rate in research studies, because it is easy to obtain high agreement between immittance and otoscopy when many normal subjects are examined. The low specificity rates of immittance audiometry are due to the use of too-rigid failure criteria for peaked negative pressure curves. Adherence to middle ear pressure failure criterion of − 200 mm daPa alleviates the overreferral and low specificity problems.

Of course, the ultimate validation technique for middle ear effusion is myringotomy (see Chapter 3). The studies reported by Orchik, Dunn, & McNutt (1978a) and Orchik, Moroff, & Dunn (1978b) with acoustic immittance and myringotomy have shown that the combined use of tympanometry and acoustic reflex measurement showed a statistically significant correlation with the presence of middle ear fluid. The studies showed the correlation between "flat" impedance curves and the presence of effusion proven by myringotomy to be 82–90% accurate. This high correlation between flat impedance curves and absent acoustic reflexes speaks highly for referral and medical evaluation of such children.

Guidelines for screening for outer and middle ear disorders were published by ASHA in 1997. The single set of guidelines can serve for all age groups of children, including the developmentally delayed, with the following steps:

- A careful case history, when possible, through the verbal report of a parent or guardian.

- A visual inspection of the ears to identify risk factors for outer and middle ear disease and to ensure that no contraindications exist for performing tympanometry (e.g., drainage, foreign bodies, tympanostomy tubes).

- The use of a lighted otoscope or video otoscope to examine the external ear canal and tympanic membrane for obvious obstructions or structural defects.

- Performance of tympanometry with a low-frequency (220 or 226 Hz) probe tone and a positive to negative air pressure sweep.

- Acoustic reflex measurements should not be used as screening pass/refer criteria.

Children with results that fall within normal limits for all procedures will pass the screening for outer and middle ear disorders. Children should be referred for medical evaluation if ear drainage is observed, ear canal abnormalities (such as obstructions, impacted cerumen, or foreign objects) are noted, blood or other secretions are present, stenosis or atresia are observed, otitis externa is present, or when perforations or other abnormalities of the tympanic membrane are apparent. If the tympanic equivalent ear canal volume is greater than 1.0 cm^3 and accompanied by a flat tympanogram, the child is likely to have an opening in the tympanic membrane. Referral is not necessary if a tympanostomy tube is in place (usually visible by otoscopic examination) or if the patient is already receiving medical care for perforation. Most investigators have concluded that the acoustic reflex measurement is too variable to be useful in acoustic immittance screening programs.

Tympanometric criteria for referral when screening for middle ear effusion vary depending on factors related to the population screened. Tympanometric peak pressure (TPP) is not recommended in the criteria for identifying children at risk for otitis media. Negative TPP associated with an otherwise normal tympanogram is a poor determinant of middle ear effusion (ASHA, 1990). For infants and children from 1 year to school age, tympanometric width (TW) greater than 200 daPa is the recommended screening criterion. This value is just outside the normal range for infants younger than 30 months and has been shown to have high specificity and good sensitivity in children of school age (Roush, Bryant, Mundy, Zeisel, & Roberts, 1995; Nozza, 1995). In children with a history of chronic middle ear effusion and scheduled for myringotomy and tube surgery, a more severe criterion of TW >300 daPa is recommended (Nozza, Bluestone, Kardatzke, & Bachman, 1994).

The ASHA (1997) guidelines recommend that a child with a unilateral or bilateral tympanogram meeting referral criteria (other than those findings consistent with a previously unidentified perforation of the tympanic membrane) should be rescreened 6–8 weeks after the initial test. Because middle ear disease often resolves without treatment, referral based on a single screening is generally not recommended. Various schemes for a two-stage acoustic immittance screening protocol have been suggested (Roush, 1990; Northern, 1992).

AUDITORY SCREENING OF THE DEVELOPMENTALLY DELAYED CHILD

Standards for institutions serving the developmentally delayed generally recommend that all new residents, children younger than 10 at annual intervals, and other residents at regular intervals receive hearing screenings. Whenever possible, conditioning techniques (including VRA) are the methods of choice for determining auditory thresholds under earphones, insert phones, or in the sound field. Modified speech audiometry using developmentally appropriate vocal commands at various hearing levels can help estimate hearing thresholds in each ear when necessary. Acoustic immittance and EOAEs testing should be an integral part of every hearing screening for this special needs population (Northern, 1977a, 1978c, 1980d). The presence of EOAEs may be used to confirm the presence of normal hearing. If the acoustic immittance battery suggests conductive hearing loss, EOAEs will likely be absent. ABR testing is not recommended as an initial screening procedure for this population because of the likely need for sedation and possible central auditory pathway dysfunction.

Hearing screening for severely and profoundly developmentally delayed children presents a difficult situation in terms of efficiency, accuracy, and time. Limited behavioral screening may be possible for some patients with the subject seated or held in the sound suite facing one speaker. Initially the stimulus is presented through the opposite speaker so that if the subject localizes, he or she must make an overt obvious lateralization to seek the sound from the speaker furthest away. If localization to the stimulus occurs, the examiner quickly reinforces the head turn with a flashing light or noisy action toy. Conditioning trials are necessary to ensure that the response is reliable and valid. Speech is primarily used as the sound stimulus, but a variety of other stimuli can be employed. It is sometimes necessary to change the stimuli during testing to pure tones, warble tones, white noise, or complex noise. Obviously, success in conditioning depends on the severity of developmental disability of the patient.

Behavioral observations may include some or all of the following responses to auditory stimuli: (1) responses that indicate sound awareness such as eye opening, quieting, assuming a listening attitude, smiling, laughing, and ceasing activity; (2) localization responses; and (3) startle responses, which are the involuntary reflexive responses that are expected 65–85 dB above threshold and include eyeblink, orientation reflex, tonic neck reflex, and the full-body Moro reflex.

Recommended Protocol for Auditory Screening of Developmentally Delayed Children

1. An ascending approach with speech or narrow-band noise stimuli should be used in an attempt to obtain responses from the patient at levels of 25 dB HL or better. Awareness, or preferably localization by 25 dB HL, constitutes "passing" the observational portion of the screening.

2. If no reliable responses are obtained by 25 dB, the screen should ascend in 10 dB steps in an attempt to elicit a response. If the patient shows awareness or localizes by 65 dB HL and a startle can be elicited, near normal hearing or mild to moderate hearing loss is likely.

3. Operant conditioning techniques as described in Chapter 6 are recommended when possible.

4. Each screening procedure should include acoustic immittance audiometry and EOAEs testing. These physiologic measures may rule out or establish the presence of normal hearing or conductive hearing loss as well as suggest the need for additional audiometric evaluation.

SCREENING FOLLOW-UP ISSUES

The effectiveness of any screening program is only as good as the subsequent follow-up program. If experienced audiologists are unavailable or if parents have difficulty gaining access to audiologic assistance, hearing-impaired infants and young children may not receive the necessary follow-up and intervention. The philosophical question remains, who is responsible for follow-up—the audiologist, the parents, or the institution? Who should bear the financial burden of further evaluation, the parents or the institution, when the infant or child must return for additional and possibly more expensive testing and evaluation? Audiologists responsible for hearing screening programs must also be concerned about the ever-present possibility of progressive sensorineural hearing loss in infants and young children. When babies pass the admission birth screening protocols and are later determined to have hearing loss, the question always remains, did the screening test miss this baby or did the hearing loss occur after the hearing screening was applied?

An interesting point can be made by examining the reported age of *detection* of hearing loss against the age of *confirmation* of hearing loss. Parents view the chief obstacles in confirming the hearing loss as the primary care physician's unwillingness to accept the parent's opinions, the failure of these physicians to perform simple hearing screening tests, and finally the reluctance of the physicians to arrange for referral of the child for audiologic evaluation. Detection and confirmation of a child's hearing problem depends on the astuteness and insistence of the parents as well as the alertness of the physician.

Stein et al. (1990) compared patterns of initial identification and habilitation between groups of hearing-impaired infants studied during the 1980s and found that the advantage of earlier diagnosis may easily be lost due to delays in habilitation program enrollment. The Never Too Young project of Arizona organized and distributed a questionnaire to parents of congenitally hearing-impaired children to probe for information regarding the identification and intervention processes that the parents had experienced, as well as to inquire regarding the children's birth and medical histories (Elssmann et al., 1987). The findings revealed that advice given by managing physicians in response to parental concern, whether good or poor advice, indeed had significant influence on the early identification (or lack thereof) of their child's hearing loss. The pattern of delays between the identification and confirmation of the hearing loss and the recommendation and the fitting of a hearing aid seemed to be threefold: (1) referral back to the physician for ear examinations and medical clearances, then long, silent intervals without action; (2) babies with multiple physical and developmental problems in which hearing was only part of the total concern of the parents; and (3) parental disbelief or avoidance of the fact that their child had an important hearing loss.

James Jerger relates that the clinical audiologist can make two mistakes when counseling parents of an infant or child suspected to have hearing loss. One of the mistakes, however, has considerably more serious consequences than the other mistake. The *lesser* of the two mistakes (the false positive) is for the audiologist to initially decide that the infant or young child is deaf and then subsequently to determine that the infant has normal hearing. An embarrassing mistake to be sure, but probably every experienced clinician has fallen prey to this error. In this situation, however, the final outcome of normal hearing for the infant or child is a great relief to all.

The more serious mistake is devastating to the infant or young child in question. In this grave error (the false negative) the audiologist initially informs the parent that their child has normal hearing when, in fact, the infant or young child has severe to profound hearing loss. In this situation, the parents believe the audiologist and assume with confidence that their baby hears normally. Unfortunately, by the time the mistaken diagnosis is identified and rectified, maximum habilitation for the infant or child may never be achieved.

Armed with knowledge about the potential for these two mistakes in infant hearing assessment, the audiologist must practice extreme care in pronouncing an infant to have normal hearing. When in doubt, it behooves the clinician to assume that the infant has a hearing problem until proven otherwise. The audiologist is still the best professional to serve as an advocate for the child and to be the one whose ultimate responsibility is to provide maximum support for the infant under evaluation.

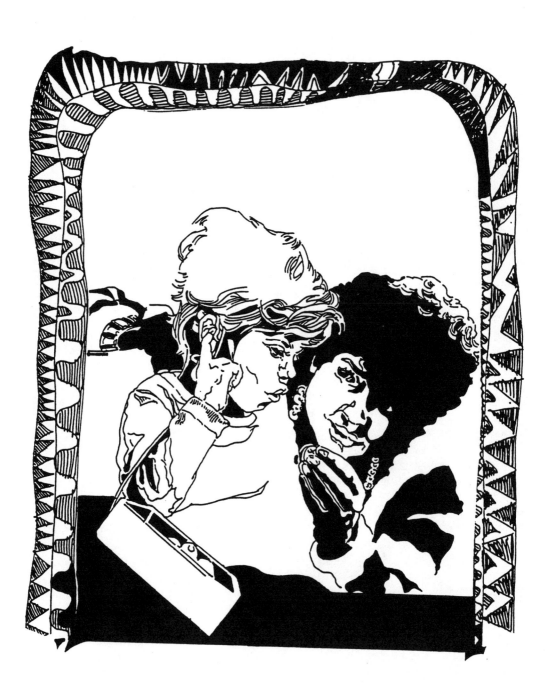

CHAPTER 9

Amplification

There is little doubt that the single most important invention to help the hearing handicapped child is the amplifying hearing aid. There is an old adage, "As we hear, so shall we speak," and it is this very close relationship between hearing, speech, and language that is so important to the hearing-impaired child. The fitting of hearing aids is the first significant step in the intervention process. Technology is now readily available to help the child with hearing impairment learn to speak through the use of voice pitch indicators, speech timing equipment, vowel indicators, voice/nonvoice meters, speech spectrum displays, and visible speech machines. None of these devices, however, is more fundamental to the hearing-impaired child's education and ability to learn speech than the properly fitted hearing aid. Hearing aids provide the hearing-impaired child with optimal use of the residual hearing so that speech and language milestones can be achieved at appropriate age levels.

The task of selecting and fitting hearing aids for a child is not to be taken lightly. The inexperienced clinician or the nonprofessionally trained individual must not undertake selection and fitting of hearing aids for the hearing-impaired or deaf child. The process of selecting hearing aids for a child is complex and requires numerous special considerations as developed and published by the Pediatric Working Group on Amplification for Children (1996) and thoroughly described by Dillon (2000). The pediatric evaluation and hearing aid fitting may involve many people including the otolaryngologist, pediatrician, audiologist/dispenser, speech/language pathologist, teacher of the deaf, and other auxiliary professionals such as the public health or school nurse and the social worker. These individuals must work together closely, in a coordinated effort, to ensure that the hearing-impaired child obtains maximal benefit from amplification.

The audiologist is clearly the individual to coordinate and guide the hearing aid selection procedure. The audiologist is able to identify the nature and degree of the child's hearing loss, which may in itself be a challenging task. The audiologist ensures that proper medical clearance is obtained before the hearing aid selection procedure. The audiologist is able to evaluate the performance of various hearing aids on the child, make an earmold impression, perform probe-microphone measurements, and select and dispense the hearing aids to obtain the best amplification available for the child's hearing loss. As part of this process, the audiologist counsels the parents about new hearing aids and their care and use and arranges for therapy for the child and special training if necessary. Finally, the audiologist is able to devote the necessary time to follow the progress of the patient and to be ever vigilant to be sure that the hearing aids are in top operating condition.

The authors' recommended protocol is to fit hearing aids on pediatric patients as soon as the presence of significant hearing loss is confirmed. Our long-term goal is to establish ear-specific auditory thresholds for all test frequencies in each ear. Obviously, this goal may not be achieved with every child during the first visit, or perhaps even the second or third visit. Although the audiologic information may be limited to only a few frequencies in each ear, the recommendation and provision of hearing aids should proceed as quickly as possible. Despite everyone's best intentions, it is not uncommon for the hearing aids to take 1–4 (or more) months to be selected, ordered, programmed, and fitted. Clinicians should keep in mind the study of Yoshinaga-Itano, Sedey, Coulter, and Mehl (1998), who found that significantly better language development is achieved when the child's hearing loss is diagnosed and early intervention is provided by the age of 6 months.

The appointment time scheduled for hearing aid evaluations with children should include ample consideration for counseling and therapy. Time for thorough preparation is involved in the preselection hearing aid workup for the hearing-impaired child. Nearly as much time may be necessary to select the proper hearing aid and earmold. Additional telephone calls and letters are usually required to be sent to appropriate agencies to obtain financial assistance for the purchase of the aid. Electroacoustic analysis of the hearing aids is important to confirm optimal operation of the hearing instrument. However, the time consumed by these procedures is only fleeting seconds when compared with the long-term therapy and follow-up programs that the child will need through the remainder of his or her life.

HEARING AIDS FOR CHILDREN

Tremendous technologic advances in the hearing aid have been made over the past three decades. Many years ago hearing aids were heavy, cumbersome units with large, unsightly battery requirements. The portable electronic hearing aid became a reality in the 1930s, and the vacuum tube became part of the system in the 1940s. Transistors permitted the hearing aid to be a much smaller unit in the 1950s. Today, tiny "solid state" computerized circuits in the devices have reduced the instrument and its power source to a practical size and weight. Developments in the microphone component of the hearing aid have extended both ends of the frequency reproduction range. Microphones are now available that are truly directional—amplifying only sounds that are immediately in front of the hearing aid and at the same time attenuating sounds emitted from the sides or back of the listener. Directional microphones also increase the signal-to-noise relationship so important for the understanding of speech in noisy environments.

The operation of the hearing aid has been likened to a miniature high-fidelity set made up of a group of tiny components that picks up sound wave vibrations from the air and converts them into electrical signals. Actually, hearing aids are much more than just ultraminiature electroacoustic amplifiers. They are sophisticated personal signal processing systems comprising not only the hearing instrument itself but also a technically elaborate acoustic coupling system while directing the signal toward the tympanic membrane. The major amplification, signal limiting, and complex controlling functions are achieved within the hearing aid itself, programmed by specialized software programs.

Hearing aids have three basic components as shown in Figure 9-1. Sound from the environment enters the hearing aid through a *microphone*, which changes the acoustic (sound) signals into electrical signals. The electrical signal is enhanced, or increased in intensity, through an *amplifier*. The amplified electrical signal is then passed through the *receiver*, which changes the signal back into amplified acoustic sound. The amplified acoustic sound is delivered into the user's ear canal through some type of earmold. A small battery powers the hearing aid system.

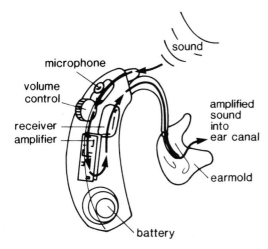

Figure 9-1. The basic anatomy of a behind-the-ear hearing aid.

The current availability of programmable and digital-based hearing aids has proven to be especially useful in fitting amplification on children. Major changes in the physical hardware and appearance of hearing aids have been seen, as well as computerized evaluation techniques to ensure improved fitting protocols. Advanced signal processing technology has improved hearing instrument performance. These high-technology hearing aids utilize programmable settings and adjustments, so that very specific prescriptive fitting can be applied to each individual hearing loss and audiometric configuration. Each programmable hearing aid is adjustable to fit nearly any degree of hearing loss and almost every audiometric hearing loss configuration. Although this new technology was initially developed for adult users, the long-term benefit to hearing-impaired children is very important. Programmable hearing aids offer the flexibility to be altered electroacoustically to fit the child's changing needs and possible fluctuations in hearing levels.

Persons working with children who use hearing aids are familiar with the wide variety of occurrences and bizarre experiences that can render the hearing aid inoperable. Just because a child wears his or her hearing aid faithfully everyday, the assumption cannot be made that the aid is functioning adequately. In the analysis of hearing aids in use and worn by children, it is not uncommon to find that the hearing aids are not working to their original specifications. It is strongly recommended that each child's amplification units receive regular longitudinal electroacoustic analysis. Potts and Greenwood (1983) described a daily hearing aid monitoring program, the results of which created a significant decrease in the incidence of hearing aid malfunction in their school. The program was based on a detailed visual-auditory inspection (Table 9-1) and routine electroacoustic analysis. The Education for All Handicapped Children Act of 1975 (Public Law 94-142) states that each public agency shall ensure that those hearing aids worn by hearing-impaired students in school are functioning properly (*Federal Register,* August 23, 1977, 121a.303).

The Food and Drug Administration (FDA) regulations of 1977 include the following rules related to hearing aids for children:

• Before purchase of a hearing aid, an individual with a hearing loss must have a medical evaluation of the hearing loss by a physician (preferably a physician specializing in diseases of the ear) within 6 months preceding the sale of the aid.

• Adult patients, under carefully defined circumstances, can sign a waiver of the medical clearance requirements. However, there is no waiver option of persons younger than 18 years of age. The physician who examines the child must provide a written statement that the patient's hearing loss has been medically evaluated.

• In addition to seeing a physician for a medical evaluation, a child with a hearing loss should be directed to an audiologist for evaluation and rehabilitation, because hearing loss may cause prob-

Table 9.1.
Total Looking/Listening Check for Hearing Aids

Component	Looking	Listening (use sounds /a/ /u/ /i/ /ʃ/ /s/)
Remove aid from child, noting "as worn" volume setting		
Earmold	Opening clear? Cracks, rough areas?	
Battery	Read voltage (replace at 1.1 or below) —compartment clean?	
Case	Cracks? Separating?	Press case gently—interruption in amplification?
Microphone	Clean? Visible damage?	
Dials	Clean? Easily rotated?	Rotate—reasonable gain variation: static?
Switches	Clean? Easy to move?	Turn on and off—static?
Tubing (ear-level aid)	Cracks? Good connection to mold and aid? Moisture? Debris?	Cover opening of earmold and turn to maximum gain—feedback?
Oscillator (bone-conduction aid)	Cracks? Plug clean? Attached well to band?	Listen with oscillator on mastoid, ears plugged to block air-conducted sound
Variable controls	Proper OSPL90, frequency response, gain setting?	Speech sounds clearly amplified? Gain sounds normal for this hearing aid?
Distortion		Clear quality?
Feedback	Recheck receiver snap, tubing, earmold	Turn to maximum gain to check— external feedback? Internal?
Replace aid and check fit of the earmold to the child's ear		

From Potts, P., & Greenwood, J. (1983). Hearing aid monitoring. *Language, Speech and Hearing Services in Schools, 14,* 163.
SSPL, saturated sound pressure level.

lems in language development and the educational and social growth of the child.

The audiologic assessment that precedes the hearing aid evaluation should be as thorough as possible given the child's age and cooperation. Children with a developmental age of 6 months or younger need confirmation of behavioral measurements with auditory brainstem response threshold assessment. In addition to ear-specific, frequency-specific auditory thresholds, evoked otoacoustic emissions and bone-conduction testing should be attempted in all children. Acoustic immittance testing or evoked otoacoustic emissions testing should precede every hearing aid evaluation session

because of the high incidence of middle ear pathology in young children.

Basic to the concept of hearing aid recommendations is a realistic understanding of what the aid can do for the patient. No hearing aid will enable a hard-of-hearing youngster to perform normally in all situations. The goal in providing amplification to the child with a hearing impairment is to make speech audible at safe and comfortable listening levels at a sensation level that provides as many acoustic speech cues as possible. This goal must be accomplished while the amplification system makes soft speech audible, speech and environmental sounds comfortably loud, and loud sounds not uncomfortable (IHAFF, 1994). Of course, the hearing aids must work equally as well in a wide variety of listening situations (e.g., in background noise, at close distances, with multiple speakers and sounds, and amplifying sounds from far away distances). The primary reason for recommending the use of amplification is to enable the child to communicate better with a hearing aid than without it. Such improvement may be possible in only a few select conditions for the child who will ultimately learn to utilize the aid to its maximal benefit. Ross (1969) stated that "merely because one can 'get along' without a hearing aid is *not* an adequate reason to discourage its use."

The selection of children's hearing aids requires special consideration. The procedures followed by the audiologist for selection of the hearing aid will be a function of the experience of the clinician. Considerable expertise is required to select the correct amount of gain, output, and frequency response curves in multiple programs. The final selection may be influenced by the age and motor skills of the child, cosmetic considerations including color selections of the cases and earmolds, availability of options such as direct audio input, and, of course, cost of the hearing instruments. Pediatric instruments should have a wide range of programmable adjustments such as saturated sound pressure level (OSPL90) reduction control, programmable frequency and gain possibilities, and choice of compression circuits and adjustments. The wide range of programmability is especially valuable in children's fittings because of the possible incomplete or tentative hearing threshold measurements and the fact that the child's listening skills will likely change over time after the hearing aids are fitted.

The hearing aids must have maximum performance flexibility, so that a significant range of adjustments and modifications can be made without the need to purchase new hearing aids as the child's needs change. *Programmable hearing aids* have numerous advantages over conventional hearing aid circuits in children because of the increased flexibility, more sophisticated technology, and enhanced sound quality. Programmable hearing aids are noted for high sound quality from an analog amplifier that is controlled by a computer programmable memory chip. The basic programmable hearing aid features an omnidirectional microphone, two memories for different listening environments, a telephone amplifier, and models with or without volume control wheels. Advanced programmable hearing aids have all of the above features plus two or more independent frequency channels that can be adjusted for precise prescriptive fitting.

Unfortunately, higher technology in hearing aids costs more, requires accurate individual threshold measurements for maximum programming benefit, and may depend on a remote control unit to operate the hearing aid. For example, *digital hearing instruments* have exceptional sound quality, multiple frequency bands, multiple memories for storing different prescriptive programs, plus a fully digital amplifier with or without an external volume control. Some models feature multiple microphones for improved speech understanding in the presence of background noise. Clearly, some of these requirements are not necessary for a young infant or toddler, and of course, cost of the higher technology instruments is a factor that may preclude purchase. Furthermore, more advanced and more expensive hearing aid technology does not always result in increased hearing benefit. Individual results depend on the type, severity, and duration of the hearing loss as well as the programming skills of the audiologist. Some parents and families may have to make the difficult decisions between conventional and high-technology hearing aids as well as whether to purchase spare or backup hearing aids, direct audio input features, separate FM systems, and insurance coverage for loss or breakage.

Telecoil circuitry allows the hearing aids to amplify sound conveyed by magnetic signals picked up from a telephone receiver or other special assistive listening aids. The telecoil microphone picks up only magnetic signals while not amplifying background noise. Some hearing aids have a special microphone-telecoil two-position switch, or a programmable parameter, to change from the normal microphone use to the special telecoil microphone when compatible telephone receivers are being used. Children's hearing aids should have the capability for direct audio input (DAI), which allows for direct connection of the hearing aid to a telephone receiver, radio, television, movie projector, stereo, or other assistive listening system. Common wisdom requires that a child's hearing aid must be exceedingly durable; of course, consideration should also be given to an insurance protection plan for extended warranty, loss, or damage.

Young children have not developed a "listening strategy," and it is important to reemphasize that the hearing aid evaluation in children is a continuing process. Other factors to be considered require the best possible amplified signal with good quality and clear sound. The hearing aids' performance must be checked electroacoustically and with probe-microphone measurements by the audiologist for every child at every clinic visit. New hearing aid instruments should be checked before they are dispensed to the patient to be sure that they meet the manufacturer's performance specifications.

TYPES OF HEARING AIDS

Ear-Level Hearing Aids. Ear-level hearing aids are the amplification instruments of choice for adults and children. Ear-level instruments include behind-the-ear (BTE) models as well as in-the-ear (ITE), in-the-canal (ITC), and completely-in-the-canal (CIC) hearing instruments (Fig. 9-2). The ITE and ITC models have no external wires or tubes and are very lightweight. The ear-level

hearing aids may be used for patients with all degrees of hearing loss, from mild to severe.

The BTE model has all its components housed in one curved case that fits neatly behind the pinna and rests against the mastoid surface. A short clear plastic tube connects the earmold to the hearing aid case. BTE hearing aids may deliver up to 80 dB full-on gain and 125–140 dB OSPL90. Because the microphone and receiver of the BTE are in very close proximity to the earmold, increased opportunity exists for acoustic feedback (Fig. 9-3).

The BTE hearing aid has many advantages over the seldom recommended and older style body-worn hearing aid. The BTE hearing aid is much less conspicuous and does not amplify clothing noise because it is worn on the head and not on the body. Most importantly from the audiologist's point of view, the child's hearing reception is at a more natural position on the head. The authors' success with ear-level hearing aids in children has been very good, and this type of aid is recommended for the majority of their pediatric patients. They have recommended and fit ear-level instruments on infants as soon as the hearing impairment is identified (Fig. 9-3).

As children grow older they become more concerned about the cosmetic appear-

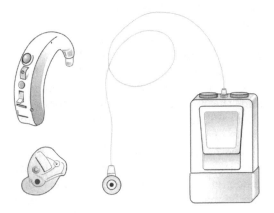

Figure 9-2. Illustrative styles of hearing aids: a body-worn instrument, an all-in-the-ear hearing aid, and a behind-the-ear hearing aid.

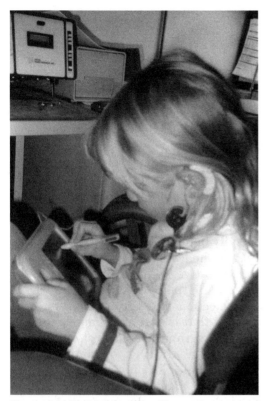

Figure 9-3. Ear-level hearing aids are the preferred style for young children.

ance of their hearing aid. As they reach those trying teen years, they often demand smaller, less visible, ear-level (or especially in-the-canal) hearing instruments, and the authors willingly follow this recommendation whenever possible. It is better to fit the growing pediatric patient with a hearing aid that will be willingly worn and used daily, than to force the use of an unwanted hearing aid that will not be worn.

Bone-Conduction Hearing Aids. Bone-conduction hearing aids are used in selected children with significant conductive hearing loss who cannot (for whatever reason) use an air-conduction hearing aid. The bone-conduction hearing aid has a vibratory flat surface that rests on the mastoid and transduces sound waves into vibrotactile sensation, thereby stimulating the cochlear cells via the bone-conduction auditory pathway. Bone-conduction hearing

aids are not commonly used today except in infants and young children with maximum conductive hearing loss due to congenital anomalies such as severe microtia of the pinnae or atresia of the external ear canal. The authors have placed bone-conduction hearing aids on infants as young as 1 month of age. Soft material can be used to pad the headband for a small child or infant if necessary. The bone oscillator can be used any place on the infant's skull, including the mastoid area behind the ear, the forehead, or at the back or top of the skull when the infant is placed stomach-down.

Everyone involved must understand that the bone-conduction hearing aid fitting is not permanent. Chances are quite good that the cause of the conductive-type hearing problem will ultimately be alleviated through surgical intervention. Successful surgical treatment will permit the fitting of a traditional air-conduction ear-level hearing aid.

Body-Type Hearing Aids. The on-the-body model of hearing aids has a relatively large microphone, amplifier, and power supply enclosed in a case attached to the clothing, placed in a pocket, or carried in a harness around the chest. An external receiver attaches directly to the earmold and is driven by power supplied through a thin flexible wire from the instrument case. Body-type hearing aids provide stronger gain and power output than ear-level instruments. Since the microphone and receiver are separated by considerable distance, the probability of acoustic feedback (or squeal) from amplified sound that leaks out around the earmold and "feeds back" into the microphone of the hearing aid is reduced.

The authors reserve the fitting of body-type hearing aids to children with congenital anomalies of the pinna and ear canal, children with multiple handicaps in addition to hearing loss, and other special situations in which ear-level hearing aids cannot be used. Despite their size, bulk, and cord, body aids can be firmly carried by young children in garment-type carrier harnesses. The body aid is considered by some clinicians to be more durable and less likely to be broken than ear-level instruments. The external controls are easier to adjust, although this often creates problems with children who play with the aids or inadvertently turn the hearing aid volume down or shut it off.

Extended-Frequency Hearing Aids. Conventional hearing aids attempt to provide optimal amplification for the speech frequency range between 200 and 5000 Hz. For years, however, attempts have been made to produce amplification systems that can provide supplemental speech cues for the profoundly hearing-impaired. In recent years, special amplification systems have been developed to enable hearing-impaired children with residual hearing in the low frequencies to use amplification. These special hearing aids provide greater low-frequency acoustic stimulation than does the conventional hearing aid. Initial evaluations of these amplification systems by their proponents were reported to be favorable, but later studies have produced conflicting results.

Berlin (1982) described hearing loss in which hearing is poor in the standard audiometric ranges but nearly normal at frequencies between 8000 and 15,000 Hz. In his report, Berlin described the development of an upward-shifting translating hearing aid that has a frequency response extending well beyond 10,000 Hz. Candidates for his special translating hearing aid are difficult to diagnose. They typically have unusually good speech and sensitivity to environmental sounds in the presence of poor speech perception and severe pure tone hearing losses with unusually good speech-detection thresholds. Their audiograms suggest severe to profound deafness, poor speech understanding, and good speech production. Many of these patients reject standard

hearing aids and may function intermittently well without them.

HEARING AID FITTINGS

According to Ross and Tomassetti (1980), "the early and appropriate selection and use of amplification is the single most important habilitation tool available." The goals for pediatric hearing aid fitting are for comfort and audibility of speech and environmental sounds. This requires properly programmed and adjusted ear-level hearing aids. It should be fully understood by all that initial pediatric hearing aid recommendations are tentative and will likely need to be altered in time. The pediatric hearing aid selection and fitting is an ongoing process that is part of a complete habilitation program. The focus of routine audiologic monitoring of amplification must include not only the child's auditory status and the function of the hearing aids, but also the function of the direct auditory input system used in the school as well as the parent's participation in the habilitation program.

Mueller and Hall (1998) describe a six-step protocol for organizing hearing aid fittings:

- Step 1: Assessment. The extent and cause of the hearing loss as well as candidacy for hearing aids are determined.

- Step 2: Treatment Planning. Audiologist, patient, and family members review the results of the hearing assessment and identify areas of difficulty and need.

- Step 3: Selection. The needed amplification characteristics, including the style and technology of the hearing aids as well as the electroacoustic requirements, are determined.

- Step 4: Verification. The audiologist determines that the hearing aids meet standardized measures that include basic electroacoustic performance, cosmetic appeal, comfortable fit, and real-ear performance.

- Step 5: Orientation. A formal procedure for counseling the patient and family on the use and care of the hearing aids and expected hearing aid performance is performed.

- Step 6: Validation. The effects of amplification intervention and verification of the aided improvement as discerned by family members, teachers, and therapists are determined.

Whenever possible an ear-level type aid is the aid of choice for a child. For some very active children of age 3 or so, the parents may not be able to maintain an ear-level aid. On the other hand, a well-behaved 2.5-year-old may be given consideration for an ear-level aid. The authors have, on numerous occasions, fitted a small ear-level hearing aid on young infants as soon as a diagnosis of hearing loss is strongly suspected or confirmed. Parents should be warned that the hearing aids might end up flushed down a toilet, chewed up by the family dog, thrown out of a window, or used as a pacifier. The parents must be willing to handle the problems of the ear-level aid. They will then assume the responsibility of seeing that it is cared for and protected against loss or damage.

The selection of a specific hearing aid for a hearing-impaired child challenges the skills of even the most experienced audiologists. When a child has both receptive and expressive speech and language, the selection of a hearing aid is certainly easier. It is the nonverbal child who poses problems, because this youngster is not capable of communicating with the audiologist about the quality of various hearing aids. Appropriate selection of the frequency response and output characteristics must be carefully considered in fitting amplification to children. A number of techniques, both behavioral and electroacoustic, have evolved as a

means to select the optimal hearing aid for each patient. None of the methods provides exact, precise information that is valid for every hearing aid fitting, but each procedure provides direction about the appropriate range of performance that the hearing aid must encompass. In many cases, more than one hearing aid instrument will meet the appropriate gain and output requirements, and selection is then based on other considerations such as hearing aid size, durability, cosmetics, ease of use, cost, and availability of service and insurance.

Audibility. A simple technique for demonstrating the "audibility" provided by hearing aids, based on the traditional articulation index (AI) concept, was described by Mueller and Killion (1990). Their suggested procedure, known as the count-the-dots method, uses a template of 100 dots weighted and fitted into the speech spectrum on an audiogram (Fig. 9-4). The AI is a measure of the proportion of speech cues that are audible and therefore closely related to the intelligibility of

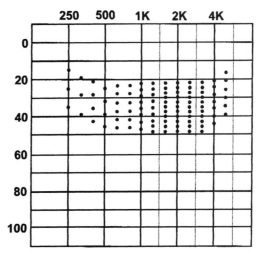

Figure 9-4. The count-the-dots audiogram template for calculation of the articulation index and the display of "audibility" for audiograms and hearing aids. The dots represent the contribution of different frequencies according to their importance for the understanding of normal speech. (From Mueller, G., & Killion, M. (1990). An easy method for calculating the articulation index. *The Hearing Journal*, 43, 9.)

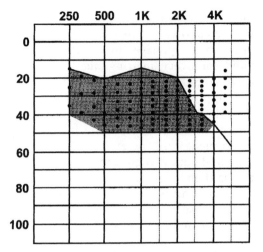

Figure 9-5. A count-the-dot template overlaid with a high-frequency sloping sensorineural hearing loss. The shaded area represents the portion of the speech spectrum that is audible. Amplification with hearing instruments would move the aided audiogram line further to the right of the template, allowing more of the speech spectrum to be audible.

speech. The patient's hearing thresholds are plotted on the count-the-dots template, and the number of dots under the audiogram, representing speech sounds that the patient can hear, are counted and multiplied by 100 to express the value as a percentage. The count-the-dots AI template presents a visual method that can demonstrate the potential benefit that will be obtained from hearing aids as well as to show the amount of communication handicap for normal-level speech that might be experienced by the patient in an aided or unaided situation (Fig. 9-5). Most of probe-microphone equipment will calculate the AI automatically. The 100-dot template of the speech spectrum is a useful tool to make the standard audiogram more meaningful to both clinicians and patients and is valuable as a counseling and teaching aid for parents and families.

The Selection Process. The selection procedure begins with consideration of the type of hearing aids to be utilized. Body-type hearing aids are now seldom recommended for children because of technologic improvements in ear-level

hearing aids, especially in terms of programmable adjustments, flexibility, and output power. Ear-level aids are lightweight and provide hearing reception at the natural position of the head. Ear-level hearing aids are the choice for most children, with the exception of the multiply handicapped child with poor head control that may lead to persistent feedback problems when ear-level aids are used. Color of the hearing aids and earmolds may be selected to please the younger pediatric patient or to be more cosmetically appropriate for the older child. Earmolds for children are typically constructed of soft materials.

Tremendous strides have been made in the technology of ITE hearing aids. Selection of a particular make and model of hearing aids for the pediatric patient requires a DAI feature and strong telecoil microphone with a microphone/telephone option. These features enable the use of personal FM systems and assistive listening devices with the child's hearing aid. Increased attention of the manufacturers to the importance of DAI and improved telecoil response of ITE hearing aids increases the likelihood that ear-level hearing aids will be recommended more often for children. Safety factors and other practical issues that the audiologist must keep in mind in selecting a child's hearing aids are the provision of child-proof battery doors, volume control covers, and a multiyear warranty (Stelmachowicz, 1996). Simple recasing of the ITE instrument as often as necessary by the manufacturer readily solves the problem of a child outgrowing their custom molded and fitted hearing aids.

Binaural Hearing Aids. The critical need for optimal hearing by infants, toddlers, and children demands the use of binaural hearing aids. The authors' policy is that *all children should be fitted with binaural hearing aids whenever possible* to maximize auditory potential. The fitting of binaural amplification with all hearing-impaired children should prevail unless an absolute contraindication (such as total deafness in one ear) is determined. A binaural hearing aid system consists of two complete hearing aids worn simultaneously— one in each ear. Fortunately, most third-party payers now recognize the importance of two hearing aids for hearing-impaired children to achieve their highest learning potentials.

Common wisdom prevails that two ears are better than one; thus, two hearing aids must be better than one hearing aid. Obviously, the binaural hearing system is twice as expensive as a single, monaural system. Hearing-impaired adults often prefer binaural systems. It is of interest that an audiologist can often successfully add a second hearing aid to a monaural hearing aid user, but the reverse is never true. That is, a binaural hearing aid user will never change to a monaural listening system. Despite the additional expense of two hearing aids, there is obviously something about using binaural hearing aids that makes better listening for hearing-impaired users.

Mueller and Hawkins (1990) presented an up-to-date review of the advantages of binaural hearing aid systems. They described three main advantages for binaural hearing aids: *binaural summation, elimination of head shadow,* and *binaural squelch.* These three factors work together to improve speech recognition for the hearing-impaired binaural amplification user.

- Binaural Summation. When a sound is presented binaurally, it is perceived louder than if the same sound is presented monaurally. Hawkins, Prosek, Walden, and Montgomery (1987) demonstrated that persons with bilateral sensorineural hearing loss have 6–10 dB of binaural summation. This loudness summation has significant benefit to hearing-impaired amplification users, since they can have equivalent perceived loudness at lower volume control set-

tings, thus reducing potential feedback problems and prolonging battery life.

- Elimination of Head Shadow. Head shadow occurs when an individual is wearing a single hearing aid and speech is presented from the nonaided side. Head shadow can attenuate the speech signal 6–12 dB as sound "bends" around the head to reach the hearing aid on the opposite ear. Thus, the binaurally hearing-impaired patient who is unfortunately wearing only one hearing aid is constantly attempting to manipulate the hearing aid to be on the side of the speech signal. This situation adds increased stress to the monaural hearing aid user who is often in situations in which it is not easy to continually turn the hearing aid toward the signal of interest, as might be encountered in theater seats, at a dinner party, or in a car. According to Mueller and Hawkins (1990), the monaural hearing aid user may lose as much as 10–18 dB of gain compared with the binaural hearing aid wearer in the same situation because of the head shadow effect.

- Binaural Squelch. Binaural squelch is the term applied to the reported ability of the auditory system to diminish noise or reverberation more efficiently when input is received from two ears rather than one ear. The immediate effect of this phenomenon is to increase speech recognition in background noise for the binaural hearing aid user.

Other advantages attributed to binaural hearing aids include increased auditory localization abilities, improved sound quality (fidelity), spatial balance, and ease of listening.

It may be difficult to demonstrate empirically the improvement provided by binaural hearing aids versus a monaural fitting, especially in sound-treated test rooms. Traditional hearing aid evaluation procedures using functional gain measurements at threshold levels are hard-pressed to show superior performance of binaural hearing aids. As audiologists have gained first-hand experience in dispensing, fitting, and managing patients with hearing aids, the improvement in speech recognition in noise created by binaural hearing aids has proven the superiority of listening with two ears rather than one ear.

Traditionally, the only pediatric patients fitted with binaural hearing aids were those children with bilateral, symmetrical hearing loss. However, asymmetrical hearing loss should not be a contraindication to binaural amplification. The challenge for the audiologist is to balance the performance of the two hearing aids until aided symmetry is achieved. The use of computerized probe-microphone–aided measurements from each ear canal is critical to achieve symmetry in a binaural hearing aid fitting for a child with asymmetrical bilateral hearing loss.

Auditory Deprivation. Intriguing research projects were reported by Silman, Gelfand, and Silverman (1984) and Gelfand (1987) to evaluate the phenomenon of auditory deprivation in monaural and binaural aided adult subjects. The auditory performance of the subjects before the use of hearing aids was compared with their auditory performance after 4–5 years of hearing aid use to determine whether the unaided ears showed effects of auditory deprivation. The most revealing finding was that the speech recognition scores remained stable in both ears of the binaurally fitted patients, while the unaided scores of the monaurally fitted patients showed a significant reduction, apparently the result of auditory deprivation. Later studies showed that the deprivation from lack of amplification could be overcome with resultant increase in speech understanding scores when amplification was added to the previously unaided ears (Silverman & Silman, 1990; Silverman & Emmer, 1993; Boothroyd, 1993). These studies show that auditory function does

indeed deteriorate in the unaided ears of patients with bilateral sensorineural hearing loss who wear monaural hearing aid fittings. The results of these studies have important implications that aid in understanding the necessity of binaural hearing aids for all children with hearing impairment.

Frequency Response. The frequency response of a hearing instrument is defined as the output of the transducer in cycles per second across time. Early in the history of hearing aid fitting a controversy arose between the "selective" frequency response proponents and those preferring a "flat," more uniform response curve. The controversy soon became rather one-sided, with the selective fitting proponents enjoying the recognition and acceptance of the majority. The selective method was based on the patient's audiogram and provided amplification only where most needed. Amplification was restricted to the frequency areas in which the user still had residual hearing to be reached.

There has been a reevaluation of the importance of low-frequency hearing aid amplification, suggesting that the relative intensity level of the low-frequency band is critical. Danaher and Pickett (1975) clearly demonstrated that when a low-frequency sound is presented at high-intensity levels, a type of masking is produced that reduces the person's ability to detect sounds in the higher-frequency regions. This effect is termed *upward spread of masking* and occurs in normal-hearing persons and most persons with sensorineural loss. When amplified with a low-frequency emphasis aid, moderate levels of environmental noise may be sufficiently intense to produce spread of masking, making speech intelligibility frustratingly difficult for the hearing-impaired listener.

The audiologist's task is to discover an acoustic system that will provide the pediatric patient with all the acoustic cues necessary to achieve maximum use of his or her residual hearing for daily real-world communication, while minimizing the degradation of the speech signal through upward spread of masking or too much compression. This task is confounded when the patient is very young, nonverbal, or noncooperative.

Output. The maximum power output of the hearing aid describes the decibel level of the greatest possible intensity that a hearing aid is capable of producing through amplification. Mueller and Bright (1994) argue that measuring a patient's tolerance for loud sounds and the subsequent selection of a hearing aid's maximum saturation sound pressure level (OSPL90) may be the two most critical measurements of the hearing aid selection procedure. The authors believe that hearing aids should not be selected because of their power output alone. The output range of the hearing aid fixes the minimum-to-maximum decibel levels of the receiver when sound enters the microphone. Various electronic compression circuits may be used to suppress automatically loud sound picked up by the hearing aid. Programmable and digital hearing instruments may provide a selection of more than one type of compression circuit within the same hearing aid.

Typically, the audiologist adjusts the hearing aid output control so that sound is limited below the child's level of discomfort. If the OSPL90 is too high, intense sounds will cause physical discomfort to the child and may be the cause of additional hearing loss. If the OSPL90 setting is too low, the child will not receive sounds at an adequate sensation level to understand speech clearly, and the hearing aid output will become saturated and possibly introduce the compression circuit more often than necessary (Dillon & Storey, 1998). Although one would not purposefully choose hearing aids with inadequate output, a common error is to "overfit" by selecting hearing aids with too much power. Seewald, Ross, and Spiro (1985) pointed out that the selection of real-ear

OSPL90 is a nearly always a compromise. The hearing aid's power output must be high enough to provide adequate amplification without exceeding the saturation level frequently (which drives the hearing aid into compression mode), yet the OSPL90 must not exceed the child's loudness discomfort level.

Establishing loudness discomfort levels in children can be a challenge. Kawell et al. (1988) described a technique for use with children that uses a set of illustrations that represent various levels of loudness (Fig. 9-6). The child's task is simply to point to the drawing that most closely represents his or her perception of the loudness of the sound. This procedure can be used under earphones, with insert earphones, or in aided conditions.

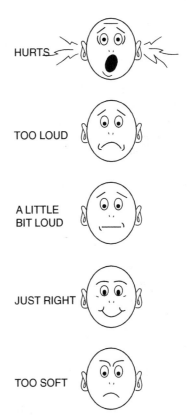

Figure 9-6. Pediatric loudness level identification chart for determining loudness discomfort levels in children. (Adapted from Kawell, M., Kopun, J., & Stelmachowicz, P. (1988). Loudness discomfort levels in children. *Ear and Hearing, 9,*).

Gain. Hearing aid gain is defined as the difference in amplitude between the input signal and the output signal. The authors attempt to assure optimal audibility of the speech spectrum between 750 and 3000 Hz while avoiding overamplification of the low-frequency energy found in background noise. Gain adjustment may be accomplished to a limited degree through the gain controls of the hearing aid or by programming advanced technology hearing aids.

The selection of appropriate gain in children's hearing aids is an especially difficult task, as the youngsters often cannot verbalize their perceptions of the amplified sound quality. Thus, we use a number of *prescriptive formulae* to determine target gain requirements relative to the patient's auditory thresholds. There are different prescriptive rules to be used with various types of hearing loss, but all are based on auditory thresholds in each ear. Obviously, in infants and young children, the auditory thresholds established may be rather tentative. Then the selection of an appropriate formula and prescriptive protocol depends on the personal preference and experience of the audiologist. Knowledgeable audiologists agree that none of the prescriptive rules provide a precise prediction of appropriate hearing aid performance, but rather since each rule varies by formula and methodology, there is little to suggest that one prescriptive technique is intrinsically superior to another. Hawkins (1992) provides a thorough discussion of the advantages and limitations of each of the prescriptive rules described below.

- Berger Rule. This prescriptive fitting formula is a half-gain rule with more emphasis around the speech frequency of 2000 Hz.

- POGO Rule. This technique (*p*rescription *o*f *g*ain and *o*utput) is based on the half-gain rule but provides reduction amplification for the low frequencies. A POGO II rule has also been described

with a special correction factor for hearing losses greater than 65 dB HL.

- One-Third Gain Rule. This prescriptive fitting rule uses less amplification gain than the other methods and is thus especially useful with mild hearing impairment.

- NAL, NAL-NL1, and NAL-RP Rules. These methods developed at the National Acoustic Laboratories in Sydney, Australia, may be the most popular prescription for determining appropriate hearing aid gain. The techniques are an attempt to amplify all the frequency bands of speech to equal loudness.

- Desired Sensation Level (DSL). This hearing aid fitting method was specifically developed for use with children. All measures are defined in dB SPL as measured in the ear canal to allow direct comparison among all audiometric, acoustic, and electroacoustic variables that pertain to the hearing instrument fitting. A computerized version of the procedure used for fitting nonlinear amplification instruments is known as DSL.

Although these formulae can be calculated manually for each hearing aid patient to determine target gain values at each frequency, this requires complex calculations. Most audiologists rely on manufacturer's software programs or automated probe-microphone instruments to calculate the gain values based on any of the target rules at each frequency. Typically the automatic calculation results in a display of the target on the video monitor.

HEARING AID VERIFICATION METHODS

Hearing aid fittings in children may be accomplished through a number of different techniques. Historically, the most popular procedure for verifying hearing aid fittings in children was the functional gain method. Functional gain has been generally replaced by computerized probe-microphone techniques, but the knowledgeable audiologist is always prepared to utilize behavioral measurements to verify the benefits of the selected amplification system. The steps of the various procedures do have some elements in common, such as preselection of the hearing aid(s), determination of frequency response, output characteristics, and acoustic or electronic adjustments and modifications. Every fitting should incorporate some procedure to verify or validate the final fitting. The material presented below is not intended to be a complete treatise on hearing aid selection and fitting, but rather an overview of the special considerations that must be incorporated in the pediatric hearing aid evaluation. Readers interested in more complete information about hearing aids are referred to the textbooks edited by Valente (1994, 1996; Dillon, 2000).

Parents of young children must understand that the hearing aid fitting process is an ongoing activity to be analyzed and reconsidered at each clinic visit (Fig. 9-7). As more audiometric information is obtained and careful observation of the child's behavior and development is noted with the hearing aids in place, the audiologist may decide to modify or adjust the hearing aids when necessary. When available, computerized probe-microphone measurements should be conducted at each clinic visit as a means of monitoring the performance of the child's hearing aids as they are worn. Permanent hard copy of these real-ear measurements will permit comparative evaluation of the hearing aids' performance from visit to visit. Probe-microphone measurements should be used to identify malfunctioning hearing aids that need repair or adjustment, particularly in children who are too young or unsophisticated to voice complaint.

Especially important in working with hearing-impaired children and their hearing aids is the concept of a "target" fitting. The prescriptive formula, based on auditory threshold measures in quiet, serves as the basis for defining target gain of the

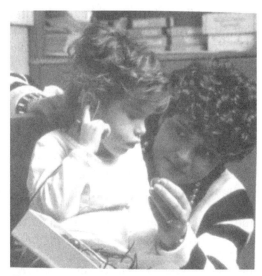

Figure 9-7. Hearing-impaired children have special needs and require considerable clinical attention to obtain maximum benefit from their hearing aids.

hearing aid. When insertion gain of the hearing aid matches the prescriptive target gain within some definable degree of accuracy at each test frequency, the procedure is considered successful (Fabry & Schum, 1994). The target fitting technique, either with behavioral measurements or the preferred probe-microphone measurements, is the audiologist's best prediction for final optimal amplification, taking into account the patient's audiometric configuration, the hearing aid frequency response, and its gain and output characteristics. It is often possible, once the target fitting has been ascertained, to modify or adjust the frequency response of the hearing aids to approximate or overlay, as closely as possible, the desired (target) amplified configuration. To be sure, all facts and data concerning the critical factors of successful hearing aid fittings are not yet available. Although audiologists can now control the shape, smoothness, and bandwidth of the amplified frequency response precisely with programmable instruments, there has yet to emerge a "best" way to determine insertion gain or output levels necessary to achieve optimal speech intelligibility.

Probe-Microphone Measurements.

Computerized probe-microphone hearing aid measurement and analysis is the method of choice in fitting hearing aids on infants, toddlers, and older children (Fig. 9-8). This technique utilizes a soft silicone tube that is inserted into the ear canal, under the earmold, with the hearing aid turned on and properly seated in the ear canal. The amplified sound in the ear canal is picked up by the silicone tube probe-microphone, subjected to signal processing by a special-purpose computer, and presented on a computer monitor and/or hard copy printout. Real-ear probe-microphone measurements permit the audiologist to know precisely the aided frequency response and output levels of the amplified signal intensity at the child's eardrum. Hawkins and Northern (1992) have published a thorough discussion of the use of probe-microphone measurements with hearing instruments in pediatric patients with hearing loss.

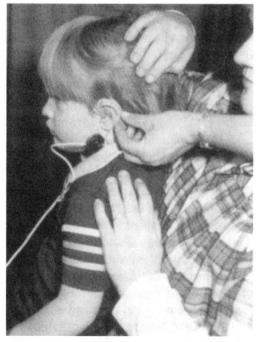

Figure 9-8. Computerized probe-microphone measurements provide real-ear electroacoustic information about hearing aid performance that is especially valuable during the fitting and verification process.

Dalsgaard and Dyrlund-Jensen (1976) used a probe-microphone in the ear canal to demonstrate that a natural resonance in adult ears occurs at 2700 Hz with 17 dB of amplification. Thus, nature has provided a natural amplifier based on the size and shape of the ear canal that actually helps amplify the frequency spectrum of speech. The natural resonance peak is termed *the real-ear unaided gain* (REUG) and is expressed in dB SPL at the highest frequency peak in the unoccluded ear canal. It is critical to be aware that the REUG in infant ear canals occurs at a much higher frequency (6000–7200 Hz) than in adults. In fact, studies have documented that the resonance frequency of the external ear decreases gradually with age from 7200 Hz at birth until the adult resonance value of 2700 Hz is reached when the child reaches the second year of life (Kruger, 1987). The higher resonance in the infant is due to a smaller concha and shorter ear canal length. This information is important in selecting appropriate hearing aid frequency characteristics in babies.

Unfortunately, when an earmold or ITE hearing aid is placed into the ear canal, the acoustic properties of the system are disrupted, the natural ear canal resonance is altered in frequency, and sound is diminished. The presence of the earmold or custom hearing aid in the ear canal creates an obstruction that tends to keep natural sound out of the ear canal, an effect called *insertion loss.* One must be sure that the recommended amplification has sufficient gain to overcome the insertion loss provided by the earmold or hearing instrument's obstruction of the ear canal.

A major advantage of the computerized probe-microphone real-ear measuring device is that the entire amplification system is evaluated so the effects of programming changes, tubing, earmold, vents, and filters can be measured precisely. Physiologic differences among children, such as the length, diameter, and shape of the ear canal, are extremely important fitting considerations and are taken into account in probe-microphone measurements. Computerized probe-microphone measurements provide quick, objective data regarding insertion gain, ear canal sound pressure levels, and the telemagnetic response of the hearing aid. The measurements may be read in 1 dB intervals so that every acoustic modification or electroacoustic adjustment made with the hearing aids will be noted clearly.

Most probe-microphone equipment includes a "listening" circuit and lightweight earphones, so that the amplified sound can be heard by the child's parents and family, who thereby gain full appreciation of exactly how their youngster's hearing aids amplify environmental and speech sounds (Northern, 1992). Sullivan (1985) suggested that predrilling a 1.5-mm hole in the earmold, which is then sealed with a removal plug, could accommodate the probe-tube microphone. The plug may be removed when future probe-microphone measurements are desired.

Computerized probe-microphone measurements have numerous distinct advantages over functional gain measurements as a method of assessing hearing aid performance, especially with hearing-impaired children. These advantages include: (1) elimination of dependency on the behavioral threshold responses; (2) electroacoustic information across the entire frequency range of interest rather than only octave or half-octave intervals; (3) no contamination of aided threshold measures by internal hearing aid and/or room noise, a significant problem with functional gain measurements when hearing thresholds are in the normal or near-normal range; and (4) considerable savings in time and efficiency, with improved accuracy and reliability in the electroacoustic analysis of the hearing aid under evaluation (Fig. 9-9).

A valuable aspect of this technique is the ability to plot hearing aid responses visually on the video screen target. The audiologist selects a prescriptive method

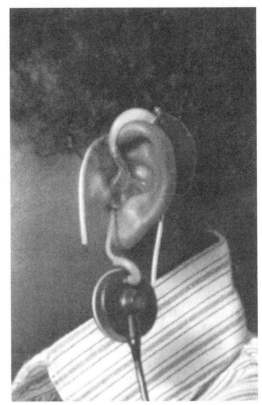

Figure 9-9. Close-up view of computerized probe-microphone system in place.

of gain prediction (e.g., DSL, NAL-NL1) to achieve the best amplified responses for each child. Then, acoustic measurements are performed in the ear with probe-microphone systems to provide information regarding the total effect of the amplified hearing aids with minimal patient cooperation. Comparison of the probe-microphone responses with the target amplification response permits an immediate comparison of the hearing instrument performance and the desired target fit. The hearing aid can be reprogrammed as often as necessary until the best fit to the target gain or output is achieved.

An especially important concept used in pediatric hearing aid measurements is the real-ear to coupler difference (RECD). The RECD, as it implies, is the difference in dB between the output of a hearing aid (or insert earphone) in the real ear versus a 2-

cc coupler. Because there is considerable variability in children's ear canal volumes, it is best to measure the RECD for each individual. Before probe-microphone tests, there was no way to know what the actual output of a hearing aid might be in a child's small ear canal. The probe-microphone technique allows the audiologist to determine the actual SPL that exists in the ear canal for each hearing instrument setting. This knowledge has important implications for setting the OSPL90 of the hearing aid as well as determining the appropriate gain and frequency response (Mueller, 1996).

A recommended procedure for probe-microphone real-ear hearing aid fittings in hearing-impaired infants and children is as follows:

- Examine the child with an otoscope to be sure ear canals are clear of cerumen or other debris.

- Situate infant or child in the parent's lap approximately 1 m from the loudspeaker.

- Set marker on silicone probe tube at 5 mm longer than earmold canal.

- Insert probe into child's open ear canal with marker at tragus so that marker is observable.

- Measure "open" real-ear unaided response (REUR) as the baseline for the insertion gain measure (this step is not necessary in the DSL or DSL[i/o] procedures).

- Enter hearing minimal response data or hearing threshold data into the probe-microphone computer program.

- Select the prescriptive fitting formula of choice to establish the target goal at each frequency to be achieved with "ideal" amplification response.

- Place hearing aid and earmold in the infant's or child's ear; a silicone probe-microphone is placed in the ear canal under the earmold with marker observable at the same initial tragus location used for REUR.

- Measure real-ear insertion gain (REIG) and compare to target insertion gain response on the video monitor.

- Make acoustic modifications or adjust the hearing aid response programs as necessary to achieve "ideal" amplification response and remeasure REIG.

- Measure in situ real-ear response (REAR) to monitor the overall SPL of the amplification system in the ear canal; be sure that output measures do not exceed loudness discomfort levels.

- Establish the child's RECE to estimate OSPL90 values.

- Attempt to achieve smooth response curves for all measurements with minimal peaks and valleys across the frequency response range.

- Print out results of each measurement for future comparative evaluations of the hearing aid's performance.

The use of probe-microphone measurements in fitting hearing aids and managing amplification with hearing-impaired children provides the audiologist with objective and reliable data. The audiologist and parents must be aware, however, that the REAR should not be misconstrued to represent what the child "hears." Hearing, of course, requires cerebral integration of speech and environmental sounds. Probe-microphone evaluation gives audiologists confidence in their selection and fitting of hearing aids for this difficult-to-test population, provides objective information to resolve hearing aid problems, and permits in-office adjustments, reprogramming, and modifications to hearing instruments.

DSL. The DSL is a method for fitting hearing aids developed specifically for determining amplified speech targets for linear and nonlinear gain hearing aids in children (Seewald, Zelisko, Ramji, & Jamieson, 1991). The DSL procedure requires a series of calculations best per-

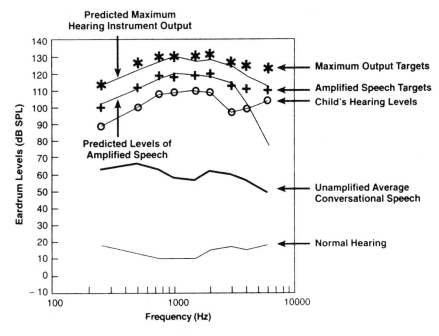

Figure 9-10. Overview of the DSL hearing aid fitting protocol displayed on a SPLogram. Note the maximum output targets and amplified speech targets. The required hearing aid gain is the difference between the average speech spectrum and the amplified speech targets. (With permission from Seewald, R., Ross, M., & Stelmachowicz, P. (1987). Selecting and verifying hearing aid performance characteristics for children. *Journal of the Academy of Rehabilitative Audiology,* 20:25–38.

formed with computer-assisted software (1996). DSL is based on a systematic protocol to provide amplified speech signals that are audible, comfortable, and undistorted across a broad frequency range. The method applies age-appropriate individual or average values for relevant acoustic characteristics that are known to vary as a function of age—specifically, external ear resonance characteristics and real-ear to 2-cc coupler differences. A special advantage to the DSL method is that all measurements are made or converted to ear canal SPL. The real-ear SPL values of the residual auditory area and hearing aid targets are displayed on an SPLogram graph. An algorithm of the protocol has been developed for nonlinear hearing aids and is known as DSL[i/o] (Seewald et al., 1997). Figure 9-10 shows a schematic representation of the DSL method.

Lewis (1999) points out that (1) children typically wear their hearing instruments at fixed settings, (2) the amplification characteristics selected are important in the acquisition of speech and language, (3) the amplification characteristics may be based on limited audiologic information, and (4) a number of age factors are included in the DSL approach that are important to consider in fitting amplification to children. The computerized DSL program allows the audiologist to enter threshold information obtained by probe-microphone thresholds in SPL, insert earphones, TDH earphones, or sound field measurements. All threshold information is converted to ear canal SPL using specific coupler to real-ear transforms as individually measured or by using age-appropriate transforms for REUR and RECD. Corrections may be inserted into the program for the style of hearing instrument to be fitted. The most recent version of the DSL [i/o] was developed to provide an algorithm for fitting wide dynamic range compression instruments with fixed and variable compression ratios.

Mueller and Hall (1998) describe the DSL method in three general steps:

- The residual auditory area is measured as the difference between the upper limit of comfort level and the child's auditory thresholds. The real-ear SPL of the upper limit of comfort is predicted from the real-ear SPL of the hearing thresholds using RECD measures.

- The targets for amplified speech are defined. The amplified speech targets are approximately midway between the hearing thresholds and the upper limit of comfort contours. The target gain for linear hearing aids is determined by calculating the difference between the one-third octave band level of the long-term average speech spectrum and the SPL from the real-ear target output SPL for speech. The calculated amount of linear gain is then applied over a range of input levels.

  - The target maximum output is defined. The target real-ear maximum output is set to the predicted upper limit of the comfort level. The predicted upper limit of comfort levels used to set the real-ear maximum output are 1 standard deviation below mean loudness discomfort levels (LDL).

After determining the selected hearing aid frequency response, gain values, and maximum output levels, it is critical to verify the amplification parameters in the ear canal of the pediatric patient. Probe-microphone measurements are the procedure of choice for verification of the electroacoustic characteristics of the hearing aids. Because of the large variability in RECD that exists among young children, all measurements should be made with custom fit earmolds in place. The Pediatric Working Group (1996) emphatically recommended that no facility or audiologist should fit hearing aids to young children if the proper equipment for electroacoustic evaluation and verification is not readily available.

Functional Gain. Functional gain is the difference between *unaided* and *aided* minimal response levels obtained through behavioral threshold measurements. The purpose of functional gain measurements is to compare unaided and aided responses under identical conditions. The young child is typically seated on the parent's lap between two sound field speakers. Through visual response audiometry (VRA), minimal response levels are obtained for speech signals and narrow bands of noise, 250–8000 Hz, without the hearing aids. Then with the hearing aids in place on the child and the gain controls set at preselected levels, minimal response levels are again obtained for speech and narrow bands of noise. The difference between the aided and unaided minimal response levels is the functional gain. If the functional gain measurements are different from the target gain, appropriate adjustments should be made.

Because functional gain measures are based on behavioral responses, caution must be exercised in interpreting results. Behavioral audiometry techniques consistent with the child's chronologic and mental ages should be used as described in Chapter 6. The variable factors are the degree of hearing loss, the level of language skills, and the intellectual function of the child. A mentally retarded child of 9 years, for example, may need to be managed with techniques designed for a 3-year-old. Uses for functional gain measurements include (1) comparing the performance of hearing aids with different internal settings, (2) obtaining information regarding various types of earmolds, (3) monitoring stability of the young child's amplification system over time, and (4) demonstrating improvement in unaided versus aided conditions. However, since functional gain measurements are typically made in 5 dB intervals, smaller differences due to minor hearing aid adjustment may not be noticeable with functional gain measurements.

Some clinicians believe that "reasonable" aided hearing levels can be estimated in relation to the degree of hearing loss. A child with greater than 100 dB of average hearing loss should be responsive with hearing aids to sound field presentations at approximately 35 dB HL; in a similar fashion, the child with hearing loss of greater than 75 dB can be expected to show aided responses of 25 dB HL; hearing loss of 50 dB or less should have near normal hearing aided responses to sound field stimuli. Greater hearing aid gain can be tolerated by the child with a conductive or mixed loss than by the child with a sensorineural loss. For example, a child with a conductive loss of 60 dB HL (average) can easily be fit with hearing aid gain that brings his or her awareness level to 20 dB HL or even less. A child with a sensorineural loss of 60 dB may be fit successfully with a gain that brings the aided speech threshold to 20 dB HL. The authors recommend evaluation of the hearing aid fitting and settings in the sound booth by the audiologist every 3 months until the child is 2 years of age and thereafter at least every 6 months.

Major disadvantages occur during functional gain procedures in young children, as pointed out by Stelmachowicz, Seewald, and Gorga (1998). Functional gain measurements reflect performance only at minimal response or threshold levels, with no information about the input/output characteristics or the output limiting performance of the hearing aids. Thus, there is no assurance that the child will receive meaningful perception of speech at intensities sufficiently above threshold with appropriate output limiting to prevent overamplification. Minimal response levels established in the sound field might underestimate functional gain when low-frequency unaided hearing lev-

els are near normal limits. Of course, the success of functional gain measurements rests with the audiologist's abilities to determine accurate measurements in the sound field — which may be difficult to do in the case of young infant patients or other difficult-to-test youngsters.

Infants are difficult to test behaviorally with hearing aids. Initially, the hearing aids are set and fitted using behavioral measurements in the sound booth to speech stimuli or narrow band noise signals. Aided behavioral responses, unconditioned or conditioned, are observed from infants and small children by the audiologist and or his or her assistant as well as the child's parents. The child is tested with various levels of gross speech through a loudspeaker. Hearing thresholds of should be established as well as behavioral measurements of the child's reactions to sounds presented at higher levels. Ongoing evaluation of the hearing aid fitting is done while the child is in the home environment or in therapy sessions.

The child of 2 or 3 years and older who can be play conditioned or taught hand-raising responses to sounds can be given a satisfactory functional gain hearing aid evaluation. It may be necessary to schedule more than one testing session for the 2- or 3-year-old. The child's tolerance for testing has a limited time span, and it is fruitless to try to extend it. Some bright children between 24 and 36 months of age are capable of learning play conditioning techniques for speech or pure tones that can sustain their interest for a reasonable time. A 2-year-old may learn play conditioning long enough to give a speech awareness level or a threshold at one frequency before quitting the task. Two or three frequencies are sufficient to approximate the hearing loss: 500 and 2000 Hz, or 500, 1000, 2000 Hz. Measures of 3000 Hz should be included if possible. These frequencies will represent the major frequency range of hearing aid amplification for speech. The variable factors are the degree of hearing loss, the level of language skills, and the intellectual function of the child. A developmentally delayed child of 9 chronologic years, for example, may need to be managed with techniques designed for a 3-year-old. The variable factors are the degree of hearing loss, the level of language skills, and the intellectual function of the child.

When receptive language is present in the child, testing can be accomplished easily through functional gain measures with hearing aids. When there is expressive language present, finer word recognition tests such as the Pediatric Speech Intelligibility (PSI) test (described in Chapter 6) are applicable. The cooperative older child, between ages 6 and 10 years, can be given more sophisticated behavioral audiology tests.

One should always keep in mind the audiologist's adage: "The best hearing aids are the ones that are worn." The pediatric hearing aid evaluation procedure is nearly always an ongoing process, and parents must be aware that changes will probably be made in the hearing aid fitting as more accurate and detailed information is determined regarding the child's hearing loss, development, social-educational needs, and special circumstances. Occasionally, the audiologist should be prepared to accept a temporary compromise hearing aid fitting to maintain the child's and parent's interest and cooperation, knowing full well that modifications to the hearing aids or finer acoustic tuning can be accomplished at a near-future appointment session.

In general, the principles behind the selection of hearing aids for children are no different from hearing aid characteristics used by adults. Libby (1982) summarized these considerations as follows: (1) an amplification system with a smooth frequency response and no sharp peaks is selected; (2) plans are made to compensate for the 10–15 dB insertion loss at 2700 Hz created by the occluding earmold; (3) a wide-frequency bandwidth ensures greater fidelity for speech and music; (4) an appropriate balance between high-frequency amplification for speech recognition and low-frequency energy for intelligibility and sound quality is preserved; and (5) the output of the hearing aid does not exceed the patient's loudness discomfort level.

Aided Auditory Brainstem Evoked Response. Some authors have suggested using ABR measurements for hearing aid evaluation in young children because patient participation is not necessary. However, questions have been raised about the accuracy of ABR hearing aid measurements as well as genuine concerns about the lengthy time and high expense of the procedure. A major limiting factor is that the ABR technique does not provide specific frequency information. Mahoney (1985) proposed a hearing aid-ABR testing protocol and Cox and Metz (1980) suggested simply that the gain of the hearing aid be adjusted to the level at which additional increases in gain no longer produce further decreases in ABR wave V latency. Seitz and Kisiel (1990) published an extensive discussion of hearing aid assessment and ABR. The availability of probe-microphone measurements and the development of the DSL protocols make aided ABR evaluation superfluous.

Acoustic Reflex Method. McCandless and Miller (1972) described a technique for establishing hearing aid gain by use of acoustic reflex thresholds as measured with an immittance meter. With this procedure, the patient is fitted with a hearing aid to one ear and an immittance probe tip is placed in the contralateral ear. Using constant sound pressure input of average environmental sounds or conversational speech, the gain control of the hearing aid is slowly raised until the acoustic reflex is barely observed in the contralateral ear. A gain setting is accomplished by adjusting the controls just below this level, which will be safely under the patient's loudness discomfort level. Ross and Tomassetti (1980) indicate that the OSPL90 of the hearing aid should not exceed the SPL that elicits an aided stapedial reflex. The acoustic reflex will not be present in patients with severe to profound sensorineural hearing loss or in patients with unilateral or bilateral middle ear effusion.

HEARING AID COUPLING AND MODIFICATIONS

Today's audiologist/dispenser must be cognizant of the methods of hearing aid response modification technology. Level and spectral modifications can be implemented to produce a uniform effect over the entire spectrum or to effect selectively the frequency ranges of the overall spectrum. Modifications to the hearing aid response can be influenced by a number of factors including the microphone location, frequency response adjustments, the earhook and tubing length, diameter, configuration and filter characteristics, the earmold shape and size, the seal or openness of the earmold (which can strongly influence low-frequency amplification), and the ear canal space between the tip of the earmold and the tympanic membrane. One of the most important electroacoustic characteristics of a hearing aid is the absence of "peaks and valleys" in the frequency response curve.

The acoustic coupling of the hearing aid refers to the "plumbing" of the system (i.e., all of the external components that convey sound from the hearing aid itself into the ear canal of the user). With BTE hearing aids, the acoustic coupling refers to the earmold, tubing, and earhook. Audiologists now understand the importance of the acoustic coupling in modifying the performance of the hearing aid. Inadequate acoustic coupling efforts can essentially ruin the performance of even the best of hearing aids.

The earmold itself is an essential feature of the hearing aid system (Fig. 9-11). It

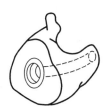
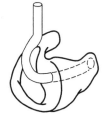

TYPICAL STANDARD MOLD   **TYPICAL SKELETON MOLD**

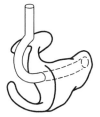
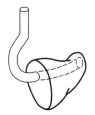

Figure 9-11. Illustrative earmold styles including basic full standard mold, skeletal molds, and a canal mold.

provides support for the hearing aid on or in the patient's external ear while directing the sound into the ear canal and, if properly fitted, prevents acoustic feedback. Because even minor variations in the fitting and configuration of the earmold can alter the electroacoustic parameters of the hearing aid, it is important to evaluate each hearing aid with the earmold that is to be used with it. This may require two or more sessions for fitting hearing aids on children—one session during which the earmold impression is obtained, and an additional session after the permanent custom earmold has been fabricated. It is particularly difficult to conduct hearing aid evaluations with children using stock earmolds, since the stock earmolds often do not fit well in the child's ear canals and most certainly do not represent how the hearing aid will perform when the child has his or her own earmold. The pinna continues to grow and the concha changes shape until the child reaches approximately 9 years of age. Thus, earmolds and custom ITE hearing aids should routinely be reevaluated and remade every 3–6 months during the child's early years and once a year after age 5 to ensure satisfactory fit.

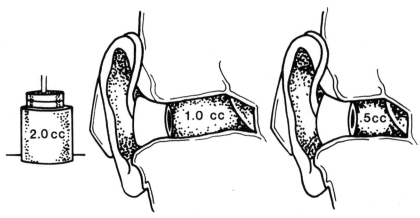

Figure 9-12. Consideration must be given to the child's small ear canal volume, relative to the hearing aid specifications measured in a 2-cc coupler, to avoid overamplification.

The earmold may be crafted in many ways (with open vents, various tubing, filters, and so on) to enhance the hearing aid. The material of the earmold is relatively insignificant in terms of general acoustics. The most important factor about the earmold is that acoustic feedback must be prevented if the child is to obtain maximum benefit from the hearing aid. Programmable circuits in high-technology hearing aids often include a special circuit for "sensing" the presence of feedback and making automatic frequency response changes to eliminate the feedback immediately.

EAR CANAL VOLUME AND HEARING AIDS

Hearing aid technical specifications are reported in decibels measured in a hard-walled 2-cc coupler. The hearing aid specifications relative to a 2-cc cavity are altered significantly when the hearing aid is coupled tightly to an ear canal that is less than 2 cc in volume. In fact, each time the cavity volume is reduced by one-half, sound pressure is increased by 6 dB. It can be expected that hearing aid sound pressures measured in a 2-cc cavity will be delivered to an adult 1 cc canal with 6 dB more intensity than that shown on the standard hearing aid frequency response curve. Infants with very small ear canal volumes of 0.5 cc or less may actually receive as much as 12–15 dB more

amplification than that shown on hearing aid technical specification sheets (Fig. 9-12).

The most common problem in pediatric hearing aid fitting is overamplification. Clinicians who select hearing aids based on 2-cc coupler measurements must be aware, therefore, that overamplification may result from coupling an aid and a full earmold to an ear having a volume of less than 2.0 cc. The 2-cc coupler underestimates aided SPL relative to the human ear canal by as much as 15 dB in the higher frequencies. The acoustic immittance meter can provide important information if the physical volume test (PVT) is conducted to estimate ear canal volume before the hearing aid is selected. More importantly, each pediatric hearing aid evaluation must include a probe-microphone real-ear aided response (REAR) measurement of the overall SPL in the child's ear canal to verify in situ amplification levels.

CAN HEARING AIDS DAMAGE HEARING?

Clinicians often worry that powerful hearing aids fitted to children may cause additional hearing damage due to overamplification. Indeed, case studies suggest that the use of hearing aids may cause temporary and permanent threshold shift, resulting in further hearing loss. Based on their experiences with two patients who exhibited temporary increases in hearing loss following hearing aid use, Heffernan and Simons (1979) suggested the following routine pediatric protocol: (1) check performance with the new hearing aid within 30 days of purchase, (2) electroacoustic analysis of the new aid within 30 days of purchase, (3) monthly appointments thereafter to monitor hearing thresholds until the hearing levels have stabilized for at least 3 months of continual hearing aid use, (4) reevaluation at least every 3 months for the next calendar year, and (5) annual otologic and audiologic evaluations as long as the aid is worn.

Macrae and Farrant (1965) evaluated changes in the aided and unaided ears of 87 children and concluded that individuals with sensorineural hearing loss should be fitted with limited maximal power output hearing aids, and frequent audiologic follow-up of aided children should be required. Macrae (1968a,b) found temporary threshold shift in the aided ears of children with sensorineural deafness following use of powerful hearing aids. He measured the hearing levels of children from a school for the deaf on Friday afternoon after the youngsters had worn their hearing aids all week and then deprived the children of amplification over the weekend until the following Monday morning. Hearing levels in the children showed improvement on Monday morning but again deteriorated after 4 hours of hearing aid use. A comprehensive review of the literature by Mills (1975) concluded that "the results of all studies indicate that habitual use of a hearing aid is not associated with additional deterioration of hearing in a large majority of persons tested. In some subjects, however, decreases in auditory sensitivity are observed." Rintelmann and Bess (1988) summarized details of several experimental investigations regarding the use of amplification and its effect on residual hearing.

After considerable study of the possible deleterious effect of hearing aids on children, the authors offer the following considerations to alleviate or lessen the possibility of inadvertent traumatic hearing loss related to overamplification:

- Additional hearing loss is most likely related to the use of extremely high levels of maximal power output that exceed 130 dB SPL that could result in levels as high as 150 dB SPL in a child's ear canal. Hearing aid recommendations for children with sensorineural hearing loss should include only hearing aids with less than 130 dB as determined by probe-microphone measurements in the ear canal.

- Although we recognize that traumatic hearing loss may be related to hearing aid use, the incidence seems quite small, and our concern is by no means to be interpreted as contradictory to amplification. In fact, the authors believe that denying a child a hearing aid during the critical language years may only be saving his or her hearing for no good purpose. If the aid is fitted too late, it will not help.

- Frequent follow-up audiometric and hearing aid evaluation is an absolute must for all children with sensorineural hearing loss who wear hearing aids. These children should be evaluated at least twice a year.

AMPLIFICATION IN THE CLASSROOM

One of the most important aspects of amplification is its use in the school or educational setting. Important technological advancements have occurred in the past few years that make amplification in the classroom an essential component in the education of hearing-impaired children. Excellent reviews of classroom amplification have been written by Ross (1992), Lewis (1994a) and Crandell, Smaldino, and Flexer (1995).

The acoustic environment in which hearing-impaired students learn typically has high noise levels and poor acoustic reverberation conditions. Studies conducted by Finitzo-Hieber (1981a) have shown that classroom acoustics are an important consideration that can be deleterious to the hearing-impaired student. The three critical factors are the level of noise in the classroom, the level of speech or the desired signal, and the amount of room acoustic reverberation. To be sure, certain architectural improvements, such as acoustically treated walls and ceilings, can be made in schoolrooms to help reduce unwanted noise and limit reverberation (Berg, 1993). In these days of mainstreaming disabled children, however, it is unlikely that all school classrooms can be modified to meet the needs of students with hearing impairment. Sanders (1965) reported the mean noise values of normal school classrooms to be between 55 and 65 dBA or as high as 69 dBA. In a normal setting, the teacher's voice measures approximately 65 dB, perhaps 5 dB louder than the background noise. For the student with a hearing impairment to hear the teacher's voice adequately, the speech signal should be 15–20 dB louder than the background noise. Bess and McConnell (1981) stated that the highest acceptable noise level in classrooms used by hearing-impaired children should not exceed 35 dBA.

Hearing aid users complain about the difficulty of understanding speech in the presence of background noise. It is well known that the noise in the environment is the most significant factor limiting benefit from the use of personal amplification. The challenge of helping hearing-impaired children who wear hearing aids in the typical noisy classroom situation creates serious problems for the teacher and the educational audiologist.

The personal hearing aid is, of course, the most common means of providing schoolroom amplification. The major drawback to the personal unit is its dependence on close distance to the speaker to achieve a high signal-to-noise effect. Unfortunately, this is difficult to control in the typical classroom. As the teacher moves away from the child, the increase in distance contributes quickly to the demise of signal amplification. When faced with a weak sound signal, the hearing aid user must turn up the gain of the unit, which also increases the background noise, creating unavoidable masking effects.

These problems led to the development of radio frequency transmission units (FM) with wireless microphones (Lewis, 1994b). FM amplification represents the best means of combating poor classroom acoustics. The teacher simply clips a transmitter to his or her belt or slips it into a pocket, positions the wireless microphone approximately 6 inches from the mouth, and speaks normally. The student wears a receiver to collect the speaker's voice while simultaneously minimizing the effect of background sounds. External receivers may be coupled to the personal earmolds or hearing aids worn by the hearing-impaired child. The student receivers can be adjusted to make them adaptable to a wide range of individual frequency responses. The American Speech-Language-Hearing Association (1994) developed guidelines for fitting and monitoring FM systems.

The major benefit of FM sound field amplification is that the system "amplifies" or "projects" the teacher's voice an average of +6–+10 dB above the classroom background noise by simply bridging the distance gap to the student. The FM system produces a uniform loudness level in the classroom that is unaffected by the teacher's location, while reducing the effects of noise, reverberation, and distance. The Improving Classroom Acoustics Project in Florida, reported by Rosenberg (1995), showed that FM sound field systems substantially improve the performance and behavior of normal-hearing children in regular school classrooms while enhancing their learning skills.

Although historically the FM system was a body-worn device, today's FM systems are typically coupled with a BTE hearing aid. A number of newer techniques permit the dovetailing of the personal hearing aid to the FM system through electrical, induction, or acoustical techniques. The advantages of an FM radio transmission through a wireless microphone attached close to the mouth of the speaker, sending high-fidelity signals to the personal hearing aid of the hearing-impaired child (who may be as far as 200 m [650 ft] away), are obvious. With the help of an FM system, the distance between the primary signal and the listener becomes effectively no more than 6 inches, the distance between the microphone and the speaker's mouth.

Hawkins (1984) states that the optimum classroom amplification system using the personal FM system concept would consist of (1) a directional microphone as close as possible to the teacher's mouth, (2) FM receiver coupled via direct input to binaural hearing aids on each hearing-impaired child, and (3) switch positions on the hearing aids allowing for choice of hearing aids only, FM reception only, or FM plus hearing aid microphones. Hawkins showed that the advantage of the FM system over hearing aids alone is substantial, equivalent to a 12 to 18 dB improvement in signal-to-noise ratio, when the child is in an optimal classroom position. For the child with less-than-optimal classroom position, the FM advantage over hearing aids alone is even greater. It is important to conduct a performance assessment of the FM system with the individual user. The use of probe-microphone measurements, behavioral audiometry, and 2-cc coupler measurements should be used to document improvement in hearing aid only, FM only, and FM plus hearing aid conditions.

The applications of the assistive personal listening system are much broader than just schoolroom use. Lewis (1994a) describes the benefits and limitations of large-area induction-loop-amplification systems and sound field amplification systems as alternatives to FM amplification. These assistive listening systems are practical for at-home use, learning sports activities, driver's education, and large group theater or auditorium activities. The assistive listening device or system should no longer be a "special instrument" consideration, but an important part of every hearing-impaired child's daily life (Fig. 9-13).

TACTILE SENSORY AIDS

Interest in tactile sensory aids for the hearing impaired has been a long-time research activity, although wide acceptance and utilization of these devices has not occurred. Levitt (1988) reviewed the issues underlying the development of tactile sensory aids and pointed out that interest in cochlear implants has stimulated new research in alternatives to traditional amplification instruments. Amid concern for the surgical intervention and finality of cochlear implants, many have questioned whether hearing-impaired persons could do just as well with a technologically advanced, noninvasive sensory aid.

Tactile aids change auditory signals into either vibratory or electrical patterns on the skin. The vibrotactile approach presents a vibration to the skin through a bone-conduction vibrator, a small solenoid, or other mechanical transducer. The electrotactile approach presents the acoustic signal through the skin via a tiny electrical current. As Roeser (1985) described it, "The goal of a tactile communication system is to extract relevant information from the acoustic signal and to present it to the individual as a means of supplementing or replacing the auditory reception of speech as the ultimate challenge." These devices are also used to teach and reinforce speech production.

Vibrotactile devices have been preferred over electrotactile instruments due to the availability of vibrators and difficulties of applying electrical current to the skin. Vibrotactile devices, however, have generally

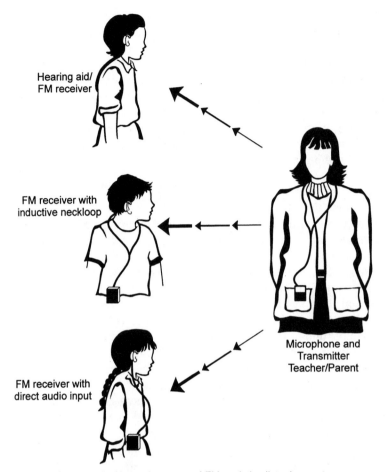

Hearing aid/
FM receiver

FM receiver with
inductive neckloop

FM receiver with
direct audio input

Microphone and
Transmitter
Teacher/Parent

Figure 9-13. Alternative types of FM assistive listening systems.

poor frequency response and high power requirements; in addition, users have difficulties in background noise environments. Sachs, Miller, and Grant (1980) compared vibrotactile and electrotactile devices and showed that the vibrotactile instruments were more efficient in transmitting lower frequencies, while the electrotactile devices were more efficient with higher frequency signals. Technological advances have resulted in tactile aids that include spectral displays in which the spectrum of the encoded sound is represented with a one- or two-dimensional array of stimulators, as well as speech-processing tactile devices in which features of the speech signal are displayed visually.

Research results obtained with tactile aids during the 1980s were modestly en-

couraging. Oller, Payne, and Gavin (1986) showed improvement in pronunciation of fricative and nasal consonants attributed to the use of tactile aids. Friel-Patti and Roeser (1985) reported increased vocalization and sign language communication in deaf children using the vibrotactile aid as well as decreased vocalization and sign language without the tactile aid. Other studies suggested that children with hearing impairment who wear tactile aids are helped at the syllable level in recognizing supersegmental features of speech such as rhythm, number of syllables, contrasting voiced/unvoiced sounds, nasal versus oral production, and stop continuants (Franklin, 1988).

Since 1990, truly wearable, commercially produced multichannel tactile aids have been available for use by deaf children. The most widely used vibrotactile device is the Tactaid VII (Franklin, 1991), which features a seven-transducer vibratory display attached to a body-worn processor. The encoding strategy of the Tactaid VII delivers energy from the acoustic signal to the seven transducers that are tuned to seven individual filtered frequency bands between 200 and 7000 Hz. The display system of the Tactaid VII is flexible and may be worn at any of several body sites including the sternum, abdomen, neck, or arm. Children are usually fitted to wear the display on the flat surface of their sternum, permitting the device to be monitored and adjusted easily if necessary.

Early advocates of vibrotactile aids claimed that these devices perform comparably to results obtained with single-channel cochlear implants. However, a carefully controlled 3-year study of hearing-impaired school-aged children who wore a vibrotactile aid and received intensive auditory training showed that the children were still unable to recognize recorded words. The study concluded that the vibrotactile aid provided sufficient pattern sequence information to be beneficial to children who were unable to discriminate prosodic stress or duration cues in speech. However, the vibrotactile aid did not compare to the positive results in the acquisition of speech or spoken language obtained by matched children wearing multichannel cochlear implants (Geers & Moog, 1994).

COCHLEAR IMPLANTS FOR CHILDREN

One of the most dramatic and exciting developments in hearing and deafness has been the cochlear implant. Over the past 25 years, the idea of restoring hearing to profoundly deaf patients by artificially stimulating the sensory system has progressed from a futuristic possibility to reality (Koch, 1996a). The cochlear implant is a surgically inserted device that delivers electrical stimulation to the inner ear and eighth cranial nerve. The device has both internal and external components. A cochlear implant relies on the fact that many auditory nerve fibers remain viable in patients with cochlear-type deafness. The surviving neurons of the eighth nerve can be stimulated to excitation by applying external electric currents of the proper strength, duration, and orientation, resulting in actively propagating neural impulses. These evoked electrical neural potentials arrive at the temporal lobes of the cortex just like the normal neural impulses generated by acoustic signals that intact cochlear hair cells transduce. The brain interprets these artificial induced potentials as sound (Figs. 9-14a and 9-14b).

Although the value of the cochlear implant in children with deafness has often been exceptional, the literature on pediatric implant patients has also cited significant individual differences in success among implanted children. Some prelinguistically deaf children do exceptionally well with their cochlear implants and progress to acquire spoken language and produce intelligible speech. Other children, however, develop only an awareness of sound and never appear to acquire language fully or produce intelligible speech to the same degree or proficiency as the exceptionally good users (Pisoni, 2000). Researchers are just beginning to analyze and understand the factors that may predict success with a cochlear implant in a young child (Waltzman & Cohen, 2000).

Several paradigms have been developed into various types of cochlear implants to create direct stimulation of the eighth nerve. Sophisticated single- and multi-channel devices have been manufactured in the United States, Australia, and Europe and have undergone considerable animal and human research. The cochlear implant devices consist of external and internal components. A tiny audio receiver is implanted behind the pinna, and a special wire array of electrodes is

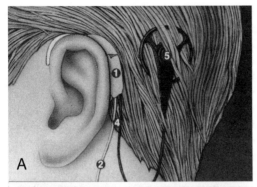

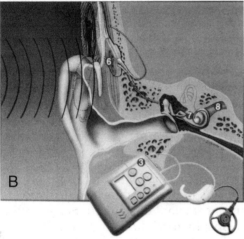

Figure 9-14a and b. Operation of the cochlear implant. (1) Directional microphone (2) sound is carried from the microphone by a cord to the speech processor worn on the belt or pocket. (3) The speech processor filters, analyzes, and digitizes the sound into coded signals and sends it (4) to the transmitting coil (5). The coil sends the coded signals as FM radio signals to the cochlear implant inserted under the skin. (Photograph provided by Cochlear Corporation, Englewood, CO.) The cochlear implant (6) delivers the electrical energy to the array of electrodes surgically inserted into the cochlea (7). The electrodes stimulate the remaining auditory nerve fibers (8), and sound information is sent to the brain for interpretation. (Photograph provided by Cochlear Corporation, Englewood, CO.)

the internal component surgically inserted into the cochlea. Allowing a month for healing of the surgical incision, the patient is then fitted with the system's external parts (a microphone and a transmitter connected by wires to a computerized speech processor worn in a shoulder pouch, in a pocket, or on a belt). A microphone within a BTE case picks up external sounds and relays them to a speech processor, which amplifies and filters the signal, then converts it into a digital code. The encoded information is modulated by a radio-frequency signal and sent across the skin via inductive coupling. The implanted receiver demodulates and decodes the signal and sends the appropriate stimulation patterns to the electrodes implanted in the cochlea. The electrodes stimulate the auditory nerve fibers, thereby providing a sensation of hearing.

Each device has a microphone for picking up external sounds and a microelectronic processor for converting the sound into electrical signals. The processor analyses and digitizes sounds into coded signals that are sent to a transmitter attached magnetically to the mastoid or through a percutaneous plug. The transmitter sends the code across the skin to the receiver/stimulator, which sends instructions to the internal tiny electrode array, surgically inserted into the cochlea to stimulate auditory nerve fibers (Fig. 9-15). Only carefully selected patients benefit from cochlear implants, in particular, those deafened individuals who have defective sensory elements (hair cells) in the cochlea with surviving intact fibers of the auditory (VIII) nerve. The cochlear implant replaces the defective hair cells of the inner ear with an array of stimulation electrodes. An excellent overview of cochlear implants is provided in the text edited by Clark, Cowan, and Dowell (1997).

Loeb (1985a) described the operation of the cochlear implant:

The loudness of the sound perceived depends roughly on the number of nerve fibers activated and their rates of firing. Both variables are functions of the amplitude of the stimulus current. The pitch is related to the place on the basilar membrane from which those nerve fibers once derived their acoustic input, in agreement with the place-pitch theory. In principle, with enough independent channels of stimulation, each controlling the activity of a small, local subset of the auditory nerve fibers, one could recreate the normal neural response to acoustic stimuli of any spectral composition. The brain would then process that information in its usual manner and the subject "hear" the "sounds."

Cochlear implants have been used successfully with adult deaf patients since the mid-1970s and in children since 1982. All the early cochlear implants in the United States used the 3M/House single channel device (Loeb, 1985b). Although the early 3M/House single channel device could not actually reproduce speech sounds to the patient, the implant provided important and useful sound cues to aid in speech reading and in the identification of environmental sounds. In 1982, federal investigation device exemption was granted for the 3M/House single channel device to be implanted into profoundly deaf children.

Subsequent advances in technology led to the development of more sophisticated multichannel cochlear implants that enabled adult users to recognize more environmental sounds, provided more speech reading enhancement, and enabled users to understand more open speech materials than provided by single-channel implants (Gantz, Tyler, Knutson, Woodworth, et al., 1988). Based on the success of their multichannel cochlear implant with adults, the federal government approved controlled studies with profoundly deaf children. Because of the concern and need for thorough evaluations of child candidates for cochlear implants, only approved implant centers with an active children's cochlear implant team (composed of an otologist, audiologist, speech/language pathologist, psychologist, deaf educator, and pediatrician) can perform the surgery and carry out the critical extensive follow-up. The candidacy process is individualized for each child, and the cochlear implant team evaluates specific criteria such as amount of residual hearing, age of the child, length of deafness, availability of appropriate educational options, communication methodology, and parent commitment to success with the implant. If the child is approved as a candidate for a cochlear implant, the surgery is followed 3–4 years later by the programming of the external equipment and initial stimulation of the device is begun. One of the most important components of the cochlear implant procedure is the ongoing, follow-up habilitation, with close coordination among parents, educators, therapists, and the implant center staff.

In the early years, the use of cochlear implants in children raised concerns related to the long-term effects of the implant in the child's body. Yet it was agreed among professionals that maximum benefit afforded by these surgically implanted devices, if successful, would be most valuable to young deaf children in their quest to learn speech and develop social communication skills. In 1995, the National Institutes of Health (NIH) sponsored a national consensus conference on cochlear implants to summarize current knowledge on the benefits and limitations of the devices as well as technical and safety issues. Factors that the consensus panel evaluated that affect the auditory performance of the cochlear implantation included the etiology and the age of onset of the deafness, age at implantation, duration of the deafness and the remaining residual hearing, electrophysiologic factors, and differences among the available devices. The panel concluded that cochlear implantation definitely improves communication abilities in the majority of children, although outcomes are more variable than noted in adults. Nonetheless, gradual, steady improvement in speech perception, speech production, and language does occur following implantation. Access to optimal educational and habilitation services is critical for children to maximize the benefits available from cochlear implantation.

It is important to point out that the amount of benefit from the cochlear implant varies greatly among children. A child's ability to use the cochlear implant for communication appears to be dependent on a variety of factors including the amount of time the device is used each day, the extent to which sound is integrated meaningfully into the child's daily life, the habilitation services the child receives, the degree of parental involvement and support, the degree of remaining auditory nerve survival, the duration of the deafness, and the age at implantation. Children with successful cochlear implants show a significant increase in speech intelligibility and speech perception as well as continued growth and increases in receptive and expressive language. The tremendous growth in use of the cochlear implant is reflected by the fact that by 1998 more than 18,000 people worldwide, including more than 6500 hearing-impaired pediatric patients, had undergone implantation (Cochlear Corporation, Personal Communication. Denver, Co, 1998).

The FDA approved the Clarion Multi-Strategy Cochlear Implant System in 1991. The Clarion implant system uses 16 electrodes arranged in 8 bipolar pairs. The Clarion provides a choice of speech

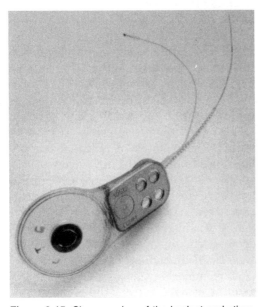

Figure 9-15. Close-up view of the implant and stimulating electrode array and ground electrode and the ESPrit, multichannel ear level speech processor in a small BTE package. (Photograph provided by Cochlear Corporation, Englewood, CO.)

processing options, and the speech processor can store several customized programs for the wearer. The Clarion has a two-way telemetry system that allows information about the internal cochlear stimulator and electrodes to be read by the speech processor, thereby providing a means for assessing electrode impedance and function (Koch, 1996b).

The implanted device is capable of delivering biphasic stimulus current pulses between any pair of electrodes or between any one electrode and the remaining linked electrodes. This system requires postsurgical programming that permits individual electrodes to be "tuned" to fit the specific hearing loss pattern of the patient. The device is programmed through a sophisticated computerized system, usually based on audiologic behavioral hearing responses from the newly implanted patient. If changes in hearing occur over time, or as newer speech processing algorithms are developed, the speech processor and electrodes can be reprogrammed as many times as needed with no disturbance to the implant or the patient. The speech processor may be a body-worn or ear-level device. Typically, the audiologist is the cochlear implant team member responsible for programming the implant device to the individual child's needs (Fig. 9-16).

Extensive training is necessary to teach the young deaf child to give reliable, time-locked behavioral responses to discrete electrical stimulation of the electrodes. Special procedures are taught to each child, before implant placement, to serve for initial programming and later fine-tuning of the speech processor. It is possible to teach young children to respond to electrode threshold levels, to establish loudness comfort levels across frequency, and to comprehend loudness concepts to determine effective electrical dynamic range (Firszt & Reeder, 1996). Once children have experience listening to sound through the implant, they can be taught to perform loudness scaling to assess loud-

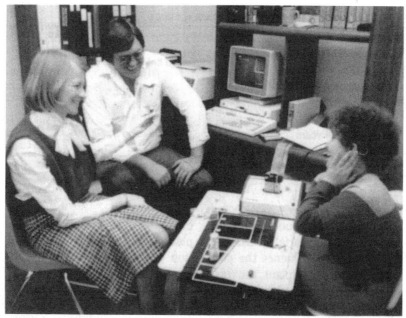

Figure 9-16. An audiologist programs and "tunes" a child's cochlear implant. (Photograph provided by Jon Shallop, PhD.)

ness growth relative to electrical current levels. Before the initiation of the children's implant study program, concern was expressed by professionals that deaf children could not be taught to respond to such subtle differences in the acoustic stimuli necessary to program the multichannel cochlear implant. It is to the credit of the skilled audiologists involved in these early children's implant programs that techniques were successfully developed, even with the youngest of deaf children, to measure the various psychophysical parameters necessary for the accurate programming of the cochlear implant.

Selection of Children for Cochlear Implants. The minimal criteria for pediatric patient selection for cochlear implantation is summarized in Table 9-2. The recommended minimum age constraint of 18 months is imposed not for technical surgical considerations, but rather to permit sufficient time to establish the diagnosis of deafness, with full audiologic information and hearing aid performance evaluation. An important consideration in selecting child implant patients is evidence of strong family support exemplified by an understanding of the problems that may be associated with the implant device. It is necessary that the immediate family of the child have appropriate expectations and a strong commitment to the responsibilities of postimplant auditory training with the child.

The American Academy of Audiology (1995) defines the criteria for "limited functional hearing aid benefit" by a child before cochlear implantation decisions. The audiologist is responsible for evaluating the hearing aid benefit obtained by the candidate in terms of (1) aided thresholds with conventional hearing aids relative to aided results reported for multichannel cochlear implant users, including aided results in the high frequencies at which important consonant cures occur; and (2) performance on word recognition tasks, administered with auditory cues only in a closed- or open-response set.

Guidelines for selecting children for cochlear implantation are as follows:

Table 9.1.
Minimum Requirements for Children for Cochlear Implants

Minimum 18 months of age

Bilateral, profound, sensorineural deafness

Completion of all preevaluation procedures

No additional handicaps that might adversely affect potential success with the implant

Strong evidence of family support

Satisfactory progress in auditory development not being made despite effective training and appropriately fitted hearing aids

From Northern, J.L. (1986). Selection of children for cochlear implantation. *Seminars in Hearing, 7* (4), 342.

- Age 18 months to 17 years with bilateral profound sensorineural deafness. Patients with onset of deafness from birth to 2 years of age are considered to be *prelinguistically* deafened; those patients with an onset of deafness from 2–5 years of age are considered to be *perilinguistically* deafened; and patients deafened after 5 years of age are considered *postlinguistically* deafened.

- The child demonstrates little or no benefit from appropriately fitted binaural hearing aids. In younger children, little or no benefit is defined as lack of progress in the development of simple auditory skills in conjunction with appropriate amplification and participation in intensive aural habilitation over 3–6 months. A 3- to 6-month hearing aid trial is required for children without previous hearing aid experience.

- Contraindications for cochlear implants in children include deafness due to lesions of the acoustic nerve or central auditory pathway, active middle ear infections, absence of cochlear development, or tympanic membrane perforation in the presence of active middle ear disease.

- Families of children under consideration for cochlear implantation should receive extensive counseling regarding the limited nature of expected postoperative benefits. Prelinguistic and perilinguistic deafened patients are at higher risk for nonuse of the implant than postlinguistic patients. However, many prelinguistically and perilinguistically deafened patients demonstrate improved detection of medium to loud environmental sounds, including speech. A few patients demonstrate improved lip reading abilities following implantation and extensive training.

In 1995, the NIH Consensus Panel recognized that cochlear implants had been successful in meningitic pediatric patients and approved implantation in younger children in part to overcome the risk of new bone formation that might preclude implantation at a later date. Although improvements in speech perception, speech production, and language acquisition in children are often reported as primary benefits, the NIH Panel noted that performance variability across children is substantial. Using tests of pattern perception, closed-set word identification, and open-set perception, the performance of children with implants increases on average with each succeeding year after implantation. Shortly following implantation, performance may be broadly comparable to that of some children with hearing aids. Over time, implant performance may improve to match that of children who are highly successful hearing aid users. Children who undergo implantation at younger ages are on average more accurate in their production of consonants, vowels, intonation, and rhythm. Speech produced by children with implants is more accurate than speech produced by children with comparable hearing losses using other devices. One year after implantation, speech intelligibility is twice that typically reported for children with profound hearing impairments and continues to improve with time. Oral language development in deaf children with cochlear implants remains a slow, training-intensive process.

Success With Cochlear Implants. Deaf children are not a homogeneous population, and there are numerous variables associated with each child that may influence the potential success of a cochlear implant. A child's success with a cochlear implant depends on the age of deafness onset, the duration of auditory deprivation due to deafness, and the type of educational training the child has been given since the onset of the deafness. In general terms, children with acquired deafness are better candidates for cochlear implants than children with congenital deafness; children who have been deaf for only a short time do better with cochlear implants than children who have been deaf for an extended length of time; and deaf children from auditory-oral educational training backgrounds are more likely to achieve success with a cochlear implant than deaf children from total communication (manual) educational settings. When clinically appropriate, the poorer ear is always selected for implantation, as surgical placement of the device will result in complete loss of hearing in the implanted ear. These general guidelines have proven useful in counseling parents and educators about the relative potential for a child's success with a cochlear implant.

Geers and Moog (1994) conducted an important research project at the Central Institute for the Deaf for 3 years. Their study compared the use of traditional hearing aids, vibrotactile aids, and cochlear implants in matched triad sets of children with hearing impairment. Analysis of data showed that the children with cochlear implants outperformed their matched peers in every area of evaluation. The children with cochlear implants showed significantly faster growth in speech and language acquisition than the matched children wearing other sensory aids. The researchers reported that the children with cochlear implants were able to identify words based on spectral, rather than temporal, cues after 1 year of implant use. Following 2 years of cochlear implant use, the children showed a dramatic increase in perception and production of the suprasegmental and vowel features of spoken speech.

Parents' attitudes are especially revealing when they are asked about their children with cochlear implants. Tucker (1999) reported a survey of 176 parents. The cochlear implant children were largely prelingually deaf (86%) and had been fit with a variety of implant devices. An amazing 100% of parents said they were glad that their children received cochlear implants, and 86% rated their children's implants as very successful, 10% as moderately successful, and 2% as mildly successful. Most of the postlingual deafened children, especially those deafened from meningitis, understood some open-set speech without visual clues with multichannel cochlear implants. The survey of parental attitudes supports the view that the earlier a child receives a cochlear implant, the more open-speech discrimination and eventual language development the child will acquire.

It has been a full decade since the first clinical trials began with cochlear implants in deaf children. The FDA has expanded the original rigid criteria for implant candidacy to include younger children with less profound hearing losses. The results of children's cochlear implant programs have been so encouraging that the application of the technology has now been extended to include prelingual deafened children who lost their hearing before developing speech and language. Increasingly, parents and cochlear implant teams have pressed for implantations in children younger than 2 years of age when appropriate diagnostic considerations are met and the children demonstrate lack of auditory development. Device modifications have allowed implantation in younger children as the hardware becomes thinner, smaller, and with more flexible receiver/stimulators. Cohen and Waltzman (1996) reported successful implant results in children younger than 2 years of age. Surgical techniques require minimal surgical modification because the cochlea is full adult size at birth. Initial progress reviews of these children have shown positive results, and there is little doubt that more children will be candidates for cochlear implants at earlier ages.

Current results in young children with profound deafness have exceeded the expectations of most professionals. The technology and surgery is expensive, although private insurance or Medicaid may cover most costs. The future for cochlear implants in children is especially bright, and technology is continually improving in terms of better speech processing paradigms and hardware design. It is likely that as more experience is gained with today's cochlear implants, future candidates will have lesser degrees of sensorineural loss.

FAMILY MANAGEMENT

The importance of parental involvement in the habilitation process of their hearing-impaired children is absolutely crucial to the child's success with amplification. Unfortunately, there are no specific guidelines that can always be followed when dealing with parents. Just like children, parents are unique and have backgrounds, attitudes, and needs that must be dealt with on a very personal basis. The audiologist may be well advised to plan on spending at least as much time talking with parents as working with the child. Often the parents develop a special relationship with the audiologist, as it is the audiologist who probably confirmed the presence of hearing loss in the child.

Pratt (1999) points out that a relatively consistent finding in the literature is that hearing loss in children substantively increases stress levels in normal-hearing families, and that this situation can have deleterious effects on parent-child interac-

tions. The increase in stress levels puts the children at risk for attachment problems and has implications for emotional, cognitive, and linguistic development—all of which may affect the stability of the family. Pratt describes the audiologist as working "beyond the audiology clinic doors" to provide an accepting and supportive environment for parents and families of children with hearing impairment.

Traditionally, the audiologist acted as an outside expert in the hearing aid fitting process who imparted selected information to the parents and then made decisions on behalf of the child. However, there has been an important change in the role of the parents and family in the recognition that the child cannot be viewed apart from the family. The audiologist's role is to be involved in a collaborative process with the parents to determine what is best for both the child and the family. This family-centered philosophy assumes that the child's needs are best met by meeting family needs and that families have the right to retain as much control as they desire over the intervention process (Roush & McWilliam, 1994; Roush & Matkin, 1994).

The prognosis for the hearing-handicapped child to obtain maximum benefit from amplification has a direct relation to the level of support provided by the immediate family. Evidence of strong family support can actually be noted with empiric observation by the audiologist and is not just based on subjective intuition. Family behavior can be observed over time and modified when necessary through careful and appropriate counseling. Behaviors that may have influenced the child's use of amplification include the following:

- Family accepts and understands the child's hearing loss.

- Family shows responsibility for scheduling and keeping all medical and educational appointments on behalf of the child.

- Family is knowledgeable about the etiology of and the prognosis for the child's hearing loss.

- Family communicates well with the child by encouraging conversation under all circumstances.

- Family has appropriate expectations about the amplification devices used by the child.

- Family displays high interest and motivational levels in child-related activities.

- Family spends ample, constructive time with the child.

- Family has genuine concern for the child's educational and physical development.

In Luterman's book, "Counseling Parents of Hearing-Impaired Children" (1979), he describes different approaches for the audiologist to use in order for parents to cope with their child's special needs. It is the parents, not the professional, who must make the decisions regarding the child's habilitation because they must accept and take the ultimate responsibility. Certainly, parents must accept and understand the need for amplification before hearing aids can be placed and used successfully by the hearing-impaired youngster.

More recently, Luterman, Kurtzer-White, and Seewald (1999), in writing about the young deaf child, included a chapter on parental counseling that the current authors believe should be required reading for every audiologist who works with pediatric patients. Luterman described the feelings that parents go through after learning the diagnosis of their child's deafness. Parents' feelings are often below the level of awareness, and except for denial and shock, may not be able to express themselves until the emotions come in a flood. Feelings of inadequacy, anger, guilt, vulnerability, and confusion are certain to surface with time. Luterman's view is that these feelings are neither good nor bad, but need to be acknowledged and accepted. The audiologist must be nonjudgmental toward the parent's emotional behaviors and expressions and be prepared to participate in these normal processes, providing support through empathetic listening.

Once hearing aids have been recommended and selected, it is important for parents to observe the child's aided and unaided responses in a sound field situation to see for themselves that their child benefits from using personal amplification. Once convinced of the need and benefits provided by amplification, the parents would likely not be embarrassed or apologetic about the hearing aids. The parents must understand that although personal amplification is absolutely necessary for the development of their child, it may require extensive auditory therapy before these newly amplified sounds will be meaningful to the child. The parents should also be made aware of the number of important assistive listening devices that are available to help the hearing-impaired child gain maximum benefit and relate effectively with daily communication and listening tasks.

The audiologist's role in parental management of their child's personal amplification and assistive listening devices has a great deal to do with the ultimate successful acceptance and utilization of these hearing instruments. That role should include education, guidance, and counseling, because the parents' attitude regarding amplification may be the single most important factor in successful hearing aid use by the hearing-impaired child.

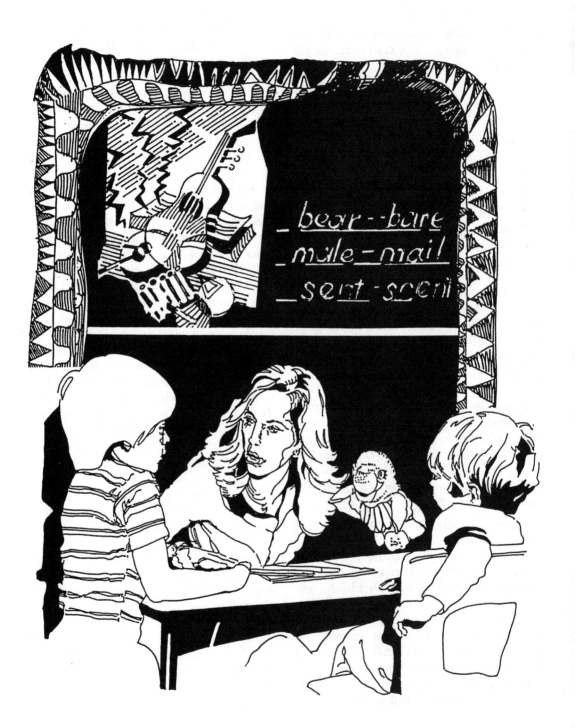

CHAPTER 10

Education of Hearing-Impaired Children

One of the first issues to be clarified in this chapter is that of terminology and definitions. The authors' definition of "hearing-impaired children" includes *all* children with hearing loss who are handicapped to such an extent that some form of special education is required. Obviously, this broad definition includes those with profound hearing loss that is traditionally defined as "deaf." The Conference of Executives of American Schools for the Deaf defines "the deaf" as having a hearing loss of 70 dB hearing level (HL) or greater in their better ear, while the "hard-of-hearing" student has a loss of 35–69 dB HL in the better hearing ear. In fact, the definition of deaf describes a hearing impairment so severe that a child experiences difficulty in processing linguistic information through hearing, with or without amplification. Although it is easy to speak in general terms about the education of students with various degrees of hearing impairment or deafness, the point must be made that these groups are by no means homogeneous. Further, it must be realized that there is no single educational method, system, or approach that is uniformly applicable to all children with varying degrees of hearing impairment or deafness. This chapter orients students toward the single most important aspect of management of the child with hearing impairment—achieving the maximum potential of the child through education.

Matkin and Wilcox (1999) point out that it is a common misconception to equate the term *hearing impairment* only with severe to profound bilateral hearing loss. Although children with severe hearing loss receive the largest share of education attention, children with minimal hearing loss deserve equal educational opportunity (see Chapter 1). Fortunately, schools are beginning to extend support services to include children with mild to moderate bilateral sensorineural hearing losses, those with permanent unilateral hearing loss, younger children with bilateral conductive losses, and even high-frequency losses identified through screening of school-aged children. According to Matkin and Wilcox (1999) these children with mild to moderate hearing losses are best described as having *educationally significant hearing loss* (Table 10-1).

The audiologist is often hard-pressed to maintain the distinction between being an expert in the measurement and management of hearing and hearing disorders and the necessary role of serving as an advocate for the child with hearing impairment. When the audiologist expresses an objective statement within the field of hearing measurement, the facts are based on standardized and solid data. However, when the audiologist expresses a viewpoint or an opinion advocating a position on questions of general policy not directly related to audiology (i.e., approaches to education of hearing-impaired children), the stated opinion is often based on limited knowledge and information. In the area of education of hearing-impaired children, it behooves the audiologist to know as much as possible about all avenues, methodologies, techniques, and

Table 10.1.
Guidelines for Educationally Significant Hearing Loss

An average pure-tone hearing loss in the speech range (0.5–2 kHz) of 20 dB HL in the better ear, which is not reversible within a reasonable period

An average high-frequency pure tone hearing loss of 35 dB HL or greater in the better ear at two or more of the following frequencies: 2, 3, 4, and 6 kHz

A permanent unilateral hearing loss of 35 dB HL or greater in the speech range (0.5–2 kHz)

Any hearing impairment that significantly affects communication with others and in which the individual requires supplemental assistance or modification of instructional methods to achieve optimum performance

Adapted from the Colorado Department of Education (1991). *Effectiveness indicators for audiological services.* Denver, CO: CDE, 1991.

systems for teaching this special population. It is obligatory that the audiologist who specializes in pediatric hearing evaluation also be knowledgeable and well informed on the current status of education for hearing-impaired children.

The educational audiologist is the appropriate intermediary trained in deafness education methodologies and management of children with hearing impairments. As defined by the Educational Audiology Association, an educational audiologist is a specialist who ensures that all aspects of children's hearing and learning are maximized so that their educational and real-life capabilities can be met. The educational audiologist is the person responsible for the child with hearing difficulties. In many instances, the role could be the case manager. The educational audiologist is qualified in the overall ramifications of sound, hearing, hearing loss, hearing aids, auditory perception (including central auditory abilities), and their impact on development, learning, and life. The educational audiologist is responsible for identification, diagnosis, assessment, amplification programming, aural rehabilitation programming (and training when feasible), and central auditory processing disorders (CAPD) programming. In addition, this specialty area audiologist is responsible for support personnel training, parent training and support, specialist coordination, listening training, hearing conservation programming, supervision of specialized testing, otologic referral, and ongoing evaluations of the child's classroom and educational functioning.

The audiologist is the professional best able to manage the complete hearing care of a child who experiences hearing loss of any degree (Flexer, 1990). Even a "mild" hearing loss can sabotage the development of academic competencies, and there is a growing population of school children with mild to moderate hearing loss. Unfortunately, there are far too few audiologists employed in educational settings (approximately 700 nationally), with an average ratio of 1 audiologist for every 12,000 children (Blair, Wilson-Vlotman, & Von Almen, 1989). Ross and Calvert (1977) recommended a minimum ratio of 1 audiologist to every 75 hearing-impaired children in school programs, in addition to necessary support personnel, to exploit the residual hearing of children effectively.

This book has described objective tests and behavioral measures that have been adequately standardized and has also outlined subjective assessments that lend themselves to some measurable degree of judgment. Within these topics, the audiologist has a fair amount of control. However, in the field of directing children with hearing impairment into educational channels, the audiologist becomes an "advocate of a cause." Many audiologists do not have knowledge or experience with various educational training methods, nor do audiologists necessarily have an understanding of all the variables that will affect the child's functioning in a given training method. To rectify these inadequacies, the audiologist must (in addition to personal empirical testing) seek the opinions of various members of the deafness team, including the child's parents, physicians, educators, psychologists, sociologists, and others. With these specialists the audiologist must evolve a decision concerning the direction of management of the child—a decision that is flexible enough to change with the further accumulation of information.

Certainly there is a need for a variety of experts in the field of pediatric deafness. The difficulty comes from the fact that few "experts" have the important ingredient of objectivity when it comes to evaluating the field of deaf education. The professional groups that know most about this area are the teachers themselves or program administrators. Yet these people are limited in number and isolated from new parents of a deaf child. It is the author's philosophy that the audiologist should operate as an "advocate without a cause" in the field of educational management for the child. The audiologist should not be biased in the direction of any training method or philosophy and should consider only what will best ensure the child's maximal ultimate development. In this book the authors try to give the audiologist the tools to arrive at a working construct concerning the direction of management of a child.

In another sense, however, the audiologist can espouse advocacy for principle or cause alone. This is in the sense of fighting for the child's right to be given a chance to show what he or she can do despite contrary information, differences in personal opinions, and even in light of questionable evidence. Audiologists must be sufficiently sensitive to let hope play a part in the judgments for the prognosis of a disabled child. Audiologists would be less than human if they failed to glow with satisfaction when a child develops useful speech with hearing aids and hearing therapy, or when an infant with hearing impairment becomes in every way a hearing child with continually improving speech and language skills.

Among the fundamental rights that audiologists (as surrogates for children) should demand from society is a child's right to achieve his or her maximal potential communication abilities. Society should make special provisions to help the hearing-impaired child override the disability and become as "normal" as individual limitations will allow. The world-famous child psychologist, A.L. Gesell (1956), said, "The aim should not be to convert the deaf child into a somewhat fictitious version of a normal hearing child, but into a well-adjusted non-hearing child who is completely managing the limitations of his [or her] sensory deficit."

EDUCATION GOALS FOR THE CHILD WITH HEARING IMPAIRMENT

Obviously, there are many goals to be achieved in educating hearing-impaired and deaf children, but only the four most important are highlighted here. These goals, presented in order of importance, include achievement of adequate language skills, establishment of sound mental health, establishment of intelligible speech, and establishment of easy communication with peers. These goals are by no means to be interpreted as limiting the range of objectives that one might have for the hard-of-hearing or deaf child. However, other goals that might be enumerated—high employability, job satisfaction, and enrichment of life—all depend on the success of achieving the four goals described below.

Language. The importance of language cannot be denied. Language comes so easily to normal-hearing children and is a giant stone wall for children with significant hearing impairment. Educators of hearing-impaired students realize the long-term commitment and years of diligent work needed to establish communicative competence based on adequate linguistic abilities. The process of developing language competency is very difficult for the child who has significant hearing impairment, and all children who are prelingually deaf will experience serious difficulties and delays in acquiring language skills. For some children, full language acquisition may be a feasible goal; for other children, lesser language skills will have to be acceptable. The hearing-impaired child with limited language skills will have additional difficulties in subjects other than language studies, because each new step in education requires mastery of the previous steps. It is the role of the school or program to create an environment for learning that maximizes the language acquisition process of children with hearing impairments.

Montgomery and Matkin (1992) stated that successful language learning for a child with a hearing loss depends on several variables:

- The type, severity, and configuration of the hearing loss in each ear.
- The effects of the hearing loss on the child's ability to detect and discriminate the key acoustic components of the speech signal.
- Consistency in the use of amplification to provide optimal recognition and discrimination of auditory signals.

Reading ability is highly correlated with language skills, so many hearing-impaired students also have difficulty in becoming proficient readers. The ability to express or comprehend language in written form is closely allied with the ability to express and comprehend language through face-to-face spoken communication. Historically, deaf education programs have not been very successful in assisting the majority of hearing-impaired students to achieve age-level reading skills. Some believe that it is the inherent weakness in English grammar that is the primary block to reading for the deaf child.

Osberger and Hesketh (1988) described the language difficulties experienced by hearing-impaired and deaf children in terms of language form (syntax), content (semantics), and function (pragmatics). According to these au-

thors, hearing-impaired children may have only minor difficulties in acquiring the basic rules of English, compared with the profoundly deaf child who has a great deal of difficulty in syntax acquisition because of his or her dependence on learning language through the visual modality. Language content as reflected by word knowledge is commonly limited and delayed even in children with mild hearing losses. Hearing-impaired children have a restricted knowledge of synonyms and special difficulties in recognizing relationships between words. In terms of language function, children with hearing impairment must be taught directly the rules that govern conversations, such as turn-taking and topic negotiation.

From the author's point of view, we have been misled into placing oral speech as the primary goals for deaf children, never realizing that the enrichment of their lives may be sacrificed for the simple ability to mouth words. What words? And in what relationships and context? The primary goal in education of the hearing-impaired child must be to develop linguistic abilities and ensure communication development by whatever means possible. A secondary goal should be to develop intelligible oral expression of that language—a skill that itself depends on the acquisition of a high degree of language competence through auditory or visual input.

An important question that has been debated for years centers on whether combining signing with spoken language contributes to or interferes with the development of spoken language. Geers, Moog, and Schick (1984) attempted to answer this question by testing a nationwide sample of 327 congenital, profoundly deaf children from 13 oral/aural programs and 15 total communication programs through their own tool, the Grammatical Analysis of Elicited Language-Simple Sentence Level (GAEL-S). The GAEL-S measures production of selected English language structures in a standardized manner, so that each child's "spontaneous" language sample is evoked in precisely the same manner. In their study, Geers et al. examined their data separately for four different response modes: the oral productions of the oral/aural children, the oral productions of the total communication children, the manual productions of the total communication children, and the combined productions of the total communication children. The results showed that the percentage of correct scores for the oral productions of the total communication children were substantially below the scores for their manual productions and below scores of the oral/aural children in all grammatical categories sampled on the GAEL-S. Most of the children in the total communication programs tested in this study did not simultaneously talk and sign, and their signed productions were far superior to their spoken productions. Thus, based on this study, the children in total communication programs did not develop competence with selected simple sentence structures at a rate faster than those children trained in the oral/aural programs. The authors point out that both groups of children showed relatively poor performance in language production and urged that more emphasis on systematic instruction in English be included in all training programs regardless of the mode of communication.

Sound Mental Health. The most effective learning takes place in the context of warm, nurturing relationships within the family. This is particularly important for the very young child during the critical years for language development. Whatever type of educational program a child is receiving, the parents should be given close emotional support and guidance in their management of the child's disability. The results should be the development of the child's self-confidence, high self-esteem, and the ability to relate well to people in the environment.

The warm relationship between parents and child can be fostered by helpful, supportive communications from the physician and educational personnel. The initial phase of reporting the child's deafness to the parents is crucial to the parents' attitude toward the problem (see Chapter 6). Time should be allowed for the parents to air their feelings and their sorrow over having an "imperfect" child. Grief must be expressed if acceptance of the disability is to come. These natural feelings should be shared with empathy and understanding. The physician and the audiologist can create the kind of atmosphere out of which nurturing attitudes can grow.

Together with the parents, the audiologist can help guide decisions about an educational program for the child that will allow the continuation of good parent nurturing. As Schlesinger (1973) pointed out, "Early parent-child communication is a traumatic issue between hearing parents and their deaf children. Although the hearing parents talk to and in front of the child, they can only guess at the level of understanding." Frustration results, for both parents and child. Thus it is important that an educational program be chosen that minimizes this frustration. It should be noted that such problems are minimized in the relationships of deaf parents to their deaf children. Denton, Brill, Kemp, et al. (1974) stated, "Deaf parents, as they communicate to and in front of the child, can test the child's understanding more easily. The child . . . can learn the symbols, the signs the parents use, and learn to understand and reproduce them more easily." It is estimated that 3% of all congenitally deaf children are born to deaf parents.

Intelligible Speech. Certainly an important goal in the education of deaf children is intelligible speech. However, caution should be used when placing this skill too high in the hierarchy of educational goals. Intelligible speech without good language skills is an exercise in futility; intelligible speech in an emotionally disordered mind is a useless function. Articulate speech is greatly to be desired, but a program producing excellence only in this skill and not in language or emotional stability cannot be highly rated. Clear oral speech is greatly to be desired but should not become the mainstay of the child's educational efforts. So-called "deaf speech" is characterized by a significantly higher fundamental frequency, a slower speaking rate than found in normal-hearing persons, and typical increased voice intensity with abnormally large amplitude fluctuations.

Oral production of speech for the deaf child is a problem that stems from inadequate control at nearly all levels of production. In addition, there is a systematic relationship between the degree of hearing impairment and the intelligibility of the child's speech so that the greater the hearing loss, the more unintelligible the child's speech is likely to be. Although exceptions to this rule do exist, for whatever unknown reasons, all audiologists have seen children with profound hearing loss and exceptionally clear oral speech.

Parents of a newly diagnosed hearing-impaired child must decide whether their child will be taught to communicate with manual signs, by speech reading and producing speech, or by some combination of methods. The choice is a difficult one. In general, parents can be advised that children with greater hearing loss will be less likely to succeed in speech reading and will most likely benefit from sign language. The disadvantages of sign language are obvious and compelling to hearing parents. Because it is not the language of society or the family, parents worry that their child will be difficult to communicate with, and they will naturally be worried abut learning a new language to communicate with their own child. On the other hand, the most important advantage of sign language is that it is easily learned. Children whose parents sign acquire sign language at the same rate that hearing

children acquire spoken language. For instance, they begin a "sign babble" of repetitive hand motions by 10 months, just as hearing infants begin to babble in sound at that same age (Petitto & Marentette, 1991). A hearing-impaired infant who understands and learns signs can achieve the same level of language production as the normal-hearing child at the same age milestones. The audiologist can encourage parents who feel intimidated about learning signs by assuring them that they have years to become really fluent, but that it is extremely valuable to use a limited vocabulary of "baby signs" while the child is young.

One of the major factors that opened up the education potential of children with profound deafness has been the cochlear implant (see Chapter 9). Carefully documented prospective and long-term studies of children with cochlear implants have provided a volume of information about the development of learning, speech recognition, and speech production in young children with hearing impairment. Increased awareness of the precise parameters of the speech of deaf individuals has accompanied the development of the cochlear implant. In general, the immediate effect of the cochlear implant is that the patient has an improved ability to monitor and adjust vocal output as well as an increased clarity of oral speech. Admittedly, even with the best of personal amplification or a cochlear implant, the deafened child is destined to spend long hours in speech therapy. It is to be remembered, however, that the goal of clear oral speech is secondary to the goal of developing a strong language base, so that when the deaf child speaks, something of value will have been spoken. When the desire to communicate is instilled in deaf children and the necessary language skills to do so are provided, teaching speech will become a far easier task.

The family, particularly the parents, is the most important part of the child's support system. Families need assistance in understanding the problems of deafness and in learning those skills that will, in turn, be of benefit to the hearing-impaired child. The family must be inherently involved in all decisions regarding their child and must believe positively about the child's potential. Many parents of deaf children complain that their concerns and desires were not given consideration when their child was beginning special education programs. It is essential that parents be committed to, and trained in the use of, whichever communication system is used by their child. Behind many successful deaf children will be found devoted and concerned parents.

For any child, disabled or not, a positive self-concept is crucial. Emotional stability and maturity are often problem areas for children who are deaf. When a child has low self-esteem, has tendencies to be withdrawn, or exhibits inappropriate behaviors, strategies must be established to improve the child's emotional well being. Both the home and the school environment should be evaluated, and everyone concerned must be flexible to make the necessary adjustments for the good of the child. The goal of sound mental health is essential to any successful achievement that can be desired for the hearing-impaired child.

Communication With Peers. Humans have a special need for communication, and happiness and satisfaction go hand-in-hand with the ease by which we transmit and receive information. It is too often the case that without careful guidance and intervention that the child with hearing impairment or deafness can become isolated from family and friends. Interaction with peers is an important part of normal development, and it is critical that deaf children be able to communicate freely and easily with children of their own age. Peer relationships serve as models for appropriate behavior and self-identity. It is recommended that deaf children be exposed to older, same-gender role models

who are also deaf, as recognition of deafness in others provides a sense of belonging for the child, rather than a feeling of pure isolation in a world of hearing people.

Children have cultural needs. Culture is knowledge that gives individuals a shared understanding of the world and accepted behaviors and values. Culture enables us to know what is expected and anticipated and permits individuals to gauge their place within the group. When not recognized, differing cultural standards can interfere with the learning process in the classroom and in the home. Recently, there has been a strong movement among deaf adults to recognize their unique needs and their accommodation to the world around them as *deaf culture.* Edward Dolnick wrote explicitly about the deaf culture movement in the "Atlantic Monthly" (1993). He points out that the view of deafness as a culture is held vehemently by many deaf adults. So strong is the feeling of deaf cultural solidarity that many deaf parents cheer on discovering that their newborn is also deaf. Thus, the well-meaning efforts to integrate deaf children into conventional schools and to help them learn to speak provokes fierce resistance from activists who favor sign language and argue that the world of deafness is distinctive, rewarding, and worth preserving.

The deaf child, who most of the time has two hearing parents, may experience rejection through dislike, pity, and misunderstanding from the hearing world. It is thus not surprising that the deaf child of deaf parents seems to be much happier and better adjusted than the deaf child of hearing parents. Many deaf children have social problems that complicate their language disability. Accordingly, the frustrated deaf child is noted to show outbursts of anger and rage throughout the school years. In schools and classes for the hearing-impaired taught only by hearing teachers, children with hearing impairment and deafness may develop strong emotional ties and loyalties to each other as classmates, which leads them to the exclusive and excluded community of the deaf as adults. This presents a difficult position for audiologists to accept and advocate when faced with management of the future of a deaf child born into a family of "deaf culturists."

Schwartz (1987) stated that no method for teaching hearing-impaired children can completely make up for a lack of communication at home. In a classic comment, Schwartz says that "staunch advocates of Oralism, of Total Communication, and of Cued Speech, alternately inspire and terrify parents with various tales of triumph and tragedy." Obviously, success in communication for the hearing-impaired child will be enhanced when the particular methodology used at home is also used at school. Cornett (1985) charges that few hearing parents of profoundly deaf children actually become competent in manual communication. Hearing parents, according to Cornett, tend to learn a few signs and do reasonably well in communicating until the child starts school. As the child's signing sophistication increases, communication with the parents may become more and more limited. Certainly, in today's environment, ample books, videos, and classes are readily available to teach parents and other interested persons how to communicate in standard American Sign Language (ASL). It is important that when parents make a choice and commitment to communication that the choice be made for the benefit of the entire family and not just for one parent to be able to talk to the hearing-impaired youngster.

The degree to which hearing-impaired children of hearing-impaired parents demonstrate an advantage in their acquisition of signed and spoken English when compared to hearing-impaired children of hearing parents was studied by Geers and Schick (1988). Their results indicated that by ages 7 and 8, the hearing-impaired children of hearing-impaired parents demonstrated a significant linguistic advantage in both spoken and signed English over hearing-impaired children of normal-hearing parents. The hearing-impaired children of hearing-impaired parents appeared better able to utilize a language training program to produce linguistic structures of English in both manual and oral modes than the hearing-impaired children of hearing parents.

The authors strongly believe that it is unfair to force a child into a peer relationship in which the hearing disability is such a detriment that the child cannot compete or be accepted fully. The hearing-impaired child must be in an environment in which communication can be accomplished successfully, without stress or censure. Because the child has a strong vested interest in placement decisions, the child's opinions and preferences should be given ample consideration whenever possible. The real world of normal-hearing, fast-talking adults and children is a difficult environment for the deaf child to understand and overcome without achieving some means of easy communication. At the same time, the culture of the deaf community and the possible positive role it can play in the lives of children with profound hearing loss must be taken into account.

FEDERAL LEGISLATIVE ACTS

The passage of the Education for All Handicapped Children Act of 1975 (otherwise known as Public Law 94-142) represented a landmark in federal recognition of their responsibility to provide funding for the costs of special education that ensures a basic minimum level of program quality for handicapped children and their parents. The importance of this legislation was to assure the right of all children to be educated in the school districts in which they live. Federal legislation since 1975 has changed focus from the concept of *handicap* to that of *disability*.

The basic purposes of the law are to ensure that every disabled child in the United States receives a free, appropriate public education. This free (at no cost to the child or parents) education is to be appropriately designed to fit the special needs of the child and public (i.e., the state education department has the legal responsibility to provide appropriate educational services under public auspices at public expense). The basic goals of this legislation broaden the options available to educate deaf students, recognize the diverse needs of individual children, and support the need for early identification and diagnosis.

The specific provisions of the law include (1) a free, appropriate public education for all handicapped children; (2) the identification, location, and evaluation of all handicapped children; (3) the preparation and implementation of an individualized education program (IEP) for each involved child; (4) assurance of education in the least restrictive environment; (5) procedural safeguards for parents—"due process"; (6) maintenance of rights for children placed by the state in private schools; (7) in-service training; and (8) related services (including some health-related services). Although the 1970s will be remembered for this encompassing law, the economic conditions of the 1980s created challenges for the enactment and fulfillment of the law's provisions. The "education of all handicapped children" is a multibillion-dollar per year undertaking for which most funding has been allocated to the state and local communities.

It should not be necessary to point out that the law itself is not a panacea, but it has served to substantially improve services and education for deaf students since its enactment. The limited numbers of deaf students may make it difficult to group deaf children with other deaf children in day programs in smaller school districts. The law does not necessarily mean that "least restrictive environment" and "maximal integration" are synony-

mous terms or concepts. Considering the ultimate objective of producing well-educated, socially adjusted, and responsible adults, the least restrictive environment is also not necessarily the one that is closest to home or the one that has maximum integration in schools.

In many ways, the law was enacted before answers were available to meet the educational mandates. In fact, many questions and procedural ramifications still exist regarding identification, evaluation, and education of hearing-impaired and deaf children. One of the major tenets of the legislation related to the placement of children in the least restrictive environment. Although "mainstreamed children" experienced some of the obvious benefits of association with age-similar peers, they have also experienced isolation and rejection within the classroom. Bess and McConnell (1981) summarized the factors associated with a higher degree of success in mainstream programs to include the onset of hearing loss after oral language has been established, middle- or upper-income-family background, and an ability to speak intelligibly.

Mainstreaming has become a reality for a high percentage of hearing-impaired students, as discussed later in this chapter. The intent of PL 94-142 was not to force mainstreaming on local school districts, but to ensure that a range of placement options be made available to disabled children. Improvements in technology (such as programmable hearing aids, personal FM systems and other assistive devices, and cochlear implants) have positively influenced mainstream programs.

Since passage in 1975 of what is now the Individuals with Disabilities Education Act (IDEA), a number of important judicial interpretations of this special education law have been issued. The U.S. Supreme Court issued its first decision providing a definitive answer to the most central question raised by the law in 1982: "What, exactly, is an "appropriate" education for children with disabilities?" Although in this specific suit *(Board of Education, Hendrick Hudson Central School District v. Rowley, 458 U.S. 176, 181)* the Court found that a young deaf student did not require a sign language interpreter in school, it affirmed the right of all handicapped children to receive personalized instruction and the supportive services they need to benefit from their IEP. In this decision, however, the amount and quality of services to which children with disabilities are entitled vs. those that are necessary so that the children receive an education that is good enough to enable them to make passing grades, is open to interpretation. Obviously, this is a lower standard than many advocates wish had been set. The Court upheld the basics of the law that parents are to share in the planning and development of their child's IEP and that if the parents are not satisfied, they can appeal through the due process of law. An interesting story about this landmark case has been written by R.C. Smith (1996) and is entitled, "A Case About Amy."

Schildroth (1988) reports a definite shift in the educational placement of hearing-impaired students since implementation of Public Law 94-142. A significant decrease in the number of hearing-impaired children receiving special education services is attributed to the departure from the secondary schools of the large number of hearing-impaired students born during the 1964–1965 maternal rubella epidemic. With a drop in enrollment of deaf students from special day schools and residential schools, the number of hearing-impaired students enrolled in local school districts has increased 16% in just the past few years. However, a new concern is emerging based on the fact that an increasing number of local school districts report having only one or two hearing-impaired students in their schools. In fact, more than 52% of the 8428 schools reporting data to the 1985–1986 Annual Survey of Hearing-Impaired Children and Youth enrolled only one hearing-impaired student.

The proliferation of local schools enrolling hearing-impaired students has resulted in a dispersion of these children away from the special schools in which they were grouped together, usually at one location. These circumstances may be cause for concern regarding special staffing and support services not available or available only on an itinerant basis. The communication and socialization limits resulting from this isolation and dispersion may effect the hearing-impaired student's emotional and behavioral development. The profound effect of a serious hearing impairment on the communication, social, and academic achievement of deaf children is often not realized by many school officials, boards of education, or lawmakers.

In 1997, Congress passed the IDEA Amendments (PL 105-17) to reauthorize and make improvements to the original IDEA. Major revisions in the language of the law changed wording from "handicapped" to "child/student/individual with a disability." The IDEA Amendments required inclusion of children with autism and traumatic brain injury as a distinct class to benefit from the law. A final important point is that the Amendments now require a written plan for transition of these special needs children into general education classes by the age of 16 years. In 1999, Part B of IDEA was expanded to permit the use of school-purchased assistive technology outside school premises.

During 1986, Congress enacted Public Law 99-457, known as the Education of the Handicapped Act Amendments. The Amendments reauthorized the Education of the Handicapped Act (PL 94-142) and included a rigorous national agenda pertaining to more and better services to young special-needs children and their families. This legislation requires states receiving federal funds to extend the benefits of a "free appropriate public education to children ages 3 through 5 years." Specifically, these amendments expanded Public Law 94-142 to include handicapped infants from birth to age 2 years as well as preschool children. The new amendments challenge professionals in the field of deaf education to reexamine basic assumptions and develop a new range of services for this population, as well as incorporate and develop the role of families who have children with hearing impairments. This new federal funding presents an opportunity for innovative programs, research and development in early intervention programs, and cooperative working relationships between related-service professionals outside the discipline of deafness. In 1990, amendments to the Education for All Handicapped Children Act (EAHCA) officially changed the name to the Individuals with Disabilities Education Act (IDEA, PL 101-476).

PL 99-457 also called for an individualized family service plan (IFSP) for infants and their families, and in this way changed the focus to the family for very young children. The IFSP is the core of the recent family-centered approaches to early interventions for children and their families. The IFSP ensures that the family's strengths, beliefs, and values will be recognized, respected, and built on in the development of their disabled child. In most cases, the family into which a deaf child is born typically has no experience in interacting with deaf individuals and has no first-hand knowledge of the problems that lie ahead. Today single parenthood is common, and more and more families have two parents in the workforce. These changes in the family have tremendous implications for the early education and living environments for young deaf children.

CURRENT STATUS OF EDUCATION OF THE DEAF

The Babbidge Committee met in 1965 and reported that "the American people have no reason to be satisfied with their limited success in educating deaf children and preparing them for full participation in our society." The Babbidge report cited the underlying cause of this poor result as the failure to launch an aggressive assault on the basic problems of language learning by the deaf. Further, there was an urgent need for substantial progress in the development of improved systematic and adequate programs for educating the deaf at all grade and age levels.

In 1988 a blue ribbon Commission on Education of the Deaf met and published a comprehensive report on the status of education of the deaf in the United States. The report, "Toward Equality: Education of the Deaf," stated the primary and inescapable conclusion that the present status of education for persons who are deaf is "unacceptably unsatisfactory." The report points out that although we have had the knowledge available to improve the situation, our good intentions alone have not been sufficient. Granted that it will be an expensive effort to improve the current education of children with hearing impairment, but we really cannot afford not to remediate existing problems. The report called for action and prevention, rather than reaction and remediation, to enhance the well-being of the deaf and their families. The 1988 Commission believed that significant strides in educating persons who are deaf had been made during the intervening years since the Babbidge report, but that actual implementation of many initiatives had been inadequate. The Commission's report to the President and the Congress of the United States included 52 recommendations dealing with all aspects of deafness and education. "Toward Equality: Education of the Deaf" was aimed at federal government agencies to expend funds and establish the deaf as a priority to increase their present status quo situation.

Manual signing was first acknowledged as a language and incorporated into deaf education in 18th century France. Early educators of the deaf, Abbé de L'Epée and Thomas Hopkins Gallaudet, brought sign-based education for deaf children into the United States early in the 19th century. At the same time, Alexander Graham Bell was advocating auditory/oral education inspired by the communication success of his deaf wife. So began the often emotional and totally unresolved 200-year-old debate of which method of educating deaf children should prevail. During the 1960s, ASL was revived and widely used in deaf education in the United States. Today, ASL is said to be the third most used language in the United States, following Spanish and Italian. ASL, also known as "Ameslan," is the native language of the majority of the early-onset deaf population (Lotke, 1995).

Morres (1996) summarized the current situation in education of the deaf by indicating that three basic questions have yet to be resolved completely: (1) How shall we teach deaf children? (2) Where should we teach deaf children? and (3) What should we teach children? The answers to these questions will depend, of course, on whom is asked. It is likely that the answers will be greatly influenced by the emotional factors and associated biases within the various communities of professionals and concerned consumers who care about education of the deaf. The "how shall we teach" question addresses the oral versus manual controversy (signed or spoken language). The "where shall we teach" question concerns actual academic placement (residential schools, day school programs, or mainstreamed public schools). The "what should we teach" question relates to exactly what should be taught to a deaf student on any typical day (focus on academic content or speech production, speech reading, and auditory training?).

The most important consideration in the education of these special needs children is that the answers to these questions must lead to overcoming their difficulties in mastering language skills. For deaf children, it is that language barrier that stands between them and the full realization of their academic, intellectual, emotional, and social development.

Traditionally, residential schools have been aligned with manual-type communication in their education system, while private day schools tend to be auditory/oral in nature. Such dichotomy, however, is no longer so specific. With increased individualization of academic placement, more complex patterns of teaching and communication are available, and teachers are realizing that the use of FM amplification systems and classroom sign language interpreters have, in some locations, distorted the pure boundaries of the oralism and manualism controversy. The deinstitutionalization movement has dropped residential school enrollment considerably, while local school attendance now accounts for nearly 70% of attendance by deaf and hearing-impaired students. Special schools now enroll a higher percentage of the more seriously hearing-impaired students than did previous placement patterns (Schildroth, 1988). It can be seen that education of the deaf has undergone tremendous changes in recent years. Since 1975, classroom instruction in programs for the deaf has, interestingly, evolved to primarily total communication techniques at every education level, from primary grades to secondary school classes (Schildroth & Hotto, 1994).

The selection of an appropriate educational setting is not a simple decision. Although practical considerations (such as cost, geographic location, and transportation) must be taken into account and may play important roles, the best decisions are based on two primary knowledge bases: (1) a thorough understanding of the child's unique needs and (2) an awareness of the educational facilities and personnel available to meet those needs (Palmer & Yantis, 1990). Parents usually lack sufficient information to make these judgments independently. In urban communities, consultation is normally provided by many agencies serving the needs of communicatively impaired children and adults. Internet website searches are often the basis of information-gathering.

Because of the growth in educational options, Moores (1996) categorized and described the most common types of placement programs for students with hearing-impairment and deafness as follows:

- Residential Schools. The historic placement for deaf students into educational facilities that provide total living accommodations in addition to all of the required educational needs. Traditionally, each state supported at least one large residential school. More recently, the residential school has evolved to accommodate day students who live within commuting distance or weekday residents who return home for weekends and holidays. The effect of Public Law 94-142 was to change the scope of the residential school. The current status is that these programs are much smaller in total attendance with more day students rather than resident students.

- Day Schools. Generally found in larger metropolitan areas, these educational programs are typically established in separate and special school facilities. Children commute to these programs daily, and no normal-hearing students are included in classes.

- Resource Rooms. Most resource room programs are planned so that children spend most of their day in the regular classroom with normal-hearing classmates, returning to the resource room for special and or supplemental education activities. Special skills teacher(s) in the resource room are expected to provide individualized services to students varying in age, hearing loss, and academic achievement.

- Itinerant Programs. In this setting, children with hearing disabilities attend regular classes full-time and receive support services from an "itinerant" teacher who travels to work with children from several schools. The support education services may vary from daily to weekly lessons, depending on the child's needs and the teacher's availability.

An evaluation of the education cost for children with hearing impairment is shown in Table 10-2. A detailed analysis performed for the Colorado Department of Education concluded that every hearing-impaired child who is educated in a special self-contained classroom costs $6306 per year more than the child who is mainstreamed into regular classrooms. Hearing-impaired children educated in state residential programs cost $32,397 per child per year more than children educated in regular classrooms. The Educational Audiology Association (Von Almen et al., 1994) states that early identification is a bargain as educational costs increase significantly with the intensity of services required. Children with mild to moderate degrees of hearing impairment have the potential to be educated in regular classrooms with minimal extra support. The EEA concluded that taxpayers should be willing to pay a little more earlier in a child's life (i.e., cost of hearing screening and early intervention services) rather than paying a lot more later due to the specialized educational requirements for children identified with hearing loss at an older age.

Table 10.2.
Comparison of Education Costs

Placement	Annual Cost
Regular education (no special services)	$4064
Itinerant/consultant (up to 5 hr/wk)	$5767
Resource teacher (usually 20 hr/wk)	$6397
Self-contained classroom (more than 20 hr/wk)	$12,389
Preschool (special education 3 days/wk)	$8193
Residential (Room and board)	$31,139
Early home intervention program (90 min/wk)	$2600

Source: Von Almen et al., Educational Audiology Association (1994). [Letters to the Editor]. *Pediatrics, 94* (6), 957.

CHALLENGES IN TEACHING THE DEAF

All educators would agree that the most vital aspect of any child's intellectual development is language. For the deaf child, language is not a facilitating system for acquiring knowledge. The child's successful learning of language skills paves the road of progress in school and throughout life. The ability to communicate thoughts, wants, and needs to others and, in turn, the understanding of thoughts and feelings of others depends on crucial language skills. The deaf child's problem is that hearing plays a vital role in language development to build concepts and clarify them. The deaf child lacks this valuable input channel and accordingly throughout life has trouble developing and clarifying concepts. The entire process is slowed down and becomes laborious. Although deafness itself has no effect on intellectual potential, it may lead to impoverished communication skills that can limit development severely, unless the children are provided with some compensatory tools (Moores, 1996).

Language and concept developments clearly proceed hand-in-hand with communication. For the hearing child, the early states of communication are primarily via speech and hearing and may be categorized into five components:

- Reception. Sensory data are fed into the brain via the senses.

- Symbols. Words, signs, gestures that are used in *reception.*

- Encoding. Meaningful arrangement of symbols.

- Transmission. Meaningful sending of encoded material to someone else.

- Decoding. The receiver's mind utilizes the message and extracts meaning from it.

For smooth, free-flowing communication, all five components must be operating efficiently. There must be a sufficient

number of symbols to represent the message (vocabulary). There must be sufficient skill to encode the symbols (grammar). There must be sufficient mechanisms for transmission, such as speech and writing. The process of decoding involves understanding the vocabulary and grammar that form the very basis of the most important factor, the substance or content of the message itself. Incomplete communication and frustration result from a breakdown anywhere along the line.

The educator of the deaf faces the problem with every deaf child who may be stuck at the very first element of the communication process. The deaf child's mind is deprived of the rich sensory data supplied normally through the auditory mechanism and depends only on a meager supply of symbols to use for labeling, categorizing, and storing. New symbols are difficult to come by. The deaf child functions on the concrete level of mental operations; thus, abstract operations are most difficult because they are performed with words—the very commodity of which the deaf child never has enough. Abstract operations demand precise encoding and decoding and mastery of "word" concepts. Deaf children seldom attain sufficient language skills to master abstract operations even after arduous effort.

The usual process of trial and error learning—or teaching for that matter—is seriously hampered for the deaf child. The deaf child cannot hear errors of vocabulary or grammar. Attempts to correct the deaf child's errors are chancy undertakings. Because of the often indistinct transmissions (speech), the listener cannot be certain that the child made an error in the use of words or grammar or whether the listener just did not understand the spoken phrase. Suppose the listener thinks an error was indeed committed; imagine the task of trying to correct the error. Or suppose an error was committed but the listener is unsure and, because of the problems in trying to correct the error situation, is content to deduce an answer and let the error go. Thus, the child's error is reinforced and will surely be perpetuated.

One is never really sure what the hearing-impaired child is thinking because of difficulties in communication. Consider this example relayed to the authors by a teacher of the deaf. In her classroom of hard-of-hearing preschoolers, when some object would drop accidentally on the floor with a loud noise, the concept was conveyed to the children by the teacher who quickly held her hands over her ears and showed exaggerated facial expression of disdain. The children could see the situation clearly and quickly followed example, with similar behavior each time an object was dropped. A few days after this lesson, a pencil was dropped on a soft carpet accidentally. As expected, the preschoolers clapped their hands over their ears and made exaggerated faces! To what were they reacting? Surely not "noise" as the teacher thought she was teaching a few days previously. And so every concept must be carefully considered by the deaf educator from the eyes and mind of the hearing-impaired child.

Today, the problems of teaching the deaf are further complicated by the fact that a greater proportion of deaf young people are born deaf, or lose their hearing before the acquisition of language, than was the case 25 years ago. In fact, today, with medical achievements creating more control over the various etiologies of deafness, there are fewer adventitiously deaf children (who might have some language acquisition before their deafness) entering deaf education programs. Today's hearing-impaired child is usually congenitally deaf (at least, prelinguistic) and exhibits many more difficulties and frustrations in meeting language needs and speech skills than the child who may have lost hearing after the critical language age of 2 years. Further, many of today's deaf children, if born 30 or 40 years ago, might not have survived to enter school. Today they live, perhaps exhibiting addi-tional disabilities, significantly adding to the complexity of the education issue.

Legislation has influenced, and been influenced by, public perceptions of deafness and deaf individuals. It is an important sign that increasing numbers of deaf adults are entering the professions and taking advantage of more and more business opportunities. Deaf teachers, psychologists, counselors, researchers, and administrators are now having great influence on the education of deaf children. However, the irony of a field of communication specialists locked in seemingly intractable problems and conflicts cannot be overlooked. Despite overall documented improvements in education of the deaf, the academic achievement of deaf children remains unacceptably low. Limitations on literacy—reading and writing—continue to block achievement of reaching full potential for many deaf students. Opportunities for economically deprived deaf children, with less than adequate family environments, are still woefully inadequate. It is hoped that increased emphasis on early detection of hearing loss in newborns and early intervention will positively influence successful outcomes for children with severe to profound hearing impairments.

Individualized Educational Plan (IEP) . One of the key factors in successful mainstreaming is the guarantee that hearing-impaired students will not be "dumped and forgotten" into the regular classroom. This proviso is covered by the requirement in Public Law 94-142 for all handicapped children to receive personalized instruction and supportive services they need to benefit from an individualized educational program. The IEP is confirmation for hearing-impaired children that a more objective and scientific educational decision-making process will be followed. Through the use of IEPs, educators no longer rely on personal biases and preconceived ideas of what is best for the hearing-impaired child.

The term IEP means a written statement for each disabled child that is developed in any meeting by a representative of the local educational agency or an intermediate educational unit who shall be qualified to provide, or supervise the provision of, specially designed instruction to meet the unique needs of handicapped children, the teacher, the parents, or guardian of such child, and, wherever appropriate. The statement shall include (1) a statement of the present level of educational performance of such child, (2) a statement of annual goals including short-term instructional objectives, (3) a statement of the specific educational services to be provided to such child, and the extent to which such child will be able to participate in regular educational programs, (4) the projected date for initiation and anticipated duration of such services, and appropriate objective criteria and evaluation procedures and schedules for determining, on at least an annual basis, whether instructional objectives are being achieved (Johnson, Benson and Seaton, 1997).

Flexer (1990) points out that it is the school audiologist's role to actively integrate hearing services into the overall educational program of the hearing-impaired child in a manner consistent with the philosophy, goals, and objectives of the child's IEP. If the provision of hearing services or auditory pieces of equipment is not mentioned in the IEP, there is no assurance that the child's hearing needs will be met. When the audiologist is included as an IEP team member and a signatory of the IEP, there is greater probability that the hearing needs will be noted, understood, and appropriately managed.

No one is more important to the success of today's mainstreamed hearing-impaired student than well-informed and assertive parents who are intimately involved in their child's mainstreamed program on a regular basis and are serving as IEP team members. Hearing-impaired children must have strong advocates if they are to be educated successfully in public schools. Most regular teachers, special educators, and administrators receive little training in the effects of hearing loss. Moreover, administrators are responsible for a wide variety of students and programs under their jurisdiction. Their problem is to stretch inadequate resources to cover many programs, and they cannot serve as effective advocates for individual or small groups of special needs children (Davis, 1988).

Data regarding the psychoeducational status of children with mild and moderate hearing loss are scarce. Despite the limited data base, audiologists and speech/language pathologists often counsel parents regarding the possible deleterious effects of hearing loss and must help establish IEPs to enhance communication with these children and thus enrich their academic achievement. A project conducted by the University of Iowa (Davis, Elfenbein, Schum, & Bentler, 1986) attempted to evaluate the psychoeducational performance of 40 hearing-impaired children to study the effects of degree of hearing loss, age, and other factors on intellectual, social, academic, and language behavior. Their data did not predict the hearing-impaired children's language or educational performance on the basis of the degree of hearing impairment alone. Although some children evaluated in this study were performing exceptionally well, as a group the children fell into three major categories of significant delay: verbal skills, academic achievement, and social development. Some of these deficits did not manifest themselves until the child was in school for several years. The differences exhibited by the hearing-impaired children on the personality inventories suggest that these children are more likely to show aggressive tendencies, to express physical complaints, and to show significant behavior difficulties, especially social problems involving isolation and adjustment to school. It must be pointed out, however, that the individual results of this study confirmed the heterogeneity of hearing-impaired children and that the effects of hearing loss vary from child to child. The study did conclude that children with any degree of hearing loss appear to be at risk for delayed development of verbal skills and reduced academic achievement.

PREDICTING SUCCESS FOR HEARING-IMPAIRED CHILDREN

The prognosis for educational success for any child is nearly impossible to predict with any degree of accuracy. However, attempts have been made to identify the personal characteristics that may help parents and teachers identify the appropriate educational approach to facilitate learning for each child.

The Deafness Management Quotient (DMQ) was developed by Marion Downs (1974) to predict which children might be more successful in auditory/oral programs or need the supplemental information provided by the total communication approach. Her proposed formula consisted of five weighted scales based on the child's residual hearing, central processing intactness, intellectual factors, family constellation and support, and socioeconomic status. Lurterman and Chasin (1981) applied the DMQ scale retrospectively to a school-aged group of severely hearing-impaired children. The children with high DMQ scores were found to be in mainstream classes, whereas those children with lower DMQ scores had been placed in total communication classrooms. The authors suggested the addition of a measure of the child's use and acceptance of amplification as being more important than the audiometric hearing threshold pure tone averages.

The Spoken Language Predictor (SLP), devised by Geers and Moog (1987), attempted to improve on the concept of Down's DMQ scale by (1) selecting factors that better reflect a hearing-impaired child's potential for acquiring spoken language, (2) specifying more precisely the procedures for assigning weights to the factors, and (3) providing an option for a diagnostic category for those children for whom intensive instruction and periodic reevaluations will be required. Five factors were selected in the SLP that were judged to contribute significantly to a child's success in oral instruction and that could be estimated reliably in clinical evaluations of hearing-impaired children as young as 3 years of age. The five factors are hearing capacity, language competence, nonverbal intelligence, family support, and speech communication attitude. Geers and Moog described in detail all the tests used in each category to determine the point rating awarded to the hearing-impaired child in terms of educational recommendations. The SLP scale was validated in a sample of students at the Central Institute for the Deaf who were between 11 and 16 years of age. Each child's hearing, language, intelligence, family support, and communication attitude were obtained from test results and clinician ratings in their file that had been obtained between the ages of 3 and 5 years during their initial evaluation for school placement. The results suggest that children with high SLP scores have excellent potential for acquiring spoken language and should be enrolled in programs emphasizing oral communication. Children with low SLP scores are not likely to develop communicative competence with spoken language even with intensive oral instruction.

These suggested predictive formulae are somewhat dated in their utilization, but the concepts behind their development can still be applied today. Additional studies are underway to predict the educational success of children who are candidates for cochlear implants. The concept of the indices described above may be too simple for such a complex problem as education in childhood deafness, but the guidelines offered can tune the audiologist to those important variables that are necessary for successful educational outcomes.

EDUCATIONAL METHODOLOGIES

Many claims have been made about success of education of the deaf. Many claims, however, are from teachers of the deaf who have a strong personal belief in their own teaching techniques. Most claims, furthermore, are testimonials supported by a demonstration from one or two deaf children who have performed exceedingly well under the advocated, or advertised, method. During the past decade, more and better research efforts have been conducted to evaluate various methodologies used to teach deaf children. Most knowledgeable professionals agree, however, that *no single methodology works for all deaf children.* In this section, the discussion is limited to the oral, manual, and total communications philosophies of deaf education and a few of the most significant variations of these three major categories. Although virtually volumes of material have been written on the methodologies in education of the deaf, only a basic, and necessarily shallow, synopsis can be provided in these pages.

The terminology *auditory/oral* is used to describe programs that depend on spoken language alone for communication and teaching. A more recent development and specialized approach to the oral approach is known as *auditory-verbal* and is based on the expectation that young children who are deaf or hearing impaired can be educated through use of their own residual hearing, however slight. The descriptor *manual communication* is used to refer to programs that incorporate signs and/or fingerspelling. The term *total communication* is used to describe programs in which communication is accomplished by the simultaneous use of speech and signs with fingerspelling.

Although an enormous amount of research effort has been expended to determine the "best" communication mode for hearing-impaired children, the overall results have been inconsistent. Contrary to the expectations of proponents for each of the deaf education methods, there are no widespread and consistent interactions between the degree of a child's hearing loss and communication mode or between the child's intelligence and preferred communication mode. Some studies have shown the superiority of auditory/oral programs, whereas other studies favor total communication systems. Obviously a number of factors, which may or may not be interrelated, influence the results as well as the interpretation of the results among these many studies.

Auditory/Oral Method. The fundamental assumption of auditory/oral (also termed oral-aural) methods is that every deaf child should be given an opportunity to communicate by speech. Advocates of this method believe that children who are deaf or hearing impaired should be educated in regular learning and living environments, and that this will enable them to become independent, participating, and contributing adults. Within the spirit of this philosophy, advocates believe that an employer is more inclined to hire a deaf person to whom he or she can give oral instructions rather than an equally capable deaf person to whom the employer must communicate in gestures and writing. Proponents of this approach believe that orally trained children do very well in life and that training in speech and speechreading permits an earlier adjustment to a world in which speech is the chief means of communication.

In terms of preschool hearing-impaired children, there has been a shift from the number of children in total communication programs to more children in auditory/oral programs. This shift has, no doubt, been a byproduct of successful utilization of cochlear implants in young hearing-impaired and deaf children. Further, the success of legislative mandates in terms of early identification of disabled children has been largely responsible for the decrease in the age of intervention for younger and younger children with hearing losses. Clearly there has been an increase in the number of school-aged hearing-impaired children who are integrated (mainstreamed) with normal-hearing peers and an increased emphasis on parental involvement. These programs represent the oral/verbal approach to education of deaf children.

The auditory/oral systems teach that children who are to become good listeners also must use their vision to become good speechreaders. Since the two events do not happen simultaneously, it is necessary to establish the acoustic channel as the primary input means whenever possible. The use and development of the visual channel then seems to come naturally as needed. Conversely, auditory/oral proponents would suggest that if the visual channel is established first as the main source of the child's perceptions and information, then the use of hearing will not come naturally but only laboriously and slowly and with much intensive training.

An interesting study of 139 preschool children with severe to profound hearing loss from Ontario, Canada, attempted to investigate the relationship of several background and educational variables with the linguistic, academic, and social aspects of the children over a 4-year period (Musselman, Lindsay, & Wilson, 1988). Despite their careful analysis, they concluded that those unequivocal statements about the value of particular approaches or the consequences of not following one approach or another were unwarranted. They did state strongly, however, that no approach succeeded in reversing the devastating effects on language of severe to profound hearing impairment. As they tracked the children's movement among programs, it was found that auditory/oral

programs and IEPs were the programs of choice, whereas the children in total communication programs and group education programs tended to do less well. Musselman et al. (1988) noted that language itself is not a unitary ability but consists of a number of skills that respond differently to different interventions. In particular, it is necessary to distinguish among spoken language, receptive language, and mother-child communication. Despite the placement factors that operated in their study, these researchers found those children in total communication programs scored higher on measures of receptive language and mother-child communication, whereas children in auditory/oral programs had better spoken language.

Essentially three methods of auditory/oral education for deaf children are in use in the United States today, with a fourth methodology gaining new attention. All the auditory/oral methods have the commonality that they depend on speechreading and audition and wholly exclude the use of any natural signs or gestures. At times it is difficult to separate these auditory/oral education approaches, and some eclectic programs choose to utilize the best from all three methods. It would seem that the children who do best in such programs are those with good residual hearing and good listening skills. The main aim of these auditory/oral methods is to make the youngsters with hearing impairment or deafness an integral part of the hearing society through good speechreading and hearing aid use.

The first and primary oral method is *pure oralism* or *auditory stimulation*. It was developed in the United States at the Clarke School for the Deaf during the late 19th century. All sign language is discouraged, and the child is exposed to sounds and spoken language at every opportunity. The child is fitted with hearing aids and every excuse for auditory stimulation is utilized. In theory, the deaf youngster is to "hear" everything that a youngster with normal hearing might be exposed to, only the auditory stimulation must be conducted with more deliberate action and intensity than usual circumstances might dictate. The method starts with visual attention to speechreading and includes isolated sound elements, sound combinations, words, and finally speech. Much of the work is done at home, and if a nearby preschool for the hearing handicapped is not available, the John Tracy Clinic in Los Angeles offers a home-study course designed for parents.

When auditory stimulation alone or speechreading is not sufficient to initiate satisfactory speech and language development, a second oral method known as the *multisensory/syllable unit method* may be used. It is essentially the same as the pure oral procedure with speechreading, except that reading and writing of orthographic forms of English are included. Sight and touch are used as well as sound. This system is probably the most widely used oral method. Everything in the deaf child's environment is labeled, and his or her attention is drawn to the relation between the written form and the object as well as the relation between the written form and the spoken word. The teacher may use the motokinesthetic approach to learning speech, where the child mimics speech production by feeling the teacher's face and reproducing the same breathing and vibration effects.

The third oral method is called the *language association-element method* or *"natural language" method*. It was proposed and developed by the long-time principal of the Lexington School for the Deaf in New York City, Mildred Groht, who believed that the deaf child should learn to speak through normal living and daily activities. This type of program is developed around ordinary learning activities, and the teachers continually talk to the deaf children and encourage them to ask questions through vocalized speech. Activities are supplemented with specialized instruction in speechreading and speech production.

A well-recognized variant of the auditory/oral method is the so-called "unisensory" or "aural approach" to education of the deaf (Pollack, 1971). Rupp (1971) cites the features of an auditory emphasis program: (1) audition is the most suitable perceptual modality by which a child learns speech and language, (2) the unisensory approach develops the impaired-hearing modality to its fullest by focusing attention on audition, (3) the unisensory approach has applicability to the very young child, and (4) normalcy of environmental contacts at all levels is necessary for success of the method. The unisensory approach is dependent on very early identification, early parental guidance, early amplification, and total exposure to normal language stimulation. The unisensory approach to deaf education has numerous advocates and is practiced throughout the United States. Pollack (1982) published a most informative "how-to" article dealing with early amplification and auditory/verbal training of hearing-impaired infants.

The principles of the Pollack approach have been incorporated into the fourth general type of oral/verbal program known as the *auditory-verbal practice method*. The auditory-verbal practice method has achieved increased popularity in recent years from the need for cochlear implant recipients to receive an intensive auditory therapy program in order to maximize their newly acquired auditory potential. The auditory-verbal philosophy is a critical set of guidelines that focuses on listening as the major force in nurturing the development of the child's personal, social, and academic life. It is based on the belief that the use of amplified residual hearing permits children who are deaf or hearing impaired to learn to listen, process verbal language, and speak within their family and community constellations (Estabrooks, 2000). Verbal-auditory training goals and activities are tied to the developmental stages of each child and incorporated into ordinary daily routines, in song, educational activities, and play. An active international nonprofit organization, with stringent certification requirements for teachers, has been established as Auditory-Verbal International, Inc. to support professionals, parents, and persons who are deaf or hard of hearing.

According to Luterman (1976), the auditory/oral approach presupposes that speechreading or visual awareness of the face need not be taught; rather, the impaired auditory modality must be trained while allowing the child to use visual information as he or she needs it. This approach differs from the multisensory (visual/oral) system in which no formal work is attempted in speechreading, nor is the child's attention deliberately directed toward the speaker's face. While all agree that auditory training is an important part of the auditory/oral and the visual/oral program, the visual/oral proponents view auditory training as a supplement to vision.

Opponents argue against the aural/verbal methods citing several objections to the approach. In general, the complaints are against speechreading as a basic skill and the dependence on residual hearing to pick up auditory cues. They cite the fact that the oral method depends too heavily on the development of speechreading skills that are difficult for many to achieve at any level of proficiency. Speechreading is notoriously ambiguous because (1) many sounds and words look alike on the lips (homophonous words such as [mat], [pan], and [bat]; (2) many sounds are not visible because they are made in the back of the throat such as [k], [g], and [ng]; (3) many people do not speak clearly and distinctly; and (4) speaking styles among persons vary tremendously. In fact, speechreading is an art mastered by very few. Those who have the talent do very well and serve as demonstration students. Speechreading depends on good language skills, acute vision, good lighting, and exposure of the lips and is limited by distance between speakers. Speechreading is less useful in dimly lit environments, within groups of talkers, or for speaker-audience formats.

Critical Appraisal of the Auditory/Oral Methods. Eric Greenway (1964), a well-known British educator of the deaf, indicted oralism with the following comments:

> For almost a century we have witnessed the great oral experiment. . . . In theory it is ideal and there are essential virtues in its principles. In many respects it has been a courageous attempt to bring the deaf into the world of the hearing by simulation of the normal means of communication. But an honest appraisal of the results shows plainly that it has not met with the overall success that teachers hope for or that the deaf themselves desire and demand. It cannot be denied that there have been some outstanding successes with an exclusive oral system, but for the majority it fails because it is unable to provide the fullest and most congenial means of communication.

A classic study initiated at the University of Minnesota (Weiss, Goodwin, & Moores, 1975) intensively evaluated children in seven well-known programs for the deaf and hard-of-hearing. The programs provided a diverse representation of approaches to deaf education, ranging from auditory/oral to visual/oral. One of the findings regarding children who were integrated into mainstream education was that these children had had better hearing acuity and superior articulation before integration. It seemed conclusively evident that children do not speak better because of integration but are integrated because they speak better. Other measures in the 6-year Minnesota study compared relative communication efficiency between modes of training. Children were found to receive communication most efficiently when stimuli were presented simultaneously through speech and signs. Next were simultaneous speech and fingerspelling, followed by speechreading and sound. The least efficient means was sound alone. In the area of expressive speech, the better-hearing students had better articulation scores. The type of

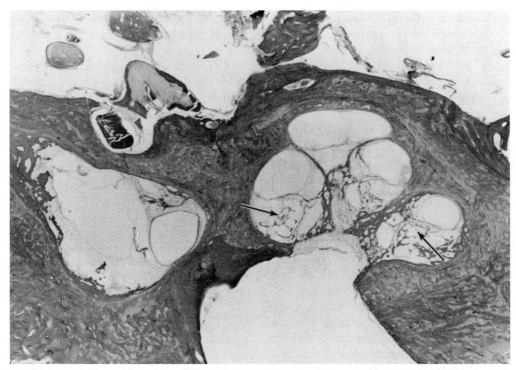

Figure 10-1. Midmodiolar section from the temporal bone of a patient whose deafness was caused by meningitis. Note the partial ossification that has taken place in the scala vestibuli portion of the cochlea (*arrows*) and the lack of eighth nerve fibers and spiral ganglia. This patient had no measurable hearing. The absence of essential sensory and neural structures makes amplification with a hearing aid useless. (Courtesy of I. Sando, MD, University of Colorado Medical Center.)

training seemed not to affect articulation scores; rather, skill in articulation related purely to the emphasis on auditory training and articulation given by a program.

It has been the authors' experience that despite the best of altruistic expectations, the auditory/oral methods cannot be successful with every deaf child. For example, some deaf children have no measurable hearing for one reason or another. Temporal bone studies from children with profound deafness have been reported with total absence of the cochlear structures or eighth nerve fibers (Fig. 10-1). Cochlear implants may not be recommended for certain deaf children for any one of a variety of reasons. Amplification, through personal hearing aids, may provide little or no substantive benefit. For the deaf and hearing-impaired children who fall into these categories, some other educational method may be the appropriate choice.

Visual/Oral Methods

The visual/oral methods are contrasted with the auditory/oral methods by their inclusion of manual signs and fingerspelling and, in fact, are most commonly known as *manual communication systems.* The basic philosophy behind these teaching techniques is that the visual aspect of signing and fingerspelling adds a component to the process that makes communication considerably easier. The children receive input through a standardized system of signs and fingerspelling and are taught to express themselves through speech, signs, and fingerspelling. The visual/oral methods do not exclude speechreading training and speech production, but they do not make these facets of the educational method the main focus. The primary goal in visual/oral education is to provide deaf and hearing-impaired children with a strong knowledge base, with production and reception of speech per se as a secondary goal. Manualists believe that their methods provide an education to the deaf child that is equal to the education of a normal-hearing child. Auditory/oral proponents question the emphasis on speechreading as a major component to the curriculum to the diminution of the three "R"s. Manual education specialists believe that language skills are paramount to speech production or speechreading, both educationally and socially.

American Sign Language (ASL). It is said by many, including the vast majority of deaf adults, that sign language is the common, natural language of the deaf. The signs have concrete meanings. Words can be spelled on the fingers to connect the signs into sentences. According to Ridgeway (1969), "the sign language with deaf children is part mime; it is beautiful to watch, highly expressive and receptive." The manual ASL serves communication purposes with far more than just signs and fingerspelling, as facial expression and body language convey much of the content of the communication.

The beginnings of ASL are said to lie with the work of L'Abbé de L'Epée, a French priest, who undertook the education of two deaf sisters in 1750. Fingerspelling had been used earlier to teach language to the deaf in France, but to it L'Epée added a "natural language of gestures." He established a school to teach the deaf in Paris in 1760 and was later succeeded by his equally famous pupil, L'Abbé Sicard. In 1815, an American named Thomas Hopkins Gallaudet, a minister from Hartford, Connecticut, met a young deaf neighbor girl, Alice Cogswell. Gallaudet was deeply taken by Alice's plight of "mutism" and the fact that she had no place to go to school. He sought support from families of other deaf children and ultimately went to Europe to study methods of teaching the deaf. He visited London and was refused access to Watson's Asylum, where secret and expensive educational methods were jealously guarded. However, he met L'Abbé Sicard and was invited to Paris to learn L'Epée's system of sign language. From this warm welcome in France, he returned to America with a young deaf teacher, Laurent Clerc, and established the first school for the deaf in the United States in 1817, the American School for the Deaf in Hartford. The school was replicated throughout the United States, and L'Epée's sign language was fused with the natural gestures used in America and became the basis for present-day sign language.

Years later, Thomas Hopkins Gallaudet, enjoying the success of establishing schools for the deaf across the United States, was still not satisfied. As an old man he passed his vision on to his son, Edward Miner Gallaudet, and his dream was realized with the establishment of Gallaudet College in 1864, the world's first college of the deaf, in Washington, DC. The establishment of the National Technical Institute for the Deaf, associated with Rochester Institute of Technology in New York, was the second full college program for the deaf—more than 100 years following the dedication of Gallaudet College.

The language of signs has been subjected to systematic analysis by several investigators including Tervoort (1964), Bornstein (1973, 1978, 1979), and Wilber (1987). Their conclusion is that sign language is an independent language that is not just a translation of oral language. Natural gestures and fingerspelling depend on situational understanding; when a sign has a tendency to become repeated and understood by more than one person, the sign is "formalized" and is no longer a natural gesture. The manual alphabet and samples of sign language are shown in Figures 10-2 and 10-3. Users of ASL understand the importance of facial expression in effective communication. In fact, the face carries much of the meaning and many of the subtleties needed to enrich communication. The limitations of sign language are also recognized and acknowledged by the experts. It is limited in scope and expressive

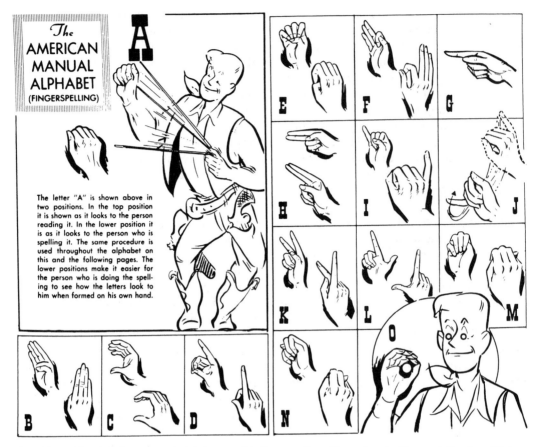

Figure 10-2. The American manual alphabet used in fingerspelling. (Reproduced with permission from Watson, D.O. (1964). *Talk with Your Hands* (pp. 185–189). Winneconne, WI.)

power when compared with oral language. Sign language is bound to the concrete and limited in expression of abstractions, metaphor, irony, and humor.

The standardization of ASL was enhanced by two important developments: the valuable contribution of Stokoe's (1965) "Dictionary of American Sign Language" and the establishment of a National Registry of Interpreters for the Deaf (RID). Garretson (1963), a respected deaf educator and long-time advocate of the use of fingerspelling and signs even though he was brought up in the oral tradition, cites the following factors as assets for the manual method:

- Denying a child the right to use his or her hands along with speech and

lipreading creates anxiety and emotional stress on the pupil.

- With the use of fingerspelling, signs, and speech, there is no doubt as to what is being communicated.

- Signs on the hands are considerably larger and clearer than lip movements.

- Fingerspelling and signs do not discriminate against anyone, and all have equal opportunity to participate and learn from classroom activities.

Certainly the major drawback to ASL is that its syntax is not particularly conducive to the development of standard English. With the ASL system it is difficult to express pronouns; verb tense is indicated by context; signs follow each other according to

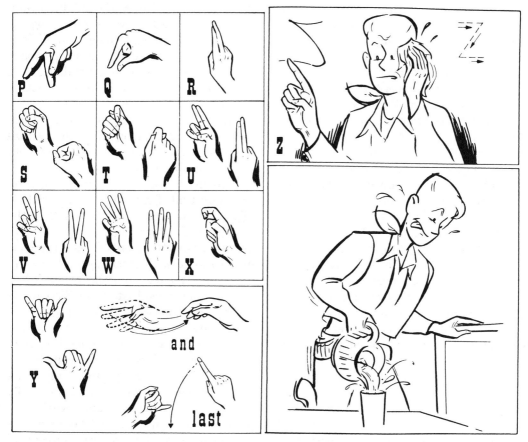

Figure 10-3. Signs and fingerspelling used in the sentence, "Please, would you like to dance with me?" (Reproduced with permission from Watson, D. O. (1964). *Talk with Your Hands* (p. 220). Winneconne, WI.)

convenience and not necessarily in accepted English order; and what is acceptable and utilized for social communication is the transmission of general concepts and not necessarily the specific content.

Mention should be made of two early variants of the manual system known as the *combined method* and the *simultaneous method*. The combined method uses speech, speechreading, hearing aids, and fingerspelling. The simultaneous method is essentially the same as the combined method with the addition of the language of signs.

Rochester Method. The New York State deaf residential school staff questioned the educational validity of signed English. They noted that deaf children, who had been taught in the auditory/oral method during primary school years and then introduced to Ameslan in later years, were still were not acquiring educationally acceptable English. There arose subsequently the *Rochester method*, which is the simultaneous use of speech and fingerspelling—a sort of "writing in air" technique superimposed on normal speech. This technique is also known as "visible speech" because the teacher is able to face the class and synchronize what is said and shown on the lips with a more visible form of English as spelled on the hands. The more visible approach of the Rochester method is thought to be a good supplement to the auditory/oral approach, because it is a pure, visible, English medium. It represents a multisensory visible oral-plus approach to language development. The Rochester method continuously emphasizes the traditional oral approach, while being supplemented by simultaneous visible fingerspelling.

Total Communication

Comparatively recently, in terms of deaf education tradition, a philosophy termed *total communication* has arisen. The proponents of total communication recognized the educational advantages of visible speech, yet they also noted certain difficulties. The manual dexterity of the preschool child limits his or her ability to fingerspell quickly, and the child's limited attention span makes it difficult to attend intensely on "flying fingers and fleeting flexible faces" for an all-day instruction session. Total communication is a philosophy that requires the incorporation of appropriate aural, manual, and oral modes of communication to ensure effective communication with and among hearing-impaired persons.

Total communication, as it is stressed by its advocates, is a *philosophy* and not simply another method for teaching deaf children. The basic premise is to use every and all means to communicate with deaf children from infancy to school age. No particular method or system is to be omitted or stressed. The student is exposed to natural gestures, ASL, fingerspelling, facial expression, and body English, all accompanied simultaneously with speech heard through hearing aids. The idea is to use any means that works to convey vocabulary, language, and idea concepts between the deaf child and everyone to whom he or she is exposed. The important concept is to provide an easy, free, two-way communication means between the deaf child and his or her family, teacher, and schoolmates. In some environments and educational facilities, total communication is practiced continually with all pupils throughout their school years.

For years, the approach to deaf education has been to start all children in an oral-type program for their early years of school. At some point, in second or third grade or at age 7 or 8, the child is evaluated with regard to educational progress and the oral method. As long as the child is progressing well, the oral/verbal approach is continued. If the child is not doing well, consideration is given for transfer into a manually oriented class. For most children, this timing of selecting their educational method so long after the critical years of language and speech development makes education prognosis very poor.

Opponents of total communication complain that if a teacher of the deaf really favors one method over another, the teacher will unwittingly move the students in the direction of that approach under the guise of teaching total communication. Some educators believe that it is not possible to evaluate the effectiveness of any one approach while using all the approaches at the same time. These arguments, however, seem to miss the main concept of total communication, which says that it is paramount to communicate without regard for which method is really achieving it. The total communication approach has been criticized because it is too much of a shotgun approach to education of the deaf. Critics argue that the overstimulation of the deaf child with speech and signs is actually detrimental to learning communication. On the other hand, new interest in total communication was the result of several research studies reporting the superiority of deaf children of deaf parents who were exposed to manual communication over deaf children of hearing parents in English skills, academic achievement, writing, reading, and social maturity. The two groups showed no differences in speech skills.

Total communication is an important concept in behalf of the deaf child and should provide years of a "head start" toward formal education. The concept of total communication has caught on and spread quickly in the United States. The progress thus far is encouraging, and the change in attitude from stressing a particular "method" to overall concern for the deaf child's needs to be immersed in two-way communication may turn out to be the most significant change in deaf education more than 100 years.

An interesting survey was conducted by Matkin and Matkin (1985) of parents whose hearing-impaired children had initially been enrolled in an aural/oral program for a minimum of 2 years and then subsequently enrolled in a total communication class in a day school setting for at least 2 years. The parents were asked a series of questions concerning the social, emotional, and educational growth of their child as well as the impact of the change in school communication system on their speech, speechreading, and hearing aid use. The study found a significant positive correlation between parents' overall perception as to the benefits of total communication and their perception of their children's educational and emotional growth. In addition, the parents did not perceive the use of total communication as adversely affecting speechreading, speech production, or hearing aid use.

OTHER SIGN SYSTEMS

During the past few years, several manual sign systems have been developed as improvements to ASL, since their design is such that they represent spoken or written English. These sign systems are described here to orient readers to the basic philosophies, approaches, nomenclature, and differences, because these approaches have been developed to overcome apparent inadequacies of the ASL. The other sign systems have as their premise that Ameslan, with linguistically generated variations, can be the visual equivalent of spoken English. Furthermore, they share the idea that if this type of system is introduced to the deaf child at a very early age, the language skills, total experiences, mental health, and communicative abilities will be improved over traditional approaches.

The sign systems discussed below have several principles in common. The basic premise is that deaf children need a visual symbol system to develop their language competency to its fullest potential. Manual communication proponents assume that the more syntactically correct the symbols, the more it will aid in development of language in the deaf child. Apparently, all agree that although ASL is an adequate communication tool, its syntax is such that it is not necessarily related to the grammatical structure of English. Finally, with exception of "cued speech" (described below), each manual method is based on the belief that a visual symbol system can be developed with basic ASL sign modifications that encourage the use of meaning through context that is more consistent with the form of spoken English.

Cued Speech. Cued speech is a method of communication developed by R. Orin Cornett for the hearing-impaired in which eight hand configurations and four hand placements are used to supplement the visible manifestations of natural speech. Cued speech was hailed in 1967 as a possible answer to the oralism versus manualism controversy. The 12 cues described above are used around the chin, cheek, and neck, drawing attention to the speaker's face and lips. The cued speech system provides a visible phonetic analog of speech in the form of lip movements supplemented by hand cues with both vowel and consonant cues.

According to Cornett (1985), most users of the auditory-only and multisensory approaches do not introduce written language until there is sufficient foundation in the basic oral skills to permit mutually supportive use of oral communication and written language. He believes that cued speech offers specific advantages for supportive use in oral programs. The greatest advantage of cued speech is that it facilitates the acquisition of the vocabulary and the syllabic-phonemic-rhythmic patterns of the spoken language without interrupting the natural process of communication to interpolate the written form. Cornett argues that cued speech meets the objections of total communication and other manual-language advocates that early communication through exclusively oral methods is insufficient to meet the psychosocial needs of the child. Cued speech forces the use of information on the lips by the hearing-impaired child without subjecting the child to the confusion of speechreading. The cues are not intelligible without proper mouth motions. Because "cueing" is completely dependent on spoken language and speechreading, it helps satisfy the auditory/oralist's demand that emphasis be placed on learning to communicate with those who do not know sign language.

Seeing Essential English. Seeing Essential English (SEE$_1$), a sign system originated by David Anthony in 1962 and developed in Southern California, uses modifications of Ameslan to resemble English. SEE$_1$ is intended for use by all age groups and now has as its basis an impressive two-volume manual that includes an introduction to the system, how it is used, grammar and syntax guidelines, and well over 5000 vocabulary entries (Anthony et al., 1971). The SEE$_1$ system has the largest vocabulary of any of the new systems. SEE$_1$ signs represent word forms or word parts such as roots, prefixes, or suffixes. The signs are used in combinations to form any desired word. To reflect English syntax, SEE$_1$ emphasizes complete English word order. Verb tense is clearly indicated and irregular verb forms have signed representation. In general, English words are represented by the traditional American sign word plus a suffix and/or prefix. English compound words are often made up of elements different from the single sign element often used in ASL. As a result, SEE$_1$ words often do not closely resemble the original source sign in ASL. SEE$_1$ is similar enough to ASL so that users can almost read it in context but may not be able to identify specific SEE$_1$ signs without previous exposure or explanation.

Signing Exact English. Signing Exact English (SEE$_2$) was a sign system developed in 1972 by a group of former members of the Seeing Essential English group. The notations SEE$_1$ and SEE$_2$ are used to differentiate the two systems. According to Bornstein (1973), the reasons leading to the development of Signing Exact English is that SEE$_1$ used many signs that were too distant from ASL, that it was too radical in its use of the root word, and that it was too complex for the needs of parents and teachers. Accordingly, SEE$_2$ uses signs that represent words rather than roots, as well as basic affixes as needed. SEE$_2$ has a vocabulary of some 2800 words published in booklet form. SEE$_2$ is also intended to be used by young children.

It is readily apparent that a situation can develop whereby parents and children who interact with persons trained in another system will use different signs for the same word. According to calculations reported in Bornstein (1973), 61% of the SEE$_2$ vocabulary is based on traditional ASL signs, 18% is based on modified ASL signs, and 21% consists of entirely new signs. When SEE$_2$ signs were compared with SEE$_1$ signs, some 80% of the traditional sign group were identical in both systems. Bornstein, Saulnier, and Hamilton (1980) and Bornstein and Saulnier (1981) concluded that difficulties created by these sign word differences are relatively minor.

VERBOTONAL METHOD

Around 1952, Professor Petar Guberina from the University of Zagreb, Yugoslavia, began developing a method to improve foreign language teaching through emphasis on the spoken rhythm of the language to be learned. He later applied his theory and methods to teaching deaf children and adults, still with emphasis on the rhythm of spoken language and on speech perception and production as an interacting loop system. According to Craig and Craig (1972), the verbotonal approach is characterized by (1) emphasis on low frequencies (below 500 Hz) and on vibratory clues in perception of spoken language patterns, (2) matching of special amplification devices known as SUVAG to the deaf person's optimum "field of hearing," (3) use of body movements to assist both in production and perception of speech, (4) emphasis on acoustic memory for language patterns aided by body movements and by articulatory movements from the production of speech, (5) providing speech and language work in active "play"-type situations so that much longer periods of concentrated work on spoken language are possible, and (6) emphasis on language in meaningful context of "situations."

Guberina's concept is based on his theory that the low frequencies of spoken language do not mask the high spoken frequencies. He believes that amplifications of auditory clues below 500 Hz, to include rhythmic patterns and the sound fundamentals, can actually help the deaf person to perceive the higher speech frequencies. In an additional effort to reach the low-frequency residual hearing of profoundly deaf children, the verbotonal approach includes the use of vibrators, or bone oscillators, to provide vibratory cues in the perception of language rhythms and sound patterns. Body movements are an important part of the technique, and speechreading is taught only incidentally. Asp (1985) reported that in the University of Tennessee verbotonal preschool program, between 65 and 75% of the hearing-impaired children (average hearing loss of 90 dB HL in the better ear) have been successfully integrated into regular public school classrooms. Guberina and Asp (1981) summarized a number of studies of international verbotonal programs.

MAINSTREAMING

Mainstreaming may be the single most important issue in education of deaf children in the past few decades. According to Madell (1984) mainstreaming is an educational programming option for handicapped youth which provides support to the handicapped student(s) and his teacher(s) while he pursues all or a majority of his education within a regular school program with nonhandicapped students." In short, mainstreaming is the current term for the practice that used to be known as "integration" of the hearing-impaired student into regular classrooms with hearing children. Mainstreaming is a procedure that is already well established in the United States and is the crest of a fast-moving wave in education circles. The real push for mainstreaming has been the stimulation provided by the "least restrictive" portion of the new federal law known as the Education for All Handicapped Children Act of 1975.

The organization of educational programs for hearing-impaired students is undergoing considerable change in many states. The change is from serving only a few students, mainly in residential schools, toward serving many deaf students in local community programs with a system that provides a variety of educational opportunities to the hearing-disabled child and his or her parents. It has become apparent over time, however, that partial or full-time integration for hearing-impaired students into regular classes is not a realistic goal for every child, nor is the policy of self-containment classes suitable for all hearing-impaired children. The integration of hearing disabled students into the regular classroom is a means of eliminating the deleterious effects of segregation and the stigma often attached to the "handicapped" student. Normal children are thus exposed to disabled children, resulting in positive and enlightened responses toward the integrated person. Of course, a negative response to the integrated child or disability condition is also possible, with devastating results to the integrated child.

Birch (1976) suggested that mainstreaming deaf children should be done only after thorough preparation, with sensitivity to the needs of all parties and with careful monitoring and support. Birch stated that degree and onset of hearing loss are not the primary factors in selecting children for mainstreaming. Regular classroom teachers are very accepting of hearing-impaired pupils and are willing to design programs for complete or partial mainstreaming, depending on the child's capabilities, requirements, and the school's resources. Mainstreaming has been tried for years, and its ultimate success for both normal-hearing and hearing-disabled children is the reason for its continued survival and growth.

In one scenario of mainstreaming, the deaf child is put into a class with hearing children only when a tutor-interpreter is available to translate everything said in the classroom into sign language and fingerspelling. The tutor-interpreter is a trained teacher of the deaf so that the teacher aide function is utilized constantly to help the hearing-impaired student. The tutor helps the deaf child to keep up with the rest of the class and grasp fully what is going on at all times. Acceptance of such a program in the regular school is enhanced by teaching all normal-hearing students and classroom teachers elements of sign language and fingerspelling.

Special consideration must be given when hearing aids are worn by the hearing-impaired child mainstreamed into the regular classroom without regard for the acoustic characteristics of the normal schoolroom. Poor signal-to-noise ratios produce detrimental effects on speech discrimination and understanding by the hearing-impaired student using amplifi-

cation aids. A study of this problem in the Detroit metropolitan area indicated that hearing-impaired children with malfunctioning hearing aids studying in regular classrooms suffered a high scholastic failure rate (Robinson & Sterling, 1980).

Madell (1984) and the staff at the New York League for the Hard of Hearing published a monograph based on their years of experience in helping hearing-impaired children succeed in mainstreamed educational settings. Their monograph, "Mainstreaming," offered excellent practical information to help any audiologist meet the challenge of assisting an auditory-handicapped child in a regular school setting, as well as suggestions to adapt the school environment to achieve optimal opportunities for the integrated children and the normal-hearing students.

Brackett and Maxon (1986) published a useful listing of services for hearing-impaired mainstreamed children that might be provided by the educational audiologist in the public school setting (Table 10-3).

A thought-provoking essay questioning the quality of a mainstreamed education for prelingually deaf children was published by Brill (1975), a veteran of 25 years as the Superintendent of the California School for the Deaf in Riverside. Until a few years ago many deaf children were postlingually deafened as a result of some childhood illness. However, today's deaf children are mostly *prelingually* deaf and present different educational problems. Brill points out that the deaf child learns best when in a small class composed of children who are about the same age and educational level. It is likely that a limited geographic area will contain only a small number of deaf children of about the same age and educational level. Brill cautions that the integration of deaf children into a class with hearing children is sometimes only token integration. The deaf child with communication disability may not be best placed in a regular hearing classroom. The teacher in the regular classroom often does

Table 10.3.
Suggested Responsibilities for Educational Audiologists

Comprehensive audiologic and amplification evaluation

Unaided: pure tone air- and bone-conduction thresholds

Unaided: speech reception and speech discrimination

Electroacoustic impedance measures

Aided (aids and FM): sound field warble tone thresholds

Aided (aids and FM): sound field speech measures

Electroacoustic analysis of hearing aids and FM system

Thorough report from evaluator

Comprehensive communication evaluation

Preferred receptive mode: auditory only, visual only, auditory-visual combined

Comprehension of spoken language: vocabulary level, sentence level, connected discourse

Production of spoken language: vocabulary level, sentence level, connected discourse

Speech intelligibility

Written language

Annual reevaluation

Educational evaluation

Skill differentiation within subtests important

Test presentation and format to be considered during interpretation of results

Annual reevaluation

Psychosocial evaluation

Performance subtests used as an estimate of potential

Verbal subtests measure language ability

Triennial reevaluation

Classroom observation

Child/teacher interaction

Child/child interaction

Child participation

Classroom modifications

Learning strategies

Use of FM systems

Analysis of noise sources

Visual distractions

Use of classroom aide/interpreter

Audiologic management

Improving classroom acoustics

Recommending and using FM systems

Daily troubleshooting of personal aids and FM system

Assessing use of FM system within various settings

Monitoring of middle ear problems with appropriate referrals

Speech-language management

Focus on deficit areas that affect academic performance and social interaction

Coordination with other support personnel and classroom teacher

Educational management

Favorable seating

Buddy system

Notetaker

Discussion of hearing impairment/amplification

Improving classroom presentation: characteristics of teacher's speech, paraphrasing of content, directing classroom discussion using visual aids

Improving the use of classroom amplification

Improving classroom flexibility

Discussing teacher's expectations

Facilitating teacher/tutor exchange

Preview/review tutoring

Academic vocabulary

Academic content

Classroom aide/interpreter

Psychosocial management

Adolescent group, including career information

Parent support group

Extracurricular social activities

Parent involvement

Home support

Program planning

Regular contact with school personnel

In-service training

Staff: whole school: once each year

Direct service personnel: twice per year

Individual as needed

Peers: once per year

Alternative educational placement

Full mainstreaming

Partial mainstreaming

Social mainstreaming

Self-contained class in regular school

Adapted from Brackett, D. and Maxon, A.B. Service delivery alternatives for the mainstreamed hearing impaired child. *Language, Speech and Hearing Services in Schools, 17*,115–125, 1986.

not have the competencies to meet the child's special needs.

In view of the current social climate, mainstreaming is here to stay. Nevertheless, caution must be exercised so that professionals and parents do not perceive mainstreaming as "the only way to go." The most important issue is to ensure that parents have the option of choice and that they fully understand all of the possible educational placements available for their hearing-disabled child. Ling (1975) likens the deaf education controversy to cyclic sunspot activity. It has flared up on numerous occasions in the past and abates only when the protagonists realize that there is no one method or mixture of methods that can possibly meet all the needs of hearing-impaired children and their parents.

Julia Davis and colleagues (Davis, Shepard, Stelmachowicz, et al., 1981) describe the population of hearing-impaired children as "vastly heterogeneous" and correctly point out that the best use of the residual hearing in each child will require different procedures and emphasis. These authors provide a strong summary statement for this topic by stating, "We really must stop arguing over whether children use the auditory system *alone* or in conjunction with visual or tactual information during educational endeavors. If the energy spent in futile attempts to convince each other of the supremacy of one educational method over another had been spent in devising ways to maximize reception through *all* modalities, including hearing, it is unlikely that the educational achievement levels of hearing-impaired children would be as low as they are today."

DEAFNESS AND VISUAL ACUITY

As the education of children with hearing impairment depends a great deal on vision, concern for visual acuity in deaf children is crucial. It is recommended that every child with hearing loss undergo routine ophthalmologic examinations. It is vitally important that information concerning the importance of visual assessment for persons with hearing loss be provided to parents of hearing-impaired children and to professionals (Johnson & Caccamise, 1981).

Clinicians should be well acquainted with the symptoms of *retinitis pigmentosa*. Retinitis pigmentosa is characterized by an initial loss of night vision, or blind spots, followed by loss of peripheral field vision. Retinitis pigmentosa in the form of night blindness usually begins during puberty,

with blind spots appearing by the late teenage years. Retinitis pigmentosa is defined as a disorder associated with a group of diseases that are frequently hereditary, marked by progressive loss of retinal response (as elicited by electroretinogram), retinal atrophy, attenuation of the retinal vessels, and clumping of the pigment, with contraction of the field of vision. Retinitis pigmentosa may be transmitted as a dominant, recessive, or X-linked trait.

The combination of retinitis pigmentosa and deafness is known as Usher's syndrome. Of the almost 16,000 deaf and blind people in the United States, more than half are believed to have Usher's syndrome. Vernon (1969) and Vernon and Pickett (1976) noted that Usher's syndrome is the leading cause of deaf-blindness. The incidence of Usher's syndrome among the congenitally deaf if approximately 3–6%, whereas its occurrence in the general population is 3/100,000. The concern for identification of Usher's syndrome in the congenitally deaf child is very important, because the child will need extensive special education, counseling, social-emotional support, and vocational consideration. Although most hearing loss associated with retinitis pigmentosa is severe to profound, some moderate sensorineural hearing loss patients have been reported. Unfortunately, there is no current cure for Usher's syndrome, although at least eight different genes have been identified as the locus of the disorder.

Currently, there are three generally recognized types of Usher's syndrome. Children with Usher's syndrome 1 are profoundly deaf from birth and have severe balance problems. They are typically slow to sit and walk without support and usually develop severe vision problems by the age of 10 years. Children with Usher's syndrome 2 are born with moderate to severe hearing impairment and normal balance. These children tend to do well in regular classrooms and benefit from hearing aids. Retinitis pigmentosa, characterized by blind spots, begins to appear shortly after the teenage years. The visual problems associated with Usher's syndrome 2 tend to progress more slowly than those in Usher's syndrome 1. Children with Usher's syndrome 3 are born with normal hearing, balance, and vision. However, Usher's syndrome 3 victims are usually blind by mid-adulthood (Kimberling & Pieke-Dahl, 1998).

Hicks and Hicks (1981) presented a five-stage program for dealing with deaf youngsters with symptoms of retinitis pigmentosa. Stage I is an *awareness period* between the ages of 6 and 12 years and consists of a comprehensive diagnosis and explanation of the disease to the child and parents. Stage II involves *general counseling* including genetic counseling and educational and career planning. Stage III is the *general planning and community resource identification* stage, during which the child is established with an appropriate resource agency that can assume primary responsibility for case management. By this period, the deaf patient has probably suffered considerable loss of vision. Stage IV consists of the *specific planning and adjustment counseling* stage and deals with the middle adult years and stresses. Finally, Stage V, the *adjustment stage,* deals with the later adult years when Usher's syndrome has caused a complete loss of usable vision in the deaf client. This is an extremely important article written to acquaint the uninitiated with the real world severity and traumatic experiences for those involved with this problem. It is hoped that the current genetic analysis of the many types of Usher's syndrome will yield treatments and prevention of the various vision disorders associated with deafness.

PARENT TRAINING

Perhaps no calling is more important than that of being a parent, and no job is more challenging. For most parents, raising children is a trial-and-error process marked by countless frustrations. This is especially challenging for parents of children with hearing disabilities. When asked, most parents readily admit that they would benefit from learning more about children and parenting. Fortunately, numerous education and training programs are available to help parents of hearing-impaired children. Parent support programs seek to provide basic education while striving to improve parental attitudes and behavior toward their disabled child. Researchers have found that parent training programs have consistent and persistent influence on both parental behavior and the intellectual development of the young child. Training program participants express more confidence and satisfaction with parenting. According to the Carnegie Task Force on Meeting the Needs of Young Children (Carnegie Corporation, 1994), these findings confirm that improved interactions within the family system indeed have a substantial and lasting influence on the family environment and the child's long-term development.

For too many years, the attention of professionals has been devoted to the hard-of-hearing or deaf child and little consideration has been given to the parents. The parents of the deaf child may be the keys to one of the most significant factors in the deaf youngster's development. Fortunately, during the past few years, parent-oriented habilitation programs for children with hearing impairment have emerged. The importance of families of hearing-impaired children and the role they play in the development of the handicapped child is the subject of an excellent textbook by Schuyler and Rushmer (1987).

The major emphasis of parent training includes emotional support for the parents by helping them recognize, realize, accept, and understand the implications of their child's hearing problem. This increased awareness should help reduce anxiety and worry often expressed by parents of hearing-disabled children. Education for the parents is important so that they might fully understand the nature of their child's hearing loss with realistic expectations of the educational future for their youngster. The parent is taught to understand child growth and development as well as the need for communication skills, social contact, and emotional expression.

Horton (1975) summarized the objectives of parent training programs into categories:

- To teach parents to optimize the auditory environment for their child.
- To teach parents how to talk with their child.
- To teach parents strategies of behavior management.
- To familiarize parents with the principles, stages, and sequence of normal development (including language development) and apply this frame of reference to stimulating their child.
- To supply effective support to aid parents in coping with their feelings about their child and to reduce the stresses that a hearing-disabled child places on the integrity of the family.

Parents must be involved in the choice of the communication system used with the hearing-handicapped child. The communication system itself is secondary to parental agreement, enthusiasm, and commitment to the system. Professionals can provide guidance, exposure, and background to the parents, but the final choice should be made with full cooperation and agreement with the parents. Imposing the use of signs on parents who lack confidence in their ability to interact with the child is a common cause of failure. If the parents choose to use signs, the entire family must develop fluency with this means of communication.

It is vitally important to teach the parents how to utilize and adapt daily activities of the home as experiential teaching events for the preschool child. It is hoped that the result is a stimulating home environment for the hearing-impaired child where auditory, speech, and language development is a daily, ongoing, and natural activity. Some programs have a model home completely furnished and operational with kitchen, bathroom, bedroom, and playroom. The home is stocked with typical utensils and furnishings. Parents spend time with the parent-training supervisor to learn how to develop a repertoire of experiences and activities to stimulate interaction with their children. Videotape is used extensively to observe parent-child interaction, with immediate feedback to the parents to increase their abilities with their children.

Major cities and most large clinic programs have parent-centered projects underway, and it would appear that the deaf child will be the ultimate beneficiary of the support and education aimed at his or her parents during the initial stages of discovery of the hearing loss. Meadow and Trybus (1979), in a review of emotional problems of the deaf, report three family variables of importance to a deaf child's mental health: (1) degree of parental overprotectiveness, (2) development of unrealistic expectations for the child's progress, and (3) effectiveness of parent-child communication.

Greenberg (1975) published an important study that examined the attitudes and stress of hearing families with a profoundly deaf preschool child. The author studied 28 families that were equally divided into two groups: those using oral and those using simultaneous communication. These groups were further subdivided based on communicative ability (high versus low). Mothers completed questionnaires and interviews on stress concerns, parent attitudes, and their child's developmental level. Results showed few differences between families using simultaneous and oral communication. However, comparison of the four subgroups indicated that those with high-competence simultaneous communication skills had more positive attitudes and less stress than highly competent oral communication families.

The parents of children who are hearing impaired or deaf are likely to be bombarded with well-intended but conflicting messages from everyone, ranging from helpful friends to experts in various fields. Monitoring the child's development during those early years is essential, because good communication will continue to be the key to development as the child gets older.

Brothers and sisters as well as extended family members are important components of the communication network. Support groups are available to help families be in touch with others who share similar problems, but support groups need to be selected carefully in the beginning as they often come with a strong bias for one or another point of view. Parents need exposure to various advocates of all points of view, but in the end the parent must make decisions based on what is best for the child and the family.

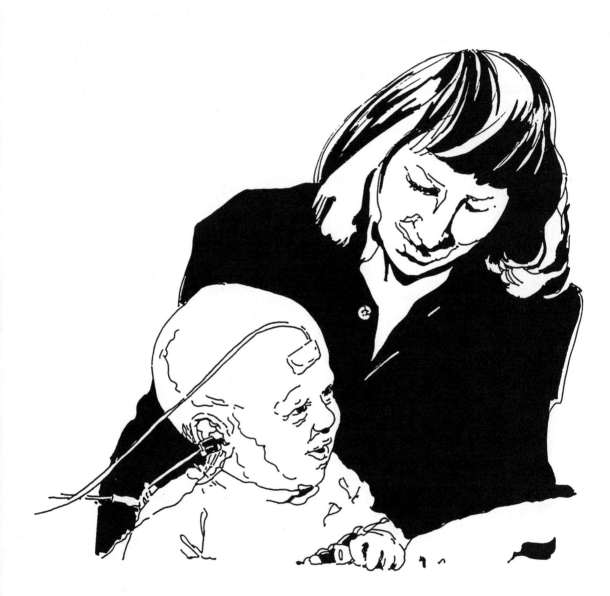

Appendix of Hearing Disorders

This appendix presents synopses of various syndromes and disorders associated with congenital deafness. A *syndrome* is a pattern of anomalies with a specific cause, a *sequence* represents a pattern of anomalies that directly results from a primary anomaly, and an *association* is a heterogeneous group of anomalies that occur together more often than expected by chance (Toriello, 1995). The majority of the 200 types of hereditary hearing loss occur without clinical indicators, leaving a remaining one-third with recognizable physical characteristics. During the late 1960s and early 1970s, considerable effort was devoted to the classification and identification of children with syndromes and the associated disorders and manifestations; the majority of classic references are from that era. Today, the technological advances in human genetics have turned attention to chromosome mapping and genetic-linkage analysis of inherited syndromes.

The materials presented here provide brief summaries of information believed to be pertinent to the audiologist. To be sure, these are not everyday patients; their presence in the general pediatric population is rare. However, because these children are highly likely to have associated hearing disorders, it is also likely that their treatment and management will involve audiologic evaluations and management. The information in this appendix is by no means intended to be exhaustive or even complete; the intent is to provide a concise, clear, and informative reference regarding special patients who have an inordinately high risk for hearing impairment. The authors recognize that children with symptoms that are variants from the generalized information about each disorder will be seen, and that readers will immediately wish to revise the summary presented here. So be it. The intent is to provide an orientation or a guide to help understand those children who demonstrate these disorders and to instill a desire to learn more about the syndromes and diseases. An accurate identification and diagnosis of a specific genetic disorder in a child may be helpful in anticipation of associated complications. More knowledge regarding a specific diagnosis will aid in long-term management decisions that will benefit the patient.

When the first edition of this textbook was produced in 1973–1974, few reference sources were available regarding syndromes that include hearing impairment or deafness as a key characteristic. Since 1976, the number of syndromes associated with hearing loss has burgeoned. Fortunately, interest in genetic deafness has also grown, and there is now a multitude of reference materials to research. Some students may wish to consult those more complete reference sources for detailed accounts of syndromes included in this section or to pursue information on syndromes not included here. Such references cover much more than individual articles and may touch on many aspects of the disorders not covered in these necessarily brief summaries. Accordingly, a list of recommended readings is presented at the end of this appendix. The authors have found these resources to be immeasurably useful in reviewing and updating birth defects, syndromes, and diseases associated with hearing loss.

Absence of the Tibia and Congenital Hearing Loss

Carraro Syndrome

Rare skeletal disorder; recessive trait; characterized by congenital absence of one or both tibias (lower legs), shortened malformed fibulas, and severe congenital sensorineural hearing loss (Pashayan, et. al., 1974; Richieri-Costa, et al., 1990).

Achondroplasia

A congenital skeletal anomaly characterized by slow growth of cartilage, retarded endochondral ossification, and almost normal periosteal bone formation (Fig. A-1). As a result, those affected are very short in stature with disproportionately short limbs, large heads with prominent foreheads, depressed nasal bridge, and "button" nose. Mentality is usually normal, but retarda-

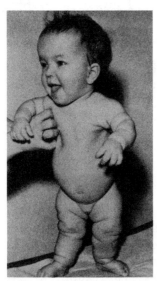

Figure A-1. Achondroplasia. (Reproduced with permission from Shepard, T.H., & Graham, B. (1967). The congenitally malformed: achondroplastic dwarfism: diagnosis and management. *Northwest Medicine, 66,* 451–456).

tion may appear secondary to hydrocephalus and increased cranial pressure. Deafness may be present. Respiratory, pulmonary, and other complications increase with age. Diagnosis may be suspected by clinical examination but is confirmed by radiographic evaluation. Autosomal dominant inheritance; however, more than 80% of cases are due to fresh mutation, with both parents being normal. Incidence increases with increasing parental age. Both conductive and/or sensorineural loss may be present. Middle ear anomalies include fusion of ossicles to surrounding bony structures as well as dense thick trabeculae without islands of cartilage in the endochondral and periosteal bone. Associated anomalies of the inner ear include deformed cochlea and thickened intercochlear partitions. High incidence of otitis. General treatment consists of genetic counseling, amplification, and surgical treatment as indicated (Cohen, 1967; Glass et al., 1981; Shohat et al., 1993).

Acoustic Neuroma

See Neurofibromatosis.

Albers-Schönberg Disease of Osteopetrosis

Chalk Bone Disease; Ivory Bone Disease; Marble Bone Disease

Craniofacial and skeletal disorder; recessive form associated with deafness. Brittle but paradoxically sclerotic thickened bones. Head may be somewhat enlarged; retarded growth in one-third of cases. Visual loss noted in approximately 80% of cases, which may lead to blindness. Mental retardation in 20% of cases; facial palsy, unilateral or bilateral. Little detailed

audiometric data available, but 25–50% of patients are reported to have mild to moderate, progressive sensorineural or conductive hearing loss (Johnston, Lawy, & Lord, 1968; Myers & Stool, 1969; Bollerslev et al., 1987).

Albinism With Blue Irides

Tietz-Smith Syndrome; Oculocutaneous Albinism

Integumentary and pigmentary disorder; dominant; scalp hair white, fine, and silky, sometimes with patches of pigmentation. Fair skin. Possible heterochromia of iris. Severe sensorineural congenital deafness (Tietz, 1963; Reed, Store, Boder, et al., 1967).

Alport Syndrome

Hereditary Nephritis With |Sensorineural Hearing Loss

Renal disorder associated with progressive sensorineural hearing loss and ocular anomalies. Genetically heterogeneous group of as many as six different disorders with an overall incidence of 1:200,000. Characteristics include autosomal dominant inheritance with men being more severely affected than women, progressive nephritis with uremia, ocular lens abnormalities such as cataracts, and progressive sensorineural hearing loss. Hearing loss with variable expressivity occurs in 40–60% of cases; ocular defects in 15%. Hearing impairment is typically mild to severe, high frequency, usually bilaterally symmetrical, and may occur alone or in combination with the renal disease. Onset of hearing impairment occurs in preadolescence (Bergstrom, Jenkins, Sando, & English, 1973; Rintelmann, 1976; Johnson & Arenberg, 1981; M'Rad et al., 1992; Wester, Atkin, & Gregory, 1995).

Amyloidosis, Nephritis, and Urticaria

Muckle-Wells Syndrome

Dominant. Onset in teens of recurrent urticaria (vascular reaction of skin with elevated patches and itching) with malaise and chills with onset of recurrent limb and joint pain. Amyloidosis (starchy-like substance in the blood) precedes nephropathy and renal failure. Progression of sensorineural hearing loss parallels progression of renal failure, resulting in severe hearing impairment by third or fourth decade of life. Endocrine and metabolic disorder with progressive sensorineural hearing loss of adolescent onset (Muckle, 1979; Champion, 1989).

Apert Syndrome

Acrocephalosyndactyly

Skeletal and associated skull malformations that include craniofacial dysostosis, syndactyly, brachiocephaly, hypertelorism, bilateral proptosis, saddle nose, high arched palate, ankylosis of joints,

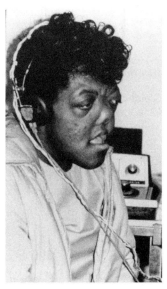

Figure A-2. Apert syndrome.

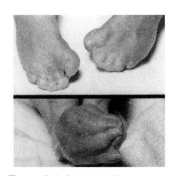

Figure A-3. Apert syndrome.

spinal bifida, and mental retardation (Figs. A-2 and A-3). Syndactyly (fusion of fingers and toes) is complete on both hands and feet. Hearing loss common. Characteristic "tower skull," with flat forehead. Most reported cases appear sporadic. When reproduction is possible, the disorder is apparently of autosomal dominant transmission. There also appears to be a high mutation rate related to increasing parent age. Manifestation present at birth. Audiometric findings usually show conductive loss. Surgical explorations have revealed congenital stapedial footplate fixation, abnormal patency of cochlear aqueduct, and enlarged internal auditory meatus (Bergstrom, Neblet, & Hemenway, 1972; Lindsay et al., 1975).

Atopic Dermatitis

Recessive. Congenital, mild to moderate, nonprogressive sensorineural hearing loss that may not be detected until school years. At about age 10, affected persons develop lichenified skin eruptions especially on forearms, hands, elbows, and trunk and arms. Very rare. Integumentary and pigmentary disorder with congenital sensorineural hearing loss (Konigsmark, Hollander, & Berlin, 1968; Konigsmark, Mengel, & Haskins, 1970; Frentz et al., 1976; Schultz et al., 1978).

Bjornstad Syndrome

Pili Torti

Recessive integumentary disorder. Dry, brittle, flat, twisted hair (pili torti) of scalp, eyebrows, and eyelashes accompanied by moderate to severe bilateral severe sensorineural hearing loss (Singh & Bresman, 1973).

Branchio-Oto-Renal Syndrome (BOR)

Branchio-oto-renal (BOR) syndrome is an autosomal-dominant form of inherited hearing impairment characterized by conductive, sensorineural, or mixed hearing loss; preauricular pits; auricular malformations of the outer ear and structural defects of the middle and inner ear; branchial fistulae or cysts; and renal anomalies ranging from mild hypoplasia to a lethal condition of bilateral renal agenesis. Like Treacher Collins syndrome, BOR results from abnormal development of the first and second branchial arches (Coppage & Smith, 1995).

Camurati-Engelmann Disease

Craniodiaphyseal Dysplasia; Progressive Diaphyseal Dysplasia

Skeletal disorder; dominant or recessive transmission. Radiologically, this syndrome is characterized by bilateral fusiform enlargement of the diaphyses of the long bones. Skull base may be sclerotic. Deafness may appear as progressive sensorineural, mixed, or conductive along with vestibular disturbance (Nelson & Scott, 1969; Sparkes & Graham, 1972; Yoshioka et al., 1980).

Cardioauditory Syndrome

See Jervell and Lang Nielsen Syndrome

Cerebral Palsy

Recessive, sporadic trait; 1 of 330 babies is born with cerebral palsy. Paralysis is due to a defect or lesion of the developing brain and is characterized by uncontrollable motor spasms. Cerebral palsy involves a wide range of severity of paralysis, weakness, incoordination, or other abnormality of motor function due to pathology of the motor control centers of the brain. Damage to the brain may occur during embryonic, fetal, or early infantile life. Essentially nonprogressive, clinical symptoms of the disorder include spasticity (40%), athetosis (40%), ataxia (10%), or combinations of these basic motor dysfunctions. Mental deficiency and convulsive disorders are common. Feeding problems, retarded growth, eye difficulties such as strabismus and nystagmus, developmental delay, orthopedic problems, communication disorders, and educational problems are often evidenced in varying degrees. Damage to the brain may occur during embryonic, fetal, or early infantile life and may result from an antecedent disorder such as trauma, metabolic disorder of infection, destructive intercranial cerebral processes, or developmental defects of the brain. Location of the lesion may be in cerebral cortex, basal ganglia, or other sites in the pyramidal or extrapyramidal systems (coexistent involvement in both systems is observed). Cerebellar damage may be evident less frequently. Management is a multidisciplinary process, and patients may have mild to moderate

sensorineural hearing loss, typically more severe in high frequencies (Stanley & Blair, 1994; Goulden & Hodge, 1998).

Cervico-oculo-acoustic Dysplasia

See Klippel-Feil Sydrome

CHARGE Association

The various abnormalities that make up CHARGE association are coloboma (*C*), heart defects (*H*), atresia of choanae (*A*), retarded growth and development (*R*), genital hypoplasia (*G*), and ear anomalies and/or deafness (*E*). Although the most consistent features are included by the mnemonic, CHARGE, additional abnormalities have been reported including facial palsy, renal abnormalities, orofacial clefts, and tracheoesophageal fistulas. The etiology is unknown, with most cases being sporadic. Approximately 30–35% of patients die within the first 3 months of life. Hearing loss may be progressive and present in 85% of reported cases, mild to profound in degree, and conductive, sensorineural, or mixed. Abnormalities of the pinnae, with or without hearing loss are a cardinal feature Dobrowski et al., 1985; Davenport et al., 1986; Thelin et al., 1986; Lin et al., 1990; Toriello, 1995).

Cleft Palate or Lip

Relatively common birth defects resulting from multifactorial inheritance; cleft lip occurs in about 1 in 1000 births and cleft palate occurs in about 1 per 2500 births. Cleft lip almost always occurs as fissure in the upper lip and may be unilateral or bilateral. Cleft palate may involve only

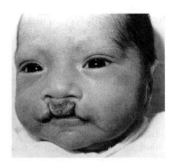

Figure A-4. Bilateral cleft palate and lip.

the uvula or both the hard and soft palate. The anatomic and physiologic derangement of a cleft palate predisposes patients to a high incidence of recurrent middle ear effusion episodes. Otorrhea is a frequent complication during the first year of life. Middle ear disease generally stabilizes or improves by the end of the first decade. Tympanic membrane (TM) perforations and cholesteatoma usually present after preschool age. Approximately 35–50% of babies with cleft palate have associated anomalies (Fig. A-4). Cleft lip and/or palate is a common anomaly found in many syndromes. See Chapter 3 for additional information (Paradise, 1976; Paradise & Bluestone, 1974; Bzoch, 1979; Bent & Smith, 1998).

Cleidocranial Dysostosis

Cleidocranial Dysplasia; Osteodental Dysplasia

A general disorder of the skeleton due to retarded ossification of membranous and cartilaginous precursors of bone characterized by congenital absence of clavicles, softness of skull, and irregular ossification of bones (Fig. A-5). In addition, shortness of stature, narrow drooping shoulders, widely spaced eyes, irregular or absent teeth, and high arched palate

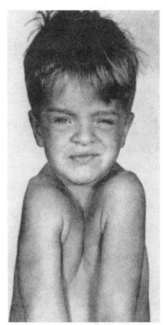

Figure A-5. Cleidocranial dysostosis. (Reproduced with permission from Jaffee, I.S. (1968). Congenital shoulder-neck-auditory anomalies. *Laryngoscope, 58,* 2119–2139).

or submucous cleft have been noted. Concentric narrowing of external auditory canals is present. Mental development is usually normal. Chromosome analyses show normal karyotypes. Autosomal dominant with high percentage and wide variability in expression. About one-third of the cases appear to be sporadic. Progressive deafness is occasionally reported. May be conductive or sensorineural due to retarded bone ossification (Hawkins et al., 1975; Jensen, 1990).

Cockayne's Syndrome

Recessive. Generally rare syndrome of progressive growth failure and neurologic deterioration, with about 50 cases described in the literature. Dwarfism, mental retardation, retinal atrophy, and motor disturbances are present. Appearance is normal at birth. Growth and development are normal through the first year. During the second year, growth falls below normal range and mental-motor development becomes abnormal. Minimal diagnostic characteristics include dwarfism, retinal degeneration, microcephaly, cataracts, neurologic impairment including progressive mental retardation, sun-sensitive skin, thickening of the skull bones, disproportionately long extremities with large hands and feet, eye disorder, and progressive sensorineural hearing loss of later onset, usually of moderate to severe degree. Prognosis is poor with severe blindness and deafness. Hearing aid is possible; however, mental retardation precludes much success (Riggs & Seibert, 1972; Shemen, Mitchell, & Farkashidy, 1984; Nance & Berry, 1992).

Cornelia de Lange Syndrome

Polygenic, multifactorial syndrome characterized by severe to profound mental and growth retardation, hirsutism, microcephaly, and confluent eyebrows often accompanied by anomalies of the external ear, including low-set auricles and small external auditory canals. Usually, full-term infants although they may be small at birth. The upper limbs are severely malformed; there may be missing toes or fingers and possible webbing between toes. Cardiac defects are common; possible cleft palate accompanied by neonatal feeding and respiratory difficulties. Speech and language problems are severe, and hearing losses attributed to conductive, sensorineural, and mixed etiologies have been reported. Prognosis is poor with diminished life expectancy (Silver, 1964; Moore, 1970; Fraser & Cambell, 1978; Hall, Prentice, Smiley, & Werkhaven, 1995).

Crouzon's Syndrome

Craniofacial Dysostosis

Abnormally shaped head characterized by a central prominence in the frontal region, a peculiar nose resembling a beak, and marked bilateral exophthalmos caused by premature closure of cranial sutures (Fig. A-6). Shape of the skull depends on which sutures are involved. Mentality may be low but usually is not unless there is brain damage secondary to increased intracranial pressure. Bifid uvula and cleft palate may be present. Autosomal dominant with variable expression. Approximately one-fourth of reported cases arise as fresh mutations. Detected at birth or during the first year. Ears may be low set. Approximately 50% of patients have nonprogressive conductive hearing impairment; may have mixed-type deafness. Middle ear manifestations include deformed stapes with bony fusion of promontory, ankylosis of malleus to outer wall of the epitympanum, distortion and narrowing of middle ear space, absence of the tympanic membrane, and

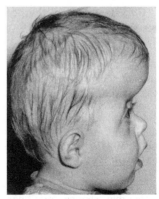

Figure A-6. Crouzon's syndrome.

perhaps bilateral atresia. Stenosis or atresia of external canal common. Early surgical intervention is usually recommended to prevent damage to the brain and eyes. Genetic counseling is recommended (Dodge, Wood, & Kennedy, 1959; Vulliamy & Normandale, 1966; Baldwin, 1968; Cohen, 1986).

Cryptophthalmus

Fraser Syndrome

Eye disorder. Recessive. Adherent eyelids that hide the eyes often accompanied by external ear malformations. In its most severe form, unilateral or (more often) bilateral extension of skin of the forehead completely covers eye or eyes to the cheeks. In less severe form, the upper or lower eyelid may be absent. Syndactyly of fingers and/or toes may be present. Laryngeal atresia has been reported. Cleft lip and palate are not uncommon. Hearing loss is mostly conductive; malformed middle ear ossicles, small and poorly formed pinnae, with stenosis of external auditory canals (Fraser, 1962; Ide & Wollschlaeger, 1969; Gattuso et al., 1987).

Cytomegalovirus (CMV) Disease

CMV is a virus of the herpes group that is the leading cause of fetal viral infection in the United States and accounts for more than 6000 cases of sensorineural hearing loss per year. More than 97% of congenitally infected infants show no signs of disease in the neonatal period. Approximately10–15% of infected children will eventually demonstrate adverse sequelae such as mental retardation, coordination disturbances, and hearing loss. Clinical manifesta-

tions include microcephaly, mental retardation, hepatosplenomegaly, and deafness. Typically the mother is asymptomatic. There is no vaccination against the disorder, and prevention of CMV infection consists of avoidance of exposure during pregnancy. See Chapters 4 and 8 for additional information (Strasnick & Jacobson, 1995; McCollister, Simpson, Dahl, et al., 1996).

Diastrophic Dwarfism

Craniofacial disorder. Recessive trait. Marked shortness of stature, characteristic hand deformity with short fingers, and severe bilateral clubfoot. The auricles show cystic swellings in infancy that later develop into cauliflower-like deformities that may calcify. There is 25% incidence of cleft palate. Congenital sensorineural hearing loss (Langer, 1965).

Down Syndrome

Trisomy 21 Syndrome

Down syndrome (Fig. A-7) is one of the most common forms of mental disability in the United States. Down syndrome is the result of a chromosomal abnormality—a 21 trisomy, translocation trisomy (Fig. A-8), or mosaicism. High incidence of occurrence (1 in

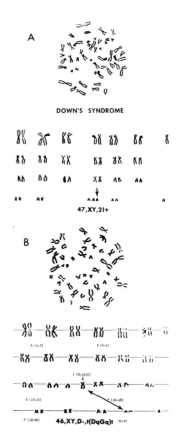

Figure A-8. Karyotypes of Down syndrome. (**A**) Note extra 21st chromosome. (**B**) Note translocation. (Courtesy of A. Robinson, MD, Cytogenetics Laboratory, University of Colorado Medical Center, Denver, CO.)

700 live births) with approximately 5000 new Down syndrome births each year in the United States. Clinical findings include a list of 50 features with varying penetrance. Mental retardation is almost universal. Characteristic personality that is warm, friendly, and affectionate. Common diagnostic features include flattened facial features, oblique palpebral fissures, flat occiput, short limbs, short broad hands, short fingers (especially the fifth finger), depressed nasal bridge, congenital hearing defects, absent Moro reflex in infancy, mouth breathing, dental abnormalities, and

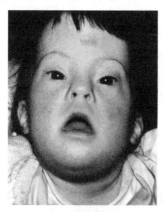

Figure A-7. Down syndrome.

mental retardation. Ear symptoms include small pinnae, narrow external ear canals, abnormal ear configuration, and a strong tendency for repeated bouts of otitis media. Incidence of hearing loss is very high with implications of sensorineural, conductive, and mixed hearing problems. Anomalies of middle ear ossicles have been reported. Risk of occurrence increases with the age of the mother: 1 in 1200 at age 25 increasing to 1 in 100 at age 40. Can be identified in early pregnancy with amniocentesis. See Chapter 4 for additional information (Balkany, Mischke, Downs, et al., 1979; Roizen, Walters, Nicol, & Blondis, 1993; Diefendorf, Bull, Casey-Harvey, Miyamoto, et al., 1995).

Duane Syndrome

Cervico-oculo-acoustic Dysplasia

Eye disorder seen as an anomaly in Wildervanck syndrome. Recessive. Congenital paralysis of the sixth cranial nerve (abducens palsy) with retracted globe and severe congenital sensorineural or conductive deafness in 15% of cases. Striking appearance because head seems to sit directly on trunk. The abducens paralysis prevents external rotation of eyes may be unilateral or bilateral; occasional cleft palate. Various ear anomalies have been described, including periauricular tags, malformation, atresia or absence of external ear canal, and abnormal ossicles. Congenital and nonprogressive (Kirkham, 1969; Singh, Rock, & Shulman, 1969; Cross & Pfaffenbach, 1972).

Dyschondrosteosis

See Madelung Deformity.

Fanconi's Anemia Syndrome

Infantile or Adolescent Renal Tubular Acidosis

A syndrome of many causes, some of which are inherited, yet often unidentified. Exposure to toxic agents directly precedes most acquired cases. The clinical manifestations are dependent on the causes of the syndrome. All aspects of the disorder reflect impaired renal tubular transport. Growth retardation is common. In the infantile form, high-frequency sensorineural deafness is noted in infancy; in the adolescent form, slowly progressive sensorineural deafness is noted during the teen years (McDonough, 1970; Walker, 1971).

Fetal Alcohol Syndrome (FAS)

Neuroectoderm syndrome that includes a combination of low birthweight, failure to thrive, and mental retardation seen in children of women who abuse alcohol during pregnancy. Occurrence is 2:1000 births. Full or partial expression of congenital malformations is associated with prenatal and postnatal growth deficiencies, central nervous system dysfunctions, and anomalies of the skeletal system and internal organs. Characterized by a variety of craniofacial disorders such as micrognathia, cleft palate, and abnormal pinnae and hearing loss. Frequently includes congenital abnormalities of the heart and eyes. Church and Gerkin (1987) noted hearing disorders in 13 of 14 children affected by FAS. Of the 14 study children, 13 had significant recurrent otitis media histories, including 4 with sensorineural hearing loss. Sparks (1984) described FAS speech and language disorders (Church, Edlis, Blakley, & Bawle, 1997).

Fragile X Syndrome

Fragile X syndrome is an inherited abnormality of the X chromosome that causes disabilities ranging from varying degrees of learning problems to mental retardation. Features commonly associated with the syndrome include severe language delay, behavior problems, autism or autistic-like behaviors (including poor eye contact and hand-flapping), macroorchidism, large prominent ears, hyperactivity, delayed motor development, and poor sensory skills. Hearing loss has seldom been associated with fragile X syndrome. Fragile X syndrome affects approximately 1 in 1000 persons. Most children affected with fragile X syndrome will have some form of speech or language delay. Because they do not speak in short phrases until 2.5 years of age, these children should have routine auditory evaluations. The speech of fragile X children has been described as compulsive, narrative, and perseverative. Fragile X speech has been described as "cluttered" and "mumbled" with poor topic maintenance; frequent tangential comments may occur. Syntax is usually appropriate for mental age; a high receptive vocabulary score is usually seen, although auditory memory and processing skills are weak (Paul, Cohen, Berg, Watson, & Herman, 1984; Wolf-Schein, Sudhalter, Cohen, et al., 1987).

Friedreich Ataxia

Nervous system disorder. Recessive. Progressive spinocerebellar ataxia appearing between the ages of 7 and 18 years. Nystagmus, optic atrophy, oculomotor paralysis, retinitis pigmentosa, cataracts, cardiac complications, and organic psychological problems are seen. Progressive sensorineural deafness of early childhood that may progressive, symmetric, or asymmetric with better hearing in the middle frequencies (Sylvester, 1958, 1972; Shanon, Himelfarb, & Gold, 1981).

Goldenhar Syndrome

Oculo-auriculo-vertebral Dysplasia

Unilateral malformation of craniofacial structures including eye, oral, and musculoskeletal anomalies (Fig. A-9). Eye abnormalities include cleft or upper lid, epibulbar dermoids, extraocular muscle defects, and antimongoloid obliquity. Auricular abnormalities include auricular appendices, unilateral posteriorly placed ear, unilateral microtia, atresia of external auditory meatus (40%), and blind-ended fistulas. Oral abnormalities include unilateral facial hypoplasia of ramus and condyle, high arched palate, and open bite. Musculoskeletal abnormalities such as hemivertebrae and clubfoot are seen. May include congenital heart disease. Mental retardation is not common. The etiology is unknown but may not be hereditary. Most cases are sporadic with a wide spectrum of anomalies. Possibly secondary to vascular abnormality during embryologic de-

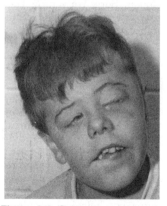

Figure A-9. Goldenhar syndrome.

velopment of first and second arches. Conductive hearing loss is present in 40–50% of reported cases as a result of atresia of external auditory canals (Shokeir, 1977; Feingold & Baum, 1978; Bassila & Goldberg, 1989).

Hallgren Syndrome

Eye disorder, very similar to Usher's syndrome. Recessive. Congenital sensorineural hearing loss. Retinitis pigmentosa, progressive ataxia, and mental retardation are seen in 25% of cases. Some patients show later psychosis; 90% have profound deafness (Hallgren, 1959).

Hand-Hearing Syndrome

Hand Muscle Wasting and Sensorineural Deafness

Dominant inheritance. Patients manifest familial congenital bilateral or unilateral sensorineural hearing loss of varying degrees. A congenital hand abnormality is seen in both normal-hearing and deaf patients (Fig. A-10). Congenital contractures of the digits and wasting of finger muscles are seen. No pain and no other deficits are present (Stewart & Bergstrom, 1971).

Harboyan Syndrome

Corneal Dystrophy

Eye disorder. Recessive. Age of detectability is usually between 10 and 25 years. Con-

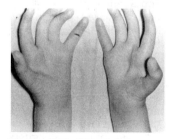

Figure A-10. Hand-hearing syndrome.

genital corneal dystrophy with slow progression leading to blindness at age 40. Progressive sensorineural deafness of delayed onset (Maumenee, 1960; Harboyan, Mamo, der Kalonstian, et al., 1971).

Hemifacial Microsomia

Craniofacial disorder with unknown etiology. Abnormalities are unilateral and include ear aplasia and hypoplasia with various pinna malformations. Preauricular tags are present in nearly all cases. External ear canals may be absent or present with the opening covered with skin. Other characteristics include eye abnormalities, such as lower palpebral fissure in the affected side, microphthalmia, cysts, iris, and choroid colobomas and strabismus, hypoplastic facial muscles, malocclusion (90%), and hypoplasia of the maxilla and mandible (95%). Unilateral conductive hearing loss may be present.

Herrmann Syndrome

Photomyoclonus, Diabetes Mellitus, Nephropathy, and Sensorineural Deafness

Nervous system disorder; dominant inheritance. Photomyoclonic and grand mal epilepsy. Later course of syndrome includes personality changes leading to severe dementia, slurring of speech, progressive hemiparesis, and mild ataxia, renal disease, and diabetes. Age of detectability is third or fourth decade. Progressive sensorineural hearing loss of late origin (Herrmann, Aguilar, & Sacks, 1964).

Hurler's Syndrome-Hunter's Syndrome

Mucopolysaccharidosis I and II (MPS I and II)

Hurler's syndrome is thought to be autosomal reces-

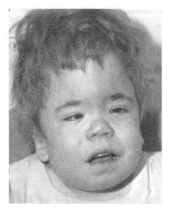

Figure A-11. Hurler's syndrome.

sive, and Hunter's syndrome is X-linked recessive (Figs. A-11 and A-12). Although the two disorders are clinically identical, Hunter's is generally less severe and affects only males. Hurler's can affect both sexes. In contrast to patients with Hurler's syndrome, patients with Hunter's syndrome usually do not show gross evidence of corneal clouding. Patients have a normal appearance at birth, but during the early months of life there is onset of progressive abnormal traits. Often described as an "inborn error of metabolism." Diagnostic features include growth failure, marked mental retardation, progressive coarsening of facial features, chronic nasal discharge, joint stiffness, and biochemical evidence of intracellular storage and acid mucopolysaccharides. Death usually occurs at

10–14 years of age. Most patients with Hurler's syndrome have some degree of progressive deafness. Hunter's syndrome has been accompanied by deafness in about half the cases, although the loss is usually not severe and most likely mixed sensorineural and conductive. Otolaryngologic manifestations include upper and lower respiratory infections, narrow nasal passages, hypertrophied adenoids, mucopurulent rhinorrhea, and noisy breathing. Affected individuals are prone to eustachian tube dysfunction and middle ear effusions (Keleman, 1966; Leroy & Crocker, 1966; Hayes, Babin, & Platz, 1980; Peck, 1984).

Hydrocephalus

A condition characterized by abnormal accumulation of fluid in and around the brain (Fig. A-13). May be congenital or acquired; typically detected at birth or within first 3 months of life. Mental retardation occurs if the condition is not treated. Risk of occurrence is 1 in 2000. Accompanied by enlargement of the head, prominence of the brain, mental deterioration, and convulsions. With successful shunt treatment, 80% of children reach 5 years of age, and 80% of survivors are normal or ed-

ucable. No data are available regarding hearing impairment, although Walker, Cervette, Newberg, Moss, and Storrs (1987) discuss auditory evoked brainstem response measurement in neonatal hydrocephalus (Shulman, 1973).

Hyperuricemia

Endocrine-metabolic problem. Dominant transmission with variable expressivity. Slowly progressive ataxia beginning in the second decade of life. Renal insufficiency. Cardiopathy, myopathy, and gout have been noted in some patients. Progressive sensorineural hearing loss of late onset, usually high frequency; may progress to total hearing loss with vestibular abnormalities (Rosenberg, Berstrom, Troost, et al., 1970).

Jervell and Lange-Nielsen Syndrome

Cardioauditory Syndrome

Cardiovascular disorder affecting 0.3% of congenitally deaf persons. Autosomal recessive trait. Consanguinity is common. Profound congenital bilateral sensorineural deafness accompanied by electrocardiographic abnormalities, fainting attacks, and occasionally sudden death in childhood. Death usually occurs between 3 and 14 years of age in more than 70% of patients. Hearing loss is usually symmetric. Often erroneously diagnosed as a seizure disorder and thus improperly treated (Jervell & Lange-Nielsen, 1957; Friedmann, Fraser, & Froggatt, 1966; Cusimano et al., 1991).

Klippel-Feil Syndrome

Craniofacial disorder (Fig. A-14) of debatable etiology. Involves fusion of some or all

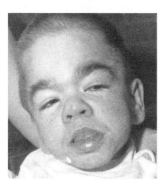

Figure A-12. Hunter's syndrome.

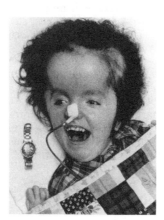

Figure A-13. Hydrocephalus.

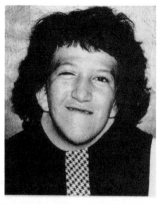

Figure A-14. Klippel-Feil syndrome with right facial paralysis.

cervical vertebrae and is characterized by a short neck with limited mobility, which gives the impression that the head sits on the shoulders. Diagnostic criteria include involvement of ear, eye, and neck. Other malformations may occur such as clubfoot and cleft palate. Associated neurologic disturbances. If familial, there is autosomal dominance with poor penetrance and variable expression. Faulty segmentation of mesodermal somites in utero, defects in maternal intestinal tract, and environmental factors have been suggested. Summary of syndrome characteristics includes multifactorial inheritance, fusion of cervical vertebrae, abducens nerve palsy, occasional cleft palate, torticollis, and severe sensorineural or conductive hearing loss. May range from mild conductive to profound sensorineural. Ear deformities occur in one-third of cases; temporal bone and roentgenogram findings include narrow to absent external auditory meatus and/or middle ear space, deformed ossicles, narrow oval window niche, underdevelopment of cochlea and vestibular structures (electronystagmograms abnormal), absence of semi-

circular canals, and absence of eighth cranial nerve. Central nervous system involvement is also frequently described and may contribute to audiologic findings. This syndrome is much more common in females (McLay & Maran, 1969; Windle-Taylor, Emery, & Phelps, 1981; Miyamoto, Yune, & Rosevear, 1983; Nagib et al., 1985; Stewart & O'Reilly, 1989).

Laurence-Moon-Biedl-Bardet Syndrome

Eye disorder with progressive sensorineural hearing loss of recessive inheritance. Patients with Laurence-Moon syndrome have retinitis pigmentosa, mental retardation, hypogenitalism, and spastic paraplegia. Patients with Biedl-Bardet syndrome show obesity and retinitis pigmentosa in association with polydactyly, hypogonadism, and mental retardation (Weinstein, Kliman, & Scully, 1969; Konigsmark & Gorlin, 1976).

LEOPARD Syndrome

Multiple Lentigines Syndrome

Integumentary-pigmentary disorder. Dominant trait. Freckly, dark brown, small spots concentrated on the neck and upper trunk. LEOPARD syndrome is an acronym derived from *l*entigines, *e*lectrocardiographic defects, *o*cular hypertelorism, *p*ulmonary stenosis, *a*bnormalities of genitalia, *r*etardation of growth, and sensorineural *d*eafness in 25% of cases. Hearing loss of marked variation and expressivity is usually detected in childhood (Gorlin, Anderson, & Blaw, 1969; Voron, Hatfield, & Kalkhoff, 1976).

Leri-Weill Disease

See Madelung Deformity.

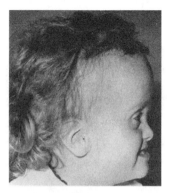

Figure A-15. Long arm 18 deletion syndrome. (Reproduced with permission from Bergsma, B. (1979). *Birth defects compendium* (2nd ed.). The National Foundation-March of Dimes. New York: Alan R. Liss.)

Long Arm 18 Deletion Syndrome

Abnormalities include mental retardation, microcephaly, short stature, hearing impairment with malformations of auricles and external auditory canals, retinal changes, facial peculiarities, and a high count of whorls on the fingers (Fig. A-15). Congenital heart disease, horseshoe kidney, cryptorchidism, spinal defects, and foot abnormalities have also been described. Genetic imbalance syndrome involving partial deletion of the long arm of the 18th chromosome (Fig. A-16). If translocation is responsible for deletion, transmission to children is possi-

PARTIAL DELETION OF 18 LONG ARM

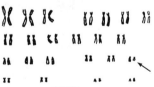

46,XX,18q−

Figure A-16. Karyotype of partial deletion of the long arm of the 18th chromosome. (Courtesy of A. Robinson, MD, Cytogenetics Laboratory, University of Colorado Medical Center, Denver, CO.)

ble. Conductive hearing loss associated with external and middle ear anomalies most frequently reported. Temporal bone study has shown collapsed Reissner's membrane in all turns of the cochlea, rolled and retracted tectorial membrane, and hypoplastic cochlear aqueduct (Smith, 1962; Kos, Schuknecht, & Singer, 1966; Bergstrom, Stewart, & Kenyon, 1974).

Madelung Deformity

Dyschondrosteosis; Leri-Weill Disease

Craniofacial-skeletal disorder. Dominant. Characterized by deformity of the distal radius and ulna bones and mild dwarfism. Congenital bilateral conductive loss with abnormal ossicles and narrow external auditory canals (Nassif & Harboyan, 1970).

Marshall Syndrome

Saddle Nose and Myopia

Dominant transmission. Characterized by short stature, severe myopia, saddle-nose defect, various skeletal defects, congenital or juvenile cataracts, and early onset, congenital progressive sensorineural hearing loss of moderate degree (Ruppert Buerk, & Pfordresher, 1970; Zellweger, Smith, & Grutzner, 1974).

Measles

A highly contagious viral infection involving the respiratory tract. The skin becomes covered with red papules that appear behind the ears and on the face before spreading rapidly down the trunk and onto the arms and legs. Measles may be complicated by bacterial pneumonia, otitis media, and demyelinating encephali-

tis. Measles may cause hearing loss as a result of invasion of the inner ear via the bloodstream or central nervous system or through purulent labyrinthitis secondary to suppurative otitis media. Hearing loss from measles is now rare due to the use of the measles, mumps, and rubella (MMR) vaccine. See Rubella, Congenital and Chapters 4 and 8.

Meningitis

Bacterial meningitis was the leading cause of acquired childhood sensorineural hearing loss until the introduction of the HIB vaccine in 1985. The disease is due to an infection of the meningeal membrane surrounding the brain and spinal cord. May result as a complication of untreated otitis media. Etiology of meningitis is varied and may be due to bacteria, virus, or fungi. Symptoms include stiff neck, headache, high fever, nausea, vomiting, and sometimes coma. Approximately 40% of children with deafness due to meningitis have at least one other major handicapping condition. It remains a common cause of sudden, severe to profound sensorineural deafness in developing countries without widespread vaccine programs. Deafness is usually bilateral but may be unilateral. See Chapter 4 (Finitzo-Hieber, Simhadri, & Hieber, 1981; Stein & Boyer, 1994; Liptak, McConnochie, & Roghmann, 1997).

Möbius' Syndrome

Facial Dysplasia

Dominant. Craniofacial nervous system disorder (Fig. A-17). Bilateral congenital facial paralysis, due to paralysis of cranial nerves VI and VII, severe but incomplete, with varying degrees of ophthalmoplegia, external ear malforma-

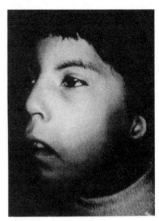

Figure A-17. Möbius' syndrome.

tions, micrognathia. Hands, feet, or digits may be missing; tongue paralysis and mental retardation may be present. Middle ear anomalies may be associated, as well as aberrant facial nerve. The syndrome presents with an expressionless face and dysarthria, but additional disabilities secondary to acquired hypoxic brain injury or associated brain dysgenesis are possible. Congenital sensorineural or conductive hearing loss (Kahane, 1979; Goulden & Hodge, 1998).

Muckle-Wells Syndrome

See Amyloidosis, Nephritis, and Urticaria.

Mucopolysaccharidosis

See Hurler's Syndrome-Hunter's Syndrome.

Mumps

A contagious viral disease occurring mainly in children characterized by swelling of the salivary and parotid glands. It is acquired by aspiration. The incubation period is 18–22 days, with fever and painful inflammation of the involved glands. Symptoms are most pronounced during the first 2 days and subside slowly over the next 4 or 5 days. Classic symptoms involve fever, headache, anorexia, malaise, earache, and enlargement of parotids. Previously a common cause of sudden, total unilateral sensorineural hearing loss. Bilateral total deafness has been reported, but only in rare instances. Approximately one-third of infections are subclinical and nearly asymptomatic. Mumps is now a rare cause of deafness in the United States due to the introduction of the measles, mumps, and rubella (MMR) vaccine. (Roizen, 1999).

Muscular Dystrophy

Recessive or X-linked. Muscle wasting of various types classified by transmission mode, age of onset, damaged muscle set, rate of disease development, and associated problems. *Pseudohypertrophic* muscular dystrophy usually begins before age 5 and affects most body muscles including cardiac and pulmonary systems. *Facioscapulohumeral* type affects face, shoulder, and upper arm muscles; slowly progressive with age of onset at 13–14 years. *Limb-girdle* type initially affects muscles of hips and shoulders. *Myotonic* muscular dystrophy associated with diabetes mellitus and cataracts, usually of late onset at age 30–40 or older. Severe infantile muscular dystrophy noted to be accompanied by sloping, sensorineural hearing loss of mild to moderate degree. Risk of occurrence is 1 in 100,000; childhood form is usually noted during the initial 3 years of life. Extremely rare in females (Black, Sando, Wagner, et al., 1971).

Myoclonic Epilepsy

Dominant nervous system disorder with variable expressivity. Seizure disorder characterized by myoclonic movements that include jerking motions involving head, trunk, and limbs. Slowly progressive ataxia. No mental retardation. Progressive sensorineural hearing loss of late onset (May & White, 1968).

Neurofibromatosis Types 1 and 2 (NF-1, NF-2)

NF-2, Vestibular Schwannomas, and Sensorineural Hearing Loss

Autosomal dominant inheritance; slowly progressive disorder. NF-1 is a multisystem progressive disorder that can frequently involve portions of the auditory system in diverse and subtle ways for which no characteristic audiologic findings are related. Diagnostic criteria for NF-2 include bilateral eighth nerve tumors and a first-degree relative with NF-2 symptoms. Tumors of the central or peripheral nervous system are hallmarks of the disorder. In addition to hearing loss due to eighth nerve tumors, other common symptoms include headaches, facial weakness, sensory or visual changes, and/or unsteadiness. In most patients, symptoms begin in the teens or twenties. The most common type of tumor is the vestibular schwannoma that may be unilateral but is mostly bilateral. Palsies of the fifth, sixth, seventh, ninth, and tenth cranial nerves as well as cerebellar ataxia may develop. Progressive visual loss is common. NF-1 is characterized with six or more café-au-lait spots and subcutaneous neurofibromas. NF-1 occurs in about 1:4000 persons, whereas NF2 affects 1:40,000 persons (Pastores et al., 1991; Pikus, 1995; NIH Consensus Conference, 1991).

Norrie's Syndrome

Oculo-acoustico-cerebral Degeneration

X-linked recessive with progressive eye degeneration leading to total blindness. Approximately one-third of persons who have this syndrome are severely mentally retarded, one-third are mildly retarded, and one-third are of normal intelligence. Auditory impairment is progressive, of late onset, and usually bilaterally symmetric sensorineural hearing loss in one-third of cases (Holmes, 1971).

Optic Atrophy and Polyneuropathy

Recessive or X-linked transmission. Symptoms include progressive visual loss with bilateral and symmetric optic atrophy beginning in second decade and leading to rapid deterioration of vision. Polyneuropathy from childhood. Progressive severe sensorineural deafness in childhood that tends to affect high frequencies. Risk of occurrence is 1 in 100,000 or less (Iwashita, Inoune, Araki, et al., 1970).

Opticocochleodentate Degeneration

Eye and nervous system disorder. Recessive trait. This fairly rare syndrome is characterized by progressive visual and sensorineural hearing loss and progressive spastic quadriplegia. Vision is normal until about 1 year of age, with total blindness occurring at about age 3 years. Microcephaly, mental deterioration, and speech problems may be evident, with death in later childhood (Konigsmark & Gorlin, 1976).

Oral-Facial-Digital (OFD) Syndrome

OFD I

Remarkably distinctive deformities of face, mouth, and fingers transmitted as recessive trait. Characterized by cleft lip and lobulated tongue, broad nasal root, hypoplasia of the mandible, polydactyly, and syndactyly. Oral deformities may cause speech problems and conductive hearing loss associated with malformed ossicles. Mild mental retardation occurs in approximately 40% of cases (Rimoin & Edgerton, 1967).

Osteogenesis Imperfecta

Van Der Hoeve's Syndrome

Heterogeneous group of at least seven types of disorders of connective tissue characterized by bone fragility. High percentage of infant death. Multiple fractures may be present at birth. Weak joints, blue sclera, thin and translucent skin, yellowish-brown and easily broken teeth, and deafness are seen. Deformities such as kyphoscoliosis and pectus excavation (Fig. A-18), internal hydrocephalus, nerve root compression, cardiovascular lesions, and thin atrophic skin may also occur. Also known as "brittle bone" disease. Etiology is hereditary autosomal dominant, present at birth. The majority of se-

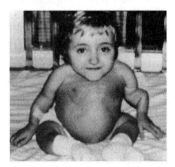

Figure A-18. Osteogenesis imperfecta.

vere cases are sporadic, and because of clinical variability, detection may range from birth through adulthood. Of reported cases, 60% have conductive hearing loss reportedly due to otosclerotic changes, the footplate of the stapes, and the posterior semicircular canal. Temporal bone findings show diminished or immature bone formation in otic capsule and ossicles. Because of the degeneration of stapes crura, no contact is possible between crura and footplate. Sensorineural hearing loss has also been demonstrated in high frequencies. Genetic counseling, magnesium therapy, and orthopedic correction are recommended. Rate of occurrence is about 2–5 per 100,000 births. Otologic surgery is usually successful. Estimates of hearing loss range between 26 and 60% of cases (Hall & Rohrt, 1968; Bretlau, Jorgensen, & Johansen, 1970; Quisling, Moore, Jahrsdoerfer, et al., 1979; Riedner, Levin, & Holliday, 1980; Cole, 1991).

Osteopetrosis

See Albers-Schönberg Disease.

Otopalatodigital Syndrome (OPD I and II)

Sex-linked recessive craniofacial-skeletal disorder with distinctive facial appearance. Features include cleft palate, stubby clubbed fingers and toes, wide-spaced nasal bridge giving pugilistic facies, low-set and small ears, winged scapulae, downward obliquity of the eyes, downturned mouth, and generalized bone dysplasia. Mild mental retardation and congenital conductive-type hearing loss due to ossicular abnormalities are seen. OPD II

has more severe skeletal manifestations (Pazzaglia & Giampiero, 1986; Schaefer, Kolodziej, & Olney, 1998; Buran & Duvall, 1967; Hall et al., 1995).

Paget's Disease (Juvenile)

Hereditary Hyperphosphatasia

Recessive skeletal disorder with fever, bone pain, and swelling. Juvenile form is characterized by progressive skeletal deformities that become apparent during the second or third year of life. May result in sporadic cranial nerve involvement. Progressive enlargement of the head and long bones. Progressive mixed-type hearing disorder due to continued new bone formation at the skull base (Thompson, Gaull, Horowitz, et al., 1969; Desai et al., 1973).

Pendred Syndrome

Goiter and Profound Deafness

Recessive endocrine-metabolic disorder. The goiter is usually apparent by age 8 years but may be noted at birth in some cases. Auditory manifestations are variable but usually demonstrate a moderate to profound sensorineural hearing loss. Age of hearing loss detection is variable. Risk of occurrence is about 1 in 14,500. Fairly common disorder related to profound deafness (Batsakis & Nishiyama, 1962; Fraser, 1965; Illum, Kaier, Hvidberg-Hansen, et al., 1972; Johnson et al., 1987; Kabakkaya et al., 1993).

Piebaldness

Divided into three integumentary-pigmentary syndromes by Konigsmark and Gorlin (1976). (1) Recessive piebaldness and profound congenital sensorineural deafness (Woolf syndrome) . Head, hair, upper chest, and both arms show substantial depigmentation. Normal vision with blue irides. (2) X-linked pigmentary abnormalities and congenital sensorineural deafness. Similar pigmentary skin changes as seen in recessive piebaldness. Profound deafness. (3) Dominant piebaldism (Telfer syndrome), ataxia, and sensorineural hearing loss. Approximately 80% of these patients have ataxia and mental retardation, and 60% have progressive sensorineural deafness (Woolf, Dolowitz, & Aldous, 1965).

Pierre Robin Sequence

Cleft Palate, Micrognathia, and Glossoptosis

Dominant, craniofacial-skeletal disorder. Oral findings include cleft palate, smallness of jaw and chin, and downward displacement or retraction of the tongue. Ears may be low-set. About 20% of cases are associated with mental retardation. Congenital amputations, hip dislocation, sternal anomalies, spina bifida, hydrocephaly, and microcephaly have been reported. A variety of cardiac and middle ear anomalies have been reported. Congenital conductive or sensorineural hearing loss. A 10-year follow-up study of 55 cases showed a high incidence of speech-language-hearing problems. Gould (1989) reported a 50% incidence of conductive hearing loss in a sample of 20 patients with Pierre Robin sequence. Risk of occurrence is 1 in 30,000 (Williams, Williams, Walker, et al., 1981).

Preauricular Abnormalities

These abnormalities include preauricular pits, preauricular tags (Fig. A-19),

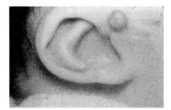

Figure A-19. Preauricular abnormalities.

and branchial fistulas, which may be multiple and are usually bilateral. This is a dominant craniofacial disorder often accompanied by conductive hearing loss or sensorineural hearing loss and sometimes by external ear canal atresia, facial paralysis, or mandibular anomalies. Preauricular tags and/or pits usually require no treatment except for cosmetic surgery or excision if draining. See Chapter 4 (Melnick, Bixler, Nance, et al., 1976; Cremers, Thijssen, & Fischer, 1981; Hayes, 1994).

Pyle's Disease

Craniometaphyseal Dysplasia

Recessive and dominant inheritance; craniofacial-skeletal disorder. Expressivity is somewhat variable; massive enlargement and sclerosis of cranial and facial bones, ribs, and clavicles. Facial features include hypertelorism, broad nasal ridge, enlarged paranasal area, and cranial sclerosis. Nystagmus is common. Progressive sensorineural or conductive hearing loss (Miller, Lehman, & Geretti, 1969; Gladney & Monteleone, 1970; Schaefer et al., 1986).

Refsum's Syndrome

Heredopathia Atactica Polyneuritiformis

Recessive eye disorder. Onset in second decade of life with visual loss, night blindness due to retinitis pigmen-

tosa, progressive ataxia, muscle wasting, obesity, ichthyosis, and polyneuritis. Major clinical symptoms include triad of retinitis pigmentosa, peripheral neuropathy, and cerebellar ataxia. May be related to enzymatic defect. Progressive sensorineural hearing loss (50%) with one side often worse than the other (Fryer et al., 1971; Nance, 1973).

Renal Tubular Acidosis

See Fanconi's Anemia Syndrome.

Richards-Rundle Syndrome

Ataxia-Hypogonadism Syndrome

Recessive trait. Nervous system disorder. Includes ataxia and muscle wasting in early childhood. Progressive severe mental retardation, absent deep tendon reflexes, and failure to develop secondary sexual characteristics are seen. Early onset of progressive, severe, sensorineural hearing loss; horizontal nystagmus (Richards & Rundle, 1959).

Rubella, Congenital

Classic triad of symptoms includes sensorineural hearing loss, congenital heart disease, and vision problems. Infants with congenital rubella virus infections have a variety of defects of varying severity depending on the embryonic stage during which the infection occurred. Maternal rubella infection within the first month of pregnancy poses a 50% chance of serious consequences which diminishes to a still high 10–15% for exposure in the 3rd month of pregnancy. Significant risk extends up to the 16th week of pregnancy. Hearing impairment can result from fetal rubella not only during the first trimester of pregnancy but also in the second and even third trimester. Several thousand persons were affected by the rubella epidemic in the United States during 1963–1965. Congenital rubella embryopathy is still a major prenatal acquired cause of profound childhood deafness in developing countries. In the United States, the measles, mumps, and rubella (MMR) vaccine program has nearly eliminated these infections.

Diagnostic features include transient neonatal manifestations of low birthweight, hepatosplenomegaly, purpura, bulging anterior suture, corneal clouding, and jaundice. Anemia, pneumonia, meningitis, and encephalitis may develop. Associated problems include hearing loss (68–90%), heart disease (50%), cataract or glaucoma (50%), psychomotor difficulties (45%), cerebral palsy (45%), and mental retardation (40%). A major feature of rubella embryopathy is a characteristic "salt and pepper" retinal pigmentation that does not interfere with visual acuity. Dental abnormalities, microcephaly, and behavioral problems are common in children with congenital rubella (Roizen et al., 1996). Rubella deafness is commonly sensorineural and often severe to profound. Variation in audiometric configuration is common. The pathology of rubella deafness includes a variety of inner ear abnormalities and middle ear and external ear anomalies. See Chapter 8 (Stuckless, 1980; Strasnick & Jacobson, 1995; Roizen, 1999).

Schwann Syndrome

Knuckle Pads and Leukonychia

Dominant. Callous-like thickening over dorsal aspects of interphalangeal joints of fingers and toes first observed in infancy and early childhood. Progressive whitening of finger and toenails (leukonychia). Integumentary-pigmentary disorder; congenital sensorineural or conductive hearing loss. Hearing loss is usually noted in infancy or early childhood. Cochlear involvement of mixed mild to moderate degree (Bart & Pumphrey, 1967; Ramer et al., 1994).

Sensory Radicular Neuropathy

Dominant trait, nervous system disorder. Onset in late teens or early adulthood of lightning pains that involve the distal extremities with painless ulcerations of feet. Progressive moderate to severe sensorineural hearing loss (Mandell & Smith, 1960; Stanley, Puritz, Birggaman, et al., 1975).

Symphalangism

Dominant skeletal disorder. Stiff fingers and toes due to bony ankylosis of the proximal interphalangeal joints. Congenital conductive hearing loss due to stapes fixation (Spoendlin, 1974).

Syphilis, Congenital

The number of cases of congenital syphilis has been increasing in the United States since 1986. This is an infectious disease contracted by the fetus from the infected mother. One-third to two-thirds of newborns are typically asymptomatic. Sensorineural hearing impairment of a slow progressive nature usually begins after 2 years of age. The pattern of deafness shows variation dependent on time of onset and rapidity of progression. The youngster may initially show normal hearing. Hearing loss usually becomes significant in the teens or later, beginning in the high frequencies and progressing to lower frequencies. Congenital syphilis is typically associated with other sensory defects. See Chapter 4 (Kerr, Smyth, & Cinnamond, 1973; Ikeda & Jensen, 1990; Strasnick & Jacobson, 1995; Roizen, 1999).

Treacher Collins Syndrome

Mandibular Dysostosis; First Arch Syndrome

Major diagnostic features include facial bone abnormalities of structures formed from the first branchial arch including downward sloping palpebral fissures, depressed cheek bones, deformed pinna, receding chin, and large fish-like mouth with frequent dental abnormalities (Fig. A-20). Atresia of auditory canal, defects of auditory canal and ossicles, and cleft palate are common. Mental deficiency is reported in about 5% of cases. Treacher Collins is a genetic defect leading to multiple congenital anomalies. Autosomal dominant with incomplete penetrance and variable expression. The incidence is 1:50,000, with more than half

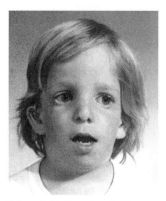

Figure A-20. Treacher Collins syndrome.

of the reported cases being fresh mutations. The external ears may be small, displaced, or simply nubbins. Atresia of the external auditory canal is common. The middle ear is often poorly developed, the tympanic ossicles being absent or deformed. Hypoplasia of the horizontal semicircular canal of the cochlea has been observed, as have branching of nerve to horizontal canal cristae bilaterally and abnormalities of bony and membranous vestibular labyrinth. Deafness is generally completely conductive but may be sensorineural. General treatment includes genetic counseling, surgical repair of ear anomalies (although severe middle ear malformations make reconstructive surgery for hearing improvement difficult, if not impossible), hearing aids, orthodontic treatment, and speech therapy if indicated (Fernandez & Ronis, 1964; Frazen, Elmore, & Nadler, 1967; Sando, Hemenway, & Morgan, 1968; Marsh et al., 1986; Richieri-Costa et al., 1993; Jahrsdoerfer & Jacobson, 1995).

Trisomy 13–15 Syndrome

Major diagnostic features include chromosomal aberration resulting in minimal characteristics of microphthalmia, cleft lip and palate, and polydactyly. A host of other abnormalities may be present, including mental retardation, deafness, broad-nose hypotelorism, microcephaly, heart and/or skin defects, retroflexed thumbs, "rocker-bottom" feet, seizures, and renal, abdominal, and genitalia abnormalities. Those affected frequently suffer feeding problems, failure to thrive, jitteriness, apneic spells, hypotonia, and jaundice. Meiotic nondisjunction appears to be the cause of the extra chromosome in the 13–15 group (Fig. A-21). Tri-

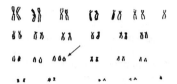

Figure A-21. Trisomy 13–15 (D₁) karyotype. (Courtesy of A. Robinson, MD, Cytogenetics Laboratory, University of Colorado Medical Center, Denver, CO.)

somy 13 syndrome with 47 chromosomes is frequently associated with increased maternal age. Low-set external ears are found in 80%, malformed ears in 80%, and cleft lip and palate in 50–80%. Middle ear findings have included deformed stapes, distorted incudostapedial joint posteriorly, and absence of stapedial muscle and tendon. Inner ear abnormalities have included distorted and shortened cochlea, shortened endolymphatic valve, abnormal branch of nerve to posterior semicircular canal crista from posterior cranial fossa, degeneration of organ of Corti, tectorial membrane, stria vascularis, and saccule. Other studies have been normal. Genetic counseling is recommended as indicated. Prognosis is poor; 95% of patients die by 3 years of age (Cohen, 1966; Maniglia, Wolff, & Herques, 1970; Black et al., 1971; Scherz, Graga, & Reichelderfer, 1972).

Trisomy 18 Syndrome

Due to chromosomal aberration, features present at birth include being underweight with an undernourished appearance and possible limpness at first, soon becoming hypertonic. Microcephaly with triangular shape due to occipital prominence and receding chin is seen. The skin is loose. Flexion of hand with overlapping of index finger

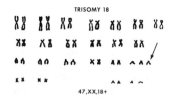

Figure A-22. Trisomy 18 karyotype. (Courtesy of A. Robinson, MD, Cytogenetics Laboratory, University of Colorado Medical Center, Denver, CO.)

over third finger, "rocker-bottom" feet, short sternum, small pelvis, and agenesis of bones of the extremities are seen. Congenital heart disease, renal abnormalities, cleft lip and palate, and deformed ears may also be present. Mental retardation is usually profound.

This syndrome is due to nondisjunction of one chromosome in the 17–18 group (Fig. A-22). Advanced maternal age is common. Possibility of recurrence in the same family is rare unless translocation is present. Audiometric testing shows failure to respond to sound. Middle ear anomalies include malformed stapes, deformed incus and malleus, exposed stapedial muscle in the middle ear cavity, absence of stapedial tendon, absence of pyramidal eminence, a split tensor tympanic muscle in separate bony canals, abnormal course of the facial and chorda tympani nerves, and underdevelopment of facial nerve. Other anomalies reported include atresia of external canals, decreased spiral ganglion cells, anomalies of cochlea, absence of utriculoendolymphatic valve, and absence of semicircular canals and cristae. Genetic counseling or other treatments are recommended as indicated. Ninety percent of patients die by 1 year of age (Smith, 1962; Kos et al., 1966;,Keleman, Hooft, & Kluyskens, 1968; Chrysostomidou, Caslaris, Alexion, et al., 1971).

Trisomy 21 Syndrome

See Down Syndrome.

Turner Syndrome

Gonadal Dysgenesis

Chromosome defect, not inherited. Low hairline, webbing of neck, widely spaced nipples, shield-like chest, and webbing of digits are seen. Chromosomal abnormality recognizable at birth by webbing or loose folds of skin of short neck, swelling of dorsa of hands and feet, deep creases on thickened palms and soles, hypertelorism, epicanthic folds, ptosis of upper lids, elongated and narrow "gothic" ears, high arched palate, micrognathia, pinpoint nipples, and enlarged clitoris. Fingernails are hypoplastic and appear small. Later manifestations include shortness of stature, ocular manifestations, hearing impairment, impairment of taste, congenital cardiovascular disease, anomalies of kidneys, and sexual infantilism. It occurs only in females. Mentality may be normal. Mild sensorineural and conductive hearing loss have been reported. Conductive hearing loss has been attributed to frequent middle ear infections in infancy and early childhood, but congenital hearing loss has also been observed (Stratton, 1965; Anderson, Lindsten, & Wedenberg, 1971; Watkin, 1989; Sculerati et al., 1990).

Usher's Syndrome

Retinitis Pigmentosa and Sensorineural Hearing Loss

Recessive, genetic condition including congenital deafness and progressive loss of vision leading to eventual blindness. The hearing loss is bilateral, moderate to severe, and sensorineural. Patient initially notices difficulty seeing at night during the early teens or twenties, narrowing of visual field (tunnel vision), and signs and symptoms of retinitis pigmentosa. May have additional disorders such as mental retardation, vertigo, psychosis, loss of smell, abnormal electroencephalograms, and epilepsy. Prevalence among profoundly deaf children has been estimated to be between 3 and 10%. Early diagnosis is important for provision of appropriate rehabilitation endeavors, genetic counseling, and screening of relatives. Can vary greatly in age of onset, severity, and speed of progression.

Vestibular response to caloric testing is generally abnormal; 90% of 177 patients (Hallgren, 1959) had severe bilateral congenital deafness, whereas 10% had moderate (30–70 dB) sensorineural hearing loss, more marked in higher frequencies. In many cases, the deafness is so profound that hearing aid use is not successful. There is no treatment for retinitis pigmentosa. Most patients are forced to retire by age 30 or 40 because of vision problems and associated disabilities. Usher's syndrome has been the subject of intense gene mapping that has identified three major phenotypic classes known as Usher I, II, and III (Kloepfer, Laguaite, & McLaurin, 1966; McLeod, McConnell, Sweeney, et al., 1971; Hicks & Hicks, 1981; Kimberling et al., 1989; Kimberling & Moller, 1995).

Van Buchem Syndrome

Hyperostosis Corticalis Generalisata

Recessive craniofacial-skeletal disorder. Generalized osteosclerotic overgrowth of the skeleton. Paralysis of cranial nerve VII and sensorineural deafness are seen frequently. Onset occurs during puberty and is demonstrated by narrowing of skull foramina causing cranial nerve paresis with visual and mixed-type hearing loss. Lion-like facial expression with square jaw; may include unilateral or rarely bilateral facial paralysis and optic atrophy (Fosmoe, Holme, & Hildreth, 1968).

Van Der Hoeve Syndrome

See Osteogenesis Imperfecta.

Vohwinkel-Nockemann Syndrome

Keratopachyderma and Digital Constrictions

Integumentary disorder, dominant trait. Hyperkeratosis involving the palms, soles, knees, and elbows. Ring-like furrows developing on fingers and toes at about 2 years of age. Mild to severe congenital sensorineural deafness, mainly for frequencies above 4000 Hz, which may be slowly progressive. May include renal disease (Bitici, 1975).

Waardenburg's Syndrome

Genetic hearing loss with integumentary system characteristics; inherited as autosomal dominant characteristic with variable penetrance. Major diagnostic features include white forelock (20%) (Fig. A-23); lateral displacement of medial canthi (95–99%); iris bicolor or heterochromia (45%); prominence of root of nose; and hyperplasia of medial portion of eyebrows (50%). Other findings include thin nose with flaring alae nasi, "cupid bow" configuration of lips, prominent mandible, and occasionally cleft palate (5%). All characteristics are not found in each patient. Mental retardation is not typical. Congenital mild to severe sensorineural hearing loss,

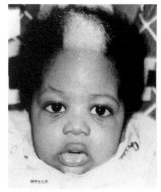

Figure A-23. Waardenburg's syndrome.

often progressive, is present in 50% of patients and may be unilateral or bilateral. Hearing impairment may be evidenced primarily in low and middle frequencies, but profound deafness may also be present. Histopathologic findings include absence of organ of Corti and atrophy of spiral ganglion. Waardenburg syndrome has been divided into types I and II (Marcus & Valvasori, 1970; Pantke & Cohen, 1971; Ambani, 1983; Nakashima et al., 1992).

Wildervanck Syndrome

Otofaciocervical Dysmorphia; Cervico-oculo-acoustic Dysplasia

Multifactorial inheritance. Depressed nasal root, protrud-ing narrow nose, narrow elongated face, flattened maxilla and zygoma, prominent ears, atresia of external ear canals, preauricular fistulas, and poorly developed neck muscles are seen. Facial asymmetry combines the Klippel-Feil characteristics with retraction of the eyeball (Duane disorder), sixth nerve paralysis, and total deafness in at lest 30% of cases that may be unilateral or bilateral. Integumentary and pigmentary disorder; fused cervical vertebrae; congenital sensorineural or mixed-type hearing loss. Female preponderance, 7:75 (Cremers, Hoogland, & Kuypers, 1984; Schild et al., 1984; Hughes et al., 1991).

Winter Syndrome

Renal-Genital Anomalies and Conductive Hearing Loss

Recessive disorder. Renal anomalies and internal genital malformations. Malformation of middle ear with low-set auricles and stenotic external canals. Moderate to severe conductive hearing loss (Winter et al., 1968; Turner, 1970).

Recommended Readings

Bergsma, D. (Ed.). (1979). *Birth defects compendium* (2nd ed.). New York: Alan R. Liss.

Fraser, G.R. (1976). *The causes of profound deafness in childhood.* Baltimore: Johns Hopkins University Press.

Gorlin, R.J., et al. (1990) *Syndromes of the head and neck* (3rd ed.). New York: Oxford University Press.

Gorlin, R.J., Toriello, H.V., & Cohen, M.M. (1995). *Hereditary hearing loss and its syndromes.* New York: Oxford University Press.

Hemenway, W.G., & Bergstrom, L. (Eds.). Symposium on congenital deafness. *Otolaryngologic Clinics of North America, 4* (2), 1–399.

Jacobson, J. (Ed.). (1995). Hereditary syndromes. *Journal of the American Academy of Audiology, 6,* 1.

Jones, K.L. (1997). *Smith's recognizable patterns of human malformation* (5th ed.). Philadelphia: WB Saunders.

Jung, J.H. (1989). *Genetic syndromes in communication disorders.* Boston: Little, Brown & Co.

Konigsmark, B.W., & Gorlin, R.J. (1976). *Genetic and metabolic deafness.* Philadelphia: WB Saunders.

Martini, A., Read, A., & Stephens, D. (1996). *Genetics and hearing impairment.* San Diego: Singular Publishing Group.

Salmon, M.A. (1978). *Developmental defects and syndromes.* Aylesbury, England: HM & M Publishers Ltd.

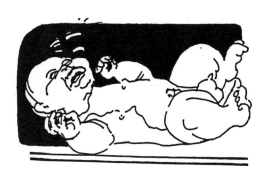

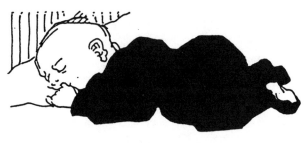

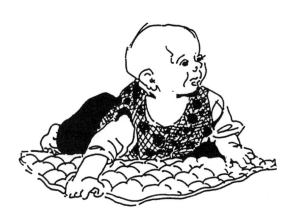

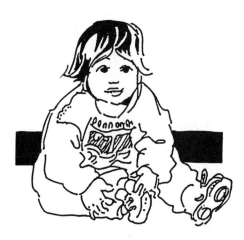

References

Accreditation Council for Facilities for the Mentally Retarded. (1971). *Standards for residential facilities for the mentally retarded.* Chicago, IL: Joint Commission on Accreditation of Hospitals.

Alberti, P.W.R.M., & Kristensen, R. (1970). The clinical application of impedance audiometry. *Laryngoscope, 80,* 735–746.

Ambani, L.M. (1983). Waardenburg and Hirschsprung syndromes. *Journal of Pediatrics, 102,* 802–806.

American Academy of Audiology. (1992). Position statement on guidelines for the diagnosis and treatment of otitis media in children. *Audiology Today, 4* (4), 23–24.

American Academy of Audiology. (1995). Position statement on cochlear implants in children. *Audiology Today, 7* (3), 14–15.

American Academy of Audiology. (1997). Identification of hearing loss and middle-ear dysfunction in preschool and school-aged children. *Audiology Today, 9* (3), 18–23.

American Academy of Otolaryngology and American Council of Otolaryngology. (1979). Guide for the evaluation of hearing handicap. *JAMA, 241,* 2055–2059.

American Academy of Otolaryngology Committee on Hearing and Equilibrium and the American Council of Otolaryngology Committee on the Medical Aspects of Noise. (1979). Guide for the evaluation of hearing handicap. *JAMA, 251* (19), 2055–2059.

American Academy of Pediatrics. (1984). Policy statement on middle ear disease and language development. *Academy of Pediatric News and Comments, 35,* 9.

American Academy of Pediatrics. (1986). Use and abuse of the Apgar score. *Pediatrics, 78* (6), 1148–1149.

American Academy of Pediatrics. (1999). Newborn and infant hearing loss: Detection and intervention task force on newborn and infant hearing. *Pediatrics, 103* (2), 527–530.

American Academy of Pediatrics, Committee on Environmental Hazards. (1974). Noise pollution: Neonatal aspects. *Pediatrics, 54,* 476.

American Academy of Pediatrics, Joint Committee on Infant Hearing. (1982). Position statement 1982. *Pediatrics, 70,* 496–497.

American National Standards Institute. (1969). *Specifications for audiometers* (ANSI S3. 6-1996). New York:Acoustical Society of America. 1996.

American National Standards Institute. (1969). *Specifications for audiometers* (ANSI S3.6-1969). New York: American National Standards Institute.

American National Standards Institute/Acoustical Society of America. (1976). *Specification of hearing aid characteristics* (ANSI S3, 22-1976). New York: American National Standards Institute.

American Psychiatric Association. (1980). *Diagnostic and statistical manual of mental disorders* (3rd ed.). Washington, DC: American Psychiatric Association.

American Psychiatric Association. (1987). *Diagnostic and statistical manual of mental disorders* (3rd ed., Rev. ed.). Washington, DC: American Psychiatric Association.

American Speech and Hearing Association. (1978). Guidelines for manual pure-tone threshold audiometry. *ASHA, 29,* 297–301.

American Speech and Hearing Association Task Force. (1981). The definition of a hearing handicap. *ASHA, 23,* 293–297.

American Speech-Language-Hearing Association. (1979). Guidelines for acoustic immittance screening of middle-ear function. *ASHA, 21,* 283–288.

American Speech-Language-Hearing Association. (1982). Joint Committee on Infant Hearing position statement. *ASHA, 24,* 1017.

American Speech-Language-Hearing Association. (1985). Guidelines for identification audiometry. *ASHA, 27* (5), 49–52.

American Speech-Language-Hearing Association. (1987, June). *The short latency auditory evoked potentials.* Rockville, MD: American Speech-Language-Hearing Association.

American Speech-Language-Hearing Association. (1989a). Audiologic screening of infants who are at risk for hearing impairment. *ASHA, 31,* 89–92.

American Speech-Language-Hearing Association. (1989b). Communication-based services for infants, toddlers, and their families. *ASHA, 31* (5), 32–34.

American Speech-Language-Hearing Association. (1990). Guidelines for screening for hearing impairments and middle ear disorders. *ASHA, 32* (Suppl. 2), 17–24.

American Speech-Language-Hearing Association. (1992, March). Sedation and topical anesthetics in audiology and speech-language pathology. *ASHA, 34* (Suppl. 7), 41.

American Speech-Language-Hearing Association. (1992, 1996). Task force on central auditory processing consensus development. *American Journal of Audiology, 5* (2), 41–54.

American Speech-Language-Hearing Association (ASHA). (1993). Guidelines for audiology services in the schools. *ASHA, 35* (Suppl. 10), 24–32.

American Speech-Language-Hearing Association. (1994). Guidelines for the audiologic management of individuals receiving cochleotoxic drug therapy. *ASHA, 36* (Suppl. 12), 11–19.

American Speech-Language-Hearing Association. (1996). Central auditory preocessing: Current status of research and implications for clinical practice. *American Journal of Audiology, 5* (2), 41–54.

American Speech-Language-Hearing Association. (1994). Guidelines for fitting and monitoring FM systems. *ASHA, 36* (Suppl. 3), 1–9.

American Speech-Language-Hearing Association. (1995). Report on audiological screening. *American Journal of Audiology, 4* (2), 24–40.

American Speech-Language-Hearing Association. (1996). Central auditory processing: current status or research and implications for clinical practice. *American Journal of Audiology, 5* (2), 41-54.

American Speech-Language-Hearing Association. (1997). Guidelines for audiologic screening: Panel on audiologic assessment. Rockville, MD: American Speech-Language-Hearing Association.

Anderson, H., Filipsson, R., Fluur, E., et al. (1969). Hearing impairment in Turner's syndrome. *Acta Oto-Laryngologica Supplement (Stockholm), 247,* 1–26.

Anderson, H., Lindsten, J., & Wedenberg, E. (1971). Hearing defects in males with sex chromosome anomalies. *Acta Oto-Laryngologica (Stockholm), 72,* 55–58.

Anderson, K.L., & Matkin, N.D. (1996). *Preschool SIFTER: Screening instrument for targeting educational risk in preschool children (age 3–kindergarten).* Tampa, FL: Educational Audiology Association.

Angeli, S.I., & Brackmann, D.E. (1998). Posterior fossa tumors. In A. Lalwani & K. Grundfast (Eds.), *Pediatric otology and neurotology* (pp. 3489–3503). Philadelphia: Lippincott-Raven.

Aniansson, G., Alm, B., & Andersson, B. (1994). A prospective cohort study on breast-feeding and otitis media in Swedish infants. *Pediatric Infectious Disease Journal, 13,* 183–188.

Anson, B.J. (1963). *An atlas of human anatomy* (2nd ed.). Philadelphia: WB Saunders.

Anson, B.J., & Donaldson, J.A. (1967). *The surgical anatomy of the temporal bone and ear.* Philadelphia: WB Saunders.

Anthony, D.A., et al. (1971). *Seeing essential English.* Greeley, CO: University of Northern Colorado.

Apgar, V. (1953). A proposal for a new method of evaluation of the newborn infant. *Anesthesiology and Analgesia, 32,* 260.

Apgar, V., & James, L. (1962). Further observations on the newborn scoring system. *American Journal of Diseases of Children, 104,* 419.

Arditi, M., Mason, E., Bradley, J., Tan, T., Barson, W., Schultze, G., Wald, E., et al. Three-year multicenter surveillance of pneumoccoccal meningitis in children: Clinical characteristics and outcome related to penicillin susceptibility and dexamethasone use. *Pediatrics, 102,* 1087–1097.

Arehart, K.H., Yoshinaga-Itano, C., Thomson, V., Gabbard, S.A., & Stredler Brown, A. (1980). State of the states: The status of universal newborn screening, assessment, and intervention systems in 16 states. *American Journal of Audiology, 7,* 101–114.

Arey, L.B. (1940). *Developmental Anatomy.* Philadelphia: WB Saunders.

Armitage, S.E., Baldwin, B.A., & Vince, M.A. (1980). The fetal sound environment of sheep. *Science, 208,* 1173–1174.

Aslin, R., Pisoni, D., & Jusczyk, P. (1983). Auditory development and speech perception in infancy. In P.H. Mussen (Series Ed.), M. Haith & J. Campos (Vol. Eds.), *Infancy and the biology of development: Vol II. Carmichael's manual of child psychology,* (4th ed.). New York: John Wiley & Sons.

Asp, C. (1985). The verbotonal method for management of young, hearing-impaired children. *Ear and Hearing, 6* (1), 39–42.

Axelsson, A., Fagerberg SE. Auditory function in diabetics. *Acta Otolaryngol* (Stockh) 66:49–64, 1968.

Axelsson, A., & Jerson, T. (1985). Noisy toys: a possible source of sensorineural hearing loss. *Pediatrics, 76* (4), 574–578.

Babbidge, H.S. (1965). *Education of the deaf. A report to the secretary of health, education, and welfare by his advisory committee on the education of the deaf* (Publication No. 0-765-119). Washington, DC: Government Printing Office.

Babson, S.G. (1980). *Diagnosis and management of the fetus and neonate at risk* (4th ed.). St. Louis: CV Mosby.

Baily, D. (1994). Forward: In J. Rouch & N. Matkin (Eds.), *Infants and toddlers with hearing loss* (p. x1). Baltimore: York Press.

Bakan, E., Yigitoglu, M.R., Gokce, G., & Dogan, M. (1993). Pendred's syndrome. *Annals of Otology, Rhinology, and Laryngology, 102,* 285–288.

Baker, D.B. (1979). Severely handicapped: Toward an inclusive definition. *AAESPH Review, 4,* 52–65.

Baker, R.B. (1992). Is ear pulling associated with ear infection? *Pediatrics, 90* (6), 1006–1007.

Baldwin, J.I. (1968). Dysostosis craniofacialis of Crouzon. *Laryngoscope, 78,* 1660–1675.

Balkany, T.J. (1980). Otologic aspects of Down's syndrome. *Seminars in Speech, Language and Hearing, 1,* 39.

Balkany, T.J., Berman, S.A., Simmons, M.A., et al. (1978). Middle ear effusion in neonates. *Laryngoscope, 88,* 398–405.

Balkany, T.J., Mischke, R.E., Downs, M.P., et al. (1979). Ossicular abnormalities in Down's syndrome. *Otolaryngology Head and Neck Surgery, 87,* 372.

Balkany, T.J., & Pashley, N.R.T. (Eds.). (1986). *Clinical pediatric otolaryngology.* St. Louis: CV Mosby.

Bart, R.S., & Pumphrey, R.E. (1967). Knuckle pads, leukonychia and deafness; a dominantly inherited syndrome. *New England Journal of Medicine, 276,* 202–207.

Basser, L.S. (1964). Benign paroxysmal vertigo of childhood: A variety of vestibular neuronitis. *Brain, 87,* 141–152.

Bassila, M.K., & Goldberg, R. (1989). The association of facial palsy and/or sensorineural hearing loss in patients with hemifacial microsomia. *American Journal of Medical Genetics, 26,* 289–291.

Batsakis, J.G., & Nishiyama, R.H. (1962). Deafness with sporadic goiter: Pendred's syndrome. *Archives of Otolaryngology, 76,* 401–406.

Battin, R.R., Young, M., & Burns, M. (2000). Use of FastForward in remediation of central auditory processing disorders. *Audiology Today, 12* (2), 13–15.

Beagley, H.A., & Fisch, L. (1981). Bio-electric potentials available for electric response audiometry: Indications and contra-indications. In H.A. Beagley (ed.). *Audiology and audiological medicine.* Oxford: Oxford University Press.

Bekesy, G. von. (1960). *Experiments in hearing.* New York: McGraw-Hill.

Bellis, T.J. (1996). *Assessment and management of central auditory processing disorders in the educational setting.* San Diego: Singular Publishing Group, Inc.

Bench, J., Collyer, D., Mentz, L., et al. (1977). Studies in behavioral audiometry. III. Six-month-old infants. *Audiology, 15,* 384–394.

Bench, R.J. (1968). Sound transmission to the human foetus through the maternal abdominal wall. *Journal of Genetic Psychology, 113,* 85–87.

Bench, R.J. (1971). Infant audiometry. *Sound, 4,* 72–74.

Bender, R., & Wig, E. (1962). Binaural hearing aids for hearing impaired children in elementary schools. *Volta Review, 64,* 537–542.

Bendet, R. (1980). A public school hearing aid maintenance program. *Volta Review, 82,* 149.

Benham-Dunster, R.A., & Dunster, J.R. (1985). Hearing loss in the developmentally handicapped: A comparison of three audiometric procedures. *Journal of Auditory Research, 25,* 175–190.

Bennett, M.J. (1984). Impedance concepts relating to the acoustic reflex. In S. Silman (Ed.). *The acoustic reflex: Basic principles and clinical applications* (pp. 35–61). New York: Academic Press.

Bennett, M.J., & Weatherby, L. (1979). Multiple probe frequency acoustic reflex measurements. *Scandinavian Audiology, 8,* 233–239.

Bennett, M.J., & Weatherby, L. (1982). Newborn acoustic reflexes to noise and pure-tone signals. *Journal of Speech and Hearing Research, 25,* 383–387.

Bent, J.P, & Smith, R.J. (1998). The cleft palate ear. In A.K. Lalwani & K. Grundfast K (Eds.), *Pediatric otology and neurotology* (pp. 627–634). Philadelphia: Lippincott-Raven.

Bentler, R.A. (1989). External ear resonance characteristics in children. *Journal of Speech and Hearing Disorders, 54,* 264–268.

Berg, F.S. (1972). *Educational audiology: Hearing and speech management* (p. 2). New York: Grune and Stratton.

Berg, F.S. (1993). *Acoustics and sound systems in schools.* San Diego: Singular Publishing Group, Inc.

Bergsma, D. (Ed.). (1979). *Birth defects compendium* (2nd ed.). The National Foundation-March of Dimes. New York: Alan R Liss.

Bergstrom, L. (1984). Congenital hearing loss. In J.L. Northern (Ed.). *Hearing disorders* (2nd ed.) (Ch.13). Boston: Little, Brown & Co.

Bergstrom, L., Hemenway, W.G., & Downs M.P. (1971). A high risk registry to find congenital deafness. *Otolaryngologic Clinics of North America, 4,* 69–399.

Bergstrom, L., Jenkins, P., Sando, I., & English, G.M. (1973). Hearing loss in renal disease: Clinical and pathological studies. *Annals of Otology, Rhinology, and Laryngology, 82,* 555–577.

Bergstrom, L., Neblett, L.M., & Hemenway, W.G. (1972). Otologic manifestations of acrocephalosyndactyly. *Archives of Otolaryngology, 96,* 117–123.

Bergstrom, L., Stewart, J., & Kenyon, B. (1974). External auditory atresia and the deletion chromosome. *Laryngoscope, 84,* 1905–1917.

Berko, J., & Brown, R. (1969). Psycholinguistic research methods. In P.H. Mussen (Ed.), *Handbook of Research Methods in Child Development.* New York: John Wiley & Sons.

Berlin, C.I. (1982). Ultra-audiometric hearing in the hearing impaired and use of upward-shifting translating hearing aids. *Volta Review, 84,* 352–363.

Berlin, C.I., & Catlin, F.I. (1965). *Manual of standard pure tone threshold procedure, programmed instruction: Tactics for obtaining valid pure tone clinical thresholds.* Baltimore: Johns Hopkins Medical Institutions.

Berman, S.A., Balkany, T.J., & Simmons, M.A. (1978). Otitis media in the neonatal intensive care unit. *Pediatrics, 62,* 198–202.

Bernstein, R.S. & Gravel, J. (1990). A method for determining hearing sensitivity in infants: The interweaving staircase procedure (ISP). *Journal American Academy of Audiology, 1,* 138–145.

Bess, F., Dodd-Murphy, J., & Parker, R. (1998). Children with minimal sensorineural hearing loss: Prevalence, educational performance, and functional status. *Ear and Hearing, 19* (5), 339–354.

Bess, F.H. (1980). Impedance screening for children: A need for more research. *Annals of Otology, Rhinology, and Laryngology, 89* (Suppl. 68), 228.

Bess, F.H., Klee, T., & Culbertson, J. L. (1986). Identification, assessment and management of children with unilateral sensorineural hearing loss. *Ear and Hearing, 7,* 43–51.

Bess, F.H., Lewis, H.D., & Cieliczka D.J. (1975). Acoustic impedance measurements in cleft-palate children. *Journal of Speech and Hearing Disorders, 40,* 13–24.

Bess, F.H., McConnell, F. (1981). *Audiology, education, and the hearing impaired child.* St. Louis: CV Mosby.

Bess, F.H., & Paradise, J.L. (1994). Universal screening for infant hearing: Not simple, not risk-free, not necessarily beneficial, and not presently justified. *Pediatrics, 98* (2), 330–334.

Bess, F.H., Peek, B., & Chapman, J. (1979). Further observations on noise levels in infant incubators. *Pediatrics, 63,* 100.

Bess, F.H., Schwartz, D.M., & Redfield, N.P. (1976). Audiometric, impedance and otoscopic findings in children with cleft palates. *Archives of Otolaryngology, 102,* 465–469.

Bess, F.H., Tharpe, A.M. (1984). Unilateral hearing impairment in children. *Pediatrics, 74,* 206–216.

Beyond "V.D." (1980). *Medical World News, 21,* 56–63. New York, NY: Medical Tribune.

Birch, J.W. (1976). Mainstream education for hearing-impaired pupils: issues and interviews. *American Annals of the Deaf, 121,* 69–71.

Birnholz, J.C., & Benacerraf, B.R. (1983). The development of human fetal hearing. *Science, 22,* 516–518.

Bitici, O.C. (1975). Familial hereditary progressive sensorineural hearing loss with keratosis and plantaris. *Journal of Laryngology and Otology, 89,* 1143–1146.

Black, F.O., Bergstrom, L., Downs, M.P., et al. (1971a). *Congenital deafness: A new approach to early detection through a high risk register.*

Boulder, CO: Colorado Associated University Press.

Black, F.O., Sando, I., Wagner, J.A., et al. (1971). Middle and inner ear abnormalities, 13–15 (D_1) trisomy. *Archives of Otolaryngology, 93,* 615–619.

Blair, J.C., Perterson, M.E., & Vieweg, S.H. (1985). The effects of mild sensorineural hearing loss on academic performance of young school-age children. *Volta Review, 87* (2), 87–93.

Blair, J.C., Wilson-Vlotman, A., & Almen, P. von. (1989). Educational audiologists: Practices, problems, directions, recommendations. *Education Audiology Monographs, 1,* 2–14. Educational Audiology Association, Tampa, FL.

Blennow, F., Svenningsen, N., & Almquist, B. (1974). Noise levels in infant incubators (adverse effects?). *Pediatrics, 53,* 29.

Bloom, L., & Lahey, M. (1978). *Language development and language disorders.* New York: John Wiley & Sons.

Bluestone, C., Klein, J., Paradise, J., et al. (1983). Workshop on the effects of otitis media on the child. *Pediatrics, 71,* 639–652.

Bluestone, C.D. (1998). Otitis media: A spectrum of diseases. In A. Lalwani & K. Grundfast (Eds.), *Pediatric otology and neurotology* (pp. 233–240). Philadelphia: Lippincott-Raven.

Bluestone, C.D., Beery, Q.C., & Paradise, J. (1973). Audiometry and tympanometry in relation to middle ear effusions in children. *Laryngoscope, 83,* 594–604.

Bluestone, C.D., Fria, T.J., Arjona, S.K., et al. (1986). Controversies in screening for middle ear disease and hearing loss in children. *Pediatrics, 77,* 57–70.

Bluestone, C.D., & Klein, JO. (1988). *Otitis Media in Infants and Children.* Philadelphia: WB Saunders.

Bluestone, C.D., Stool, S.E., & Scheetz, M.D. (Eds.). (1990). *Pediatric otolaryngology* (2nd ed.). Philadelphia: WB Saunders.

Bobbin, R. (1996). Chemical receptors on outer hair cells and their molecular mechanisms. In C. Berlin (Ed.), *Hair cells and hearing aids.* San Diego: Singular Publishing Group.

Bollerslev, J., Grodum, E., & Grontved, A. (1987). Autosomal dominant osteopetrosis. *Journal of Laryngology and Otology, 101,* 1088–1091.

Bonfils, P., Vziel, A., & Pujol, R. (1988). Screening for auditory dysfunction in infants by evoked oto-acoustic emissions. *Otolaryngology—Head and Neck Surgery, 114,* 887–890.

Boothroyd, A. (1993). Profound deafness. In R. Tyler (Ed.). *Cochlear implants: Audiological foundations* (pp. 1–34). San Diego: Singular Publishing Group.

Bornstein, H. (1973). A description of some current sign systems designed to represent English. *American Annals of the Deaf, 188,* 454–463.

Bornstein, H. (1974). Signed English: A manual approach to English language development.

Journal of Speech and Hearing Disorders, 3, 330–343.

Bornstein, H. (1978). Sign language in the education of the deaf. In I. Schlesinger & L. Namir (Eds.), *Sign language of the deaf: Psychological linguistics and social perspectives* (pp. 333–359). New York: Academic Press.

Bornstein, H. (1979). Systems of sign. In L. Bradford & W. Hardy (Eds.), *Hearing and hearing impairment* (pp. 331–361). New York: Academic Press.

Bornstein, H., Kannapell, B.M., Saulnier, K.I., et al. (1972). *Signed English basic pres-school dictionary; Little Red Riding Hood, Goldilocks and the Three Bears, etc.* Washington, DC: Gallaudet College Press.

Bornstein, H., & Saulnier, K. (1981). Signed English: A brief follow-up to the first evaluation. *American Annals of the Deaf, 124,* 69–72.

Bornstein, H., Saulnier, K., & Hamilton, L. (1980). Signed English: a first evaluation. *American Annals of the Deaf, 125,* 467–481.

Borowitz, K.C., & Glascoe, F.P. (1986). Sensitivity of the Denver development screening test in speech and language screening. *Pediatrics, 78,* 1075–1078.

Borus, J. (1972). Acoustic impedance measurements with hard of hearing mentally retarded children. *Journal of Mental Deficiencies Research* 16:196–202, 1972.

Bower, T. (1975). Competent newborns. In R. Levin (Ed.), *Child alive.* Garden City, NY: Anchor Press/Doubleday.

Brackett, D., & Maxon, A.B. (1986). Service delivery alternatives for the mainstreamed hearing-impaired child. *Language, Speech, and Hearing Services in Schools, 17,* 115–125.

Bretlau, P., Jorgensen, M.B., & Johansen, H. (1970). Osteogenesis imperfecta. Light and electron microscopic studies of the stapes. *Acta Oto-Laryngologica (Stockholm), 69,* 172–184.

Bridger, W.H. (1961). Sensory discrimination and habituation in the human neonate. *American Journal of Psychiatry, 117,* 991–996.

Bright, K.E. (1997). Spontaneous otoacoustic emissions. In M. Robinette & T. Glattke (Eds.), *Otoacoustic emissions: Clinical applications* (pp. 46–62). New York: Thieme.

Brill, R.G. (1975). Mainstreaming: Format or quality. *American Annals of the Deaf, 120,* 377–381.

Brill, R.G. (1976). Definition of total communication. *American Annals of the Deaf, 121,* 358.

Brody, J.A. (1964). Notes on the epidemiology of draining ears and hearing loss in Alaska with comments on future studies and control measures. *Alaska Medicine, 6,* 1.

Brody, J.A., Overfield, T., & McAlister, R. (1965). Draining ears and deafness among Eskimos. *Archives of Otolaryngology, 81,* 29–33.

Brookhouser, P., Worthington, D., & Kelly, W. (1994). Fluctuating and/or progressive sensorineural hearing loss in children. *Laryngoscope, 104,* 958–964.

Brookhouser, P.E., & Moeller, M.P. (1986). Choosing the appropriate habilitative track for the newly identified hearing-impaired child. *Annals of Otology, Rhinology, and Laryngology, 95* (1), 51–59.

Brooks, D. (1968). An objective method of detecting fluid in the middle ear. *International Audiology, 7,* 280–286.

Brooks, D. (1969). The use of the electro-acoustic impedance bridge in the assessment of middle ear function. *International Audiology, 8,* 563–569.

Brooks, D. (1971). Electroacoustic impedance bridge studies on normal ears of children. *Journal of Speech and Hearing Research, 14,* 247–253.

Brooks, D.N. (1975). Middle ear effusion in children with severe hearing loss. *Impedance Newsletters, 4,* 6–7.

Brown, J.B., Fryer, M.P., & Morgan, L.R. (1969). Problems in reconstruction of the auricle. *Plastic and Reconstructive Surgery, 43,* 597–604.

Brownell, W.E. (1983). Observations on a motile response in isolated outer hair cells. In W.R. Webster & L.M. Aitken (Eds.), *Mechanisms of hearing* (pp. 5–10). Clayton, Australia: Monash University Press.

Brownell, W.E., Bader, C.R., Bertrend, D., & de Ribaupierre, Y. (1985) Evoked mechanical responses of isolated cochlear hair cells. *Science, 227,* 194–196.

Buran, D.J., & Duvall, A.J. (1967). The oto-palato-digital (OPD) syndrome. *Archives of Otolaryngology, 85,* 394–399.

Busby, P.A., Dettman, J., Altidis, P.M., Blamey, P.J., & Roberts, S.A. (1990). Assessment of communication skills in implanted deaf children. In G.M. Clark, Y.C. Tong, & J.F. Patrick (Eds.), *Cochlear prostheses.* Edinburgh: Churchill Livingstone.

Butler, K. (1983). Language processing: Selective attention and mnemonic strategies. In E. Lasky & J. Katz (Eds.), *Central auditory processing disorders.* Baltimore: University Park Press.

Butterfield, E.C. (1968). An extended version of modification of sucking with auditory feedback. Working paper 43. Kansas City, KS: Bureau of Child Research Laboratory, Children's Rehabilitation Unit, University of Kansas Medical Center.

Bzoch, K.R. (Ed.). (1979). *Communicative disorders related to cleft lip and palate* (2nd ed.). Boston: Little, Brown & Co.

Campbell, P.H., & Wilcox, M.J. (1986). In *Special needs report—a newsletter from the Akron medical center.* Akron, OH: Akron Medical Center.

Capute, A.J., Palmer, F.B., Shapiro, B.K., et al. (1986). The clinical linguistic and auditory milestone scale of infancy (CLAMS): Prediction of cognition in infancy. *Developmental Medicine and Child Neurology, 28,* 762–771.

Capute, A.J., Shapiro, B.K., Wachtel, R.C., Gunther, V.A., & Palmer, F.B. (1986). The clinical linguistic and auditory milestone scale (CLAMS). *American Journal of Diseases in Children, 140,* 694–698.

Carhart, R., & Jerger, J. (1959). Preferred method for clinical determination of pure tone thresholds. *Journal of Speech and Hearing Disorders, 24,* 330–345.

Carnegie Corporation. (1994). *Starting points: Meeting the needs of our youngest children. Report of the Carnegie Task.* New York: Author.

Carney, A. (1996). Audition and the development of oral communication competency. In F. Bess, J. Gravel, & A. Tharpe (Eds.), *Amplification for children with auditory deficits* (pp. 29–54). Nashville, TN: Bill Wilkerson Center Press.

Carney, A. (1999). Auditory system development and dysfunction: What do we really know about childhood hearing loss? *Trends in Amplification, 4* (2), 32–38.

Carney, A., & Moeller, M.P. (1998). Treatment efficiency: Hearing loss in children. *Journal of Speech, Language and Hearing Research, 41,* 61–84.

Casselbrant, M.L., Brostoff, L.M., Cantekin, E.I., et al. (1985). Otitis media with effusion in preschool children. *Laryngoscope, 95,* 428–436.

Chalmers, D., Stewart, I., Silva, P., & Mulvena, A. (1989). *Otitis media with effusion in children: The Dunedin study.* Philadelphia: JB Lippincott.

Champion, R.H.J. (1989). Muckle-Wells syndrome (urticaria, amyloidosis and deafness). *British Journal of Dermatology, 121* (Suppl. 34), 75.

Chan, Y., Adams, D., & Kerr, A. (1995). Syphilitic labyrinthitis—an update. *Journal of Laryngology and Otology, 109,* 719–725.

Chen, S.J., Yang, E.Y., Kwan, M.L., Chang, P., Shiao, A,, & Lien, C.F. (1996). Infant hearing screening with an automated auditory brainstem response screener and the auditory brainstem response. *Acta Paediatrica, 85,* 14–28.

Chermak, G.D., & Musiek, F.E. (Eds.). (1997). *Central auditory processing disorders: New perspectives.* San Diego: Singular Publishing Group.

Chermak, G.D., Pederson, C.M., & Bendel, R.B. (1984). Equivalent forms and split-half reliability of the NU-CHIPS administered in noise. *Journal of Speech and Hearing Disorders, 49,* 196–201.

Chial, M. (1998). Yet another audiogram. *ASHA Hearing and Hearing Disorders: Research and Diagnostics Newsletter, 2* (1), 2–3.

Chomsky, N. (1995, June 6). Chimp talk debate: Is it really language? *The New York Times.*

Chomsky, N. (1966). *Aspects of the theory of syntax.* Cambridge, MA: MIT Press.

Chrysostomidou, D.M., Caslaris, E., Alexion, D., et al. (1971). Trisomy 18 in Greece. *Acta Paediatrica Scandinavica, 69,* 591–593.

Chugani, H., Phelps, M., Mazziotta, J. (1987). Positron emission tomography study of human brain functional development. *Annals of Neurology, 22* (4), 495.

Chugani, H. (1993). Positron emission tomography scanning in newborns. *Clinics in Perinatology, 20* (2), 398.

Chugani, H. (1997, Spring/Summer). How to build a baby's brain. *Newsweek, Special Edition,* 29–30.

Church, M., Edlis, F., Blakley, B.W., & Bawle, E.V. (1997). Hearing, language, speech, vestibular and dentofacial disorders in fetal alcohol syndrome. *Alcoholism, Clinical and Experimental Research, 21* (3), 495–512.

Church, M., & Kaltenbach, J.A. (1997). Hearing, speech, language, and vestibular disorders in the fetal alcohol syndrome: Literature review. *Alcoholism, Clinical and Experimental Research, 21* (3), 495–512.

Church, M.W., & Gerkin, K.P. (1987). Hearing disorders in children with fetal alcohol syndrome: Findings from case reports. *Pediatrics, 82,* 147–154.

Churchland, P. (1997). *The engine of reason, the seat of the soul: Philosophical journey into the brain.* Boston: M.I.T. Press.

Clark, G.M., Cowan, R., & Dowell, R.C. (Eds.). (1997). *Cochlear implantation for infants and children.* San Diego: Singular Publishing Group.

Clifton, R.K. (1998). The development of spatial hearing in human infants. In L.A. Werner & E.W. Rubel (Eds.), *Developmental psychoacoustics.* Washington, D.C.: American Psychological Association, 135–148.

Clopton, B.M., & Silverman, M.S. (1977). Plasticity of binaural interactions, II: critical periods and changes in midline response. *Journal of Neurophysiology, 40,* 1275–1280.

Clopton, B.M., & Winfield, J.A. (1976). Effect of early exposure to patterned sound on unit activity in rat inferior colliculus. *Journal of Neurophysiology, 39,* 1081–1089.

Coats, A.C. (1986). Electrocochleography: Recording techniques and clinical applications. *Seminars in Hearing, 7* (3), 247–266.

Cochlear Implants in Adults and Children. (1995, May 15–17). *NIH Consensus Statement, 13* (2).

Cohen, D., & Sade, J. (1972). Hearing in secretory otitis media. *Canadian Journal of Otology, 1,* 27.

Cohen, M.E. (1967). Neurological abnormalities in achondroplastic children. *Journal of Pediatrics, 71,* 367.

Cohen, M.M. (1986). *Craniosynostosis: Diagnosis, evaluation and management.* New York: Raven Press.

Cohen, M.M., & Kreiborg, S. (1993). The growth pattern in the Apert syndrome. *American Journal of Medical Genetics, 47,* 617–623.

Cohen, N., & Waltzman, S. (1996). Cochlear implants in infants and young children. *Seminars in Hearing, 17* (2), 215–222.

Cohen, P.E. (1966). The "D" syndrome. *American Journal of Diseases in Children, 111,* 235.

Cole, D.E., & Cohen, M.M. (1991). Osteogenesis imperfecta: An update. *Journal of Pediatrics, 119,* 73–74.

Collet, L., Gartner, M., Moulin, A., Kauffman, I., Disant, F., & Morgon, A. (1989). Evoked otoacoustic emissions and sensorineural hearing loss. *Otolaryngology—Head and Neck Surgery, 115,* 1060–1062.

Commission on Education of the Deaf. (1988, February). *Toward equality: Education of the deaf. Report to the President and the Congress of the United States.* Washington, DC: Government Printing Office.

Compton, A. (1978). *Compton speech and language screening evaluation.* San Francisco: Carousel House.

Condon, W.S., & Sander, L.W. (1974). Neonate movement is synchronized with adult speech: Interactional participation and language structure. *Science, 183,* 99–101.

Cone-Wesson, B., Vohr, B.R., Sininger, Y.S., Widen, J.E., Folsom, R.C., Gorga, M.P., & Norton, S.J. (2000). Identification of neonatal hearing impairment: infants with hearing impairment. *Ear and Hearing, 21* (5), 488–507.

Conference on Hearing Screening Services for Preschool Children. (1977). Columbus, OH: Maternal & Child Health Bureau, Department of HEW, Washington, DC.

Cooper, J., Langley, L., Meyerhoff, W., et al. (1977). The significance of negative middle ear pressure. *Laryngoscope, 87,* 92–97.

Cooper, J.C., Gates, G.A., Owen, J.H., et al. (1975). An abbreviated impedance bridge technique for school screening. *Journal of Speech and Hearing Disorders, 40,* 260–269.

Cooper, L. (1969). Rubella: Clinical manifestations and management. *American Journal of Diseases in Children, 118,* 18–29.

Cooper, L.F., & Jabs, E.W. (1987). Aural atresia associated with multiple congenital anomalies and mental retardation: A new syndrome. *Journal of Pediatrics, 110* (5), 747–750.

Coplan, J. (1987). Deafness: Ever heard of it? Delayed recognition of permanent hearing loss. *Pediatrics, 79* (2), 206–213.

Coplan, J., & Gleason, J.R. (1988). Unclear speech: Recognition and significance of unintelligible speech in preschool children. *Pediatrics, 82* (2), 447–452.

Coplan, J., Gleason, J.R., Ryan, R., Burke, M.G., & Williams, M.L. (1982). Validation of an early language milestone scale in a high-risk population. *Pediatrics, 70* (5), 677–683.

Coppage, K.B., & Smith, R.J. (1995). Branchio-oto-renal syndrome. *Journal of the American Academy of Audiology, 6* (1), 103–110.

Cornett, R.O. (1985). Diagnostic factors bearing on the use of cued speech with hearing-impaired children. *Ear and Hearing, 6* (1), 33–35.

Cox, L.C., & Metz, A.A. (1980). ABER in the prescription of hearing aids. *Hearing Instruments, 31,* 12–15, 55.

Craig, W., & Craig, H. (1972). *Verbotonal instruction for young deaf children: Questions and replies.* [Pamphlet]. Western Pennsylvania School for the Deaf.

Craig, W.N., Craig, H., & DiJohnson, A. (1972). Preschool verbotonal instruction for deaf children. *Volta Review, 74,* 236–246.

Crandell, C., Smaldino, J., & Flexer, C. (1995). *Sound-field FM amplification: Theory and practical applications.* San Diego: Singular Publishing Group.

Cremers, C.W.R.J., Thijssen, H.O.M., & Fischer, A.J.E.M. (1981). Otological aspects of the earpit-deafness syndrome. *Journal of Otolaryngology, 43,* 223–239.

Cremers, W.R.J., Hoogland, G.A., & Kuypers, W. (1984). Hearing loss in the cervico-oculo-acoustic (Wildervanck) syndrome. *Archives of Otolaryngology, 110,* 54–57.

Cross, H.E., & Pfaffenbach, D.D. (1972). Duane's retraction syndrome and associated congenital malformations. *American Journal of Ophthalmology, 73,* 442–449.

Culpepper, B., & Thompson, G. Effects of reinforcer duration on the response behavior of pre-term 2-year-olds in visual reinforcement andrometry. *Ear and Hearing, 15,* 161–167.

Culpepper, L., & Froom, J. (1995). Otitis media with effusion in young children: Treatment in search of a problem. *Journal of the American Board of Family Practice, 8,* 305–316.

Cunningham, G.C. (1970). Biochemical screening programs and problems. In E.M. Gold (Ed.), *Earlier recognition of handicapping conditions in childhood: Proceedings of a bi-regional institute* (pp. 37–41). Berkeley, CA: University of California School of Public Health.

Curran, J.R. (1988). Hearing aids. In N. Lass, L. McReynolds, J. Northern, & D. Yoder (Eds.), *Handbook of speech-language pathology and audiology* (pp. 1293–1314). Toronto: BC Decker.

Cusimano, F., Martines, E., & Rizzo, C. (1991). The Jervell and Lang-Nielsen syndrome. *International Journal of Pediatric Otolaryngology, 22,* 49–58, 1991.

Cyr, D.G. (1983). The vestibular system: Pediatric considerations. *Seminars in Hearing, 4* (1), 33–46.

Cyr, D.G., Brookhouser, P.E., Valente, M., & Grossman, A. (1985). Vestibular evaluation of infants and preschool children. *Otolaryngology—Head and Neck Surgery, 93* (4), 463–468.

Dahl, H.A. (1979). Progressive hearing impairment in children with congenital CMV. *Journal of Speech and Hearing Disorders, 44,* 220.

Dahle, A.J., Fowler, K.B., Wright, J.D., Boppana, S.B., Britt, W.J., & Pass, R.F. (2000). Longitudinal investigation of hearing disorders in children with congenital cytomegalovirus. *Journal of the American Academy of Audiology, 11* (5) 283–290.

Dahle, A.J., & McCollister, F.P. (1983). Considerations for evaluating hearing in multiply handicapped children. *The multiply handicapped child* (Proceedings of a symposium in Edmonton, Alberta). New York: Grune & Stratton.

Dallos, P. (1973). *The auditory periphery: Biophysics and physiology.* New York: Academic Press.

Dalsgaard, S., & Dyrlund-Jensen, O. (1976). Measurement of the insertion gain of hearing aids. *Journal of Audiological Technology, 15,* 170.

Dalzell, L., Orlando, M., MacDonald, M., Berg, A., Bradley, M., Cacace, A., et al. (2000). The New York State universal newborn hearing screening demonstration project: Ages of hearing loss identification, hearing aid fitting, and enrollment in early intervention. *Ear and Hearing, 21* 2, 118–130.

Danaher, E.M., & Pickett, J.M. (1975). Some masking effects produced by low frequency vowel formats in persons with sensorineural hearing loss. *Journal of Speech and Hearing Research, 18,* 261.

Danenberg, M.A., Loos-Cosgrove, M., & LoVerde, M. (1987). Temporary hearing loss and rock music. *Language, Speech, and Hearing Services in Schools, 18,* 267–274.

Davenport, S.L., Hefner, M.A., Thelin, J.W. (1986). CHARGE syndrome: Part I: External ear anomalies. *International Journal of Pediatric Otorhinolaryngology, 12,* 137–143.

Davis, A., & Wood, S. (1992). The epidemiology of childhood hearing impairment: Factors relevant to planning of services. *British Journal of Audiology, 26,* 77–90.

Davis, H. (1961). Peripheral coding of auditory information. In W.A. Rosenblith (Ed.), *Sensory communication.* Cambridge, MA: MIT Press.

Davis, H. (1976). Brainstem and other responses in electric response audiometry. *Annals of Otology, 85,* 3–13.

Davis, H. (1983). An active process in cochlear mechanics. *Hearing Research, 9,* 79–90.

Davis, J. (1988, November/December). Developing your child's individualized educational program. [Introduction letter]. *Shhh,* 26.

Davis, J.M., Elfenbein, J., Schum, R., & Bentler, R. (1986). Effects of mild and moderate hearing impairments on language, educational, and psychosocial behavior of children. *Journal of Speech and Hearing Disorders, 51,* 53–62.

Davis, J.M., Shepard, N.T., Stelmachowicz, P.G., et al. (1981). Characteristics of hearing-impaired children in the public schools. Part II: Psychoeducational data. *Journal of Speech and Hearing Disorders, 46,* 130–137, 1981.

Davis, P.A. (1939). Effects of acoustic stimuli on the waking human brain. *Journal of Neurophysiology, 2,* 444–499.

Dawe, C., Wynne-Davies, R., & Fulford, G.E. (1982). Clinical variation in dyschondrosteosis: A report on 13 individuals in 8 families. *Journal of Bone and Joint Surgery, 64B,* 377–381.

DeCasper, A.J., & Fifer, W.P. (1980). Of human bonding: Newborns prefer their mothers' voices. *Science, 208,* 1174–1176.

Delgado, J.L., Johnson, C.L., Roy, I., & Trevino, P.M. (1990). Hispanic health and nutrition examination survey: Methodological considerations. *American Journal of Public Health, 80* (Suppl.), 6–10.

Demany, I., McKenzie, B., & Vurpillot, E. (1977). Rhythm perception in early infancy. *Nature, 266,* 718–719.

Demmler, G. (1991). Infectious diseases society of America and centers for disease control: Summary of a workshop on surveillance for congenital cytomegalovirus disease. *Review of Infectious Diseases, 13,* 315–329.

Denton, D.M., Brill, R.B., Kent, M.S., et al. (1974). Schools for deaf children. In P.J. Fine (Ed.), *Deafness in infancy and early childhood.* New York: Medicom Press.

Derbyshire, A.J., & Davis, H. (1935). The action potential of the auditory nerve. *American Journal of Physiology, 113,* 476–504.

Desai, M.P., Joshi, N.C., & Shah, K.N. (1973). Chronic idiopathic hyperphosphatasia in an Indian child. *American Journal of Diseases in Children, 126,* 626–628.

Diefendorf, A.O. (1988). Behavioral evaluation of hearing-impaired children. In F.H. Bess (Ed), *Hearing impairment in children* (pp. 133–149). Parkton, MD: York Press.

Diefendorf, A.O., Bull, M.J., Casey-Harvey, D., Miyamoto, R.T., et al. (1995). Down syndrome: A multidisciplinary perspective. *Journal of the American Academy of Audiology, 6* (1), 39–46.

Dillon, H. (2000). *Hearing aids.* Sydney, Australia: Boomerang Press.

Dillon, H., & Storey, L. (1998). National acoustic laboratories' procedures for selecting the saturation sound pressure level of hearing aids: Theoretical derivation. *Ear and Hearing, 19* (4), 255–266.

Dirks, D. (1964). Perception of dichotic and monaural verbal material and cerebral dominance for speech. *Acta Oto-Laryngologica (Stockholm), 58,* 73–80.

Dobie, R.A., & Berlin, C.I. (1979). Influence of otitis media on hearing and development. *Annals of Otology, Rhinology, and Laryngology, 88* (suppl. 60), 48–53.

Dobrowski, J.M., Grundfast, K.M., Rosenbaum, K.N., Zajtchuk J.T. (1985). Otorhinolaryngic manifestations of CHARGE association. *Oto-*

laryngology—Head and Neck Surgery, 93, 798–803.

Dodge, H.W., Jr., Wood, M.W., & Kennedy, R.J. (1959). Craniofacial dysostosis: Crouzon's disease. *Pediatrics, 23,* 98.

Dodge, P.R., Davis, H., Feigin, R.D., et al. (1984). Prospective evaluation of hearing impairment as a sequela of acute bacterial meningitis. *New England Journal of Medicine, 311* (14), 869–874.

Dolnick, E. (1993). Deafness as a culture. *The Atlantic Monthly, 272* (3), 37–53.

Douek, E., Dodson, H., Banister, L., et al. (1976). Effects of incubator noise on the cochlea of the newborn. *Lancet, 2,* 1110–1113.

Downs, M.P. (1966). The establishment of hearing aid use: A program for parents. *Maico Audiological Library Series, 4,* v.

Downs, M.P. (1970). The identification of congenital deafness. *Transactions of the American Academy of Ophthalmology and Otolaryngology, 741,* 208–214.

Downs, M.P. (1971). Maintaining children's hearing aids. The role of parents. *Maico Audiological Library Series, 10,* 1.

Downs, M.P. (1974, Jan.-Feb.). The deafness management quotient. *Hearing and Speech News.*

Downs, M.P. (Ed.). (1980). Communication disorders in Down's syndrome. *Seminars in Speech, Language, and Hearing, 1,* 1.

Downs, M.P. (1982). Early identification of hearing loss. In N.J. Lass, L.V. McReynolds, J.L. Northern, et al. (Eds.), *Speech, language & hearing* (Ch. 41). Philadelphia: WB Saunders.

Downs, M.P. (1985). The high-risk concept extended. *Recent advances in otitis media* (pp. 352–353). Toronto: BC Decker.

Downs MP. (1986). The rationale for neonatal hearing screening. In E.T. Swigard (Ed.), *Neonatal hearing screening* (pp. 3–16), San Diego: College Hill Press.

Downs, M.P., & Hemenway, W.G. (1969). Report on the hearing screening of 17,000 neonates. *International Audiology, 8,* 72–76.

Downs, M.P., & Sterritt, G.M. (1964). Identification audiometry for neonates: A preliminary report. *Journal of Auditory Research, 4,* 69–80.

Doyle, K.J., Fuikawa, S., Rogers, P., & Newman, E. (1998). Comparison of newborn hearing screening by transient otoacoustic emissions and auditory brainstem response using ALGO-2. *International Journal of Pediatric Otorhinolaryngology, 43,* 207–211.

Duncan, B., Ey, J., Holberg, C., Wright, A., Martinez, F., & Taussig, L. (1993). Exclusive breastfeeding for at least four months protects against otitis media. *Pediatrics, 91,* 867–872.

Dunst, C., Trivette, C., Starnes, A., Hamby, D., & Gordon, N. (1993). *Building and evaluating family support initiatives: A national study of programs for persons with developmental disabilities.* Baltimore: Paul H. Brookes.

Dupertius, S.M., & Musgrave, R.H. (1959). Experiences with the reconstruction of the congenitally deformed ear. *Plastic and Reconstructive Surgery, 23,* 361–373.

Eagles, E.L., Wishik, S.M., & Doerfler, L.G. (1967). Hearing sensitivity and ear disease in children: A prospective study. *Monographs in Laryngoscope* (Suppl), 1–274.

Edwards, C. (1991). Assessment and management of listening skills in school-aged children. *Seminars in Hearing, 12,* 389–401.

Edwards, C. (1996). Auditory intervention for children with mild auditory deficits. In F. Bess, J. Gravel, & A. Tharpe (Eds.), *Amplification for children with auditory deficits* (pp. 383–398). Nashville: Bill Wilkerson Center Press.

Edwards, E.P. (1968). Kindergarten is too late. *Saturday Review,* 60–79.

Eilers, R., & Oller, K. (1994). Infant vocalizations and the early diagnosis of severe hearing impairment. *Journal of Pediatrics, 124* (2), 199–203.

Eilers, R., Widen, J., Urbano, R., Hudson, T., & Gonzales, L. (1991). Optimization of automated hearing test algorithms: A comparison of data from simulations and young children. *Ear and Hearing, 12* (3), 199–203.

Eilers, R.E., Miskiel, E., Ozdamar, O., Urbano, R., & Widen, J. (1991). Optimization of automated hearing test algorithms: Simulations using an infant response model. *Ear and Hearing, 12,* 191–198.

Eilers, R.E., Wilson, W.R., & Moore, J.M. (1977). Developmental changes in speech discrimination in infants. *Journal of Speech and Hearing Research, 20* (4), 766–779.

Eimas, P.D. (1975). In L.B. Cohen & M. Salapatek (Eds.), *Infant perception: From sensation to cognition* (Vol. 2). New York: Academic Press.

Eimas, P.D., Siqueland, E.R., Juscyzk, P., et al. (1972). Speech perception in infants. *Science, 171,* 303.

Eimas, P.D., & Tartter, V.C. (1979). On the development of speech perception: mechanisms and analogies. *Advances in Child Development and Behavior, 13,* 155–193.

Eisele, W., Berry, R., & Shriner, T. (1975). Infant sucking response patterns as a conjugate function of change in the sound pressure level of auditory stimuli. *Journal of Speech and Hearing Research, 18,* 296–307.

Eisen, N.H. (1962). Some effects of early sensory deprivation on later behavior: the quondam hard-of-hearing child. *Journal of Abnormal Social Psychology, 65,* 338.

Eisenberg, R.B. (1970). The development of hearing in man: An assessment of current status. *ASHA, 12,* 119–123.

Eisenberg, R.B. (1976). *Auditory competence in early life.* Baltimore: University Park Press.

Elliot, G.B., & Elliot, K.A. (1964). Some pathological, radiological and clinical implications of the precocious development of the human ear. *Laryngoscope, 74,* 1160–1171.

Elliott, L. (1982). Effects of noise on perception of speech of children and certain handicapped individuals. *Sound Vibration, 16,* 12.

Elliott, L.L., & Katz, D.R. (1980). Children's pure-tone detection. *Journal of the Acoustical Society of America, 67,* 343–344.

Elssmann, S.F., Matkin, N.D., & Sabo, M.P. (1987). Early identification of congenital sensorineural hearing impairment. *Hearing Journal, 40* (9), 13–17.

English, G.M., Northern, J.L., & Fria, T.J. (1973). Chronic otitis media as a cause of sensorineural hearing loss. *Archives of Otolaryngology, 98,* 17–22.

Erber, N. (1982). *Auditory Training.* Wash. D.C.: Alexander Graham Bell Assoc. for the Deaf.

Erber, N.P., & Alencewicz, C.M. (1972). Audiologic evaluation of deaf children. *Journal of Speech and Hearing Disorders, 41,* 256–267.

Erber, N.P. (1980). Use of the auditory numbers test to evaluate speech perception abilities of hearing-impaired children. *Journal of Speech and Hearing Disorders, 45,* 527.

Estabrooks, W.I. (2000). Auditory-verbal practice. In S.B. Waltzman & N.L. Cohen (Eds.), *Cochlear implants.* New York: Thieme Medical Publishers.

Evans, E.F. (1975). The sharpening of cochlear frequency selectivity in the normal and abnormal cochlea. *Audiology, 14,* 419.

Ewing, I.R., & Ewing, A.W.G. (1944). The ascertainment of deafness in infancy and early childhood. *Journal of Laryngology and Otology, 59,* 309–338.

Fabry, D., & Schum, D. (1994). The role of subjective measurement technique in hearing aid fittings. In M. Valente (Ed.), *Strategies for selecting and verifying hearing aid fittings* (pp. 136–155). New York: Thieme Medical Publishers, Inc.

Falk, S., & Farmer, J. (1973). Incubator noise and possible deafness. *Archives of Otolaryngology, 97,* 385.

Falk, S.A., (1972). Combined effects of noise and ototoxic drugs. *Environmental Health Perspectives, 5*–22.

Falk, S.A., & Woods, N.F. (1973). Hospital noise-levels and potential health hazards. *New England Journal of Medicine, 289,* 774.

Fausti, S., Henry, J., & Frey, R. (1996). In J. Northern (Ed.), *Hearing disorders* (pp. 149–164). Needham Heights, MA: Allyn and Bacon.

Feigin, R.D., & Dodge, P.R. (1976). Bacterial meningitis: Newer concepts of pathophysiology and neurologic sequelae. *Pediatric Clinics of North America, 23,* 3.

Feingold, M., & Baum, J. (1978). Goldenhar's syndrome. *American Journal of Diseases in Children, 132,* 136–138.

Fernandez, A.O., & Ronis, M.L. (1964). The Treacher Collins syndrome. *Archives of Otolaryngology, 80,* 505.

Ferraro, J.A. (1986). Electrocochleography. *Seminars in Hearing, 7* (3), 239–337.

Field, T.M., Woodson, R., Greenberg, R., et al. (1982). Discrimination and imitation of facial expressions by neonates. *Science, 218,* 179–181.

Finitzo, T., Albright, K., & O'Neal, J. (1998). The newborn with hearing loss: Detection in the nursery. *Pediatrics, 102,* 1452–1460.

Finitzo, T., & Crumley, W.G. (1999). The role of the pediatrician in hearing loss. *Pediatric Clinics of North America, 46* (1), 15–26.

Finitzo-Hieber, T. (1981). Classroom acoustics. In R.J. Roeser & M.P. Downs (Eds.), *Auditory disorders in school children.* New York: Thieme-Stratton.

Finitzo-Hieber, T. (1982). Auditory brainstem response: Its place in infant audiological evaluations. *Seminars in Speech, Language, and Hearing, 3,* 76–87.

Finitzo-Hieber, T., Gerling, I.J., Matkin, N.D., et al. (1980). A sound effects recognition test for the pediatric audiologic evaluation. *Ear and Hearing, 1,* 271.

Finitzo-Hieber, T., McCracken, G., & Brown, K. (1985). Prospective controlled evaluation of auditory function in neonates given netilmicin or amikacin. *Pediatrics, 106,* 129–135.

Finitzo-Hieber, T., McCracken, G., Roeser, R., et al. (1979). Ototoxicity in neonates treated with gentamicin and kanamycin: Results of a four-year controlled follow-up study. *Pediatrics, 63,* 443.

Finitzo-Hieber, T., Simhadri, R., & Hieber, J.P. (1981). Auditory brainstem response assessment of postmeningitic infants and children. *International Journal of Pediatric Otorhinolaryngology, 3,* 275.

Finitzio, T., Albright, K., O'Neal, J. The newborn with hearing loss: detection in the nursery. *Pediatrics, 102,* 1452-1460, 1998.

Finitzio, T., Crumley, W. The role of the pediatrician in hearing loss from detection to connection. *Pediatric Clinics of North America* 46:1, 15–28, 1999.

First, L.R., & Palfrey, J.S. (1994). The infant or young child with developmental delay. *New England Journal of Medicine, 330* (7), 478–483.

Firszt, J., & Reeder, R. (1996). Cochlear implants and children: Device programming and considerations for young children. *Seminars in Hearing, 17* (4), 337–351.

Fischler, R.S., Todd, W.N., & Feldman, C.M. (1985). Otitis media and language performance in a cohort of Apache Indian children. *American Journal of Diseases in Children, 139,* 355–360.

Fletcher, H. (1929). *Speech and hearing.* New York: Van Nostrand.

Fletcher, H. (1953). *Speech and hearing in communication*. New York: Van Nostrand.

Flexer, C. (1990). Audiological rehabilitation in the schools. *ASHA, 32*, (4), 44–45.

Flexer, C., & Gans, D.P. (1982). Evaluating behavioural observation audiometry with handicapped children. *Exceptional Child, 29*, 217–224.

Flexer, C., & Gans, D.P. (1985). Comparative evaluation of the auditory responsiveness of normal infants and profoundly multihandicapped children. *Journal of Speech and Hearing Research, 28*, 163–168.

Flexer, C., & Gans, D.P. (1986). Distribution of auditory response behaviors in normal infants and profoundly multihandicapped children. *Journal of Speech and Hearing Research, 29*, 425–429.

Fluharty, N.B. (1974). *Fluharty preschool speech and language screening test*. Teaching Resources Corporation.

Fortnum, H., & Davis, A. (1997). Epidemiology of permanent childhood hearing impairment in Trent Region, 1985–1993. *British Journal of Audiology, 31*, 409–446.

Fosmoe, R.J., Holm, R.S., & Hildreth, R.C. (1968). Van Buchem's disease (hyperostosis corticalis generalisata familiaris). *Radiology, 90*, 771–774.

Fowler, F.P., & Fletcher, H. (1926). Three million deafened school children: Their detection and treatment. *JAMA, 87*, 1877–1882.

Fowler, K., McCollister, F.P., Dahle, A.J., Boppana, S., Britt, W.J., & Pass, R.F. (1997). Progressive and fluctuating sensorineural hearing loss in children with asymptomatic congenital cytomegalovirus infection. *Journal of Pediatrics, 130*, 624–630.

Fowler, K.B., Stagno, S., Pass, R.F., Brittm, W.J., Boll, T.J., & Alford, C.A. (1992). The outcome of congenital cytomegalovirus infection in relation to maternal antibody status. *New England Journal of Medicine, 326*, 663–667.

Frankenburg, W.K., & Camp, B.W. (1975). *Pediatric screening tests*. Springfield, IL: Charles C Thomas.

Frankenburg, W.K., & Dodds, J.B. (1967) The Denver developmental screening test. *Journal of Pediatrics, 71*, 181–189.

Franklin, B. (1988, May). Tactile aids: what are they? *Hearing Journal, 41* (5).

Franklin, B. (1991). *Manual for the Tactaid 7*. Somerville, MA: Andiologic Engineering Group.

Fraser, G.R. (1962). Our genetical load. *Annals of Human Genetics, 25*, 387–415.

Fraser, G.R. (1965). Association of congenital deafness with goiter (Pendred's syndrome). A study of 207 families. *Annals of Human Genetics, 28*, 201–249.

Fraser, G.R. (1976). *The causes of profound deafness in childhood*. Baltimore: The Johns Hopkins University Press.

Fraser, W.I., & Cambell, B.M. (1978). A study of six cases of de Lange Amsterdam syndrome, with special attention to voice, speech and language characteristics. *Developmental Medicine and Child Neurology, 20*,189–198.

Frazen, L.E., Elmore, J., & Nadler, H.L. (1967). Mandibulofacial dysostosis. *American Journal of Diseases in Children, 113*, 405.

Frentz, G., et al. (1976). Congenital perspective hearing loss and atopic dermatisis. *Acta Oto-Laryngologica, 82*, 242–244.

French, N.R., & Steinberg, J.C. (1979). Factors governing the intelligibility of speech sounds. *Journal of Acoustical Society of America, 19*, 90–119.

Fria, T. (1980).The auditory brain stem response: Background and clinical applications. *Monographs in Contemporary Audiology, 2* (2), 37.

Fria, T., LeBlanc, J., Kristensen, R., et al. (1975). Ipsilateral acoustic reflex stimulation in normal and sensorineural impaired ears: A preliminary report. *Canadian Journal of Otology, 4*, 695–703.

Fria, T.J., Cantekin, E.I., & Eichler, J.A. (1985). Hearing acuity of children with otitis media with effusion. *Otolaryngology—Head and Neck Surgery, 111*, 10–16.

Friedman, A., Schulman, R., & Weiss, S. (1975). Hearing and diabetic neuropathy. *Archives of Internal Medicine, 135*, 573–576.

Friedmann, I., Fraser, G.R., & Froggatt, P. (1966). Pathology of the ear in the cardioauditory syndrome of Jervell and Lange-Nielsen. *Journal of Laryngology and Otology, 80*, 451–470.

Friel-Patti, S., & Finitzo, T. (1990). Language learning in a prospective study of otitis media with effusion in the first two years of life. *Journal of Speech and Hearing Research, 33*, 188–194.

Friel-Patti, S., Finitzo, T., Meyerhoff, W., & Hieber, P.J. (1986). Speech-language learning and early middle ear disease: A procedural report. In J. Kavanaugh (Ed.), *Otitis media in child development* (pp. 129–138). Parkton, MD: York Press.

Friel-Patti, S., Finitzo-Hieber, T., Conti, F., & Brown, K.C. (1982). Language delay in infants associated with middle ear disease and mild, fluctuating hearing impairment. *Pediatric Infectious Diseases, 1* (2), 104–109.

Friel-Patti, S., & Roeser, R. (1985). Evaluating changes in the communication skills of deaf children using vibrotactile stimulation. *Ear and Hearing, 4*, 31–40.

Froding, C. (1960). Acoustic investigation of newborn infants. *Acta Oto-Laryngologica, 52*, 31–41.

Froeschels, E., & Beebe, H. (1946). Testing hearing of newborn infants. *Archives of Otolaryngology, 44*, 710–714.

Fromkin, V., Krashen, S., Curtiss, S., et al. (1974). The development of language in Genie: A case of language acquisition beyond the "critical period." *Brain and Language, 1*, 81–107.

Fryauf-Bertschy, H., Tyler, R., Kelsay, M.R., Gantz, B.J., & Woodworth, G.G. (1997). Cochlear implant use by prelingually deafened children: The influences of age at implant and length of device use. *Journal of Speech, Language, and Hearing Research, 40,* 183–199.

Fryer, D.A., Winckleman, A.C., Ways , P.O. (1971). Refsum's disease. *Neurology* (Minneap) *21,* 162–167.

Fujikawa, S., Yang, L., Waffarn, F., & Lerner, M. (1997). Persistent pulmonary hypertension of the newborn (PPHN) treated with inhaled nitric oxide: Preliminary hearing outcomes. *Journal of the American Academy of Audiology, 8,* 263–268.

Fulton, R.T., Gorzycki, P.A., & Hull, W.L. (1975). Hearing assessment with young children. *Journal of Speech and Hearing Disorders, 40,* 397–404.

Gabbard, S.A., Northern, J.L.,& Yoshinaga-Itano, C. (1999). Hearing screening in newborns under 24 hours of age. *Seminars in Hearing, 20* (3), 291–305.

Galambos, R., & Hecox, K.E. (1978). Clinical applications of the auditory brainstem response. *Otolaryngologic Clinics of North America, 11,* 709–721.

Galambos, R., Hicks, G., & Wilson, M. (1984). The auditory brainstem response reliably predicts hearing loss in graduates of a tertiary intensive care nursery. *Ear and Hearing, 5* (4), 254–260.

Gallagher, J.C. (1967). *Histology of the human temporal bone.* Washington, DC: Armed Forces Institute of Pathology.

Gallaudet University Center for Assessment and Demographic Study. (1998). Thirty years of the annual survey of deaf and hard of hearing children and youth: A glance over the decades. *American Annals of the Deaf, 142* (2), 72–76.

Gans, D.P. (1987). Improving behavioral observation audiometry testing and scoring problems. *Ear and Hearing, 8,* 92–99.

Gans, D.P., & Flexer, C. (1982). Observer bias in the hearing testing of profoundly involved multiply handicapped children. *Ear and Hearing, 3,* 309–313.

Gans, D.P., & Flexer, C. (1983). Auditory response behavior of severely and profoundly multiply handicapped children. *Journal of Auditory Research, 23,* 137–146.

Gantz, B.J., Tyler, R.S., Knutson, J.F., Woodworth, G., et al. (1988). Evaluation of five different cochlear implant designs: Audiological assessment and predictors of performance. *Laryngoscope, 98,* 1100–1106.

Garretson, M.D. (1963). The need for multiple communication skills in the education process of the deaf. *Rocky Mountain Leader, 62,* 1–8.

Gates, G.A. (1988). Adenoidectomy in the management of otitis media in children. In A. Lalwani & K. Grundfast (Eds.), *Pediatric otology and neurotology* (pp. 241–250). Philadelphia: Lippincott-Raven Publishers.

Gattuso, J., Patton, M.A., & Baraitser, M. (1987). The clinical spectrum of the Fraser syndrome: Report of three new cases and review. *Journal of Medical Genetics, 24* (9), 549-555.

Geers, A., & Moog, J. (1989). Evaluating speech perception skills: Tools for measuring benefit of cochlear implants, tactile aids, and hearing aids. In E. Owens & D. Kessler (Eds.). *Cochlear implants in young deaf children.* Boston: College Hill.

Geers, A., & Moog, J. (1990). Early speech perception test. St. Louis: Central Institute for the Deaf.

Geers, A., & Moog, J. (1994). Effectiveness of cochlear implant and tactile aids for deaf children: The sensory aids study at the Central Institute for the Deaf. *The Volta Review, 96,* 5.

Geers, A.E., Moog, J., & Schick, B. (1984). Acquisition of spoken and signed English by profoundly deaf children. *Journal of Speech and Hearing Disorders, 49,* 378–388.

Geers, A.E., & Moog, J.S. (1987). Predicting spoken language acquisition of hearing-impaired children. *Journal of Speech and Hearing Disorders, 52* (1), 84–94.

Geers, A.E., & Schick, B. (1988). Acquisition of spoken and signed English by hearing-impaired children of hearing-impaired or hearing parents. *Journal of Speech and Hearing Disorders, 53,* 136–143.

Gelfand, S.A., Silman, S., & Ross, L. (1987). Long-term effects of monaural, binaural and no amplification in subjects with bilateral hearing loss. *Scandinavian Audiology, 16,* 201–207.

Gerkin, K.P. (1984). The high risk register for deafness: A tutorial. *ASHA, 25,* 4.

Gesell, A. (1956). The psychological development of normal and deaf children in their preschool years. *Volta Review, 58,* 117–120.

Gillberg, C., Rosenhall, U., & Johansson, E. (1983). Auditory brainstem responses in childhood psychosis. *Journal of Autism and Developmental Disorders, 13,* (2), 181–195.

Gladney, J.H., & Monteleone, P.I. (1970). Metaphysical dysplasia. Genetic and otolaryngologic aspects. *Archives of Otolaryngology, 92,* 147–153.

Glass, L., Shapiro, I., Hodge, S.E., Bergstrom, L., Rimoin D.L., (1981). Audiologic findings of patients with achondroplasia. *International Journal of Pediatric Otorhinolaryngology, 3,* 129–135.

Glasscockk, M.E. III., Shambaugh, G.E., & Johnson, G.D. (Eds.). (1990). *Surgery of the ear* (4th ed.). Philadelphia: WB Saunders.

Glattke, T., & Fujikawa, S. (1991). Otoacoustic emissions. *American Journal of Audiology, 1,* 29–49.

Gold, T. (1948). Hearing II. The physical basis of the action of the cochlea. *Proceedings of the*

Royal Society of London. Series B: Biological Sciences, 135, 492–498.

Goldstein, R., & Rodman, L.B. (1967). Early components of averaged evoked responses to rapidly repeated auditory stimuli. *Journal of Speech and Hearing Research, 10,* 697–705.

Gorga, M.P., Kaminski, J.R., & Beauchaine, K.A. (1988). Auditory brainstem responses from graduates of an intensive care nursery using an insert earphone. *Ear and Hearing, 9* (3), 144–147.

Gorga, M.P., Kaminski, J.R., Beauchaine, K.L., Jesteadt, W., & Neely, S.T. (1989). Auditory brainstem responses from children three months to three years of age: Normal patterns of response II. *Journal of Speech and Hearing Research, 32,* 281–288.

Gorga, M.P., Reiland, J.K., Beauchaine, K.A., Worthington, D.W., & Jesteadt, W. (1987). Auditory brainstem responses from graduates of an intensive care nursery: Normal patterns of response. *Journal of Speech and Hearing Research, 30,* 311–318.

Gorga, M.P., Worthington, D.W., Reiland, J., Beauchaine, K.A., & Goldgar, D.E. (1985). Some comparisons between auditory brainstem response thresholds, latencies and the pure tone audiogram. *Ear and Hearing, 6* (2), 105–112.

Gorlin, R.J., Anderson, R.C., & Blaw, M. (1969). Multiple lentigines syndrome. *American Journal of Diseases in Children, 117,* 652–662.

Gorlin, R.J., Toriello, H.V., & Cohen, M.M. (1955). *Hereditary hearing loss and its syndromes.* New York: Oxford University Press.

Gould, H.J. (1989). Audiologic findings in Pierre Robin. *Ear and Hearing, 10,* 211–213.

Gould, J.H., & Caldarelli, D.D. (1982). Hearing and otopathology in Apert syndrome. *Archives of Otolaryngology, 108,* 347–349.

Goulden, K., & Hodge, M. (1998). Neurogenic communicative disorders of childhood. In A.F. Johnson & B.H. Jacobson (Eds.), *Medical speech-pathology: A practitioner's guide* (pp. 409–422). New York: Thieme Medical Publishers.

Gravel, J., Berg, A., Bradley, M., Cacace, A., Campbell, D., et al. (2000). The New York State universal newborn hearing screening demonstration project: Effects of screening protocol on inpatient outcome measures. *Ear and Hearing, 21* (2), 131–140.

Gravel, J., & Ellis, M. (1995). The auditory consequences of otitis media with effusion: The audiogram and beyond. *Seminars in Hearing, 16* (1), 44–59.

Gravel, J., & Nozza, R. (1997). Hearing loss among children with otitis media with effusion. In J. Robert, I. Wallace, & F. Henderson (Eds.), *Otitis media in young children: Medical, developmental and educational considerations* (pp. 63–92). Baltimore: Paul Brookes.

Gravel, J., & Traquina, D. (1992). Experience with the audiological assessment of infants and toddlers. *International Journal of Pediatric Otorhinology, 23* (1), 59–72.

Gravel, J., & Wallace, I. (1992). Listening and language at 4 years of age. *Journal of Speech and Hearing Research, 35,* 588–595.

Gravel, J., & Wallace, I. (1995). Early otitis media, auditory abilities and educational risk. *American Journal of Speech-Language Pathology, 4* (3), 9–94.

Gravel, J., & Wallace, I. (1998). Audiologic management of otitis media. In F. Bess (Ed.), *Children with hearing impairments: Contemporary trends* (pp. 215–227). Nashville: Vanderbilt Bill Wilkerson Center Press.

Gravel, J.S. (1989). Behavioral assessment of auditory function. *Seminars in Hearing, 10,* 217–228.

Greenberg, D., Wilson, W., Moore, J., et al. (1978). Visual reinforcement audiometry (VRA) with young Down's syndrome children. *Journal of Speech and Hearing Disorders, 43,* 448–458.

Greenberg, M.T. (1975). Hearing families with deaf children: Stress and functioning as related to communication method. *American Annals of the Deaf, 125,* 1063.

Greenberg, M.T, Calderon, R., & Kusche, C. (1984). Early intervention using simultaneous communication with deaf infants: The effect on communication development. *Child Development, 55,* 607–616.

Greenstein, J.M., Greenstein, B.B., McConville, K., et al. (1976). *Mother-infant communication and language acquisition in deaf infants.* New York: Lexington School for the Deaf.

Greenway, E.B. (1964). The communication needs of the deaf child. In *Report of the Proceedings of the International Congress on Education of the Deaf* (pp. 433–439). Washington, DC: Gallaudet College.

Griffith, S., Levine, S., & Giebink, G. (1998). Management of otitis media using Agency of Health Care Policy and Research guidelines. *Otolaryngology—Head and Neck Surgery, 118* (4), 437–443.

Groothuis, J.R., Altemeier, W.A., Wright, P.F., et al. (1978). The evolution and resolution of otitis media in infants: Tympanometric findings. In E.R. Harford, F.H. Bess, C.D. Bluestone, et al. (Eds.), *Impedance screening for middle ear disease in children* (pp. 105–109). New York: Grune and Stratton.

Groothuis, J.R., Sell, S.H.W., Wright, P.F., et al. (1979). Otitis media in infancy: Tympanometric findings. *Pediatrics, 63,* 435–442.

Grundfast, K., & Carney, C.J. (1987). *Ear infections in your child.* Hollywood, FL: Compact Books.

Guberina, P., & Asp, C. (1981). *The verbo-tonal method for rehabilitating people with communication problems.* (Monograph No. 13). International Exchange of Information in Rehabilitation. New York: World Rehabilitation Fund.

Haapaniemi, J.J. (1996). The hearing threshold levels of children at school age. *Ear and Hearing, 17* (6), 469–477.

Haber, J.S., & Norris, M.L. (1983). The Texas preschool screening inventory: A simple screening device for language and learning disorders. *Children's Health Care, 12* (1), 11–18.

Haggard, M., & Hughes, E. (1988). *Objectives, values and methods of screening children's hearing: A review of the literature.* (IHR Internal Reports, Series A, No. 4). Nottingham, England: Institute of Hearing Research.

Haggard, M.P., Birkin, J.A., Browning, G.G., et al. (1994). Behavioral problems in otitis media. *Pediatric Infectious Disease Journal, 13*, S15–S20.

Hall, J. (2000). *Handbook of otoacoustic emissions.* San Diego: Singular Publishing Group.

Hall, J.G., & Rohrt, T. (1968). The stapes in osteogenesis imperfecta. *Acta Oto-Laryngologica (Stockholm), 65*, 345–348.

Hall, J.W., Prentice, C.H., Smiley, G., & Werkhaven, J. (1995). Auditory dysfunction in selected syndromes and patterns of malformations. *Journal of the American Academy of Audiology, 6* (1), 80–92.

Hallgren, V. (1959). Retinitis pigmentosa combined with congenital deafness; with vestibulo-cerebellar ataxia and mental abnormality in a portion of cases. *Acta Psychiatrica Scandinavica Supplementum, 138*, 1–101.

Harboyan, G., Mamo, J., der Kalonstian, V., et al. (1971). Congenital corneal dystrophy. Progressive sensorineural deafness in a family. *Archives of Ophthalmology, 75,* 27–32.

Harris, J. (1998). Autoimmune inner ear diseases. In A. Lalwani & K. Grundfast (Eds.), *Pediatric Otology and Neurotology* (pp. 375–385). Philadelphia: Lippincott-Raven.

Harris, S., Ahlfors, K., Ivarsson, S., Lemmark, B., & Svanberg, L. (1984). Congenital cytomegalovirus infection and sensorineural hearing loss. *Ear and Hearing, 5,* 352–355.

Harrison, M., & Roush, J. (1996). Age of suspicion, identification and intervention of infants and young children with hearing loss: A seasonal study. *Ear and Hearing, 17,* 55–62.

Harrison, R.V. (1998). An animal model of auditory neuropathology. *Ear and Hearing, 19* (5), 355–361.

Harvey, A.S. (1991). CHARGE association: Clinical manifestations and developmental outcome. *American Journal of Medical Genetics, 39,* 48–55.

Hasenstab, M.S. (1987). *Language learning and otitis media.* Rockville, MD: Aspen Systems Corporation.

Haskins, H. (1966). A phonetically balanced test of speech discrimination for children. Unpublished MS degree thesis, 1949. (Cited in O'Neill J and Oyer H: *Applied audiometry.* New York: Dodd, Mead, 1966.)

Hawkins, D. (1992). Prescriptive approaches to selection of gain and frequency response. In G. Mueller, D. Hawkins, & J. Northern (Eds.), *Probe-microphone measurements: Hearing aid selection and assessment* (pp. 91–112). San Diego: Singular Publishing Group.

Hawkins, D., & Northern, J. (1992). Probe-microphone measurements with children. In G. Mueller, D. Hawkins, & J. Northern (Eds.), *Probe-microphone measurements: Hearing aid selection and assessment* (pp. 159–182). San Diego: Singular Publishing Group.

Hawkins, D.B. (1984). Comparisons of speech recognition in noise by mildly-to-moderately hearing impaired children using hearing aids and FM systems. *Journal of Speech and Hearing Disorders, 49,* 409–418.

Hawkins, D.B., Prosek, R., Walden, B., & Montgomery, A. (1987). Binaural loudness summation in the hearing impaired. *Journal of Speech and Hearing Research, 30,* 37–43.

Hawkins, D.B., & Schum, D.J. (1985). Some effects of FM system coupling on hearing aid characteristics. *Journal of Speech and Hearing Disorders, 50,* 132–141.

Hawkins, H.B., Shapiro, R., & Petrillo, C.J. (1975). The association of cleidocranial dysotosis with hearing loss. *American Journal of Roentgenology, 125,* 944–947.

Hayes, D. (1994). Hearing loss in infants with craniofacial anomalies. *Otolaryngology— Head and Neck Surgery, 110* (1), 39–46.

Hayes, D. (1999). State programs for universal newborn hearing screening. *Pediatric Clinics of North America, 46* (1), 89–93.

Hayes, D. (2000). The New York State Project: A leap to the future. *Ear and Hearing, 21* (2), 83.

Hayes, D., & Northern, J.L. (1996). *Infants and hearing.* San Diego: Singular Publishing Group.

Hayes, E., Babin, R., & Platz, C. (1980). The otologic manifestations of mucopolysaccharidoses. *American Journal of Otology, 2,* 65.

Hecox, K. & Jacobson, J. [1984]. Auditory evoked potentials, in J.L. Northern (Ed.), Hearing disorders. Boston: Little, Brown & Co.)

Hecox, K., Squires, N., & Galambos, R. (1976). Brainstem auditory evoked responses in man. I. Effect of stimulus rise-fall time and duration. *Journal of the Acoustical Society of America, 60,* 1187–1192.

Heffernan, H.P., & Simons, M.R. (1979). Temporary increase in sensorineural hearing loss with hearing aid use. *Annals of Otology, Rhinology, and Laryngology, 88,* 86–91.

Hegyi, T., Carbone, T., Anwar, M., Ostfeld, B., Hiatt, M., Koons, A., Pinto-Martinn, J., & Paneth, N. (1998). The Apgar score and its components in the preterm infant. *Pediatrics, 101* (1), 77–81.

Hemenway, W.G., & Berstrom, I. (1972). Dysplasias of the inner ear. In D. Bergsma (Ed.), *Birth defects, atlas and compendium.* Baltimore: Williams & Wilkins, published for the National Foundation-March of Dimes.

Hendricks-Munoz, K.D., & Walton, J.P. (1988). Hearing loss in infants with persistent fetal circulation. *Pediatrics, 81* (5), 650–656.

Herbets, G. (1962). Otological observations on the Treacher Collins syndrome. *Acta Oto-Laryngologica (Stockholm), 54*, 457.

Herrmann, C. Jr., Aguilar, M.J., & Sacks, O.W. (1964). Hereditary photomyoclonus associated with diabetes mellitus, deafness, nephropathy and cerebral dysfunction. *Neurology, 14*, 212–221.

Hicks, T., Fowler, K., Richardson, M., Dahle, A., Adams, L., & Pass, R. (1993). Congenital cytomegalovirus infection and neonatal auditory screening. *Journal of Pediatrics, 123*, 779–782.

Hicks, W.M., & Hicks, D.E. (1981). The Usher's syndrome adolescent: Programming implications for school administrators, teachers, and resident advisors. *American Annals of the Deaf, 126*, 422–431.

Hodges, A., & Ruth, R. (1987). Subject related factors influencing the acoustic reflex. *Seminars in Hearing, 8*, 339–357.

Hodgson, W.R. (1985). Testing infants and young children. In J. Katz (Ed.). *Handbook of clinical audiology* (3rd ed., p. 650), Baltimore: Williams & Wilkins.

Holm, V., & Kunze, L. (1969). Effects of chronic otitis media on language and speech development. *Pediatrics, 43*, 833.

Holmes, E.M. (1949). The microtia ear. *Archives of Otolaryngology, 49*, 243–265.

Holmes, L.B. (1971). Norrie's disease; an X-linked syndrome of retinal malformation, mental retardation, and deafness. *Journal of Pediatrics, 70*, 89–92.

Hood, D.C. (1975). Evoked cortical response audiometry. In L. Bradford (Ed.), *Physiological measures of the audio-vestibular system* (Ch. 10). New York: Academic Press.

Hood, L.J. (1998). *Clinical applications of the auditory brainstem response*. San Diego: Singular Publishing Group.

Hood, L.J., & Berlin, C.I. (1996). Central auditory function and disorders. In J.L. Northern (Ed.), *Hearing disorders* (3rd ed.). Needham Heights, MA: Allyn and Bacton.

Horton, K.B. (1975). Early intervention through parent training.*Otolaryngol Clinics of North America, 8*, 143–157.

Howie, V.M. (1975). Natural history of otitis media. *Annals of Otology, Rhinology, and Laryngology Supplement, 19*, 67–72.

Howie, V.M., Ploussard, J.H., & Sloyer, J. (1975). The "otitis-prone" condition. *American Journal of Diseases in Children, 129*, 676–678.

Hughes, G.B., & Pensak, M.L. (1997). *Clinical otology* (2nd ed.). New York: Thieme Medical Publishers.

Hughes, P.J., Davies, P.T., Roche, S.W., Matthews, T.D., & Lane, R.J. (1991). Wildervanck or cervico-oculo-acoustic syndrome and MRI findings. *Journal of Neurology, Neurosurgery and Psychiatry, 54*, 503–504.

Hull, F.M., Mielke, P.W., Timmons, R.J., et al. (1971). The national speech and hearing survey: Preliminary results. *ASHA, 13*, 501–509.

Hurley, R.M. (1999). Onset of auditory deprivation. *Journal of the American Academy of Audiology, 10*, 529–534.

Ide, C.H., & Wollschlaeger, P.P. (1969). Multiple congenital abnormalities associated with cryptophthalmia. *Archives of Ophthalmology, 81*, 640–644.

IHAFF. (1994). *Independent hearing aid fitting forum manual*. Yorba Linda, CA: Dennis Van Vliet.

Ikeda, M.K., & Jenson, H.B. (1990). Evaluation and treatment of congenital syphilis. *Journal of Pediatrics, 117*, 843.

Illum, P., Kaier, H.W., Hvidberg-Hansen, J., et al. (1972). Fifteen cases of Pendred's syndrome. *Archives of Otolaryngology, 96*, 297–304.

Ireton, H., & Thwing, E. (1972). *The Minnesota child development inventory*. Minneapolis, MN: University of Minnesota.

Irving, R.M., & Ruben, R.J. (1998). The acquired hearing losses of childhood. In A. Lalwani & K. Grundfast (Eds.), *Pediatric otology and neurotology* (pp. 375–385). Philadelphia: Lippincott-Raven.

Irwin, O.C. (1947). Infant speech: Consonantal sounds according to manner of articulation. *Journal of Speech and Hearing Disorders, 12*, 402–404.

Iwashita, H., Inoue, N., Araki, S., et al. (1970). Optic atrophy, neural deafness and distal neurogenic amyotrophy. *Archives of Neurology, 22*, 357–364.

Jacobson, J.T. (Ed.). (1985).*The auditory brainstem response*. San Diego: College-Hill Press.

Jacobson, J. (1994). *Short-latency auditory evoked potentials*. In J. Northern (Ed.), *Hearing disorders* (3rd ed., pp. 57–74). Austin: Pro-Ed.

Jacobson, J.T. (1996). *Short-latency auditory evoked potentials*. In J. Northern (Ed.), *Hearing Disorders* (3rd ed., pp. 73–97). Needham Heights, MA: Allyn and Bacon.

Jacobson, J.T., & Jacobson, C.A. (1987). Application of test performance characteristics in newborn auditory screening. *Seminars in Hearing, 8* (2), 133–141.

Jacobson, J.T., Morehouse, C.R., & Johnson, M.J. (1982). Strategies for infant auditory brain stem response assessment. *Ear and Hearing, 3*, 263–270.

Jaffe, B.F. (1968a). Congenital shoulder-neck-auditory anomalies. *Laryngoscope, 58*, 2119–2139.

Jaffe, B.F. (1968b). The incidence of ear diseases in the Navajo Indians. *Laryngoscope, 58*, 2126–2133.

Jahrsdoerfer, R.A., Hall, J.W. III. (1986). Congenital malformations of the ear. *American Journal of Otology, 7*, 267–269.

Jahrsdoerfer, R.A., & Jacobson, J.T. (1995). Treacher Collins syndrome: Otologic and auditory management. *Journal of the American Academy of Audiology, 6* (1), 93–102.

Jensen, B.L. (1990). Somatic development in cleidocranial dysplasia. *American Journal of Medical Genetics, 35,* 69–74.

Jepsen, O. (1963). Middle ear muscle reflexes in man. In J. Jerger (Ed), *Modern developments in audiology* (pp. 93–239). New York: Academic Press.

Jerger, J. (1970). Clinical experience with impedance audiometry. *Archives of Otolaryngology, 92,* 311–324.

Jerger, J. (1987). On the evaluation of hearing aid performance. *ASHA, 29* (9), 49–51.

Jerger, J., Anthony, L., Jerger, S., et al. (1974a). Studies in impedance audiometry: III. Middle ear disorders. *Archives of Otolaryngology, 99,* 165–171.

Jerger, J., Burney, P., Mauldin, L., et al. (1974b). Predicting hearing loss from the acoustic reflex. *Journal of Speech and Hearing Disorders, 39,* 11–22.

Jerger, J., Chmiel, R., Frost, J., & Coker, N. (1986). Effect of sleep on the auditory steady state evoked potential. *Ear and Hearing, 7* (4), 240–245.

Jerger, J., & Dirks, D. (1961). Binaural hearing aids: An enigma. *Journal of the Acoustical Society of America, 33,* 537–538.

Jerger, J., & Hayes, D. (1976). The cross-check principle in pediatric audiometry. *Archives of Otolaryngology, 102,* 614–620.

Jerger, J., & Hayes, D. (1980). Diagnostic applications of impedance audiometry: Middle ear disorder: Sensorineural disorder. In J. Jerger & J.L. Northern (Eds.), *Clinical impedance audiometry* (2nd ed., pp. 109–127). Acton, MA: American Electromedics Corp.

Jerger, J., Hayes, D., Anthony, L., et al. (1978). Factors influencing prediction of hearing level from the acoustic reflex. *Contemporary Monographs in Audiology, 1,* 1.

Jerger, J., Hayes, D., & Jordon, C. (1980). Clinical experience with auditory brainstem response audiometry in pediatric assessment. *Ear and Hearing, 1,* 19–25.

Jerger, J., & Jerger, S. (1970). Temporary threshold shift in rock-and-roll musicians. *Journal of Speech and Hearing Research, 13,* 218–224.

Jerger, J., & Jerger, S. (1974). Auditory findings in brainstem disorders. *Archives of Otolaryngology, 99,* 342–350.

Jerger, J., Jerger, S., & Mauldin, L. (1972). Studies in impedance audiometry: I. Normal and sensorineural ears. *Archives of Otolaryngology, 96,* 513–523.

Jerger, J., & Northern, J.L. (Eds.). (1980). *Clinical impedance audiometry* (2nd ed.). Acton, MA: American Electromedics Corp.

Jerger, J., Oliver, T., & Chmiel, R. (1988). The auditory middle latency response. *Seminars in Hearing, 9* (1), 75–86.

Jerger, J., Oliver, T., & Stach, B. (1985). Auditory brainstem response testing strategies. In J. Jacobson (Ed.), *The auditory brainstem response* (pp. 371–388). San Diego: College-Hill Press.

Jerger, J., & Thelin, J. (1968). Effects of electroacoustic characteristics of hearing aids on speech understanding. *Bulletin of Prosthetic Research, 110,* 159–197.

Jerger, S. (1983). Decision matrix and information theory analyses in the evaluation of neuroaudiologic tests. *Seminars in Hearing, 4* (2), 121–132.

Jerger, S. (1984). Speech audiometry. In J. Jerger (Ed.), *Pediatric audiology.* San Diego: College Hill Press.

Jerger, S., Jerger, J., Alford, B., Abrams, S. (1983). Development of speech intelligibility in children with recurrent otitis media. *Ear and Hearing, 4,* 138–145.

Jerger, S., & Jerger, J. (1983). Pediatric speech intelligibility test: performance-intensity characteristics. *Ear and Hearing, 4,* 138–145.

Jerger, S., Jerger, J., & Fahad, R. (1985). Pediatric hearing aid evaluation: Case reports. *Ear and Hearing, 6* (5), 240–243.

Jerger, S., Jerger, J., & Lewis, S. (1981). Pediatric speech intelligibility test: II. Effect of receptive language age and chronological age. *International Journal of Pediatric Otorhinolaryngology, 3,* 101–118.

Jerger, S., Jerger, J., Mauldin, L., et al. (1974). Studies in impedance audiometry: II. Children less than 6 years old. *Archives of Otolaryngology, 99,* 1–9.

Jerger, S., Lewis, S., Hawkins, J., et al. (1980). Pediatric speech intelligibility test: I. Generation of test materials. *International Journal of Pediatric Otorhinolaryngology, 2,* 217–230.

Jervell, A., & Lange-Nielsen, F. (1957). Congenital deaf-mutism, functional heart disease with prolongation of the QT interval, and sudden death. *American Heart Journal, 54,* 59–68.

Jewett, D., & Williston, J.S. (1971). Auditory evoked far fields averaged from the scalp of humans. *Brain, 94,* 681–696.

Johansson, B., Wedenberg, E., & Westin, B. (1964). Measurement of tone response by the human fetus. *Acta Oto-Laryngologica (Stockholm), 57,* 188–192.

Johnson, C.D., Benson, P.V., & Seaton, J.B. (1997). *Educational audiology handbook.* San Diego: Singular Publishing Group.

Johnson, D., & Caccamise, F. (1981). Hearing-impaired populations: Optimizing the use of vision for academic, career and communications program planning. *American Annals of the Deaf, 126,* 317.

Johnson, G. (1995, June 6). Chimp talk debate: Is it really language? *The New York Times.*

Johnson, J.S., & Watrous, B.S. (1978). An acoustic impedance screening program with an American Indian population. In E.R. Harford, F.H. Bess, C.D. Bluestone, et al. (Eds.), *Impedance screening for middle ear disease in children.* New York: Grune & Stratton.

Johnson, R.L. (1967). Chronic otitis media in school age Navajo Indians. *Laryngoscope, 77,* 1990–1995.

Johnson, T., et al. (1987). Pendred's syndrome: Acoustic, vestibular and radiological findings in 17 unrelated patients. *Journal of Laryngology and Otology, 101,* 1187–1192.

Johnsson, L.G., & Arenberg, K. (1981). Cochlear abnormalities in Alport's syndrome. *Otolaryngology—Head and Neck Surgery, 107,* 340–349.

Johnston, C.C., Lawy, N., Lord, T., et al. (1968). Osteopetrosis. A clinical, genetic, metabolic, and morphologic study of the dominantly inherited benign form. *Medicine, 47,* 149–167.

Joint Committee of the American Speech-Language-Hearing Association and the Council on Education of the Deaf. (1994). Service provision under the Individuals with Disabilities Act: Part H (as amended to children who are deaf and hard of hearing ages birth to 36 months). *ASHA, 36,* 117–121.

Joint Committee on Infant Hearing. (1982). Joint Committee on Infant Hearing 1982 statement. *ASHA, 24,* 1017–1018.

Joint Committee on Infant Hearing. (1995). 1994 position statement. *Audiology Today, 6,* 6–9.

Joint Committee on Infant Hearing. (2000). Year 2000 position statement: Principles and guidelines for early hearing detection and intervention program. *Audiology Today, 12,* Special Issue, August, 7–27.

Jones, F.R., & Simmons, F.B. (1977). Early identification of significant hearing loss: The Crib-o-gram. *Hearing Instruments, 28,* 8–10.

Jones, R.I. (1988). *Smith's recognizable pattens of human malformation* (4th ed.). Philadelphia: WB Saunders.

Jordan, O. (1972). Mental retardation and hearing defects. *Scandinavian Audiology, 1,* 29–32.

Jordan, R.E., & Eagles, E.L. (1961). The relation of air conduction audiometry to otologic abnormalities. *Annals of Otology, Rhinology, and*

Bakan, E., Yigitoglu, M.R., Gokce, G., Dogan M., (1993). Pendred's syndrome. *Annals of Otology, Rhinology, and Laryngology, 102,* 285–288.

Kahane, J.C. (1979). Pathophysiologic effects of Möbius syndrome on speech and hearing. *Archives of Otolaryngology—Head and Neck Surgery, 105,* 29–34.

Kamhi, A.G. (1982). Developmental vs. difference theories of mental retardation: a new look. *American Journal of Mental Deficiencies, 86,* 1–7.

Kankkunen, B., & Thuringer, R. (1987). Hearing impairment in connection with preauricular tags. *Acta Paediatrica Scandinavica, 76,* 143–146.

Kaplan, S., Goddard, J., Van Kleeck, M., et al. (1973). Ataxia and deafness in children due to bacterial meningitis. *Pediatrics, 52,* 577–585.

Kaplan, S.L., Catlin, F., Weaver, T., & Feigin, R.D. (1984). Onset of hearing loss in children with bacterial meningitis. *Pediatrics, 73,* 575–579.

Karver, S. (1998). Otitis media. *Primary Care: Clinics in Office Practice, 25,* 691–692.

Kavanagh, J.F. (Ed.). (1986). *Otitis media and child development.* Parkton, MD: York Press.

Kavanagh, K.T., Gould, H., McCormick, G., & Franks, R. (1989). Comparison of the identifiability of the low intensity ABR and MLR in the mentally handicapped patient. *Ear and Hearing, 10* (2), 124–130.

Kearsley, R., Snider, M., Richie, R., et al. (1962). Study of relations between psychologic environment and child behavior. *American Journal of Diseases in Children, 104,* 12–20.

Keats, B.J.B. (1996). Genes and hearing impairment. *Audiology Today, 8* (5), 11–13.

Keith, R. (1973). Impedance audiometry with neonates. *Archives of Otolaryngology, 97,* 465–467.

Keith, R.W. (1975). Middle ear functions in neonates. *Archives of Otolaryngology, 101,* 376–379.

Keith, R.W. (1978). Commentary. [Letter to the editor]. *Audiology Hearing Education, 4,* 28.

Keith, R.W. (Ed.). (1980a). Auditory perceptual problems in children. *Seminars in Speech, Language, and Hearing, 1,* 2.

Keith, R.W. (Ed.). (1980b). *Audiology for the physician.* Baltimore: Williams & Wilkins.

Keith, R.W. (1983). Special issue: dichotic listing tests. *Ear and Hearing, 4,* 6.

Keith, R.W. (1986). *SCAN: A screening test for auditory processing disorders.* San Antonio, TX: The Psychological Corporation/Harcourt Brace Jovanovich.

Keith, R.W. (1988). Central auditory tests. In N.J. Lass, L.V. McReynolds, J.L. Northern, et al. (Eds.), *Handbook of speech-language pathology & audiology.* Toronto: BC Decker.

Keith, R.W. (1988). Tests of central auditory function. In R. Roeser & M. Downs (Eds.), *Auditory disorders in school children.* New York: Thieme Medical Publishers.

Keith, R.W. (1999a). Diagnosing central auditory processing disorders in children. In R. Roeser, M. Hosford-Dunn, & M. Valente (Eds.), *Audiology: Diagnosis, treatment strategies and practice management* (Ch. 17). New York: Thieme Medical Publishers.

Keith, R.W. (1999b) Central auditory processing disorders. In V. Newton (Ed.), *Pediatric audiological medicine.* London: Whurr Publishers Limited.

Keith, R.W. (2000a). *SCAN-C: Test of auditory processing abilities in children* (Rev. ed.). San Antonio, TX: The Psychological Corporation.

Keith, R.W. (2000b). Development and standardization of SCAN-C test for auditory processing disorders in children. *Journal of the American Academy of Audiology, 11* (8), 438–445.

Keith, W.J., & Smith, R.P. (1987).Automated pediatric hearing assessment using interactive video images. *Hearing Instruments, 38* (9), 27–28.

Keleman, G. (1958). Toxoplasmosis and congenital deafness. *Archives of Otolaryngology, 68,* 547–561.

Keleman, G. (1966). Hurler's syndrome and the hearing organ. *Journal of Laryngology, 80,* 791–803.

Keleman, G., Hooft, C., & Kluyskens, P. (1968). The inner ear in autosomal trisomy. *Practices in Otorhinolaryngology (Basel), 30,* 251–258.

Kemp, D., & Ryan, S. (1993). The use of transient evoked otoacoustic emissions in neonatal hearing screening programs. *Seminars in Hearing, 14,* 30–45.

Kemp, D. (1997). Otoacoustic emissions in perspective. In M. Robinette & T. Glattke (Eds.), *Otoacoustic emissions: Clinical applications* (pp. 1–21). New York: Thieme Medical Publishers.

Kemp, D.T. (1978). Stimulated acoustic emissions from the human auditory system. *Journal of the Acoustical Society of America, 64,* 1386–1391.

Kemp, D.T. (1980). Towards a model for the origin of cochlear echos. *Hearing Research, 2,* 533–548.

Kent, R.D. (1976). Anatomical and neuromuscular maturation of the speech mechanism: Evidenc from acoustical studies. *Journal of Speech and Hearing Research, 19* (3), 421–427.

Kent, R.D., Osberger, M.J., Netsell, R., & Hustedde, C.G. (1987). Phonetic development in identical twins differing in auditory function. *Journal of Speech and Hearing Disorders, 52,* 64–75.

Kenworthy, O.T., Bess, F.H., Stahlman, M.T., & Lindstrom, D.P. (1987). Hearing, speech and language outcome in infants with extreme immaturity. *American Journal of Otology, 5,* 419–425.

Kerr, G., Smyth, G.D., & Cinnamond, M. (1973). Congenital syphilitic deafness. *Journal of Laryngology and Otology, 87,* 1–12.

Kessner, D.M., & Kalk, C.E. (1973). A strategy for evaluating health services. In *Contrasts in health status* (Vol. 2). Washington, DC: Institute of Medicine, National Academy of Sciences.

Kessner, D.M., Snow, C.K., & Singer, J. (1974). Assessment of medical care in children. In *Contrasts in health status* (Vol. 3). Washington, DC: Institute of Medicine, National Academy of Sciences.

Kile, J. (1993). Identification of hearing impairment in children: A 25-year review. *The Transdisciplinary Journal, 3* (3), 155–164.

Kim, D.O. (1980). Cochlear mechanics: Implications of electrophysical and acoustical observations. *Hearing Research, 2,* 297–317.

Kimberling, W.J., & Moller, C. (1995). Clinical and molecular genetics of Usher syndrome. *Journal of the American Academy of Audiology, 6* (1), 63–72.

Kimberling, W.J., & Pieke-Dahl, S. (1998). Decoding Usher syndrome. *Hearing Health,* 52–54.

Kirkham, T.H. (1969). Duane's syndrome and familial perceptive deafness. *British Journal of Ophthalmology, 53,* 335–339.

Klein, J.O. (1979). Epidemiology of otitis media. In R.J. Wiet & S.W. Coulthard SW (Eds.), *Otitis media: Proceedings of the second national conference on otitis media* (pp. 18–20). Columbus, OH: Ross Laboratories.

Klein, J.O. (1983). Epidemiology and natural history of otitis media. *Pediatrics, 71,* 639–640.

Klein, J.O., Feigin, R.D., & McCracken, G.H. (1986). Report of the task force on diagnosis and management of meningitis. *Pediatrics, 78,* 5.

Kloepfer, H.W., Laguaite, J.K., & McLaurin, J.W. (1966). The hereditary syndrome of deafness in retinitis pigmentosa. *Laryngoscope, 76,* 850–862.

Koch, D.B. (1996a). Cochlear implants: A decade of clinical experience in the United States. *Seminars in Hearing, 17* (4), 309–421.

Koch, D.B. (1996b). Commercial cochlear implants. *Seminars in Hearing, 17* (4), 317–326.

Koenig, W. (1950). Subjective effects in binaural hearing. *Journal of the Acoustical Society of America, 22,* 61–62.

Koenigsberger, M.R., Chutorian, A.M., Gold, A.P., et al. (1970). Benign paroxysmal vertigo of childhood. *Neurology, 20,* 1108–1113.

Kolb, B. (1989). Brain development, plasticity, and behavior. *American Psychologist, 44* (9), 1203–1212.

Konigsmark, B.W. (1969). Hereditary deafness in man. *New England Journal of Medicine, 281,* 713–720, 774–778, 827–832.

Konigsmark, B.W. (1972). Genetic hearing loss with no associated abnormalities: A review. *Journal of Speech and Hearing Disorders, 37,* 89–99.

Konigsmark, B.W., & Gorlin, R.J. (1976). *Genetic and metabolic deafness.* Philadelphia: WB Saunders.

Konigsmark, B.W., Hollander, M.B., & Berlin, C.I. (1968). Familial neural hearing loss and atopic dermatitis. *JAMA, 204,* 953–957.

Konigsmark, B.W., Mengel, M.C., & Haskins, H. (1970). Familial congenital moderate neural hearing loss. *Journal of Laryngology, 84,* 495–506.

Koop, C.E. (1989). Importance of Early Identification of Children with Hearing Problems. US Public Health Service, Dept. of Health and Human Resources Statement.

Kos, A.O., Schuknecht, H.F., & Singer, J.D. (1966). Temporal bone studies in 13–15 and 18 trisomy syndrome. *Archives of Otolaryngology, 83,* 439–445.

Kraus, N., McGee, T., & Comperatore, C. (1989). MLRs in children are consistently present during wakefulness, stage I, and REM sleep. *Ear and Hearing, 10* (6), 339–345.

Kruger, B.: (1987). An update on the external ear resonance in infants and young children. *Ear and Hearing, 8* (6), 333–336.

Kryter, K. (1970). *The effects of noise on man.* New York: Academic Press.

Kryter, K.D. (1973). Impairment to hearing from exposure to noise. *Journal of the Acoustical Society of America, 53,* 1211–1234.

Kryter, K.D, & Ades, H.W. (1943). Studies on the function of the higher acoustic nervous centers in the cat. *Americal Journal of Psychology, 56,* 501–536.

Kryter, K.D., Williams, C., & Green, D.M. (1962). Auditory acuity and the perception of speech. *Journal of the Acoustical Society of America, 34,* 1217–1223.

Kuczwara, L.A., Birnholz, J.C., & Klodd, D.A. (1984). Auditory responsiveness in the fetus. *National Student Speech, Language and Hearing Association Journal, 14,* 12–20.

Kuhl, P. (1979). Speech perception in early infancy: Perceptual constancy for spectrally dissimilar vowel categories. *Journal of the Acoustical Society of America, 66,* 1668–1679.

Kuhl, P., & Miller, J. (1982). Discrimination of auditory target dimensions in the presence or absence of variation in a second dimension by infants. *Perceptual Psychophysics, 31,* 279–292.

Kuhl, P., Williams, K., Lacerda, F., Stebens, K., & Lindblom, B. (1992). Lingusistic experience alters phonetic perception in infants by 6 months of age. *Science, 255,* 606–608.

Kuhl, P.K. (1988). Auditory perception and the evolution of speech. *Human Evolution* 3:19–43.

Kulig, S.G., & Bakler, K. (1973). *Physician's developmental quick screen for speech disorders.* Galveston, TX: University of Texas Medical Branch.

Lalwani, A., & Grundfast, K. (Eds.). (1998). *Pediatric otology and neurotology.* Philadelphia: Lippincott-Raven.

Lamb, L.E.., & Norris, T. (1970). Relative acoustic impedance measurements with mentally retarded children. *American Journal of Mental Deficiencies, 75,* 51–56.

Lamb, L.E. & Norris, T. (1969). Acoustic impedance measurement. In R.T. Fulton & L.I. Lloyd (Eds.), *Audiometry for the retarded* (pp. 164–209). Baltimore: Williams & Wilkins.

Lane, H. (1977). *The wild boy of Aveyron.* Cambridge, MA: Harvard University Press.

Langer, L.O., Jr. (1965). Diastrophic dwarfism in early infancy. *American Journal of Roentgenology, 93,* 399.

Langer, S.K. (1957). *Philosophy in a new key.* Cambridge, MA: Harvard University Press.

Langford, C., Bench, J., & Wilson, I. (1975). Some effects of prestimulus activity and length of prestimulus observations on judgments of newborns' responses to sounds. *Audiology, 14,* 44–52.

Laughton, J. (1994). Models and current practices in early intervention with hearing-impaired infants. *Seminars in Hearing, 15* (2), 148–158.

League, R., Parker, J., Robertson, M., et al. (1972). Acoustical environments in incubators and infant oxygen tents. *Preventive Medicine, 1,* 231.

Lee, D.J., Gomez-Marion, O., Lee, H.M. (1996). Prevalence of childhood hearing loss. The Hispanic health and nutrition examination survey and the national health and nutritional examination survey II. *American Journal of Epidemiology, 144,* 442–449.

Lee, D.J., Gomez-Marion, O., & Lee, H.M. (1998). Prevalence of unilateral hearing loss in children: The national health and nutrition examination survey II and the Hispanic health and nutrition examination survey. *Ear and Hearing, 19* (4), 329–332.

Lempert, J., Wever, E.G., & Lawrence, M. (1947). The cochleogram and its clinical application. *Archives of Otolaryngology—Head and Neck Surgery, 45,* 61–67.

Lenneberg, E.H. (1967). *Biological foundations of language.* New York: John Wiley and Sons.

Leroy, J.G., & Crocker, A.C. (1966). Clinical definition of Hunter-Hurler phenotypes. A review of 50 patients. *American Journal of Diseases in Children, 112,* 518–530.

Leske, M.C. (1981). Prevalence estimates of communicative disorders in the U.S.: Language, hearing and vestibular disorders. *ASHA, 23,* 229–236.

Levine, R.L. (1979). Bilirubin: Worked out years ago? *Pediatrics, 64,* 380–385.

Levitt, H. (1988). Recurrent issues underlying the development of tactile sensory aids. *Ear and Hearing, 9,* 301–305.

Levitt, H., McGarr, N., & Geffner, D. (1987). Development of language and communication skills in hearing-impaired children. *ASHA Monographs* (No. l26). Rockville, MD: American Speech and Hearing Association.

Levitt, H., & Nye, P.W. (1971). Sensory training aids for the hearing impaired. In *Proceedings of a Conference, Easton, MD.* Washington, DC: National Academy of Engineering, Subcommittee on Sensory Aids.

Lewis, D. (1994a). Assistive devices for classroom listening. *American Journal of Audiology, 3,* 58–69.

Lewis, D. (1994b). Assistive devices for classroom listening: FM systems. *American Journal of Audiology, 3,* 70–83.

Lewis, D. (1999). Selecting and pre-setting amplification for children: Where do we begin? *Trends in Amplification, 4* (2), 72–89.

Lewis, N. (1976). Otitis media and linguistic incompetence. *Archives of Otolaryngology, 102,* 387–390.

Libby, E.R. (1981). Achieving a transparent, smooth, wideband hearing aid response. *Hearing Instruments, 32,* 9–12.

Libby, E.R. (1982). In search of transparent insertion gain hearing aid responses. In G. Studebaker & F. Bess (Eds.), *Monographs in contemporary audiology* (pp. 112–123). Nashville, TN: The Vanderbilt Hearing Aid Report.

Liden, G., & Kankkonen, A. (1961). Visual reinforcement audiometry. *Acta Oto-Laryngologica (Stockholm), 67,* 281–292.

Lieberman, P. (1975). *On the origins of language.* New York: Macmillan.

Lim, D., Bluestone, C., & Casselbrant, M. (Eds.). (1998). Recent advances in otitis media: Report of the sixth research conference. *Annals of Otology, Rhinology, and Laryngology, 107* (10), Part 2, (Suppl. 174), 29–49.

Lim, D.J. (1989). Diagnosis and screening. In Recent advances in otitis media, report of the fourth research conference. *Annals of Otology, Rhinology, and Laryngology, 98* (4), Part 2, (Suppl. 139), 39–41.

Lin, A.E., Siebert, J.R., & Graham, J.M., Jr. (1990). Central nervous system malformations in the CHARGE association. *American Journal of Medical Genetics, 37,* 304–310.

Lindsay, J.R., Black, F.O., & Donnelly, W.N. (1975). Acrocephalosyndactyly (Apert's syndrome): Temporal bone findings. *Annals of Otology, Rhinology, and Laryngology, 84,* 174–178.

Ling, D., Ling, A.H., & Doehring, D.G. (1970). Stimulus response and observer variables in the auditory screening of newborn infants. *Journal of Speech and Hearing Research, 13,* 9–18.

Ling, D. (1975). Recent developments affecting the education of hearing-impaired children. *Public Health Review, 4,* 117–152.

Lipscomb, D. (1996). The external and middle ear. In J. Northern (Ed.), *Hearing disorders* (3rd ed.). Needham Heights, MA: Allyn and Bacon.

Liptak, G.S., McConnochie, K.M., & Roghmann, K.J. (1997). Decline of pediatric admissions with *Haemophilus influenzae* type b in New York State, 1982–1983: Relation to immunizations. *Journal of Pediatrics, 130,* 923.

Litke, R.E. (1971). Elevated high-frequency hearing in school children. *Archives of Otolaryngology, 94,* 255–257.

Littman, T., Demmoer, G., Williams, S., Istas, A., & Griesser, C. (1995). Congenital asymptomatic cytomegalovirus infection and hearing loss. *Abstracts for the Association for Research in Otolaryngology, 19,* 40.

Lloyd, L.I., Spradlin, J.E., & Reid, M.J. (1968). An operant audiometric procedure for difficult-to-test patients. *Journal of Speech and Hearing Disorders, 33,* 236–245.

Loeb, G.E. (1985a, Feb). The functional replacement of the ear. *Scientific American,* 104–111.

Loeb, G.E. (1985b). Single and multichannel cochlear prostheses: rationale, strategies, and potential. In R. Schindler & M. Merzenich (Eds.), *Cochlear implants* (pp. 17–28). New York: Raven Press.

Long, J., Lucey, J., & Philip, A. (1980). Noise and hypoxemia in the intensive care nursery. *Pediatrics, 65,* 143.

Lonsbury-Martin, B., Martin, G. (1990). The clinical utility of distortion product emissions. *Ear and Hearing, 11* (2), 144–154.

Los Angeles County, office of the Los Angeles County Superintendent of Schools, Audiology Services, and Southwest School for the Hearing-Impaired. (1980). *Test of auditory comprehension.* North Hollywood, CA: Forworks.

Lucker, J. (2000). Changing your communication style. *Advance for Audiologists, 1* (1), 47–48.

Luotonen, M., Uhari, M., Aitola, L., et al. (1996). Recurrent otitis media during infancy and linguistic skills at the age of nine years. *Pediatric Infectious Disease Journal, 15,* 854–858.

Luterman, D. (1979). *Counseling parents of hearing-impaired children.* Boston: Little, Brown & Co.

Luterman, D., & Chasin, J. (1981). The deafness management quotient as an indicator of oral success. *Volta Review, 83,* 405.

Luterman, D.M. (1976). A comparison of language skills of hearing impaired children trained in a visual/oral method and an auditory/oral method. *American Annals of the Deaf, 121,* 389–393.

Luterman, D.M. (1996). *Counseling persons with communication disorders and their families* (3rd ed.). Austin, TX: Pro-Ed.

Luterman, D.M., Kurtzer-White, E., & Seewald, R. (1999). *The young deaf child.* Baltimore: York Press.

Lutman, M., Mason, S.M., Sheppard, S., & Gibbin, K.P. (1989). Differential diagnostic potential of otoacoustic emissions: A case study. *Audiology, 28,* 205–210.

MacDonald, H.M. (1980). Neonatal asphyxia: I. Relationship of obstetric and neonatal complications to neonatal mortality in consecutive deliveries. *Journal of Pediatrics, 96,* 898–902.

MacDonald, J.T., & Feinstein, S. (1984). Hearing loss following *Haemophilus influenzae* meningitis in infancy. *Archives of Neurology, 41,* 1058–1059.

Macrae, J.H. (1968a). TTS and recovery from TTS after use of powerful hearing aids. *Journal of the Acoustical Society of America, 44,* 1445–1446.

Macrae, J.H. (1968b). Recovery from TTS in children with sensorineural deafness. *Journal of the Acoustical Society of America, 44,* 1451.

Macrae, J.H., & Farrant, R.H. (1965). The effect of hearing aid use on the residual hearing of children with sensorineural deafness. *Annals of Otology, Rhinology, and Laryngology, 74,* 407–419.

Madell, J. (1998). *Behavioral evaluation of hearing in infants and children.* New York: Thieme Medical Publishers.

Madell, J.R. (Ed.). (1984). Mainstreaming the school-aged hearing-impaired child. *Seminars in Hearing, 5,* 4.

Mahoney, T. (1985). Auditory brainstem response hearing aid applications. In J. Jacobson (Ed.), *The auditory brainstem response* (pp. 349–370). Boston: College-Hill Press.

Mandell, A.J., & Smith, C.K. (1960). Hereditary sensory radicular neuropathy. *Neurology, 10,* 627–630.

Maniglia, J.M., Wolff, D., & Herques, A.S. (1970). Congenital deafness in 13–15 syndrome. *Archives of Otolaryngology, 92,* 181–188.

Marcus, R.E., & Valvasori, G. (1970). Cochleovestibular apparatus; radiologic studies in hereditary and familial hearing loss. *International Audiology, 9,* 95–102.

Mardel, M., Hosick, E., Windman, T., et al. (1975). Audiometric comparison of the middle and late components of the adult auditory evoked potential awake and sleep. *Electroencephalography and Clinical Neurophysiology, 38,* 27–33.

Margolis, R.H. (1978). Tympanometry in infants: State-of-the-art. In E.R. Harford, F.H. Bess, C.D. Bluestone, et al. (Eds.), *Impedance screening for middle ear disease in children* (pp. 41–56). New York: Grune & Stratton.

Margolis, R.M. (1979). Tympanometry for prediction of middle ear effusion. [Letter to the editor]. *Archives of Otolaryngology, 105,* 225.

Margolis, R.H., Rykken, J.R., Hunter, L.L., et al. (1993). Effects of otitis media on extended high-frequency hearing in children. *Annals of Otology, Rhinology, and Laryngology, 102,* 1–5.

Marple, B., & Meyerhoff, W. (1998). Perilymphatic fistula. In A. Lalwani & K. Grundfast (Eds.), *Pediatric otology and neurotology* (pp. 635–644). Philadelphia: Lippincott-Raven.

Marsh, J.L., Celin, S.E., Vannier, M.W., & Gado, M. (1986). The skeletal anatomy of mandibulofacial dysostosis (Treacher Collins syndrome). *Plastic and Reconstructive Surgery, 78,* 460–468.

Martin, G., Probst, R., Lonsbury-Martin, B. (1990). Otoacoustic emissions in human ears: Normative findings. *Ear and Hearing, 11* (2), 106–120.

Mason, J.A., & Herrmann, K.R. (1998). Universal hearing screening by automated auditory brainstem response measurement. *Pediatrics, 101* (2), 221–229.

Masters, M., Stedker, N., & Katz, J. (1998). *Central auditory processing disorders: Mostly management.* Boston: Allyn and Bacon.

Matkin, A., & Matkin, N. (1985). Benefits of total communication as perceived by parents of hearing-impaired children. *Language, Speech & Hearing Services in Schools, 16,* 64–74.

Matkin, N.D. (1977). Assessment of hearing sensitivity during the preschool years. In F. Bess (Ed.), *Childhood deafness* (pp. 127–134). New York: Grune and Stratton.

Matkin, N.D. (1984). Early recognition and referral of hearing-impaired children. *Pediatrics in Review, 6* (5), 151–155.

Matkin, N.D., & Carhart, R. (1966). Auditory profiles associated with Rh incompatibility. *Archives of Otolaryngology, 84,* 502–513.

Matkin, N.D., & Wilcox, A. (1999). Considerations in the education of children with hearing loss. *Pediatric Clinics of North America, 46* (1), 143-151.

Mauk, G.W., White, K.R., Mortensen, L.B., & Behrens, T.R. (1991). The effectiveness of screening programs based on high-risk characteristics in early identification of hearing impairment. *Ear and Hearing, 12,* 312–319.

Maumenee, A.E. (1960). Congenital hereditary corneal dystrophy. *American Journal of Ophthalmology, 50,* 1114–1123.

Maxon, A., & Brackett, D. (1992). *The hearing impaired child: Infancy through high-school years.* Boston: Andover Medical Publishers.

Maxon, A.B., White, K.R., Behrens, T.R., & Vohr, B.R. (1995). Referral rates and cost efficiency in a universal newborn hearing screening program using transient evoked otoacoustic emissions. *Journal of the American Academy of Audiology, 6,* 271–277.

May, D.L., & White, H.H. (1968). Familial myoclonus, cerebellar ataxia, and deafness. *Archives of Neurology, 19,* 331–338.

McCabe, B.F. (1989). Perilymph fistula: the Iowa experience to date. *American Journal of Otology, 1* (10), 262.

McCandless, G., & Miller, D. (1972). Loudness discomfort and hearing aids. *National Hearing Aid Journal, 25,* 7–32.

McCandless, G.A., & Allred, P.L. (1978). Tympanometry and emergence of the acoustic reflex in infants. In E.R. Harford, F.H. Bess, C.D. Bluestone, et al. (Eds.), *Impedance screening for middle ear disease in children* (pp. 56–67). New York: Grune & Stratton.

McClure, W.J. (1973). The ostrich syndrome and educators of the deaf. *The Kentucky Standard* (Kentucky School for the Deaf, Danville), *100,* 5.

McCollister, F.P., Simpson, L.C., Dahle, A.J., & Pass, B.F. (1996). Hearing loss and congenital symptomatic cytomegalovirus infection. *Journal of the American Academy of Audiology, 7* (2), 57–62.

McConnel, F., & Liff, S. (1975). The rationale for early identification and intervention. *Otolaryngologic Clinics of North America, 8,* 77–87.

McDonough, E.R. (1970). Fanconi anemia syndrome. *Archives of Otolaryngology, 92,* 284–285.

McFarlan, D. (1927). The voice test of hearing. *Archives of Otolaryngology, 5,* 1–5.

McLay, K., & Maran, A.G.D. (1969). Deafness and the Klippel-Feil syndrome. *Journal of Laryngology and Otology, 83,* 175–184.

McLeod, A.C., McConnell, F., Sweeney, A., et al. (1971). Clinical variation in Usher's syndrome. *Archives of Otolaryngology, 94,* 321–334.

McMillan, P., Bennett, M., Marchant, C., & Shurin, P. (1985). Ipsilateral and contralateral acoustic reflexes in neonates. *Ear and Hearing, 6* (6), 320–324.

McNellis, E.L., & Klein, A.J. (1997). Pass/fail for repeated click-evoked otoacoustic emission and auditory brainstem response screenings in newborns. *Otolaryngology—Head and Neck Surgery, 116* (4), 431–437.

Meadow, K.P. (1968). The effect of early manual communication and family climate. Doctoral dissertation, University of California-Berkeley.

Meadow, K.P., & Trybus, R.J. (1979). Behavioral and emotional problems of deaf children: An overview. In L.J. Bradford & W.G. Hardy (Eds.), *Hearing and hearing impairment.* New York: Grune & Stratton.

Meadows-Orleans, K. (1987). An analysis of the effectiveness of early intervention programs for hearing-impaired children. In M.J. Guralnick & F.C. Bennet (Eds.), *The effectiveness of early intervention for at-risk and handicapped children* (pp. 325–357). New York: Academic Press.

Meadow-Orleans, K.P., Mertens, D.M., Sass-Lehrer, M., & Scott-Olson, K. (1997). Support services for parents and their children who are deaf or hard of hearing. *American Annals of the Deaf, 142,* 278–288.

Mehl, A., & Thomson, V. (1998). Newborn hearing screening: The great omission. *Pediatrics, 101,* 34.

Melnick, M., Bixler, D., Nance, W.E., et al. (1976). Familial branchio-oto-renal dysplasia. A new addition to the branchial arch syndrome. *Clinical Genetics, 9,* 25–34.

Melnick, W., Eagles, E.L., & Levine, H.S. (1964). Evaluation of a recommended program of identification audiometry with school-age children. *Journal of Hearing Disorders, 29,* 3–13.

Mendel, M. (1980). Clinical use of primary cortical responses. *Audiology, 19,* 1–15.

Mendel, M., & Goldstein, R. (1969). The effect of test conditions on the early components of the averaged electroencephalic response. *Journal of Speech and Hearing Research, 12,* 344.

Mendel, M., & Goldstein, R. (1971). Stability of the early components of the averaged electroencephalographic response. *Journal of Speech and Hearing Research, 14,* 829–840.

Mendel, M., Hosick, E., Windman, T., et al. (1975). Audiometric comparison of the middle and late components of the adult auditory evoked potentials awake and asleep. *Electroencephalography and Clinical Neurophysiology, 38,* 27–33.

Mendel, M.I. (1985). Middle and late auditory evoked potentials. In J. Katz (Ed.), *Handbook of clinical audiology* (3rd ed., pp. 565–581). Baltimore: Williams & Wilkins.

Menyuk, P. (1972). *The development of speech.* New York: Bobbs-Merrill.

Menyuk, P. (1986). Predicting speech and language problems with persistent otitis media. In J. Kavanagh (Ed.), *Otitis media and child development* (pp. 83–96). Parkton, MD: York Press.

Merzenich, M., Jenkins, W., Johnston, P., Schreiner, C., Miller, S.L., & Tallal, P. (1996). Temporal processing deficits of language-learning impaired children ameliorated by training. *Science, 271,* 77–81.

Metz, O. (1946). The acoustic impedance measured on normal and pathological ears. *Acta Oto-Laryngologica (Stockholm),* (Suppl. 63), 11-253.

Metz, O. (1952). Threshold of reflex contractions of muscles of middle ear and recruitment of loudness. *Archives of Otolaryngology, 55,* 536–543.

Meyer, T., & Pisoni, D. (1999) Some computational analyses of the PBK test: Effects of frequency and lexical density on spoken word recognition. *Ear and Hearing, 20* (4), 363–370.

Miller, A.L., Lehman, R.H., & Geretti, R. (1969). Unusual audiological findings in cranial-metaphysical dysplasia. *Archives of Otolaryngology, 89,* 861–864.

Mills, J.H. (1975). Noise and children: A review of literature. *Journal of the Acoustical Society of America, 58,* 768–779.

Mills, J.H., Gengel, R.W., Watson, C.S., et al. (1970). Temporary changes for the auditory system due to exposure to noise for one or two days. *Journal of the Acoustical Society of America, 48,* 524–530.

Mindel, E.D., & Vernon, M. (1971). *They grow in silence: The deaf child and his family* (p. 23). Silver Spring, MD: National Association of the Deaf.

Mitchell, O., & Richards, G. (1976). Effects of various anesthetic agents on normal and pathological middle ears. *Ear, Nose and Throat Journal, 55,* 36.

Miyamoto, R.T., Kirk, K.I., Robbins, A.M., Todd, S., & Riley, A. (1996). Speech perception and speech production in children with multichannel cochlear implants. *Acta Oto-Laryngologica, 116,* (2), 240–243.

Miyamoto, R.T., Kirk, K.I., Robbins, A.M., Todd, S., Riley, A., & Pisoni, D.B. (1997). Speech perception and speech intelligibility in children with multichannel cochlear implants. *Advances in Otology, Rhinology and Laryngology, 52,* 198–203.

Miyamoto, R.T., Yune, H.Y., & Rosevear, W.H. (1983). Klippel-Feil syndrome and associated ear deformities. *American Journal of Otology, l* (5), 113–119.

Mody, M., Schwartz, R., Gravel, J., & Ruben, R. (1999). Speech perception and verbal memory in children with and without histories of otitis media. *Journal of Speech, Language and Hearing Research, 42,* 1069–1079.

Moller, A. (1962). The sensitivity of the contraction of the tympanic muscles in man. *Annals of Otology, Rhinology and Laryngology, 71,* 86–95.

Moncur, J. (1968). Judge reliability in infant testing. *Journal of Speech and Hearing Research, 11,* 348–357.

Mondini, C. (1791). Anatomica surdi nati sectio. In *DeBononiensi scientarium et artium instituto atque academia comentarii* (Vol. VII, pp. 419–431). Bonoia.

Montgomery, D.E., & Matkin, N.D. (1992). Hearing impaired children in schools: integrated or isolated? In F.H. Bess, & J.W. Hall (Eds.). *Screening children to auditory function.* Nashville: Bill Wilkerson Center Press.

Moog, J.S., & Geers, A.E. (1979). *Grammatical analysis of elicited language—Simple sentence level.* St. Louis: Central Institute for the Deaf.

Moore, J. (1999). Comparison of risk of conductive hearing loss among three ethnic groups of Arctic audiology patients. *Journal of Speech, Language and Hearing Research, 42,* 1069–1079.

Moore, J.M., Thompson, G., & Thompson, M. (1975). Auditory localization of infants as a function of reinforcement conditions. *Journal of Speech and Hearing Disorders, 40,* 29–34.

Moore, J.M., Wilson, W.R., Lillis, K.E., et al. (1976). Earphone auditory threshold of infants utilizing visual reinforcement auditory reinforcement (VR). Poster session presented at the American Speech and Hearing Association meeting, Houston, TX.

Moore, J.M., Wilson, W.R., & Thompson, G. (1977). Visual reinforcement of head-turn responses in infants under twelve months of age. *Journal of Speech and Hearing Disorders, 42,* 328–334.

Moore, M.V. (1970). Speech, hearing and language in de Lange syndrome. *Journal of Speech and Hearing Disorders, 35,* 66–69.

Moores, D.F. (1996). *Educating the deaf: Psychology, principles and practices* (4th ed.). Boston: Houghton Mifflin Co.

Morse, P.A. (1972). The discrimination of speech and nonspeech stimuli in early infancy. *Journal of Experimental Child Psychology, 14,* 477–492.

M'Rad, R., Sanak, M., Deschenes, G., Zhou, J., Bonaiti-Pellie, C., et al. (1992). Alport syndrome: A genetic study of 31 families. *Human Genetics, 90,* 420–426.

Muckle, T.J. (1979). The "Muckle-Wells" syndrome. *British Journal of Dermatology, 100,* 87–92.

Mueller, H.G. (1996). Hearing aids and people: Strategies for a successful match. *The Hearing Journal, 49* (4), 13–24.

Mueller, H.G., & Bright, K.E. (1994). Selection and verification of maximum output. In M. Valente (Ed.), *Strategies for selecting and verifying hearing aid fittings* (pp. 38–63). New York: Thieme Medical Publishers, Inc.

Mueller, H.G., & Hall, J.W. (1998). *Audiologists' desk reference* (Vol. II). San Diego: Singular Publishing Group, Inc.

Mueller, H.G., & Hawkins, D.B. (1990). Three important considerations in hearing aid selection. In R.E. Sandlin (Ed.), *Handbook of hearing aid amplification* (Vol. II, pp. 31–60). Boston: College-Hill Press.

Mueller, H.G., Hawkins, D.B., & Northern, J.L. (1992). *Probe microphone measurements: Hearing aid selection and assessment.* San Diego: Singular Publishing Group, Inc.

Mueller, H.G., & Killion, M. (1990). An easy method for calculating the articulation index. *The Hearing Journal, 43* (9), 14–17.

Murphy, K.P. (1962). Development of hearing in babies. *Child and Family, 1.*

Murphy, K.P. (1979, September). A developmental approach to pediatric audiometry. *Hearing Aid Journal,* 6–32.

Musselman, C.R., Lindsay, P.H., & Wilson, A.K. (1988). An evaluation of recent trends in preschool programming for hearing-impaired children. *Journal of Speech and Hearing Disorders, 53,* 71–88.

Myer, C.M., Farrer, S.M., Drake, A.F., & Cotton, R.T. (1989). Perilymphatic fistulas in children: Rationale for therapy. *Ear and Hearing, 10,* 112–116.

Myers, F.N., & Stool, S. (1969). The temporal bone in osteoporosis. *Archives of Otolaryngology, 89,* 44–53.

Myklebust, H. (1954). *Auditory disorders in children.* New York: Grune & Stratton.

Nager, G.T. (1971). Congenital aural atresia: Anatomy and surgical management. In *Birth Defects, Part IX, Ear.* Baltimore: Williams & Wilkins, published for the National Foundation-March of Dimes.

Nagib, M.G., Maxwell, R.E., Chou, S.N. (1985). Klippel-Feil syndrome in children: Clinical features and management. *Childs Nervous System, 1,* 255–263.

Nahmias, A.J. (1974). The TORCH complex. *Hospital Practice, 9,* 65–72.

Nahmias, A.J., & Norrild, B. (1979). Herpes simplex virus 1 and 2, basic and clinical aspects. *Disease Monographs, 25* (10), 1–49.

Nakashima, S., Sando, I., Takahashi, H., & Hashida, Y. (1992). Temporal bone histopathologic findings of Waardenburg's syndrome. *Laryngoscope, 102,* 563–567.

Nance, M.A., & Berry, S.A. (1992). Cockayne syndrome: A review of 140 cases. *American Journal of Medical Genetics, 42,* 68–84.

Nance, W.E. (1973). Symposium on Usher's Syndrome. [Public Service Programs]. Gallaudet College, Washington, DC.

Nassif, R., & Harboyan, G. (1970). Madelung's deformity with conductive hearing loss. *Archives of Otolaryngology, 91,* 175–178.

National Advisory Committee on Education of the Deaf. (1973). *Basic education rights for the hearing impaired* (Publication No. 73-24001). Washington, DC: Office of Education, Department of HEW.

National Center for Health Statistics. *Hearing sensitivity and related findings among children* (Publication No. (HRA) 76-1046). Washington, DC: US Department of HEW.

National Center for Health Statistics. (1975). *Hearing sensitivity and related mental findings among youths 12–17 years* (Publication No. (HRS) 76-1636). Washington, DC: US Department of HEW.

National Center for Health Statistics. (1994). *Plan and operation of the third national health and nutrition examination survey, 1988–1994* (Publication No. (PHS) 94-1308). Washington, DC: US Department of Health and Human Services.

National Institutes of Health NIH Consensus Development Conference. (1991). *Acoustic Neuroma Consensus Statement,* (9) 4, Dec 11-13, Bethesda, MD.

National Institute on Deafness and Other Communication Disorders: National Institutes of Health. (1997). *Recommendation of the NIDCD working group on early identification of hearing impairment on acceptable protocols for use in state-wide universal newborn hearing screening program.* Rockville, MD: Author.

National Institute on Deafness and Other Communication Disorders: National Institutes of Health Consensus Statement. (1993). *Early identification of hearing impairment in infants and young children.* Rockville, MD: Author.

Naulty, C.M., Weiss, I.P., & Herer, G.R. (1986). Progressive sensorineural hearing loss in survivors of persistent fetal circulation. *Ear and Hearing, 7,* 74–77.

Needleman, H. (1977). Effects of hearing loss from early recurrent otitis media on speech and language development. In B. Jaffe (Ed.), *Hearing loss in children* (Ch. 44). Baltimore: University Park Press.

Neff, W.D. (1947).The effects of partial section of the auditory nerve. *Journal of Comprehensive Physiology, 40,* 203–216.

Nelson, M., & Scott, C.I. (1969). Engelmann's disease (a form of craniodiaphysial dysplasia). *Birth Defects, 5* (4):301.

Nelson, S.M., & Berry, R.I. (1984). Ear disease and hearing loss among Navajo children—A mass survey. *Laryngoscope, 94* (3), 316–323.

Nichols, P.T., Ramadan, H.H., Wax, M.K., & Santrock, R.D. (1998). Relationship between tympanic membrane perforations and retained ventilation tubes. *Archives of Otolaryngology—Head and Neck Surgery, 124,* 417–419.

Nield, T., Ramos, A.D., & Warburton, D. (1989). Late-onset hearing loss. *Pediatrics, 74,* 807–808.

Niemeyer, W., & Sesterhenn, G. (1972). Calculating the hearing threshold from the stapedius reflex threshold for different sound stimuli. *Journal of Audiological Communication, 11,* 84.

Niskar, A., Kieszak, M., Holmes, A., Esteban, E., Rubin, C., & Brody, D. (1998). Prevalence of hearing loss among children 6 to 19 years of age. *JAMA, 279,* 1071–1075.

Noback, C.R., Strominger, N.L., & Demarest, R.J. (1996). *Human nervous system: Structure and function* (5th ed.). Philadelphia: Williams & Wilkins.

Nolte, J. (1988). *The human brain: An introduction to its functional anatomy* (2nd ed.). St. Louis: CV Mosby.

Northern, J.L. (1977a). Acoustic impedance in the pediatric population. In F. Bess (Ed.), *Childhood deafness: Causation, assessment, and management.* New York: Grune & Stratton.

Northern, J.L. (1977b). Impedance audiometry for otologic diagnosis. In C. Shambaugh & J. Shea (Eds.), *Proceedings of the Shambaugh fifth international workshop on middle ear microsurgery and fluctuant hearing loss* (p. 75). Huntsville, AL: Strode Publishers.

Northern, J.L. (1978a). Advanced techniques for measuring middle ear function. *Pediatrics, 61,* 761.

Northern, J.L. (1978b). Impedance screening in special populations: state of the art. In E.R. Harford, F.H. Bess, C.D. Bluestone, et al. (Eds.), *Impedance screening for middle ear disease in children* (pp. 229–248). New York: Grune & Stratton.

Northern, J.L. (1980a). Acoustic impedance measures in the Down's population. *Seminars in Speech, Language and Hearing, 1,* 81.

Northern, J.L. (1980b). Clinical measurement procedures in impedance audiometry. In J. Jerger & J.L. Northern (Eds.), *Clinical impedance audiometry* (2nd ed.). Acton, MA: American Electromedics Corp.

Northern, J.L. (1980c). Impedance measurements with distinctive groups. In J. Jerger, & J.L. Northern (Eds.), *Clinical impedance audiometry* (2nd ed.). Acton, MA: American Electromedics Corp.

Northern, J.L. (1980d). Impedance screening: An integral part of hearing screening. *Annals of Otology, Rhinology and Laryngology, 89* (Suppl. 68), 3.

Northern, J.L. (1981). Impedance measurements in infants. In G. Mencher & S. Gerber (Eds.), *Early management of hearing loss* (p. 131). New York: Grune & Stratton.

Northern, J.L. (1986a). Selection of children for cochlear implantation. *Seminars in Hearing, 7,* 341–347.

Northern, J.L. (1986b). Acoustic immittance measurements for children. In F. Bess (Ed.),

Childhood deafness: Proceedings of the third international symposium in childhood deafness. Nashville: Vanderbilt University Press.

Northern, J.L. (1988). Recent developments in acoustic immittance measurements in children. In F. Bess (Ed.), *Hearing impairment in children.* Parkton, MD: York Press.

Northern, J.L. (1992a). Probe-microphone instrumentation. In G. Mueller, D. Hawkins, & J. Northern (Eds.), *Probe microphone measurements: Hearing aid selection and assessment* (pp. 21–40). San Diego: Singular Publishing Group, Inc.

Northern, J.L. (1992b). Special issues concerned with screening for middle ear disease in children. In F.H. Bess & J.W. Hall III (Eds.), *Screening children for auditory function* (pp. 39–60). Nashville, TN: Bill Wilkerson Center Press.

Northern, J.L. (1996). Acoustic immittance measurements. In J. Northern (Ed.), *Hearing disorders* (3rd ed.). Needham Heights, MA: Allyn and Bacon.

Northern, J.L., & Bergstrom, L. (1973). Impedance audiometry. *Eye, Ear Nose and Throat Monographs, 52,* 404–406.

Northern, J.L., Gabbard, S.A., & Kinder, D.L. (1990). Pediatric considerations in selecting and fitting hearing aids. In R.E. Sandlin (Ed.), *Handbook of hearing aid amplification* (Vol. II, pp. 113–132). Boston: College Hill Press.

Northern, J.L., & Grimes, A. (1978). Introduction to acoustic impedance. In J. Katz (Ed.), *Handbook of clinical audiology* (2nd ed.). Baltimore: Williams & Wilkins.

Northern, J.L., & Hayes, D. (1994). Universal screening for infant hearing impairment: Necessary, beneficial and justifiable. *Audiology Today, 6* (2), 10–13.

Northern, J.L., & Lemme, M. (1986). Hearing and auditory disorders. In G.H. Shames & E.H. Wiig (Eds.), *Human communication disorders: An introduction* (2nd ed., pp. 416–444). Columbus, OH: Charles E. Merrill.

Northern, J.L., Teter, D.L., & Krug, R.F. (1971). Characteristics of manually communicating deaf adults. *Journal of Speech and Hearing Disorders, 36,* 71–76.

Norton, S.J. (1993). Application of transient evoked otoacoustic emissions to pediatric populations. *Ear and Hearing, 14,* 64–73.

Norton, S.J., Gorga, M.P., Widen, J.E., Folsom, R.C., Sinninger, Y.S., Cone-Wesson, B., Vohr, B.R., & Fletcher, K. (2000). Identification of neonatal hearing impairment: a multi-center intervention. *Ear and Hearing, 21* (5), 348–356.

Norton, S.J., & Widen, J.E. (1990). Evoked otoacoustic emissions in normal-hearing infants and children: Emerging data and issues. *Ear and Hearing, 11,* 121–127.

Nozza, R.J., Bluestone, C.D., Kardatzke, D., & Bachman, R.N. (1994). Identification of middle ear effusion by aural acoustic admittance and otoscopy. *Ear and Hearing, 15,* 310–323.

Nozza, R.J. (1995). Critical issues in acoustic-immittance screening for middle-ear effusion. *Seminars in Hearing, 16* (1), 86–98.

Oller, D.K. (1978). Infant vocalizations and the development of speech. *Allied Health & Behavioral Sciences, 1,* 523–549.

Oller, D.K. (1980). The emergence of the sounds of speech in infants. In G. Komshian-Yeni, J.F. Kavanagh, & C.A. Ferguson (Eds.), *Child phonology: Production* (Vol. 1, pp. 83–112). New York: Academic Press.

Oller, D.K., & Eiler, R. (1988). The role of audition in infant babbling. *Child Development, 59,* 441–449.

Oller, D.K., Payne, S.L., & Gavin, W.J. (1986). Tactile speech perception by minimally trained deaf subjects. *Journal of Speech and Hearing Research 23,* 769–778.

Olsen, W.O., & Matkin, N.D. (1979). Speech audiometry. In W.F. Rintelmann (Ed.), *Hearing assessment.* Baltimore: University Park Press.

Omerod, F.C. (1960). The pathology of congenital deafness. *Journal of Laryngology and Otology, 74,* 919.

Opheim, O. (1968). Loss of hearing following the syndrome of Van Der Hoeve-De Kleyn. *Acta Oto-Laryngologica (Stockholm), 65,* 337.

Orchik, D.J., Dunn, J.W., & McNutt, L. (1978a). Tympanometry as a predictor of middle ear effusion. *Archives of Otolaryngology, 104,* 4–6.

Orchik, D.J., Morff, R., & Dunn, J.W. (1978b). Impedance audiometry in serous otitis media. *Archives of Otolaryngology, 104,* 409–412.

Osberger, M.J., & Hesketh, L.J. (1988). Speech and language disorders related to hearing impairment. In N. Lass, et al. (Eds.), *Handbook of speech-language pathology & audiology* (pp. 858–885). Toronto: BC Decker.

Owens, E., Kessler, D.K., Raggio, M.W., & Schubert, E.D. (1985). Analysis and revision of the minimal auditory capabilities (MAC) battery. *Ear and Hearing, 6,* 280–290.

Oyler, R.F., Oyler, A.L., & Matkin, N.D. (1987). Warning: A unilateral hearing loss may be detrimental to a child's academic career. *Hearing Journal, 40* (9),18–22.

Oyler, R.F., Oyler, A.L., & Matkin, N.D. (1988). Unilateral hearing loss: Demographics and educational impact. *Language, Speech & Hearing in Schools, 19,* 201–210.

Ozdamar, O., & Kraus, N. (1983). Auditory middle-latency response in human. *Audiology, 22,* 34–49.

Ozdamar, O., Kraus, N., & Stein, L. (1982). Auditory brainstem responses in infants recovering from bacterial meningitis: Audiological evaluation. *Otolaryngology—Head and Neck Surgery, 109,* 13–18.

Ozdamar, O., & Stein, L. (1981). Auditory brainstem response (ABR) in unilateral hearing loss. *Laryngoscope, 91,* 565–574.

Pantke, O.A., & Cohen, M.M., Jr. (1971). The Waardenburg syndrome. *Birth Defects, 7* (7), 147–152.

Paparella, M.M., & Brady, D.R. (1970). Sensorineural hearing loss in chronic otitis media and mastoiditis. *Archives of Otolaryngology, 74,* 108–115.

Pappas, D.G. (1983). Hearing impairments and vestibular abnormalities among children with subclinical cytomegalovirus. *Annals of Otology, Rhinology, and Laryngology, 92,* 552–557.

Pappas, D.G., Sr. (1998). *Diagnosis and treatment of hearing impairment in children* (2nd Ed). San Diego: Singular Publishing Group.

Paradise, J. (1995). Managing otitis media: A time for change. *Pediatrics, 96* (4), 712–715.

Paradise, J. (1997). Short-course antimicrobial treatment for acute otitis media. *Journal of the American Medical Association, 278,* 1640–1642.

Paradise, J., Elster, B., & Tan, L. (1994). Evidence in infants with cleft palate that breast milk protects against otitis media. *Pediatrics, 94,* 853–860.

Paradise, J.L. (1980). Otitis media in infants and children. *Pediatrics, 65,* 917–943.

Paradise, J.L. (1976a). Pediatrician's view of middle ear effusions: More questions than answers. *Annals of Otology, Rhinology and Laryngology, 85* (Suppl. 25), 20.

Paradise, J.L. (1976b). Management of middle ear effusions in infants with cleft palate. *Annals of Otology, Rhinology and Laryngology, 85* (Suppl. 25), 285–288.

Paradise, J.L. (1981). Otitis media during early life: How hazardous to development? A critical review of the evidence. *Pediatrics, 68* (6), 869–873.

Paradise, J.L. (1982). Editorial retrospective: Tympanometry. *New England Journal of Medicine, 307,* 1074–1076.

Paradise, J.L., & Bluestone, C.D. (1969). Diagnosis and management of ear disease in cleft palate infants. *Transactions of the American Academy of Ophthalmology and Otolaryngology, 73,* 709–714.

Paradise, J.L., & Bluestone, C.D. (1974). Early treatment of the universal otitis media of infants with cleft palate. *Pediatrics, 53,* 48–54.

Paradise, J.L., & Rogers, K.D. (1986). On otitis media, child development, and tympanostomy tubes: New answers or old questions? *Pediatrics, 77* (1), 88–91.

Paradise, J.L., & Smith, C. (1978). Impedance screening for preschool children, state of the art. In E. Harford, F. Bess, & C. Bluestone (Eds.), *Impedance screening for middle ear disease in children.* New York: Grune & Stratton.

Paradise, J.L., & Smith, C. (1979). Impedance screening for preschool children. *Annals of Otology, 88,* 56.

Paradise, J.L., Smith, C., & Bluestone, C.D. (1976). Tympanometric detection of middle ear effusion in infants and young children. *Pediatrics, 58,* 198–206.

Parnes, L.S., & McCabe, B.F. (1987). Perilymph fistula: An important cause of deafness and dizziness in children. *Pediatrics, 80* (4), 524–528.

Parring, A. (1988). Hearing disabled children: epidemiology and identification. *Scandinavian Audiology,* (Suppl. 30), 21-23.

Pashayan, H., Fraser, F.C., McIntyre, J., et al. (1971). Bilateral aplasia of the tibia, polydactyly and absent thumbs in a father and daughter. *Journal of Bone and Joint Surgery, 53B,* 495–499.

Pashayan, H.M., Pruzansky, S., & Solomon, L., (1974). The EEC syndrome. *Birth Defects, 10* (7), 105–127.

Pastores, G.M., Michels, V.V, & Jack, C.R. Jr. (1991). Early childhood diagnosis of acoustic neuromas in presymptomatic individuals at risk for neurofibromatosis. *American Journal of Medical Genetics, 41,* 325–329.

Paul, R., Cohen, D., Breg, W., Watson, M., & Herman, S. (1984). Fragile X syndrome: Its relations to speech and language disorders. *Journal of Speech and Hearing Disorders 49,* 326–336.

Pazzaglia, V.E., & Giampiero, B. (1986). Oto-palato-digital syndrome in four generations of a large family. *Clinical Genetics, 30,* 338–344.

Pearson, A.A, Jacobson, A.D., Van Calcorr, R., et al. (1970). *The Development of the Ear.* Rochester, NY. Home Study Course, American Academy of Otolaryngology and Opthalmology.

Peck, J.E. (1984). Hearing loss in Hunter's syndrome: Mucopolysaccharidosis II. *Ear and Hearing, 5* (4), 243–246.

Peckham, C.S., Stark, O., Dudgeon, J.A., et al. (1987). Congenital cytomegalovirus infection: A cause of sensorineural hearing loss. *Archives of Diseases in Childhood, 62,* 1233–1237.

Pediatric Working Group of the Conference on Amplification for Children with Auditory Deficits. (1996). Amplification for infants and children with hearing loss. *American Journal of Audiology, 5* (1), 53–68.

Pellett, F.S., Cox, L.C., & MacDonald, C.B. (1997). Use of acoustic reflectometry in the detection of middle ear effusion. *Journal of the American Academy of Audiology, 8* (3), 181–187.

Pelton, S., Shurin, P., & Klein, J. (1977). Persistence of middle ear effusion after otitis media. *Pediatric Research, 11,* 504.

Penn, T.O. (1999). School-based hearing screening in the United States. *Audiology Today, 11* (6), 20–21.

Petitto, L.A., & Marentette, P.F. (1991). Babbling in the manual mode: evidence for the ontogeny of language. *Science, 251,* 1493–1495.

Peterson, G.E., & Lehiste, I. (1962). Revised CNC lists for auditory testing. *Journal of Speech and Hearing Disorders, 27*, 62.

Peterson, R.A. (1977). Ophthalmology. In B. Jaffe (Ed.), *Hearing loss in children.* Baltimore: University Park Press.

Petroff, M.A., Simmons, F.B., & Winzelberg, J. (1986). Two emerging perilymph fistula "syndromes" in children. *Laryngoscope, 96,* 498–501.

Picton, R.W., Hillyard, S.A., Krausz, H., et al. (1974). Human auditory evoked potentials. I. Evaluation of components. *Electroencephalography and Clinical Neurophysiology, 36,* 179–190.

Pikus, A.T. (1995). Pediatric audiologic profile in type I and type 2 neurofibromatosis. *Journal of the American Academy of Audiology, 6* (1), 54–62.

Pisoni, D.B. (2000). Cognitive factors and cochlear implants: Some thoughts on perception, learning and memory in speech perception. *Ear and Hearing, 21* (1), 70–78.

Plant, G., & Spens, K.E. (Eds.). (1995). *Profound deafness and speech communication.* London: Whurr Publishers.

Pollack, D. (1971). The development of an auditory function. *Otolaryngologic Clinics of North America.* [Symposium on Congenital Deafness], *4,* 319–335.

Pollack, D. (1982). Amplification and auditory/verbal training for the limited hearing infant 0 to 30 months. *Seminars in Speech, Language and Hearing, 3,* 52–67.

Potts, P., & Greenwood, J. (1983). Hearing aid monitoring. *Language, Speech and Hearing Services in Schools, 14,* 163.

Pratt, S.R. (1999). Post-fitting issues: A need for parent counseling and instruction. *Trends in Amplification, 4* (2), 103–107.

Preus, M., & Fraser, F.C. (1973). The lobster-claw defect with ectodermal defects, cleft lip-palate, tear duct anomaly and renal anomalies. *Clinical Genetics, 4,* 369–375.

Prezant, T.R., Shohat, M., Jaber, L., et al. (1992). Biochemical characterization of a pedigree with mitochondrially inherited deafness. *American Journal of Medical Genetics, 44,* 465–472.

Prieve, B.A., Dalzell, L., Berg, A., Bradley, M., Cacace, A., et al. (2000). The New York state universal newborn hearing screening demonstration project: Outpatient outcome measures. *Ear and Hearing, 21* (2), 131–140.

Prieve, B.A., & Stevens, F. (2000). The New York state universal newborn hearing screening demonstration project: Introduction and overview. *Ear and Hearing, 21* (2), 85–91.

Primus, M. (1992). The role of localization in visual reinforcement audiometry. *ASHA, 35* (3), 1137–1141.

Primus, M.A. (1987). Response and reinforcement in operant audiometry. *Journal of Speech and Hearing Disorders, 52*, 294–299.

Primus, M.A., & Thompson, G. (1985). Response strength of young children in operant audiometry. *Journal of Speech and Hearing Research, 28*, 539–547.

Querleu, Q., Renard, Z., & Crepin, G. (1981). Perception auditive et reactivite foetale aux stimulations sonores. *Journal de Gynecologie, Obstetrique et Biologie de la Reproduction, 10*, 307–314.

Quisling, R.W., Moore, G.R., Jahrsdoerfer, R.A., et al. (1979). Osteogenesis imperfecta: A study of 160 family members. *Archives of Otolaryngology, 105*, 207–211.

Ramer, J.C., et al. (1994). Familial leukonychia, knuckle pads, hearing loss, and palmoplantar hyperkeratosis: An additional family with Bart-Pumphrey syndrome. *Journal of Medical Genetics, 31*, 68–71.

Rance, G., Beer, D.E., Cone-Wesson, B., Shepherd, R.C., et al. (1999). Clinical findings for a group of infants and young children with auditory neuropathy. *Ear and Hearing, 20* (3), 238–252.

Redding, J., Hargest, T., & Minsky, S. (1977). How noisy is intensive care? *Critical Care Medicine, 5,* 275.

Reddy, J.K., & Rao, M.S. (1977). Imitation of facial and manual gestures by human neonates. *Science, 198,* 75–79.

Reed, D., & Dunn, W. (1970). Epidemiologic studies of otitis media among Eskimo children. *Public Health Report, 85,* 699–706.

Reed, D., Struve, S., & Maynard, J.E. (1967). Otitis media and hearing deficiency among Eskimo children; a cohort study. *American Journal of Public Health, 57,* 1657–1662.

Reed, W.B., Store, V.M., Boder, E., et al. (1967). Pigmentary disorders in association with congenital deafness. *Archives of Dermatology, 95,* 176–186.

Reichert, T.J., Cantekin, E.I., Riding, K.H., et al. (1978). Diagnosis of middle ear effusions in young infants by otoscopy and tympanometry. In E.R. Harford, F.H. Bess, C.D. Bluestone, et al. (Eds.), *Impedance screening for middle ear disease in children* (pp. 69–79). New York: Grune & Stratton.

Reilly, J. (1989). Congenital perilymph fistula: A prospective study in infants and children. *Laryngoscope, 99,* 393–397.

Reisen, A.H. (1947). The development of visual perception in man and chimpanzee. *Science, 106,* 107–108.

Reisen, A.H. (1960). Effects of stimulus deprivation on the development and atrophy of the visual sensory system. *American Journal of Orthopsychiatry, 30,* 23–36.

Renshaw, J., & Diefendorf, A. (1998). Adapting the test battery for the child with special needs. In F. Bess (Ed.), *Children with hearing impairment* (pp. 83–103). Nashville: Bill Wilkerson Center Press.

Richards, B.W., & Rundle, A.T. (1959). A familial hormonal disorder associated with mental deficiency, deaf mutism and ataxia. *Journal of Mental Deficiencies Research, 3,* 33–35.

Richieri-Costa, A., Bortolozo, M.A., Lauris, J.R., R.C., Guion-Almeida, M.L., Marques, D., & Moreti, D. (1993). Mandibulofacial dysostosis: report on two Brazilian families suggesting antosomal recessive inheritance. *American Journal of Medical Genetics, 46* (6), 659–664.

Richieri-Costa, A., et al. (1990). Autosomal dominant tibial hemimelia-poly-syndactyly-triphalangeal thumbs syndrome: Report of a Brazilian family. *American Journal of Medical Genetics, 36,* 1–6.

Ridgeway, J. (1969, August). Dumb children. *Saturday Review,* pp. 19–21.

Riedner, E.D., Levin, S., & Holliday, M.J. (1980). Hearing patterns in dominant osteogenesis imperfecta. *Otolaryngology—Head and Neck Surgery, 106,* 737–740.

Ries, P. (1994). Prevalence and characteristics of persons with hearing trouble: United States, 1990–1991. *Vital Health Statistics, 10* (188) 9–10.

Riggs, W., Jr., & Seibert, J. (1972). Cockayne's syndrome; roentgen findings. *American Journal of Roentgenology, 116,* 623–633.

Rimoin, D.L., & Edgerton, M.T. (1967). Genetic and clinical heterogeneity in the oral-facial-digital syndrome. *Journal of Pediatrics, 71,* 94–102.

Rintelmann, W.F. (1976). Auditory manifestations of Alport's Disease syndrome. *Transactions of the American Academy of Ophthalmology and Otolaryngology, 82,* 375–387.

Rintelmann, W.F., & Bess, F.H. (1988). High-level amplification and potential hearing loss in children. In F.H. Bess (Ed.), *Hearing impairment in children* (pp. 278–309). Parkton, MD: York Press.

Rintelmann, W.F., & Borus, J. (1968). Noise-induced hearing loss and rock and roll music. *Archives of Otolaryngology, 88,* 57–65.

Roberts, D.B. (1980). The etiology of bullous myringitis and the role of mycoplasmas in ear disease. A review. *Pediatrics, 65,* 761–766.

Roberts, J., Burchinal, M., Zeisel, S., Neebe, E., Hooper, S., Roush, J., Bryant, D., Mundy, M., & Henderson, F. (1998). Otitis media, the caregiving environment, and language and cognitive outcomes and 2 years. *Pediatrics, 102* (2), 346–354.

Roberts, J., & Wallace, I. (1997). Language and otitis media. In J. Roberts, I. Wallace, & F. Henderson (Eds.), *Otitis media in young children: Medical, developmental and educational considerations* (pp. 133–162). Baltimore: Paul Brookes.

Roberts, J.E., Burchinal, M.R., Medley, L.P., Zeisel, S.A., Mundy, M., Roush, J., Hooper, S., Bryant, D., & Henderson, F.W. (1995). Otitis media, hearing sensitivity, and maternal responsiveness in relation to language during infancy. *Journal of Pediatrics, 126,* 481–489.

Robillard, T., & Gersdorff, M. (1986). Prevention of pre and perinatal acquired hearing defects. *Journal of Auditory Research, 26,* 207–237.

Robinette, M.S., & Glattke, T.J. (1997). *Otoacoustic emissions: Clinical applications.* New York Thieme Medical Publishers.

Robinette, M.S., Rhodes, D.P., & Marion, M.W. (1974). Effects of secobarbital on impedance audiometry. *Archives of Otolaryngology, 100,* 351–354.

Robinshaw, H.M. (1995). Early intervention for hearing impairment: Differences in the timing of communicative and linguistic development. *British Journal of Audiology, 29,* 314–334.

Robinson, A. (1972). Genetic and chromosomal disorders. In C.H. Kempe, H.K. Silver, & D. O'Brien (Eds.), *Current pediatric diagnosis and treatment.* Los Altos, CA: Lange Medical Publications.

Robinson, D.O., & Sterling, G.R. (1980). Hearing aids and children in school: A follow-up study. *Volta Review, 82,* 229.

Robinson, G.C., Wildervanck, L.S., & Chiang, T.P. (1973). Ectrodactyly, ectodermal dysplasia and cleft lip-palate. Its association with conductive hearing loss. *Journal of Pediatrics, 82,* 107–109.

Roeser, R., & Downs, M. (1995). *Auditory disorders in school children: The law, identification, remediation* (3rd ed.). New York: Thieme-Stratton.

Roeser, R.J. (1985). Tactile aids for the profoundly deaf. *Seminars in Hearing, 6,* 279–298.

Roeser, R.J., Campbell, J.C., & Daly, D. (1975). Recovery of auditory function following meningitic deafness. *Journal of Speech and Hearing Disorders, 40,* 405–411.

Roeser, R.J., Glorig, A., Gerken, G.M., et al. (1977). A hearing aid malfunction detection unit. *Journal of Speech and Hearing Disorders, 42,* 351–357.

Roizen, N.J., & Johnson, D., Congenital infections. (1996). In A.J. Capute & P.J. Accardo, (Eds.), *Developmental disabilities in infancy and childhood* (2nd ed., p. 175). Baltimore: Paul H. Brooks.

Roizen, N.J. (1999). Etiology of hearing loss in children: Nongenetic causes. In N.J. Roizen & A.O. Diefendorf (Eds.), *Pediatric Clinics of North America, 46* (1), 49–64.

Roizen, N.J., Walters, C., Nicol, T., & Blondis, T. (1993). Hearing loss in children with Down syndrome. *Journal of Pediatrics, 123* (1), 9–11.

Romer, A.S. (1986). *The vertebrate body* (5th ed.). Philadelphia: WB Saunders.

Rose, D.E., Galambos, R., & Hughes, J.R. (1959). Microelectrode studies of the cochlear nuclei of the cat. *Johns Hopkins Medical Journal, 104*, 211–251.

Rosenberg, A.L., Bergstrom, L., Troost, B.T., et al. (1970). Hyperuricemia and neurologic defects. *New England Journal of Medicine, 282*, 992–997.

Rosenberg, G.G. (1995). *The improving classroom acoustics project*. Sarastoa, FL: Florida Department of Education, Bureau of Student Services and Exceptional Education, 1993–1995.

Rosenblum, S.M., Arick, J.R., Krug, D., Stubbs, E., Young, N., & Pelson, R. (1980). Auditory brainstem evoked responses in autistic children. *Journal of Autism and Developmental Disorders, 10*, 215–225.

Rosenfeld, R. (1996). An evidence-based approach to treating otitis media. *Pediatric Clinics of North America, 43*, 1165–1181.

Rosenfeld, R. (1997). Answers to parent's questions about otitis media. *Audiology Today, 9* (3), 12–13.

Ross, M. (1969). Changing concepts in hearing aid candidacy. *Eye, Ear, Nose and Throat Monographs, 48*, 27–34.

Ross, M., & Calvert, D.R. (1977). Guidelines for audiology programs in educational settings. *Volta Review, 79*, 153–161.

Ross, M., & Lerman, J. (1970). A picture identification test for hearing-impaired children. *Journal of Speech and Hearing Research, 13*, 44–53.

Ross, M., & Seewald, R.C. (1988). Hearing aid selection and evaluation with young children. In F. Bess (Ed.), *Hearing impairment in children* (pp. 190–213). Parkton, MD: York Press.

Ross, M., & Tomassetti, C. (1980). Hearing aid selection for preverbal hearing-impaired children. In M. Pollack (Ed.), *Amplification for the hearing impaired* (2nd ed.). New York: Grune & Stratton.

Ross M. *FM Auditory Training Systems: characteristics, selection and use*. Baltimore: York Press, 1992.

Ross, N., & Giolas, T. (Eds.). (1978). *Auditory management of hearing-impaired children*. Baltimore: University Park Press.

Rossi, D.F., & Sims, D.G. (1977). Acoustic reflex measurement in the severely and profoundly deaf. *Audiology Hearing Education, 3*, 6–8.

Roswell, F., & Chall, J. (1963). *Auditory blending test*. New York: Essay Press.

Roush, J. (1990). Identification of hearing loss and middle ear disease in preschool and school-age children. *Seminars in Hearing, 11* (4), 357–371.

Roush, J., Bryant, K., Mundy, M., Zeisel, S., & Roberts, J. (1995). Developmental changes in static admittance and tympanometric width in infants and toddlers. *Journal of the American Academy of Audiology, 6* (4), 334–338.

Roush, J., & Matkin, N. (Eds.). (1994). *Infants and toddlers with hearing loss*. Baltimore: York Press.

Roush, J., & McWilliam, R.A. (1994). Family-centered early intervention: historical, philosophical and legislative issues. In J. Roush & N. Matkin (Eds.), *Infants and toddlers with hearing loss* (pp. 3–94). Baltimore: York Press.

Rovee-Collier, C. (1987). Learning and memory in infancy. In J. Osofsky Doniger (Ed.), *Handbook of infant development* (pp. 98–148). New York: John Wiley and Sons.

Ruben, R.J. (1986). Current treatment of otitis media. *Pediatrics, 77*, (1) 59–60.

Ruben, R.J. (1991). Language screening as a factor in the management of the pediatric otolaryngologic patient. *Archives of Otology—Head and Neck Surgery, 117*, 1021–1025.

Ruben, R.J., Knickerbocker, G.G., Sekula, J., et al. (1959). Cochlear microphonics in man. *Laryngoscope, 69*, 665.

Ruben, R.J., Lieberman, A.T., & Bordley, J.E. (1962). Some observations on cochlear potentials and nerve action potentials in children. *Laryngoscope, 5*, 545.

Ruben, R.J., & Rapin, I. (1980). Plasticity of the developing auditory system. *Annals of Otology, Rhinology and Laryngology, 89*, 303–311.

Rupp, R.R. (1971). An approach to the communicative needs of the very young hearing impaired child. *Journal of the Academy of Rehabilitative Audiology, 4*, 11–22.

Ruppert, E.S., Buerk, E., & Pfordresher, M.F. (1970). Hereditary hearing loss with saddle nose and myopia. *Archives of Otolaryngology, 92*, 95–98.

Rush, J., & McWilliam, R. (1994). Family-centered early intervention: Historical, philosophical, and legislative issues. In J. Roush & N. Matkin (Eds.), *Infants and toddlers with hearing loss*. Baltimore: York Press.

Rushmer, N. (1994). Supporting families of hearing-impaired infants and toddlers. *Seminars in Hearing, 15* (2), 160–171.

Rutter, M. (1978). Diagnosis and definition. In M. Rutter, & E. Schopler (Eds.), *Autism: A reappraisal of concepts and treatments* (pp 1–26). New York: Plenum Press.

Ryan, A.F., & Dallos, P. (1996). The physiology of the cochlea. In J. Northern (Ed.), *Hearing disorders* (3rd ed.). Needham Heights, MA: Allyn and Bacon.

Sachs, R.M., Miller, J.D., & Grant, K. (1980). Perceived magnitude of electroacoustic pulses. *Perspectives in Psychophysics, 28*, 255–262.

Saito, H., Kishimoto, S., & Furuta, M. (1981). Temporal bone findings in a patient with Mobius syndrome. *Annals of Otology, 90*, 80–84.

Salamy, A., Eldredge, L., & Sweeton, R. (1996). Transient evoked otoacoustic emissions: feasibility in the nursery. *Ear and Hearing, 17* (1), 42–48.

Salamy, A., Eldredge, L., & Tooley, W.H. (1989). Neonatal status and hearing loss in high-risk infants. *Journal of Pediatrics, 114,* 847–852.

Salata, J.A., Jacobson, J.T., & Strasnick, M. (1998). Distortion-product otoacoustic emissions hearing screening in high-risk newborns. *Otolaryngology—Head and Neck Surgery, 118* (1), 37-43.

Samples, J.M., & Franklin, B. (1978). Behavioral responses in 7 to 9 month old infants to speech and non-speech stimuli. *Journal of Auditory Research, 18,* 115–123.

Sanders, D. (1965). Noise conditions in normal school classrooms. *Exceptional Child, 31,* 344–353.

Sanderson-Leepa, M., & Rintelmann, W.F. (1976). Articulation functions and test-retest performance of normal-hearing children on three speech discrimination tests: WIPI, PBK-50, and NU Auditory Test No. 6. *Journal of Speech and Hearing Disorders, 41,* 503.

Sandlin, R.E. (1995). *Handbook of hearing amplification* (Vols. I and II). Boston: College-Hill Press.

Sando, I., Bergstrom, L., Wood, R.P., et al. (1968). Temporal bone findings in trisomy 18 syndrome. *Archives of Otolaryngology, 72,* 913–924.

Sando, I., Hemenway, W.G., & Morgan, R.W. (1968). Histopathology of the temporal bones in mandibulofacial dysostosis. *Transactions of the American Academy of Ophthalmology and Otolaryngology, 72,* 913–924.

Sando, I., & Wood, R.P. (1971). Congenital middle ear anomalies. *Otolaryngologic Clinics of North America.* [Symposium]. *4,* 291–318.

Savage-Rumbaugh, E., Taylor, T., & Shanker, S. (1998). *Apes, language and the human mind.* London: Oxford University Press.

Schaefer, B., et al. (1986). Dominantly inherited craniodiaphysial dysplasia. *Clinical Genetics, 30,* 381–391.

Schaefer, G.B., Kolodziej, P., & Olney, A. (1998). Oto-palatal-digital syndromes. *Ear, Nose and Throat Journal, 77* (8), 586–587.

Schafer, I.A., Scriver, C.R., & Efron, M.L. (1962). Familial hyperprolinemia, cerebral dysfunction, and renal anomalies occurring in a family with hereditary nephropathy and deafness. *New England Journal of Medicine, 267,* 51–60.

Schappert SM. (1992) Office visits for otitis media: United States, 1975–1990. Hyattville, MD: National Centers for Health Statistics, Report #214.

Schein, J.D. (1965). *The deaf community study of Washington, DC.* Washington, DC: Gallaudet College Press.

Schein, J.D., & Delk, M.T. (1974). *The deaf population of the United States.* Silver Spring, MD: National Association of the Deaf.

Scheiner, A.P. (1980). Perinatal asphyxia: Factors which predict developmental outcome. *Developmental Medicine and Child Neurology, 22,* 102–104.

Scherz, R.G., Graga, J.R., & Reichelderfer, T.E. (1972). A typical example of 13–15 trisomy in a Negro boy. *Clinical Pediatrics 11,* 246–248.

Schild, J.A., et al. (1984). Wildervanck syndrome: The external appearance and radiographic findings. *International Journal of Pediatric Otorhinolaryngology, 7,* 305–310.

Schildroth, A. (1988). Recent changes in the educational placement of deaf students. *American Annals of the Deaf, 133* (2), 61–67.

Schildroth, A., & Hotto, S. (1993). Annual survey of hearing impaired children and youth: 1991–1992 school year. *American Annals of the Deaf, 138* (2), 239–243.

Schlesinger, H.S. (1973). The deaf pre-schooler and his many faces. In L. Lloyd (Ed.), *International seminar of the vocational rehabilitation of deaf persons.* Washington, D.C.: US Dept of Health, Education, and Welfare.

Schlesinger, H.S., & Meadow, K.P. Emotional support to parents. In D.L. Lillie (Ed.), *Monograph on Parent Programs in Child Development Centers* (pp. 13–25). Chapel Hill, NC: University of North Carolina Press.

Schuknecht, H.F. (1993). *Pathology of the ear* (2nd ed.). Philadelphia: Lea and Febiger.

Schulman-Galambos, C., & Galambos, R. (1979). Brain stem evoked response audiometry in newborn hearing screening. *Archives of Otolaryngology, 105,* 86–90.

Schultz, L.F., et al. (1978). Atopic dermatitis and congenital deafness. *British Journal of Dermatology, 99,* 325–328.

Schuyler, V., & Rushmer, N. (1987). *Parent-infant habilitation.* Portland, OR: IHR Publications.

Schwartz, D.M,. & Schwartz, R.H. (1978). A comparison of tympanometry and acoustic reflex measurements for detecting middle ear effusion in infants below seven months of age. In E.R. Harford, F.H. Bess, C.D. Bluestone, et al. (Eds.), *Impedance screening for middle ear disease in children* (pp. 91–96). New York: Grune & Stratton.

Schwartz, D.M., & Schwartz, R.H. (1980). Tympanometric findings in young infants with middle ear effusion: some further observations. *International Journal of Pediatric Otolaryngology, 2,* 67–72.

Schwartz, S. (1987). *Choices in deafness: A parent's guide.* Montgomery, MD: Woodbine House.

Sculerati, N., Ledesna-Medina, J., Finegold, D.N., & Stool, S.E. (1990). Otitis media and hearing loss in Turner syndrome. *Archives of Otolaryngology—Head and Neck Surgery, 116* (4), 707.

Seewald, R., Cornelisse, L., Ramji, K., Sinclair, S., Moodie, K., & Jamieson, D. (1997). *DSL v4.1 for Windows.* London, Ontario, Canada: University of Western Ontario.

Seewald, R., Zelisko, D., Ramji, K., & Jamieson, D. (1991). *DSL 3.0 user's manual*. London, Ontario, Canada: University of Western Ontario.

Seewald, R.C., Cornelise, L.E., Ramji, K.V., Sinclair, S.T., Moodie, K.S., & Jamieson, D.G. (1996). *DSL version 4.0 for Windows, a software implementation of the desired sensational level (DSL[I/O]) method for fitting linear gain and wide-dynamic-range compression hearing instrument*. London, Ontario, Canada: Hearing Healthcare Research Unit, University of Western Ontario.

Seewald, R.C., Ross, M., & Spiro, M.K. (1985). Selecting amplification characteristics for young hearing-impaired children. *Ear and Hearing, 6* (1), 48–53.

Seitz, M.R., & Kisiel, D.L. (1990). Hearing aid assessment and the auditory brainstem response. In R.E. Sandlin (Ed.), *Handbook of hearing aid amplification* (Vol. II, pp. 203–224). Boston: College Hill Press.

Sell, E.J., Gaines, J.A., Gluckman, C., & Williams, E. (1985). Persistent fetal circulation neurodevelopmental outcome. *American Journal of Diseases of Children, 139*, 25–28.

Shanon, E., Himelfarb, M., & Gold, S. (1981). Auditory function in Friedreich's ataxia. *Otolaryngology—Head and Neck Surgery, 107*, 254–256.

Shemen, L.J., Mitchell, D.P., & Farkashidy, J. (1984). Cockayne syndrome—an audiologic and temporal bone analysis. *American Journal of Otology, 5*, 300–307.

Shimizu, H., Walters, R.J., Proctor, L.R., Kennedy, D.W., Allen, M.C., & Markowitz, R.K. (1990). Identification of hearing impairment in the neonatal intensive care unit population: Outcome of a five year project. *Seminars in Hearing, 11*, 150–160.

Shohat, M., Flaum, E., Cobb, S.R., Lachman, R., Rubin, C., Ash, C., & Rimoin, D.L. (1993). Hearing loss and temporal bone structure in achondroplasia. *American Journal of Medical Genetics, 45*, 548–551.

Shokeir, M.K. (1977). The Goldenhar syndrome: A natural history. *Birth Defects, 13* (3C), 67–83.

Shulman, K. (1973). Hydrocephaly. In D. Bergsma (Ed.), *Birth defects: Atlas and compendium*. Baltimore: Williams & Wilkins.

Shurin, P.A., Pelton, S.I., Donner, A., et al. (1979). Persistence of middle ear effusion after acute otitis media in children. *New England Journal of Medicine, 300*, 1121–1123.

Siegel, J., & McCracken, G. (1981). Aminoglycoside ototoxicity in children. In S.A. Lerner, G.J. Matz, & J.E. Hawkins (Eds.), *Aminoglycoside ototoxicity* (Ch. 24). Boston: Little, Brown & Co.

Siegel-Sadewitz, V., & Shprintzen, R. (1982). The relationship of communication disorders to syndrome identification. *Journal of Speech and Hearing Disorders, 47*, 338–354.

Siegenthaler, B., & Haspiel, G. (1996). *Development of two standardized measures of hearing for speech by children*. Washington, DC: Cooperative Research Program, Project 2372, United States Office of Education.

Silman, S. (Ed.). (1984). *The acoustic reflex: Basic principles and clinical applications*. New York: Academic Press.

Silman, S., Gelfand, S., & Silverman, C. (1984). Late-onset auditory deprivation: Effects of monaural versus bilateral hearing aids. *Journal of the Acoustical Society of America, 76* (5), 1357–1362.

Silver, H.K. (1964). The de Lange syndrome. *American Journal of Diseases of Children, 108*, 523–529.

Silverman, C.A., & Emmer, M.B. (1993). Auditory deprivation and recovery in adults with asymmetric sensorineural hearing impairment. *Journal of the American Academy of Audiology, 4*, 338–346.

Silverman, C.A., & Silman, S. (1990). Apparent auditory deprivation from monaural amplification and recovery with binaural amplification. *Journal of the American Academy of Audiology, 1*, 175–180.

Simmons, F.B. (1976). Automated hearing screening test for newborns: The crib-o-gram. In G. Mencher (Ed.), *Early identification of hearing loss* (pp. 171–180). Basel: Karger.

Simmons, F.B. (1982). Comment on hearing loss in graduates of a tertiary intensive care nursery. *Ear and Hearing, 3*, 188.

Singh, S., & Bresman, M.J. (1973). Menkes' "kinky hair syndrome" (trichopolio dystrophy). *American Journal of Diseases in Children, 125*, 572–578.

Singh, S.P., Rock, E.H., & Shulman, A. (1969). Klippel-Feil syndrome with unexplained conductive hearing loss. *Laryngoscope, 79*, 113–117.

Sininger, Y.S., Doyle, K.J., & Moore, J.K. (1999). The case for early identification of hearing loss in children. *Pediatric Clinics of North America, 46* (1), 1–13.

Sininger, Y.S., Hood, L.J., Starr, A., Berlin, C.I., & Picton, T.W. (1995). Hearing loss due to auditory neuropathy. *Audiology Today, 7* (2), 10–12.

Siqueland, E.R., & DeLucia, C.A. (1969). Visual reinforcement of nonnutritive sucking in human infants. *Science, 165*, 1144–1146.

Sitnick, V., Rushmer, N., & Arpan, R. (1978). *Parent-infant communication: A program of clinical and home training for parents and hearing-impaired infants*. Portland, OR: Good Samaritan Hospital and Medical Center.

Skinner, M.W. (1978). The hearing of speech during language acquisition. *Otolaryngologic Clinics of North America, 11*, 631–650.

Skinner, P., & Glattke, T.J. (1977). Electrophysiologic response audiometry: State-of-the-art. *Journal of Speech and Hearing Disorders, 42*, 170–198.

Smith, D.W. (1962). The number 18 trisomy syndrome. *Journal of Pediatrics, 60,* 513.

Smith, K., & Hodgson, W. (1970). The effects of systematic reinforcement on the speech discrimination responses of normal and hearing-impaired children. *Journal of Auditory Research, 10,* 110–117.

Smith, P.M. (1997, February). You are not alone: For parents when they learn that their child has a disability. *News Digest.* Washington, DC: National Information Center for Children and Youth with Disabilities.

Smith, R.C. (1996). *A case about Amy.* Philadelphia: University Press.

Smurzynski, J. (1994). Longitudinal measurements of distortion-product and click-evoked otoacoustic emissions of preterm infants: Preliminary results. *Ear and Hearing, 15* (3), 210–223.

Smurzynski, J., Jung, M.D., LaFreniere, D., Kim, D.O., Kamath, V., Rowe, J.C., Holman, M.C., & Leonard, G. (1993). Distortion-product and click evoked otoacoustic emissions of preterm and full-term infants. *Ear and Hearing, 14* (4), 258–274.

Sohmer, H., Feinmesser, M. (1967). Cochlear action potentials recorded from the external ear in man. *Annals of Otolaryngology, 76,* 427–435.

Sparkes, R.S., & Graham, C.B. (1972). Camurati-Englemann disease. Genetics and clinical manifestations with a review of the literature. *Journal of Medical Genetics, 9,* 73–85.

Sparks, S. (1984). Speech and language in fetal alcohol syndrome. *ASHA, 26,* 27–31.

Spitz, R.A. (1959). *A genetic field theory of ego formation. It's implications for pathology.* New York: International Universities Press.

Spivak, L. (1998). *Universal newborn hearing screening.* New York: Thieme Medical Publishers.

Spivak, L., Dalzell, L., Berg, A., Bradley, M.,Cacace, A., et al. (2000). The New York state universal newborn hearing screening demonstration project: Inpatient outcome measures. *Ear and Hearing, 21* (2), 131–140.

Spoendlin, H. (1967). The innervation of the organ of Corti. *Journal of Laryngology and Otology, 81,* 717–738.

Spoendlin, H. (1969). Innervation patterns in the organ of Corti of the cat. *Acta Oto-Laryngologica (Stockholm), 67,* 239–254.

Spoendlin, H. (1974). Congenital stapes ankylosis and fusion of carpal and tarsal bones as a dominant hereditary syndrome. *Acta Oto-Rhino-Laryngologica, 206,* 173–179.

Sprague, B., Wiley, T., & Goldstein, R. (1985). Tympanometric and acoustic-reflex studies in neonates. *Journal of Speech and Hearing Research, 28,* 265–272.

Spring, D.R., & Dale, P.A. (1977). Discrimination of linguistic stress in early infancy. *Journal of Speech and Hearing Research, 20,* 224–232.

Stach, B. (1998a). Central auditory disorders. In A. Lalwani & K. Grundfast (Eds.), *Pediatric otology and neurotology* (pp. 387–396). Philadelphia: Lippincott-Raven.

Stach, B.A. (1998b). *Clinical audiology: An introduction.* San Diego: Singular Publishing Group.

Stach, B.A., & Jerger, J.F. (1990). Immittance measures in auditory disorders. In J. Jacobson & J. Northern (Eds.), *Diagnostic audiology.* Boston: College-Hill Press.

Stagno, S., Pass, R.F., Dworsky, M.E., Henderson, R.E., Moore, E.G., Walton, P., & Alford, C.A. (1982). Congenital cytomegalovirus infection: the relative importance of primary and recurrent maternal infection. *New England Journal of Medicine, 306,* 945–949.

Standards and recommendations for hospital care for newborn infants (6th ed.). (1977). Evanston, IL: American Academy of Pediatrics, Committee of Fetus and Newborn.

Stanley, F.J., & Blair, E. (1994). Cerebral palsy. In I.B. Pless (Ed.), *The epidemiology of childhood disorders* (pp. 473–497). New York: Oxford University Press.

Stanley, R.J., Puritz, E.M., Birggaman, R.A., et al. (1975). Sensory radicular neuropathy. *Archives of Dermatology, 111,* 760–762.

Stark, R.E. (1996, Summer). Dysyllables as a link between babbling and first words. *ASHA,* 44–45.

Starr, A., Amlie, R.N., Martin, W.H., et al. (1977). Development of auditory function in newborn infants revealed by auditory brainstem potentials. *Pediatrics, 60,* 831–839.

Stein, L. (1999). Factors influencing the efficacy of universal newborn hearing screening. *Pediatric Clinics of North America, 46* (1), 95–105.

Stein, L., & Boyer, K. (1994). Progress in the prevention of hearing loss in infants. *Ear and Hearing, 15,* 116–124.

Stein, L., Clark, S., & Kraus, N. (1983b). The hearing-impaired infant: Patterns of identification and habilitation. *Ear and Hearing, 4* (5), 232–236.

Stein, L., Ozdamar, O., Kraus, N., et al. (1983a). Follow-up of infants screened by auditory brainstem response (ABR) in the NICU. *Journal of Pediatrics, 103,* 447–453.

Stein, L., Ozdamar, O., & Schnabel, M. (1981). Auditory brainstem responses (ABR) with suspected deaf-blind children. *Ear and Hearing, 1* (2), 30–40.

Stein, L., Tremblay, K., Pasternak, J., Banerjee, S., Lindemann, K., & Kraus, N. (1996). Brainstem abnormalities in neonates with normal otoacoustic emissions. *Seminars in Hearing, 17,* 197–213.

Stein, L.K., & Boyer, K.M. (1994). Progress in the prevention of hearing loss in infants. *Ear and Hearing, 15* (2), 116–125.

Stein, L.K., & Jabaley, T. (1981). Early identification and parent counseling. In L. Stein, E.

Mendel, & T. Jabaley (Eds.), *Deafness and mental health*. New York: Grune & Stratton.

Stein, L.K., Jabaley, T., Spitz, R., Stoakley, D., & McGee, T. (1990). The hearing-impaired infants: Patterns of identification and habilitation revisited. *Ear and Hearing, 11* (3), 201–205.

Stein, L.K., & Kraus, N. (1988). Auditory evoked potentials with special populations. *Seminars in Hearing, 9* (1), 35–46.

Stein, L.K., Kraus, N., Ozdamar, O., Cartee, C., Jabaley, T., Jeantet, C., & Reed, N. (1987). Hearing loss in an institutionalized mentally retarded population. *Otolaryngology—Head and Neck Surgery, 113,* 32–35.

Stelmachowicz, P. (1996). Current issues in pediatric amplification. *The Hearing Journal, 49* (10), 10–20.

Stelmachowicz, P., Seewald, R., & Gorga, M. (1998). Strategies for fitting amplification in early infancy. In F. Bess (Ed.), *Children with hearing impairment: Contemporary trends.* Nashville, TN: Vanderbilt Bill Wilkerson Center Press.

Stewart, E.J., & O'Reilly, B.F. (1989). Klippel-Feil syndrome and conductive deafness. *Journal of Laryngology and Otology, 103,* 947–949.

Stewart, J.M., & Bergstrom, L. (1971). Familial hand abnormality and sensorineural deafness, a new syndrome. *Journal of Pediatrics, 78,* 102–110.

Stockard, J.E., Stockard, J.J., Westmoreland, B., et al. (1979). Brainstem auditory evoked responses: Normal variation as a function of stimulus and subject characteristics. *Archives of Neurology, 36,* 823–831.

Stockard, J.E., & Westmoreland, B.F. (1981). Technical considerations in the recording and interpretation of the brainstem auditory evoked potential for neonatal neurologic diagnosis. *American Journal of EEG Technology, 21,* 31–54.

Stoel-Gammon, C., & Otomo, K. (1986). Babbling development of hearing impaired and normally hearing subjects. *Journal of Speech and Hearing Disorders, 51,* 33–41.

Stokoe, W.C., Casterline, D.C., & Croneberg, C.G. (1965). *A dictionary of American sign language on linguistic principles.* Washington, DC: Gallaudet College Press.

Stool, S.E., Berg, A.O., Carney, C.T., et al. (1994). *Otitis media and effusion in young children.* (AHCPR Publication No. 94-0622, Clinical Practice Guideline. No. 12, pp. 192–208). Rockville, MD: Agency for Health Care Policy and Research, Public Health Service, US Department of Health and Human Services.

Stool, S.E., Marshak, G., Stanievich, J., et al. (1982). *Otitis media: Current concepts, incidence, pathogenesis, diagnosis and management.* [Pamphlet companion to an exhibit]. Pittsburgh, PA: Department of Otolaryngology, Children's Hospital of Pittsburgh, PA.

Storer, T. (1979). *General zoology* (6th ed.). New York: McGraw-Hill.

Strasnick, B., & Jacobson, J.T. (1995). Teratogenic hearing loss. *Journal of the American Academy of Audiology, 6* (1), 29–38.

Stratton, H.J.M. (1965). Gonadal dysgenesis and the ears. *Journal of Laryngology and Otology, 79,* 343–346.

Strauss, M. (1985). A clinical pathologic study of the hearing loss in congenital cytomegalovirus infection. *Laryngoscope, 95,* 951–962.

Striffler, N., & Willis, S. (1981). *Communication Screen.* Tucson, AZ: Communication Skills Builder.

Strong, C.J., Clark, T.C., & Walden, B.E. (1994). The relationship of hearing loss severity to demographic, age, treatment and intervention effectiveness variables. *Ear and Hearing, 15* (2), 126–137.

Stuckless, E.R. (Ed.). (1980). Deafness and rubella: Infants in the 60's, adults in the 80's. *American Annals of the Deaf, 125,* 959.

Sturner, R.A., Layton, T.L., Evans, A.W., Funk, S.G., & Machon, M.W. (1994). Preschool speech and language screening: A review of currently available tests. *American Journal of Speech-Language Pathology, 3* (1), 25–36.

Sullivan, R.F. (1985). An acoustic coupling-based classification system for hearing aid fittings. *Hearing Instruments,* Part I, *36* (9), 25; Part II, *36* (12), 17; Part III, *36* (12), 20.

Survey of hearing impaired children and youth (Series D, Vol. 9). (1971). Washington, DC: Gallaudet College Office of Demographic Studies.

Suzuki, T., & Ogiba, Y. (1961). Conditioned orientation audiometry. *Archives of Otolaryngology, 74,* 192–198.

Sylvester, P.E. (1958). Some unusual findings in a family with Friedreich's ataxia. *Archives of Diseases in Childhood, 33,* 217–221.

Sylvester, P.E. (1972). Spino-cerebellar degeneration, hormonal disorder, hypogonadism, deafmutism, and mental deficiency. *Journal of Mental Deficiencies Research, 16,* 203–214.

Tallal, P., Miller, S., Fitch, R.H., et al. (1993). Neurobiological Basis of Speech: A Case for the Preeminence of temporal processing. *Annals of the New York Academy of Sciences, 682,* 27–46.

Tanguay, P.E., & Edwards, R.M. (1982a). Electrophysiological studies of autism: The whisper of the bang. *Journal of Autism and Developmental Disorders, 12* (2), 177–184.

Tanguay, P.E., Edwards, R.M., Buchwald, J., Schwafel, J., & Allen, V. (1982b). Auditory brainstem responses in autistic children. *Archives of General Psychiatry, 39,* 174–180.

Teele, D., & Teele, J. (1984). Detection of middle ear effusion by acoustic reflectometry. *Journal of Pediatrics, 104,* 832–838.

Teele, D.W. (1994). Long term sequela of otitis media: Fact or fiction? *Pediatric Infectious Disease Journal, 13,* 1069–1073.

Teele, D.W., Klein, J.O., & Rosner, B.A. (1980a). Epidemiology of otitis media in children. *Annals of Otology, Rhinology, and Laryngology, 89* (Suppl. 68), 5–6.

Teele, D.W., Klein, J.O., & Rosner, B. (1980b). Epidemiology of otitis media in children. [Proceedings of 2nd International Symposium: Recurrent Advances in Otitis Media with Effusion]. *Annals of Otology, Rhinology, and Laryngology, 89* (3), (Suppl. 68); Part II, 5–6.

Teele, D.W., Klein, J.O., Rosner, B.A., & Greater Boston Otitis Media Study Group. (1984). Otitis media with effusion during the first three years of life and development of speech and language. *Pediatrics, 74* (2), 282–287.

Templin, M. (1966). Vocabulary problems of the deaf child. *International Audiology, 5,* 349.

Tervoort, B. (1964). Development of languages and the critical period. The young deaf child: Identification and management. *Acta Oto-Laryngologica Supplement (Stockholm), 206,* 247–251.

Tharpe, A.M., & Ashmead, D. (1993). Computer simulation technique for assessing pediatric auditory test protocols. *Journal of the American Academy of Audiology, 4* (2), 80–90.

Tharpe, A.M., & Bess, F.H. (1999) Minimal, progressive, and fluctuating hearing losses in children: Characteristics, identification, and management. In N.J. Roizen & A.O. Diefendorf (Eds.), *Pediatric Clinics of North America, 46* (1), 65–78.

Thelin, J.W., Mitchell, J.A., Hefner, M.A., & Davenport, S.L. (1986). CHARGE syndrome: Part II. Hearing loss. *International Journal of Pediatric Otorhinolaryngology, 12,* 145–163.

Thompson, G. (1983). Structure and function of the central auditory system. *Seminars in Hearing, 4,* 81–95.

Thompson, G., & Folsom, R. (1981). Hearing assessment of at-risk infants. *Clinical Pediatrics, 20,* 257–267.

Thompson, G., & Folsom, R.C. (1984). A comparison of two conditioning procedures in the use of visual reinforcement audiometry (VRA). *Journal of Speech and Hearing Disorders, 49,* 241–245.

Thompson, G., Wilson, W., & Moore, J. (1979). Application of visual reinforcement audiometry (VRA) to low-functioning children. *Journal of Speech and Hearing Disorders, 44,* 80–90.

Thompson, M.., & Thompson, G. (1972). Responses of infants and young children as a function of auditory stimuli and test month. *Journal of Speech and Hearing Research, 15,* 699–707.

Thompson, M., Thompson, G., & Vethivelu, S. (1989). A comparison of audiometric test methods for 2-year-old children. *Journal of Speech and Hearing Disorders, 54,* 174–179.

Thompson, R.C. Jr., Gaull, G.E., Horwitz, S.J., et al. (1969). Hereditary hyperphosphatasia. Studies of three siblings. *American Journal of Medicine, 47,* 209–219.

Thomsen, K.A., Terkildsen, K., & Arnfred, J. (1965). Middle ear pressure during anesthesia. *Archives of Otolaryngology—Head and Neck Surgery, 82,* 609.

Thorner, M., & Remein, O.R. (1967). *Principles and procedures in the evaluation of screening for disease.* Public Health Service Publication #846. Washington, D.C.

Tietz, W. (1963). A syndrome of deaf-mutism associated with albinism showing dominant autosomal inheritance. *American Journal of Human Genetics, 15,* 259–264.

Toriello, H. (1995). CHARGE association. *Journal of the American Academy of Audiology, 6* (1), 47–53.

Tos, M. (1980). Spontaneous improvement of secretory otitis and impedance screening. *Otolaryngology—Head and Neck Surgery, 106,* 345–349.

Tos, M. (1983). Treatment of cholesteatoma in children. *American Journal of Otology, l* (4), 189.

Trevarthen, C. (1975). Early attempts at speech. In R. Levin (Ed.), *Child alive.* Garden City, NY: Anchor Press/Doubleday.

Trine, M.B., Hirsch, J.E., & Margolis, R.H. (1993). The effect of middle ear pressure on transient evoked otoacoustic emissions. *Ear and Hearing, 14,* 401–407.

Tucker, B.P. (1999). *Cochlear implants: A handbook.* Jefferson, NC: McFarland and Co., fInc.

Turner, G. (1970). A second family with renal, vaginal and middle ear anomalies. *Journal of Pediatrics, 76,* 641.

Turner, R.G. (1990). Recommended guidelines for infant screening: Analysis. *ASHA, 32* (9), 57–61.

Tyler, R.S. (Ed.). (1993). *Cochlear implants: Audiological foundations.* San Diego: Singular Publishing Group.

Ueda, K., Hisanaga, S., Nishida, Y., et al. (1981). Low birth-weight and congenital rubella syndrome. *Clinical Pediatrics, 20,* 730–733.

Upfold, L. (1988). Children with hearing aids in the 80's: Etiologies and severity of impairment. *Ear and Hearing, 9,* 75–80.

US Department of Health, Education, and Welfare. Rules and regulations for the administration of the education for all handicapped children act. *Federal Register* (Part IV), 42, 163, August 23, 1977.

US Department of HEW, National Center for Health Statistics. (1972). *Hearing levels of children by demographic and socioeconomic characteristics* (Publication No. (HSM) 72-1025). Washington, DC: Government Printing Office.

US Department of HEW, Office of Education: Education of Handicapped Children. (1976, November 29). Assistance to states. *Federal Register, 41* (230).

Vahava, O., Morell, R., Lynch, E., Weiss, S., Kagan, M., et al. (1998). Mutation in transcription factor POU4F3 associated with inherited progressive hearing loss in humans. *Science, 279,* 1950–1954.

Valente, M. (Ed.). (1994). *Strategies for selecting and verifying hearing aid fittings.* New York: Thieme Medical Publishers, Inc.

Valente, M. (Ed.). (1996). *Hearing aids: Standards, options, and limitations.* New York: Thieme Medical Publishers, Inc.

Van Tasell, D. (1993). Hearing loss, speech, and hearing aids. *Journal of Speech and Hearing Research, 36,* 228–244.

Vaughan, V., McKay, R.J., & Behrman, R. (1979). *Nelson textbook of pediatrics* (11th ed.). Philadelphia: WB Saunders.

Ventry, I.M. (1983). Research design issues in studies of effects of middle ear effusion. *Pediatrics, 71,* 644.

Vernon, M. (1969). *Multiply handicapped deaf children* (pp. 1–112). Research Monograph, Council for Exceptional Children.

Vernon, M., & Hicks, D. (1980). Relationship of rubella, *Herpes simplex,* cytomegalovirus and certain other viral disabilities. *American Annals of the Deaf, 125,* 529–534.

Vernon, M. & Klein, N. (1982). Hearing impairment in the 1980's. *Hearing Aid Journal, 35,* 17.

Vernon, M., & Prickett, H. (1976). Mainstreaming: Issues and a model plan. *Audiology Hearing Education, 2,* 5–11.

Vienny, H., Despland, P.A., Lutschg, J., Deonna, T., Dutoit-Marco, M.L., & Gander, C. (1984). Early diagnosis and evolution of deafness in childhood bacterial meningitis: A study using brainstem auditory evoked potentials. *Pediatrics, 73,* 579–586.

Vohr, B., Carty, L., Moore, P., & Letourneau, K. (1998). The Rhode Island hearing assessment program: Experience with statewide hearing screening. *Journal of Pediatrics, 133,* 353–357.

Vohr, B., & Maxon, A. (1996). Screening infants for hearing impairment. *Journal of Pediatrics, 128,* 710–714.

Vohr, B.R., Widen, J.E., Cone-Wesson, B., Sininger, Y.S., Gorga, M.P., Folsom, R.C., & Norton, S.J. (2000). Identification of neonatal hearing impairment: characteristics of infants in the neonatal intensive care unit (NICU) and well baby nursery. *Ear and Hearing, 21* (5), 373–382.

Von Almen, P., Allen, L., Adkins, T., Anderson, K., Blake-Rahter, T., English, K., & Johnson, C.D. (1994). Universal screening for infant hearing impairment. Executive Board of the Educational Audiology Association. *Pediatrics, 94* (6 pt 1), 957.

Von Almen, P., Allen, L., Adkins, J., Anderson, K., Blake-Rahter, T., English, K., & De Carde Johnson, C. (1994). Letter to editor. *Pediatrics, 94* (6), 957.

Voron, D.A., Hatfield, H.H., & Kalkhoff, R.K. (1976). Multiple lentigines syndrome. *American Journal of Medicine, 60,* 447–456.

Vulliamy, D.G., & Normandale, P.A. (1966). Craniofacial dysostosis in a Dorset family. *Archives of Diseases in Childhood, 41,* 375.

Walker, D., Downs, M.P., Gugenheim, S., & Northern, J.L. (1989). Early language milestone scale and language screening of young children. *Pediatrics, 83* (2), 284–288.

Walker, M.L., Cervette, M.J., Newberg, N., Moss, S.D., & Storrs, B.B. (1987). Auditory brainstem responses in neonatal hydrocephalus. *Concepts in Pediatric Neurosurgery, 7,* 142–152.

Walker, W.G. (1971). Renal tubular acidosis and deafness. *Birth Defects, 7* (4), 126.

Wallace, I.F., Gravel, J.S., McCarton, C.M., Stapells, D.R., Bernstein, R.S., & Ruben, R.J. (1988). Otitis media, auditory sensitivity, and language outcomes at one year. *Laryngoscope, 98,* 64–70.

Waltzman, S.B., & Cohen, N.L. (2000). *Cochlear implants.* New York: Thieme Medical Publishers.

Watkin, P. (1996). Neonatal acoustic emission screening and the identification of deafness. *Archives of Disease in Childhood, 74,* F16–F25.

Watkin, P.M. (1989). Otologic disease in Turner's syndrome. *Journal of Laryngology and Otology, 103,* 731–738.

Watkins, S. (1987). Long term effects of home intervention with hearing impaired children. *American Annals of the Deaf, 132,* 267–271.

Watson, D.O. (1964). *Talk with your hands.* Winneconne, WI.

Weatherby, L., & Bennett, M. (1980). The neonatal acoustic reflex. *Scandanavian Audiology, 9,* 103–110.

Weber, B. (1969). Validation of observer judgments in behavioral observation audiometry. *Journal of Speech and Hearing Disorders, 34,* 350–355.

Weber, B. (1970). Comparison of two approaches to behavioral observation audiometry. *Journal of Speech and Hearing Research, 13,* 823–825.

Weber, H.J. (1987). Colorado's statewide hearing screening program utilizing visual reinforcement audiometry. *Hearing Instruments, 38* (9), 22–24.

Weber, H.J., McGovern, F.J., & Zink, D. (1967). An evaluation of 1000 children with hearing loss. *Journal of Speech and Hearing Disorders, 32,* 343–354.

Webster, D.B., & Webster, M. (1977). Neonatal sound deprivation affects brainstem auditory nuclei. *Archives of Otolaryngology, 103,* 392–396.

Webster, D.B., & Webster, M. (1979). Effects of neonatal conductive loss on brainstem auditory nuclei. *Annals of Otology, Rhinology, and Laryngology, 88,* 684–688.

Webster, D.B., & Webster, M. (1980). Mouse brainstem auditory nuclei development. *Annals of Otology, Rhinology, and Laryngology, 89* (Suppl. 68), 254–256.

Weiner, R., & Koppelman, J. (1987). From birth to five: Serving the youngest handicapped children. Alexandria, VA: Capitol Publications.

Weinstein, R.L., Kliman, B., & Scully, R.E. (1969). Familial syndrome of primary testicular insufficiency with normal virilization, blindness, deafness, and metabolic abnormalities. *New England Journal of Medicine, 281,* 969–977.

Weir, R.H. (1966). Some questions on the child's learning of phonology. In F. Smith & G. Miller (Eds.), *The genesis of language* (pp. 153–169). Cambridge, MA: MIT Press.

Weiss, K.L., Goodwin, M.W., & Moores, D.F. (1975). Characteristics of young deaf children and early intervention programs (Research Report 91). Washington, DC: Department of HEW, Bureau of Education for the Handicapped.

Wepman, D. (1987). *Helen Keller: Humanitarian.* New York: Chelsea House Publishers.

Werner, L.A., Folsom, R.C., Mancl, L.R. (1994). The relationship between auditory brainstem response and behavioral thresholds in normal hearing infants and adults. *Hearing Research, 68,* 131–141.

Wester, D.C., Atkin, C.L., & Gregory, M.C. (1995). Alport syndrome: Clinical update. *Journal of the American Academy of Audiology, 6* (1), 73–79.

Wetherby, A.M., Koegal, R., & Mendel, M. (1981). Central auditory nervous system dysfunction in autistic individuals. *Journal of Speech and Hearing Research, 24,* 420–429.

Wever, E.G., & Bray, C.W. (1930). Auditory nerve impulses. *Science, 71,* 215.

Wever, E.G., Lawrence, M. (1954). *Physiological Acoustics* (pp 187–194). Princeton, NJ: Princeton University Press.

Wever, E.G., & Neff, W.D. (1947). A further study of the effects of partial section of the auditory nerve. *Journal of Comparative Physiology and Psychology, 40,* 217–226.

White KR, Vohr B, Maxon B, Behrens T, McPherson M, Mark G. Screening all newborns for hearing loss using transient evoked Otoacoustic emissions. Int J Pediatr Otorhinolaryngo 29(3) 203–217, 1994.

White, K.R. (1996). Universal newborn hearing screening using transient evoked otoacoustic emissions: Past, present and future. *Seminars in Hearing, 17* (2), 171–183.

White, K.R., & Behrens, T.R. (Eds.). (1993). The Rhode Island hearing assessment project: Implications for universal newborn hearing screening. *Seminars in Hearing, 14* (1), 1–122.

Widen, J.E. (1997). Evoked otoacoustic emissions in evaluating children. In M. Robinette & T. Glattke (Eds.), *Otoacoustic emissions: Clinical applications* (pp. 271–306). New York: Thieme Medical Publishers.

Wilber, R.B. (1987). *American sign language: Linguistic and applied dimensions.* Boston: Little, Brown & Co.

Wiley, T., & Fowler, C. (1997). *Acoustic immittance measures in clinical audiology: A primer.* San Diego, CA: Singular Publishing Group, Inc.

Williams, A., Williams, M., Walker, C., et al. (1981). The Robin anomaly (Pierre Robin syndrome)—follow-up study. *Archives of Diseases in Childhood, 56,* 663–668.

Williamson, W.D., Demmler, G.J., Percy, A.K., & Catlin, F.I. (1992). Progressive hearing loss in infants with asymptomatic congenital cytomegalovirus infection. *Pediatrics, 90* (6), 862–866.

Wilson, W.R., Folson, R.C., & Widen, J.E. (1982). Hearing impairment in Down's syndrome children. [Paper presented at the Elks 1982 International Symposium, The Multiply Handicapped Hearing Impaired Child]. Edmonton, Canada.

Wilson, W.R., & Thompson, G. (1984). Behavioral audiometry. In J. Jerger (Ed.), *Pediatric audiology* (pp. 1–44). San Diego: College-Hill Press.

Windle-Taylor, P., Emery, P.J., & Phelps, P.D. (1981). Ear deformities associated with the Klippel-Feil syndrome. *Annals of Otology, 90,* 210–216.

Wing, L. (1993). The definition and prevalence of autism: a review. *European Child & Adolescent Psychiatry, 2* (1), 1–14.

Wolf-Schein, E., Sudhalter, V., Cohen, I., et al. (1987). Speech-language and the fragile X syndrome: Initial findings. *ASHA, 29,* 35–38.

Woolf, C.M., Dolowitz, D.A., & Aldous, H.E. (1965). Congenital deafness associated with piebaldness. *Archives of Otolaryngology, 82,* 244–250.

Worthington, D.W., & Peters, J.F. (1980). Quantifiable hearing and no ABR: Paradox or error? *Ear and Hearing, 1,* 281–285.

Wright, L.B., & Rybak, L.P. (1983). Crib-o-gram (COG) and ABR: Effect of variables on test results. *Journal of the Acoustical Society of America, 74* (Suppl. 1), 540–544.

Wright, P., McConnell, K., Thompson, J., Vaughn, W., Sells, S. (1985). A longitudinal study of the detection of otitis media in the first two years of life. *International Journal of Pediatric Otolaryngology, 10,* 245–252.

Yoshie, N., & Ohashi, T. (1996). Clinical use of cochlear nerve action potential responses in man for differential diagnosis of hearing losses. *Acta Oto-Laryngologica* (Suppl) (Stockh) 252, 71–87.

Yoshinaga-Itano, C. (1994). Language assessment of infants and toddlers with significant hearing loss. *Seminars in Hearing, 15* (2), 128–140.

Yoshinaga-Itano, C. (1995). Efficacy of early identification and intervention. *Seminars in Hearing, 16,* 115–120.

Yoshinaga-Itano, C. (1999). Early identification: An opportunity and challenge for audiology. *Seminars in Hearing, 20* (4), 317–336.

Yoshinaga-Itano, C., & Apuzzo, M. (1995). Early identification of infants with significant hearing loss and the Minnesota child development inventory (MCDI). *Seminars in Hearing, 16* (2), 124–135.

Yoshinaga-Itano, C., Sedey, A., Coulter, D., & Mehl, A. (1998). Language of early- and later-identified children with hearing loss. *Pediatrics, 102* (5), 1161–1171.

Yoshioka, H., Mino, M., Kiyosawa, N., Hirasawa, Y., Morikora, Y., Kasubuchi, Y., & Kusunoki, T. (1980). Muscular changes in Engelmann's disease. *Archives of Diseases in Childhood, 55,* 716–719.

Yost, W.A., & Nielsen, D.W. (2000). *Fundamentals of hearing: An introduction* (4th ed.). New York: Holt, Rinehart and Winston.

Zellweger, H., Smith, J.K., & Grutzner, P. (1974). The Marshall syndrome; report of a new family. *Journal of Pediatrics, 84,* 868–871.

Zemlin, W.R. (1998). *Speech and hearing science: Anatomy and physiology* (4th ed.) Needham Heights, MA: Allyn & Bacon.

Zielhuis, G.A., Straatman, H., Rach, G.H., & van den Broek, P. (1990). Analysis and presentation of data on the natural course of otitis media with effusion in children. *International Journal of Epidemiology, 19* (4):1037–1044.

Zigler, E. (1969). Developmental versus different theories in mental retardation and the problem of motivation. *American Journal of Mental Deficiencies, 73,* 536–556.

Zwislocki, J. (1963). An acoustic method for clinical examination of the ear. *Journal of Speech and Hearing Research, 6,* 303–314.

Index

Page numbers in italics followed by f denote figures; those followed by t denote tables.

Index

Page numbers in italics followed by f denote figures; those followed by t denote tables.